Anatomy, Physiology
and
Health Education

Anatomy, Physiology and Health Education

Rohini Agrawal

M Pharm, PhD (Postdoc)

Assistant Professor
College of Pharmacy
JSS Academy of Technical Education (JSSATE)
Noida

Neeraj Agrawal

M Pharm, PhD

Director and Professor
SMS Group of Institutions
Ajmer, Rajasthan

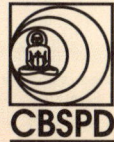

CBSPD

CBS Publishers & Distributors Pvt Ltd

New Delhi • Bengaluru • Chennai • Kochi • Kolkata • Lucknow • Mumbai
Hyderabad • Jharkhand • Nagpur • Patna • Pune • Uttarakhand

Anatomy, Physiology and Health Education

ISBN: 978-93-85915-52-9

Copyright © Authors and Publisher

CBS Reprint: 2016, 2019, 2021, 2023, **2025**
First Edition: 2012

Published by Satish Kumar Jain and produced by Varun Jain for

CBS Publishers & Distributors Pvt Ltd

4819/XI Prahlad Street, 24 Ansari Road, Daryaganj, New Delhi 110 002, India.
Ph: 011-23289259, 23266861   Website: www.cbspd.com
                                                          e-mail: delhi@cbspd.com

Corporate Office: 204 FIE, Industrial Area, Patparganj, Delhi 110 092
Ph: 011-4934 4934   Fax: 011-4934 4935   e-mail: publishing@cbspd.com;
                                                                             publicity@cbspd.com

Branches

- **Bengaluru:** Seema House 2975, 17th Cross, KR Road, Banasankari 2nd Stage, Bengaluru 560 070, Karnataka, India Ph: +91-80-26771678/79   Fax: +91-80-26771680   e-mail: bangalore@cbspd.com
- **Chennai:** 18/8B, Subbarayan Street, Shenoy Nagar, Chennai 600 030, Tamil Nadu, India Ph: +91-44-42032115, 26681266   e-mail: chennai@cbspd.com
- **Kochi:** 42/1325, 1326, Power House Road, Opp KSEB, Power House, Ernakulum Kochi 682 018, Kerala, India Ph: +91-484-4059061-65,67   Fax: +91-484-4059065   e-mail: kochi@cbspd.com
- **Kolkata:** 147, Hind Ceramics Compound, 1st Floor, Nilgunj Road, Belghoria, Kolkata-700056, West Bengal, India Ph: +033-25633055, 033-25633056   e-mail: kolkata@cbspd.com
- **Lucknow:** Basement, Khushnuma Complex, 7 Meerabai Marg (Behind Jawahar Bhawan), Lucknow-226001, UP, India Ph: +0522-4000032   e-mail: tiwari.lucknow@cbspd.com
- **Mumbai:** PWD Shed, Gala no 25/26, Ramchandra Bhatt Marg, Next to JJ Hospital Gate no. 2, Opp. Union Bank of India, Noorbaug, Mumbai-400009, Maharashtra, India
  Ph: 022-66661880/89   e-mail: mumbai@cbspd.com

Representatives

• Hyderabad	0-9885175004	• Jharkhand	0-9811541605	• Nagpur	0-8692091830
• Patna	0-9334159340	• Pune	0-9664372571	• Uttarakhand	0-9716462459

Printed at Goyal Offset Works Pvt. Ltd., Haryana (INDIA)

Preface

This textbook has been written and designed to fulfil the needs of health care professionals including pharmacists, nurses, physiotherapists, and medical and dental students. It has been written in clear, concise and easily understandable scientific language and is structured in such a way that it fulfils the requirements of the present-day curriculum.

This book encompasses the knowledge of basic principles of anatomy and physiology, and thus, will guide the students along a journey of understanding of how the human body operates on a daily basis from birth to death. The book has been structured in 15 chapters. Each chapter has been written with the aim to give a reasonable account of every topic for academicians, researchers and students in a simple, direct and clear manner. An appendix has been devoted to provide information about the health education concepts like health and disease, balanced diet, family planning techniques, communicable diseases and first aid measures.

Our objective of making this book the best in the segment has been fully achieved by systematic assemblage of the well-written chapters with neat and clean well-labelled diagrams wherever needed.

Suggestions and criticisms are always solicited to further improve the quality of the book.

Rohini Agrawal
E-mail: ahuja_rohini@yahoo.co.in

Neeraj Agrawal
E-mail: neeraj_pharm@rediffmail.com

Acknowledgements

This book would not have been possible without the efforts of many people. Accordingly, we recognize and thank the members of our editorial team, who often worked evenings and weekends, as well as days, to bring this book to you within the stipulated time. We extend our gratitude to Ms Ritu Sharma, the publishing manager, who illuminated the path with her dedication and creative ideas. We are thankful to Mr Nitin Valecha, the commissioning editor, for his expert assistance in quality publication of this book. A very special thanks is also extended to Mr Subodh Kumar, the development editor, who was always available with assistance and consistent words of encouragement. We are immensely thankful to Elsevier India for their guidance and cooperation to publish this book.

We also express our heartfelt thanks to Mr Varun Soti and Dr Komal Sharma for their helpful contributions to this textbook. Also, we convey the deep sense of gratitude to our families for their continued patience, support and acceptance of lost evenings and weekends.

Rohini Agrawal
Neeraj Agrawal

We submit this book to the Almighty, whose blessings have been with us at every step of this journey. It is by God's grace only that we are able to complete this book.

Contents

Chapter 5 The Nervous System 159

Chapter 10   The Respiratory System   337

Chapter 11   The Cardiovascular System   395

Structural and Functional Organization of Human Body

CHAPTER OUTLINE

- Introduction
- Anatomical Terminology
- Basic Processes of Human Body
- Homeostasis
- Levels of Structural Organization

- The Cellular Level of Organization
- The Tissue Level of Organization
- The System Level of Organization
- Diseases Associated with Cells and Tissues

STUDY OBJECTIVES

- ✓ To define anatomy and physiology and discuss about the subdisciplines of these sciences
- ✓ To describe the anatomical position of human body and discuss various directional terms related to it
- ✓ To describe the basic processes of human body
- ✓ To discuss about homeostasis and the operation of negative and positive feedback systems
- ✓ To describe the levels of structural organization that make up the human body
- ✓ To describe the parts of a cell
- ✓ To describe the structure and functions of the plasma membrane

- ✓ To discuss the various processes that transport substances across the plasma membrane
- ✓ To describe the structure and functions of cytoplasm, the organelles and the nucleus
- ✓ To discuss the four basic types of tissues that make up the human body
- ✓ To describe the structure, location and functions of different types of epithelial tissue and connective tissue
- ✓ To discuss the structural features and functions of muscle tissue and nervous tissue

INTRODUCTION

Human body is like a highly complicated and sophisticated machine in which various systems work interdependently to perform various functions that are required for the survival of an individual. This integrated working of various systems ensures the normal well-being of the individual.

The human body is complex in both structure and function. Anatomy and physiology are two branches of science that provide the foundation for understanding the various body parts and their functions.

- ❑ **Anatomy**: It is the study of the structure of the body and the organization of the body parts.
- ❑ **Physiology**: It is the study of the functions of body structures and the ways in which they work interdependently to maintain the life and health of an individual.

SUBDISCIPLINES OF ANATOMY AND PHYSIOLOGY

Various subdisciplines of anatomy include the following:

- **Embryology**: The science of the origin and development of the individual from fertilization of an oocyte to the end of the eighth week of development.
- **Developmental anatomy**: The study concerned with the changes that cells, tissues, organs and the body as a whole undergo from fertilization of a secondary oocyte to the resulting offspring.
- **Histology**: The science concerned with the minute structure of tissues and organs in relation to their function.
- **Radiographic anatomy**: The study of the anatomy of tissues based on their visualization on X-ray films.
- **Pathological anatomy**: The anatomy of diseased tissues.

Various subdisciplines of physiology include the following:

- **Endocrinology**: The branch of physiology and medicine concerned with endocrine glands and hormones.
- **Cardiovascular physiology**: The study of the circulatory system, that is, the heart (cardio) and blood vessels (vascular).
- **Immunology**: The study of the body's immune system or natural defence mechanisms against diseases.
- **Respiratory physiology**: The branch of human physiology focusing on respiration.
- **Renal physiology**: The study of the physiology of the kidney.
- **Exercise physiology**: The study of the function of the human body during various acute and chronic exercise conditions.
- **Pathophysiology**: The disordered physiological processes associated with a disease or an injury.

DO YOU KNOW

- There are anywhere from 75 to 100 trillion cells in the body.
- The largest cell in the human body is the female egg and the smallest is the male sperm.
- Three hundred million cells die in the human body every minute.
- Every day an adult body produces 300 billion new cells.
- There are more bacterial cells in the body than human cells.
- The longest cells in the human body are the motor neurons. They can be up to 4.5 ft (1.37 m) long and run from the lower spinal cord to the big toe.
- The longest living cells in the body are brain cells, which can live an entire lifetime.
- Our eyes are always the same size from birth, but our nose and ears never stop growing.

MEDICAL TERMINOLOGY

- **Extracellular fluid**: The body fluid outside the cell.
- **Intracellular fluid**: Liquid contained inside the cell membranes (usually containing dissolved solutes).
- **Interstitial fluid**: Liquid found between the cells of the body that provides much of the liquid environment of the body.
- **Ligands**: An ion, a molecule or a molecular group that binds to another chemical entity to form a larger complex.
- **Phagocytosis**: A cell, such as a white blood cell, that engulfs and absorbs waste material, harmful microorganisms or other foreign bodies in the bloodstream and tissues.

ANATOMICAL TERMINOLOGY

Scientists and health care professionals have adopted a common language of special terms to describe the body position and have designed a special vocabulary for relating body parts to one another. When any body part or region is described in the study of anatomy, it is assumed that the body is in a specific posture referred to as *anatomical position*. In the anatomical position, the human body is erect and facing forward. The arms are at the sides and the palms of the hand and feet are positioned towards the front (Fig. 1.1).

The position of various body parts is described in reference to the body as a whole, and specific directional terms are used to facilitate this description. The major directional terms used to describe the human body are as follows:

1. **Superior**: The upper part of a structure, for example, the head is superior to the neck.
2. **Inferior**: The lower part of a structure, for example, the foot is inferior to the ankle.
3. **Anterior (ventral)**: Towards the front of the body, for example, the sternum (breast bone) is anterior to the heart.
4. **Posterior (dorsal)**: Towards the back of the body, for example, the oesophagus (food pipe) is posterior to the trachea (wind pipe).
5. **Medial**: Near the midline of the body, for example, ulna is on the medial side of the forearm.
6. **Lateral**: Away from the midline of the body, for example, the lungs are lateral to the heart.
7. **Proximal**: Nearer to the attachment of limb to the trunk, for example, the humerus is proximal to the radius.
8. **Distal**: Away from the attachment of limb to the trunk, for example, wrist is distal to the elbow.
9. **Superficial**: Towards the surface of the body, for example, the ribs are superficial to the lungs.
10. **Deep**: Away from the surface of the body, for example, the ribs are deep to the skin of the chest.

The human body is divided into five principal regions that include the following:

1. **Head**: It consists of skull and face.
2. **Neck**: It supports head and attaches it to the trunk.
3. **Trunk**: It consists of chest, abdomen and pelvis.
4. **Upper limb**: It attaches to trunk and comprises shoulder, armpit, arm (from shoulder to elbow), forearm (from elbow to wrist), wrist and hand.
5. **Lower limb**: It comprises buttock, thigh (from buttock to knee), leg (from knee to ankle), ankle and foot.
6. **Groin**: It is the area on the front surface of the body, where the trunk attaches to the thighs.

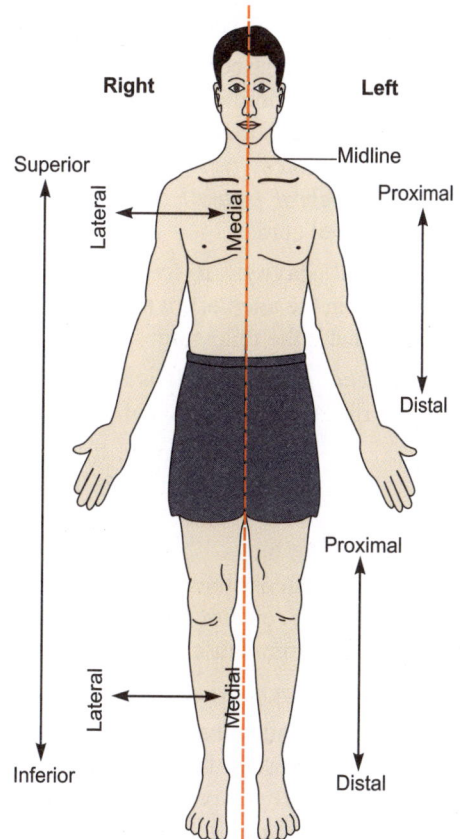

Figure 1.1 Anatomical position of the body.

The body can also be described relative to planes, that is, the imaginary flat surfaces that pass through the body parts (Fig. 1.2).

❑ **Sagittal plane**: It is a vertical plane that divides the body into right and left portions. A median plane or midsagittal plane passes through the midline of the body and divides it into equal right and left sides, whereas a parasagittal plane does not pass through the midline and divides the body into unequal right and left sides.

❑ **Frontal or coronal plane**: It divides the body into anterior (front) and posterior (back) portions.

❑ **Transverse or horizontal plane**: It divides the body into superior (upper) and inferior (lower) portions.

The body is divided into two major cavities that separate and support the internal organs. The organs present within the cavity are referred to as the *viscera*. The two major body cavities are the dorsal cavity and the ventral cavity (Fig. 1.3).

1. **Dorsal cavity**: It contains organs of the nervous system that coordinate the body's functions. It includes the following:
   (a) *Cranial cavity*: It contains the brain.
   (b) *Vertebral (spinal) cavity*: It contains the spinal cord.

2. **Ventral cavity**: It contains organs that maintain the internal environment of the body. It includes the following:

   (a) *Thoracic cavity*: It is surrounded by the rib cage and consists of the following:
      (i) Pericardial cavity: It is a fluid-filled space that surrounds the heart.
      (ii) Two pleural cavities: They consist of lungs.
      (iii) Mediastinum: It is the central part of the thoracic cavity between the two pleural cavities. It contains the heart, oesophagus, trachea, thymus and several blood vessels.

   The diaphragm muscle separates the thoracic cavity and the abdominopelvic cavity.

   (b) *Abdominopelvic cavity*: It includes the following:
      (i) Abdominal cavity: It contains the stomach, spleen, liver, gall bladder, small intestine and most of the large intestine.
      (ii) Pelvic cavity: It contains some portions of the large intestine, urinary bladder and internal organs of the reproductive system.

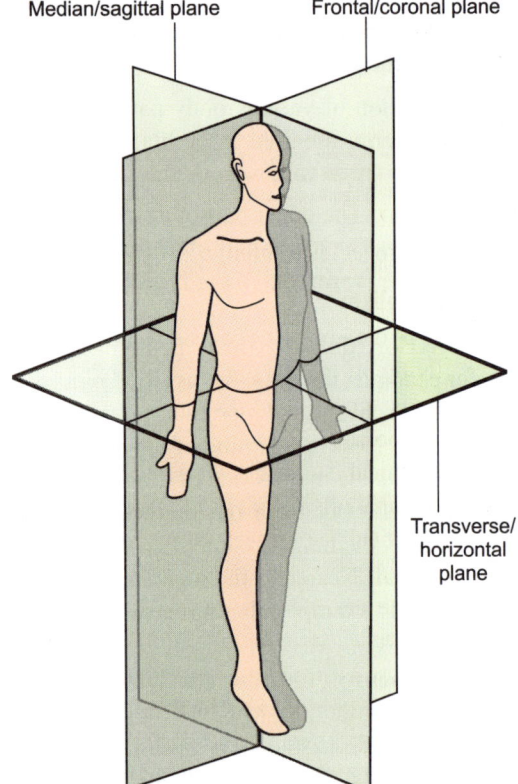

Median/sagittal plane   Frontal/coronal plane

Transverse/horizontal plane

Figure 1.2 Planes of the human body.

A double-layered serous membrane covers the internal organs of the thoracic and abdominal cavities. The parts of the serous membrane are as follows:

1. **Parietal layer**: It lines the walls of a cavity.
2. **Visceral layer**: It covers the organs (viscera) within the cavity.

Serous fluid is present between the two layers, which reduces friction during movements.

BASIC PROCESSES OF THE HUMAN BODY

The basic processes of human body are as follows:

1. **Metabolism**
   - ❑ It is the set of chemical reactions that occur in living organisms to maintain life.
   - ❑ It is generally divided into two categories: catabolism, that is, breakdown of complex chemical substances into simpler components, and anabolism, that is, the building up of complex chemical substances from smaller components. For example, the digestive processes break down the proteins into amino acids, which can be combined again to form some newer proteins.

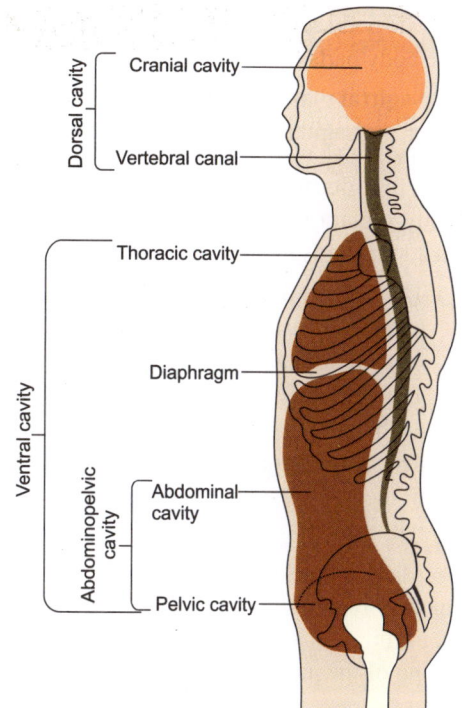

Figure 1.3 Body cavities.

2. **Movement**: It includes motion of the whole body, organs or even single cells. For example, any injury or infection stimulates the white blood cells to move from the blood towards the injured site to heal or repair the injured site.

3. **Responsiveness**: It is the ability of the body to detect and respond to changes in its internal and external environment. For example, endocrine cells in the pancreas detect the elevated blood glucose level and respond by secreting the hormone insulin, which lowers the blood glucose level to normal.

4. **Growth**: It is characterized by increase in body size owing to hypertrophy (increase in size of existing cells), hyperplasia (increase in number of cells) or both.

5. **Differentiation**: It is one of the characteristics of the cell by which it develops from an unspecialized state into a specialized state with different forms and functions than its unspecialized ancestor cells. For example, the red bone marrow contains unspecialized ancestor cells that differentiate to form red blood cells (RBCs) and different types of white blood cells (WBCs).

6. **Reproduction**: It includes cell division and the formation of new cells for growth, repair or production of a new individual. For example, epithelial cells undergo cell division throughout the lifetime for growth or to replace the worn-out cells.

HOMEOSTASIS

Homeostasis can be defined as the condition of equilibrium that is maintained by keeping the body's internal environment within narrow limits. The term *homeostasis* was coined by the American physiologist Walter B. Cannon, and the significance of homeostasis in the survival of an organism was first discussed by the French scientist Claude Bernard. Bernard proposed that the cells in the body remain in a fairly constant internal environment despite changes in the external environment that surrounds the body.

❏ The cells in the body are surrounded by the interstitial fluid, which is often referred to as the *body's internal environment* as it serves to provide substances such as glucose, oxygen and ions needed by the cells and also removes cellular waste.

❏ The composition of the interstitial fluid continuously undergoes certain changes as there is continual exchange of substances between the interstitial fluid and the plasma present in the blood capillaries. Thus, regulation of the interstitial fluid composition is very essential to maintain the proper functioning of the body cells and therefore each body structure contributes in some way to keep this composition within narrow limits.

Many factors in the internal environment must be maintained within narrow limits, and some of them include blood glucose levels, oxygen and carbon dioxide levels, blood pressure, water and electrolyte concentration and body temperature. When these limits are disturbed or imbalanced, it affects the well-being of the individual.

CONTROL OF HOMEOSTASIS

Homeostasis in the human body is continually being disturbed due to changes in the external environment (such as intense heat and lack of oxygen) or in the internal environment (e.g. changes in blood glucose level). The body regulates this through various feedback systems that continually monitor, evaluate and respond to changes to maintain the balance of the internal environment.

The feedback system has three basic components: *detector*, *control centre* and *effector*.

❏ The detector or sensor monitors the changes in the internal environment that acts as a stimulus and then sends input in the form of nerve impulses or chemical signals to the control centre.

❏ The control centre in the body sets the limits within which various factors should be maintained. It evaluates the input coming from the detector, and when certain adjustments are required, it generates the output in the form of nerve impulses or hormones and sends it to the effector.

❏ Effector is the body structure that receives output from the control centre and produces a response or an effect that brings the condition back to normal.

For example, when our body temperature drops significantly, the specialized temperature-sensitive nerve endings detect the change and send input to the control centre, that is, the hypothalamus of the brain. The control centre then sends signals to the skeletal muscles, causing the body to shiver, thereby raising the body temperature, and also causes vasoconstriction to conserve body heat.

FEEDBACK SYSTEM (Fig. 1.4)

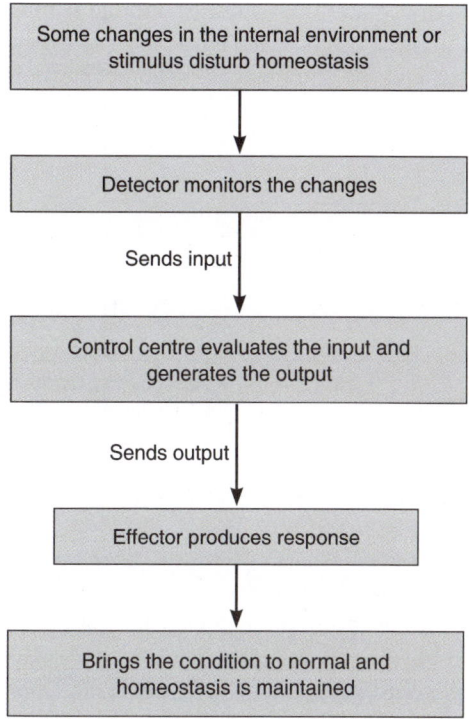

Figure 1.4 Feedback system.

The regulation of homeostasis requires different responses, which are achieved by two types of feedback systems: negative feedback system and positive feedback system.

Negative feedback system

❏ In the negative feedback system, the response generated by the effector reverses or opposes the stimulus or change and brings the condition back to its normal state (Fig. 1.5).

Example: Blood pressure is regulated by the negative feedback system. When there is increased blood pressure (stimulus), the change is detected by baroreceptors (pressure-sensitive nerve cells) located in the walls of certain blood vessels. The baroreceptors send nerve impulses (input) to the brain (control centre), which interprets the impulses and generates output by sending nerve impulses to the heart (effector). The heart (effector) receives the output and decreases the heart rate in response, which causes the blood pressure to decrease. Thus, the response generated by the effector (heart) reverses or opposes the stimulus (i.e. an increase in blood pressure) and restores the homeostasis.

❏ Most of the homeostatic controls in the body use the negative feedback system to maintain the homeostasis of the internal environment.

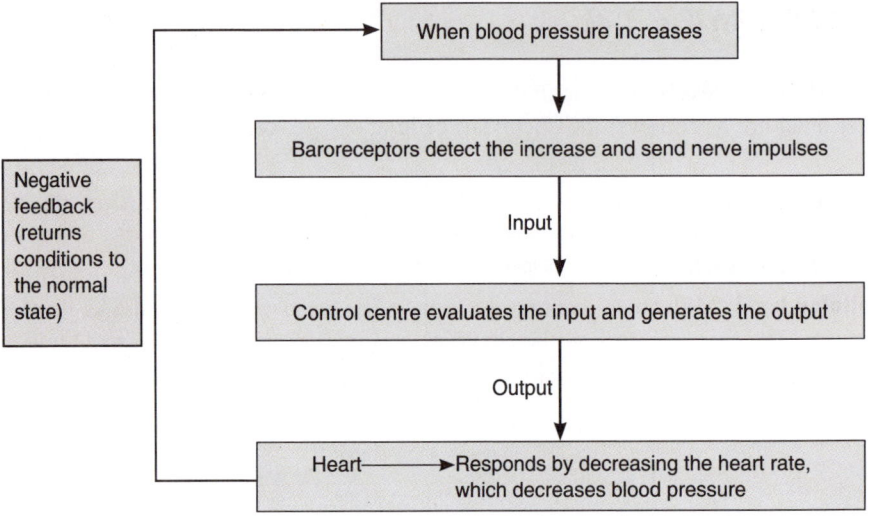

Figure 1.5 Negative feedback system.

Positive feedback system

In the positive feedback system, the response generated by the effector enhances or intensifies the change or stimulus. There are only a few conditions where the positive feedback system works to maintain homeostasis.

Example: The positive feedback system operates during uterine contractions in normal child birth. The initial contractions of labour (stimulus) push the baby's head into the cervix of the uterus, which stretches the cervix. The stretching is detected by stretch receptors (detector) that sends nerve impulses (input) to the control centre (brain), which in response releases the oxytocin hormone (output) into the blood. Oxytocin further enhances the contractions that push the baby further down the uterus, which stretches the cervix even more. This cycle of stretching (stimulus), release of hormone (output) and increased contractions (response) is interrupted only by the birth of the baby. After the baby is born, the cervix no longer stretches and thus the release of oxytocin stops. Thus, the response (uterine contractions) further reinforces the stimulus (stretching of the cervix) in the positive feedback system.

HOMEOSTATIC IMBALANCE

When the body's internal environment or homeostasis is maintained, the body cells function efficiently and the body stays healthy. Moderate homeostatic imbalance leads to an abnormal state, resulting in a disorder or disease, but the body cells try to restore this balance quickly. However, if the disorder is not controlled and severe imbalance occurs, it may be fatal.

Difference between signs and symptoms

Signs: Objective changes that a clinician can observe and measure, for example, BP and fever.

Symptoms: Subjective changes in the body functions that cannot be observed by the clinician, for example, headache, nausea and anxiety.

LEVELS OF STRUCTURAL ORGANIZATION

There are six different levels of structural organization within the human body. The smallest level to the largest level are as follows: the chemical, cellular, tissue, organ, system and organismal levels (Fig. 1.6).

1. **The chemical level**: The chemical level includes the smallest unit of the matter, *the atom,* such as carbon (C), hydrogen (H) and oxygen (O). In the chemical level, two or more atoms join together to form *molecules* such as glucose ($C_6H_{12}O_6$).

2. **The cellular level**: Molecules combine to form *cells*, the basic structural and functional unit of an organism. The cell performs all the activities necessary to maintain life, including metabolism, assimilation, digestion, excretion and reproduction (discussed later in detail).

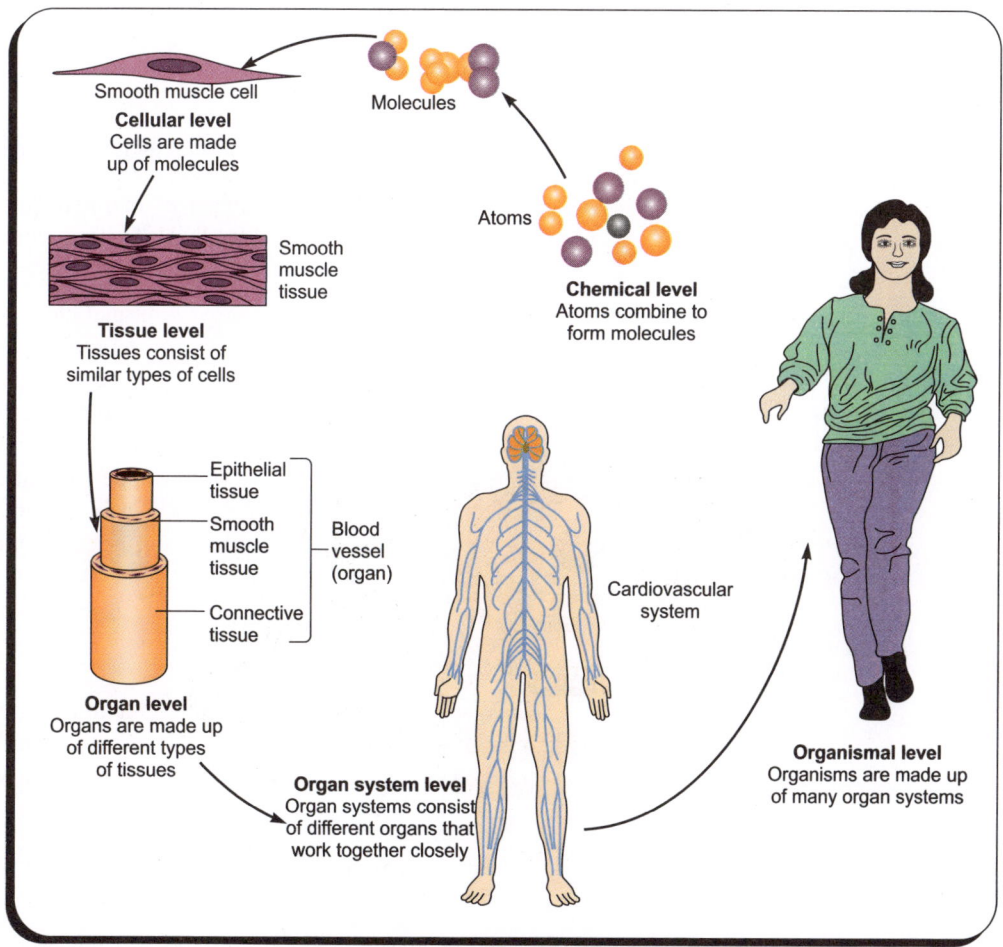

Figure 1.6 Levels of structural organization.

3. **The tissue level**: Different kinds of cells that work together to perform a particular function make up a *tissue*. There are four basic types of tissues: epithelial tissue, connective tissue, muscular tissue and nervous tissue (discussed later in detail).

4. **The organ level**: Different types of tissues are grouped together to form an *organ* that carry out a specific function, for example, stomach and heart.

5. **The system level**: A number of organs with a common function are grouped into systems. The human body has several systems, which work interdependently to carry out specific functions, for example, the digestive system, the urinary system and the skeletal system.

6. **The organismal level**: All the parts of the human body function together and constitute the total *organism*.

THE CELLULAR LEVEL OF ORGANIZATION

The cells are the basic structural and functional units of the human body. All cells arise from the preexisting cells through the process of cell division. The study of the structure and functions of the cell is called *cell biology*.

PARTS OF A CELL

The cell comprises three main parts: the plasma membrane, the cytoplasm and the nucleus. The cell is surrounded by the plasma membrane and comprises the nucleus and a number of organelles suspended in a watery fluid called *cytoplasm* (Fig. 1.7).

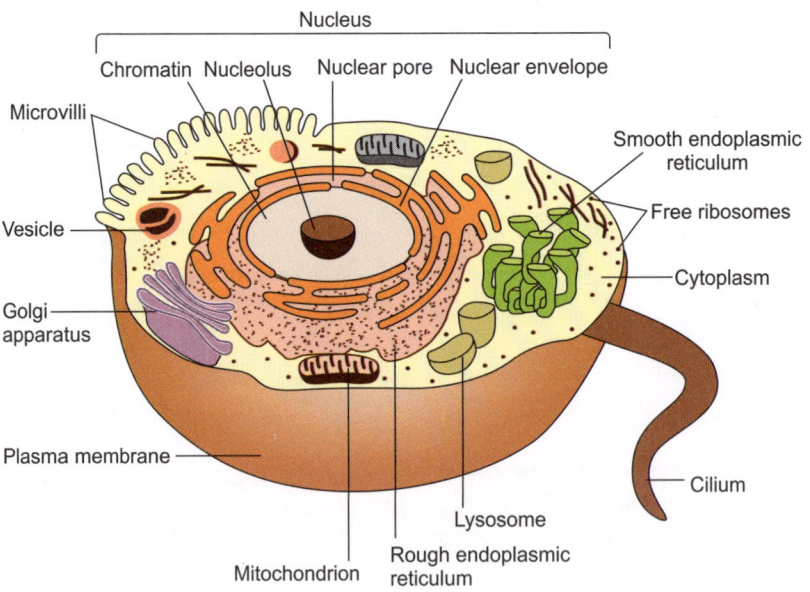

Figure 1.7 Parts of a cell.

The plasma membrane

The plasma membrane or the cell membrane is a protective semipermeable membrane that surrounds the cell. This membrane separates the extracellular fluid (fluid outside the cell) and the intracellular fluid (fluid inside the cell) and helps maintain the cell's internal environment by regulating the flow of substances into and out of the cell.

Structure of the plasma membrane

The structure of the plasma membrane is best described using a structural model called *the fluid mosaic model*. According to this model, the plasma membrane resembles a sea of fluid lipids containing various proteins floating like icebergs or anchored like boats in it. Electron microscopic study has revealed that the plasma membrane is a lipid bilayer with various proteins embedded in it (Fig. 1.8).

❑ The lipid bilayer is made up of three types of lipid molecules: phospholipids (75%), cholesterol (20%) and glycolipids (5%). As majority of the lipid molecules are phospholipids, this lipid bilayer is also referred to as the *phospholipid bilayer*.

➤ The phospholipids molecules resemble a headed pin in shape and have a *head* that is electrically charged (polar) and hydrophilic (water loving) and a *tail* that is nonpolar and hydrophobic (water repelling). The two layers of phospholipids are arranged in such a way that the hydrophilic heads face outwards and thus are close to the watery fluid on either side, that is, the cytoplasm inside and the extracellular fluid outside. The hydrophobic tails point inwards towards one another forming a nonpolar, hydrophobic region in the interior of the membrane. This arrangement allows only the nonpolar, fat-soluble substances such as steroids, oxygen and carbon dioxide to pass through the hydrophobic tail and acts as a barrier to the entry of polar, water-soluble substances such as glucose, urea and electrolytes.

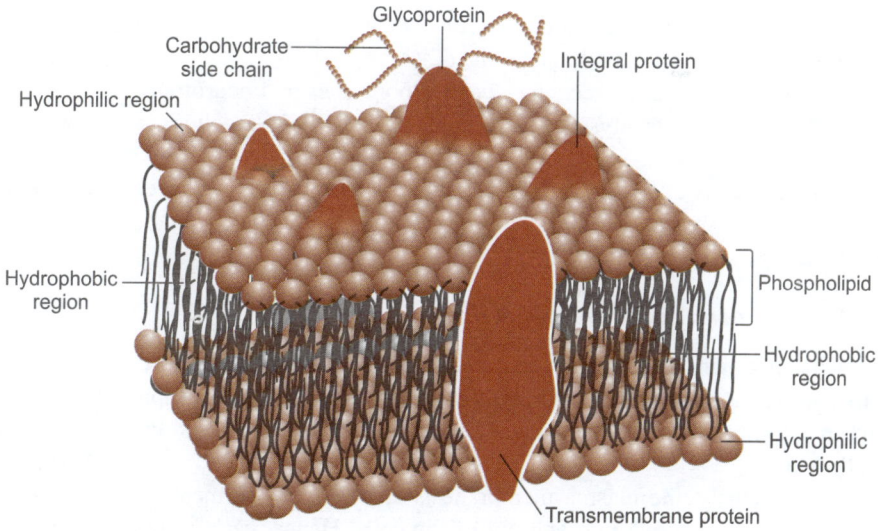

Figure 1.8 Plasma membrane (fluid mosaic membrane model).

➤ The cholesterol molecules are arranged in between the phospholipid molecules and provide structural integrity to the cell membrane.

➤ The glycolipids (i.e. the lipids with attached carbohydrate group) are present throughout the surface of the plasma membrane.

❑ The membrane proteins embedded in the lipid bilayer are of two types: integral proteins and peripheral proteins.

➤ The integral proteins are also known as *transmembrane proteins* as they pass through the entire thickness of the plasma membrane from one side to the other and are firmly embedded in the membrane.

➤ The peripheral proteins are partially embedded in the outer and inner surfaces of the plasma membrane and do not penetrate the membrane. They are loosely bound and hence can dissociate readily from the cell membrane.

❑ Most of the membrane proteins are glycoproteins (proteins with carbohydrate groups). The carbohydrate portions of glycoproteins and glycolipids form a thin loose covering over the entire surface of the cell membrane called *glycocalyx*.

Functions of plasma membrane

1. The plasma membrane protects the cytoplasm and various organelles in the cytoplasm and is responsible for maintaining the shape and size of the cell.

2. The plasma membrane is selectively permeable and thus permits only some selective substances to pass through it and acts as a barrier for other substances. Thus, it enables the cell to maintain homeostasis or a constant internal environment.

3. The membrane proteins embedded in the lipid bilayer of the plasma membrane perform several functions:

   (a) Some integral proteins form *ion channels* through which specific ions, such as potassium ions (K^+), can move in or out of the cell.

   (b) Some proteins act as *channels* and *transporters* that selectively transport the polar substance or ion from one side of the membrane to the other.

   (c) Some proteins serve as the *receptor sites* for hormones and neurotransmitters, whereas some form the enzymes that catalyse specific chemical (metabolic) reactions inside or outside the cell surface.

4. The glycocalyx acts as *cell-identity markers* and enables the cells to recognise one another. In addition, the glycocalyx acts as a cementing material for cell adhesion and helps in attaching cells to one another.

Transport of substances across the plasma membrane

Transport of substances across the plasma membrane is essential for the survival of the cell. Certain substances like nutrients, water and electrolytes must move inside the cell to support the cell's metabolic reactions, whereas other unwanted substances like cellular waste products and carbon dioxide must move out of the cell.

As discussed previously, the plasma membrane is a selectively permeable membrane and allows only selected substances to move into and out of the cells. Hence, certain transport mechanisms are involved in the transport of substances across the plasma membrane. These transport mechanisms can be classified into two types: passive transport and active transport (Fig. 1.9).

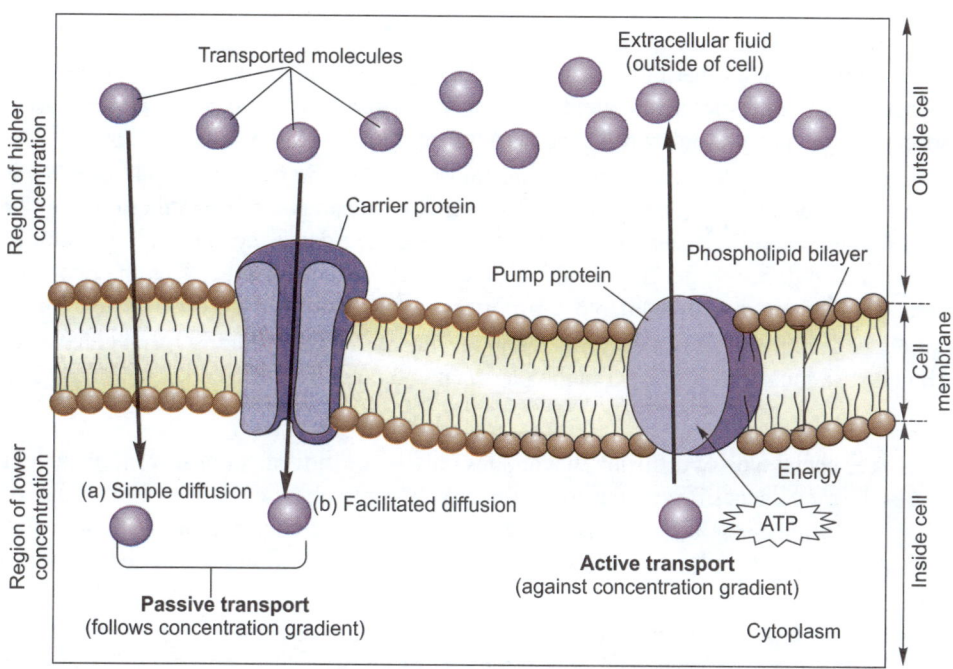

Figure 1.9 Passive and active transport.

Passive transport

❏ The movement of substances along the concentration gradient (downhill), that is, from the region of higher concentration to lower concentration without using energy, is called *passive transport* or *diffusion*.

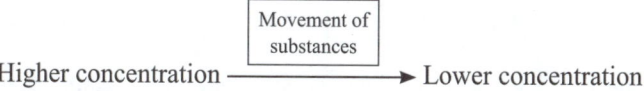

Higher concentration ⎯⎯⎯⎯⎯⎯⎯⟶ Lower concentration

❏ Diffusion is of two types, namely simple diffusion and facilitated diffusion.

Simple diffusion

❏ Simple diffusion refers to the movement of a chemical substance from an area of high concentration to an area of low concentration until it reaches equilibrium. It occurs mainly in gases, liquids and solutions. The process of diffusion is accelerated if the temperature and/or concentration of diffusing substances are increased. An important example of diffusion in the human body is the transfer of oxygen from lungs (high concentration) into the blood (low concentration) and the transfer of carbon dioxide from blood to the lungs.

❏ Substances can also diffuse through the semipermeable membrane if the membrane is permeable to them. The movement of nonpolar, lipid-soluble substances like oxygen, carbon dioxide and alcohol through the lipid bilayer of plasma membrane is one such example of diffusion. The electrolytes (K^+, Na^+, Cl^-, Ca^{2+}) diffuse through the protein layer of the plasma membrane as some integral proteins form ion channels or pores for the movement of specific ions across the lipid bilayer.

Facilitated diffusion

❏ This is a passive process that facilitates the diffusion of large molecules that are unable to diffuse through the semipermeable membrane, for example, glucose and amino acids. These substances are transported by the integral proteins that act as a transporter.

❏ In this process, the solute binds to a specific transporter on the membrane side that has a higher concentration of solute. The transporter then changes its shape and releases the solute on the other side of the membrane. In this way, the solute is transported down the concentration gradient. The rate of facilitated diffusion depends on the difference in concentration between the two sides of the membrane and the number of available transporters.

❏ An important example of facilitated diffusion in the human body is the transport of glucose inside the cells by glucose transporters present in the plasma membrane of certain cells.

Osmosis

❏ Osmosis is a special type of diffusion that applies only to the movement of solvent (water). It can be defined as the movement of water through a selectively permeable membrane from an area of higher water concentration (e.g. pure water) to an area of lower water concentration (e.g. water with salt/sugar). Osmosis occurs only when the membrane is permeable to water and is not permeable to the solutes.

❏ The force with which this diffusion occurs is called *osmotic pressure*. The osmotic pressure of a solution is directly proportional to the concentration of solute (i.e. the higher the solute concentration, the higher would be the osmotic pressure). Osmosis proceeds until equilibrium is reached, that is, the point when the solutions on each side of the membrane are of the same concentration and this state is said to be *isotonic*.

❏ The effect of osmosis can easily be demonstrated on red blood cells (RBCs) in the following ways (Fig. 1.10).

    (a) If an RBC is placed in a normal saline solution (*isotonic solution*) where the salt concentration outside the RBC equals the salt concentration inside the RBC, water molecules will pass into and out of the RBC at an equal rate and there will be no observed change in the shape of the RBC.

    (b) If, however, the RBC is placed in a *hypotonic solution* (e.g. distilled water) where the water molecules are in higher concentration outside the RBC, water will move down its concentration gradient into the RBC, causing it to swell and eventually rupture.

    (c) If the RBC is placed in a *hypertonic solution* (e.g. 5% salt solution) where there is more water inside the RBC than in the solution, the RBC will lose water and will shrink up or crenulate.

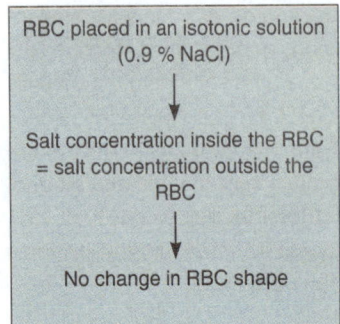

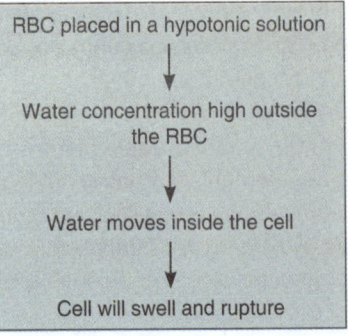

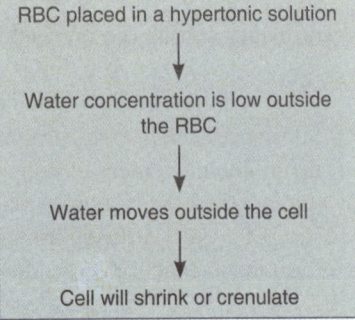

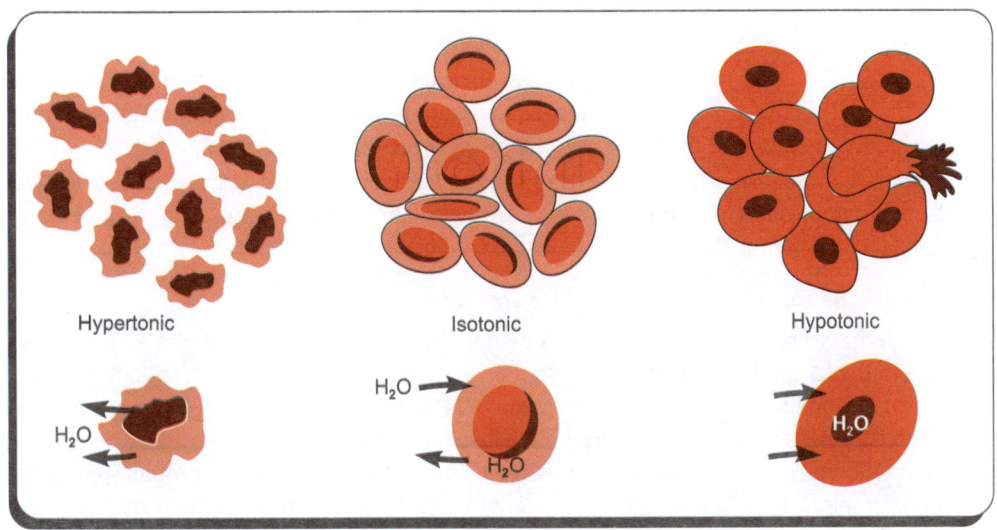

Figure 1.10 Osmosis in RBC.

Factors affecting the rate of diffusion

The rate of diffusion of substances through the plasma membrane is affected by the following factors:

1. **Concentration gradient**: Rate of diffusion is directly proportional to the concentration difference between the two sides of the membrane. The greater the concentration gradient, the higher would be the rate of diffusion.
2. **Temperature**: The rate of diffusion is directly proportional to temperature. The diffusion processes in the body occur more rapidly in a person who has fever.
3. **Size of the diffusing molecules**: Rate of diffusion is inversely proportional to the size of molecules. Thus, the smaller molecules diffuse more rapidly than the larger ones.
4. **Surface area**: Rate of diffusion is directly proportional to the surface area available for diffusion.

Active transport

❏ The movement of substances against their concentration gradient (uphill), that is, from a lower to a higher concentration, is called *active transport*. It is an active process as the specialized protein carrier molecules or transporters require energy to move the solutes across the membrane against the concentration gradient. The substances that are actively transported across the plasma membrane include several ions (such as Na^+, K^+, H^+ and Ca^+), amino acids and monosaccharides (such as glucose).
❏ There are two types of active transport: *primary active transport* and *secondary active transport*.

Primary active transport

❏ In primary active transport, the energy is obtained directly from the hydrolysis of adenosine triphosphate (ATP). The transporter proteins that carry out this transport are called *pumps*.
❏ The *sodium–potassium (Na^+/K^+) pump* is the most prevalent primary active transport mechanism in the human body. This pump is present in all the cells of the body and is responsible for the distribution of sodium and potassium ions across the plasma membrane.

❑ The plasma membrane maintains a difference in the distribution of ions between the two sides of the plasma membrane. Typically, potassium ions (K⁺) are present intracellularly and sodium ions (Na⁺) extracellularly. These ions tend to diffuse down their concentration gradients (i.e. K⁺ outwards and Na⁺ into the cell). Thus, to maintain their concentration gradients, the sodium–potassium pumps work constantly to pump out the Na⁺ across the plasma membrane in exchange for K⁺.

❑ The transporter protein involved in the Na⁺/K⁺ pump has six binding sites: three for sodium ions towards the cytoplasm (intracellular), two for potassium ions towards the extracellular fluid (extracellular) and one for the enzyme adenosine triphosphatase (ATPase).

Mechanism of the action of the Na⁺/K⁺ pump (Fig. 1.11)

1. Three sodium ions present in the cytoplasm bind to the Na⁺ binding site and two K⁺ ions outside the cell bind to the K⁺ binding site of the transporter protein.
2. Binding of Na⁺ and K⁺ ions activate the enzyme ATPase, which triggers the hydrolysis of ATP into ADP with the release of one high-energy phosphate group (Pi).
3. The energy liberated causes some conformational change in the transporter protein (pump) because of which the intracellular site (with sodium ions) faces the outer side of the cell and vice versa.
4. Now, the dissociation and release of ions take place so that Na⁺ ions are released outside the cell and K⁺ ions are released inside the cell.

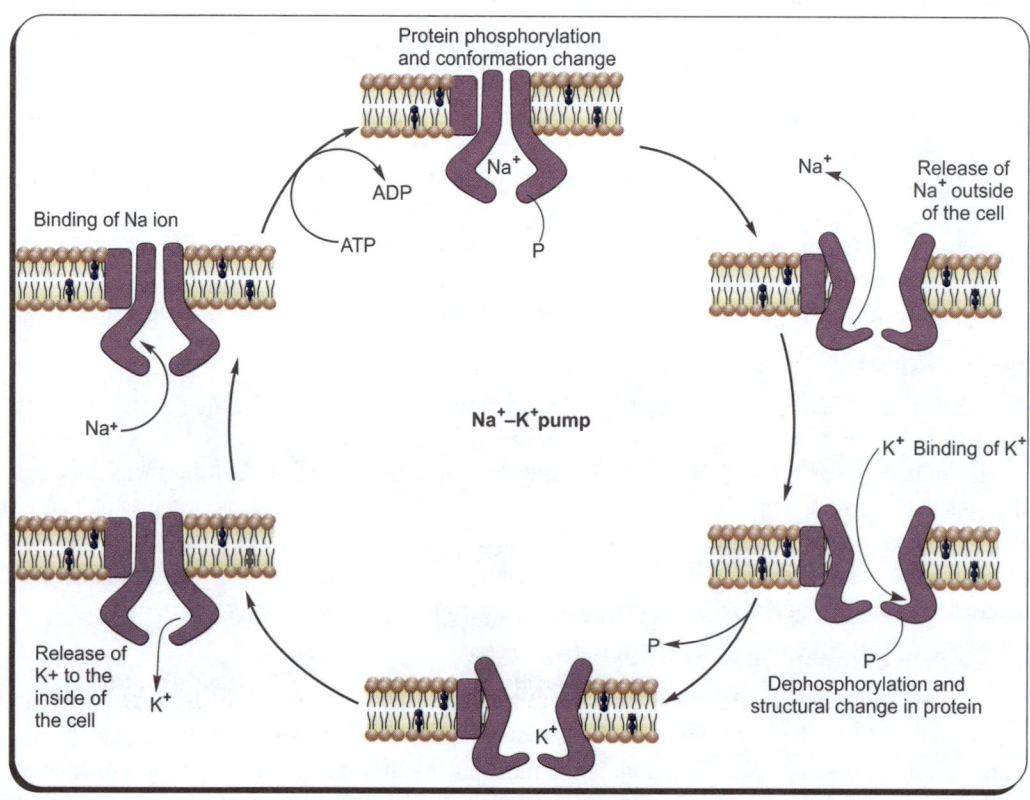

Figure 1.11 Sodium–potassium pump.

Secondary active transport

❑ As discussed previously, the Na^+/K^+ pump maintains a concentration gradient of Na^+ across the plasma membrane. However, sodium ion tends to diffuse down its concentration gradient with the help of a transporter protein.

❑ In secondary active transport, the transporter protein simultaneously binds to sodium and another substance and transports the other substance against its concentration gradient and sodium ion along its concentration gradient simultaneously. Thus, in this process, Na^+ ions move down their concentration gradient, that is, moves inside the cell whereas the other substance moves uphill against its concentration gradient.

❑ Secondary active transport is of two types:

➤ **Sodium cotransport**: If the transporter moves Na^+ and another substance in the same direction, the process is called *Na+ cotransport*, and the transporters involved are called *symporters*; for example, Na^+/glucose and Na^+/amino acid symporters help in the absorption of glucose and amino acid into the cell.

➤ **Sodium counter-transport**: If the transporter moves Na^+ and another substance in the opposite directions across the membrane, the process is called *Na+ counter-transport*, and the transporters involved are called *antiporters*; for example, the Na^+/Ca^{2+} counter-transport ejects Ca^{2+} ions from the cell; the Na^+/H^+ counter-transport regulates the pH of the cytoplasm by expelling excess H^+ while Na^+ enters the cell.

Special categories of transport mechanisms

In addition to the active and passive transport mechanisms, some special categories of transport systems also exist in the body. These special transport mechanisms include endocytosis and exocytosis. These mechanisms are used to transport large particles such as whole bacteria, red blood cells and macromolecules such as polysaccharides and proteins that cannot pass through the plasma membrane.

Endocytosis

❑ Endocytosis is the process by which large molecules enter the cell in a vesicle formed from the plasma membrane. In this process, the plasma membrane surrounds the substances to be taken inside the cell and then that area buds off inside the cell to form a vesicle.

❑ Endocytosis is of three types: pinocytosis, phagocytosis and receptor-mediated endocytosis (Fig. 1.12). The macromolecules that cannot cross the plasma membrane are transported by pinocytosis or phagocytosis.

Pinocytosis

❑ The process by which macromolecules such as bacteria or antigens are transported into the cell is called *pinocytosis* or *cell drinking*. It is also called cell drinking because it involves the uptake of tiny droplets of solutes dissolved in the extracellular fluid.

❑ In pinocytosis, the fluid droplets bind to the outer surface of the plasma membrane and then that area of the plasma membrane folds inwards around the droplets to form a vesicle. This vesicle is called *endosome*, and it detaches or 'pinches off' from the plasma membrane and enters the interior of the cell. Within the cell, the lysosomes come in contact with the endosome and adhere to it, which leads to the rupture of the lysosomal membrane. This causes release and activation of enzymes present in the lysosome. The enzymes break down the membrane of endosomes and release the substances present in the endosome into the cytoplasm.

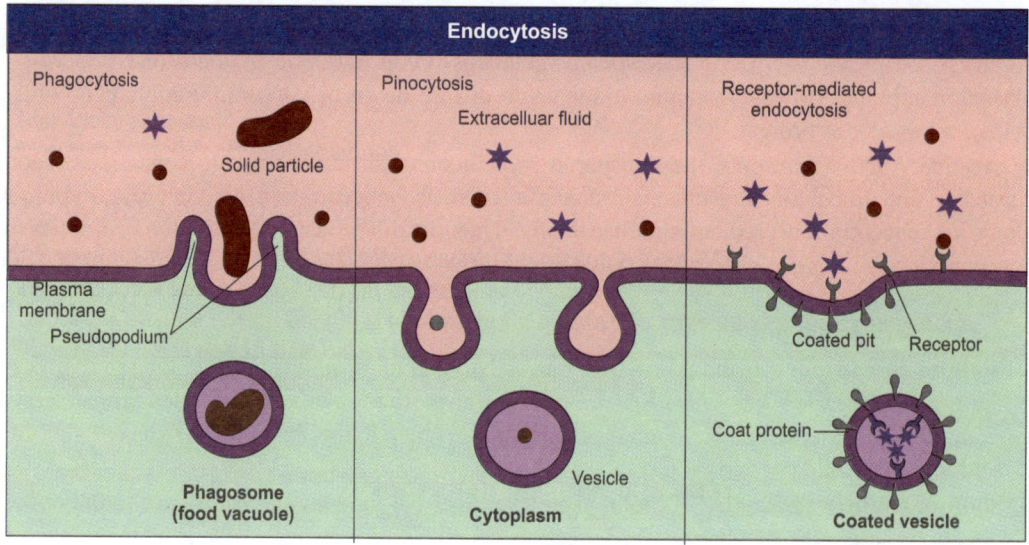

Figure 1.12 Endocytosis transport mechanism.

Phagocytosis

❑ The process by which particles larger than macromolecules such as whole bacteria or viruses are engulfed into cells is called *phagocytosis* or *cell eating*. Only few cells in the body show phagocytosis, and these cells are termed as *phagocytes*. Phagocytes include neutrophils, monocytes and tissue macrophages, and they mainly engulf and destroy bacteria and other foreign substances and help protect the body from diseases.

❑ When the bacteria or the foreign body binds to the plasma membrane, the phagocytic cell extends projections of its plasma membrane and the cytoplasm called *pseudopods* around them. The pseudopods then form a vesicle called *phagosome,* which enters the cell, and the ingested material is broken down by lysosomal enzymes.

Receptor-mediated endocytosis

❑ The process by which the ligands bind to the receptors present on the plasma membrane and are taken inside the cell is called *receptor-mediated endocytosis*. This process is used by the cells for the uptake of some vitamins, hormones such as insulin, low-density lipoproteins (LDLs) and other specific macromolecules.

❑ The receptors that bind to the ligands are concentrated in specific regions of the plasma membrane and contain a receptor protein called clathrin; hence, they are also called *clathrin-coated pits*. Binding of ligands to the receptors forms ligand–receptor complexes, which get aggregated in the clathrin-coated pit. This binding causes the edges of the membrane around the ligand–receptor complexes to invaginate (fold inwards) and detach from the plasma membrane to form a clathrin-coated vesicle. This vesicle is now called *endosome*, and it moves into the deeper part of the cell where it fuses with the lysosome. The enzymes of the lysosome digest the membrane of the endosome and release the ligand or substances present in the endosome into the cytoplasm.

Transcytosis

When the ligand–receptor complexes move across the cell inside the vesicles and undergo exocytosis on the opposite side, the process is called *transcytosis*. It usually occurs in the endothelial cells that line the blood vessels and is used to transfer substances between blood and the interstitial fluid.

Exocytosis

❑ Exocytosis is the process by which substances move out of a cell in vesicles without passing through the plasma membrane. It is mainly involved in the release of secretory substances like hormones, digestive enzymes and neurotransmitters.

❑ During exocytosis, the substances to be secreted are stored in membrane-enclosed vesicles called *secretory vesicles* in the cytoplasm. These secretory vesicles come close to the plasma membrane, fuse with it and release their contents out of the cell in the extracellular fluid.

Cytoplasm

The cytoplasm is the fluid portion present inside the cell between the plasma membrane and the nucleus. It can be divided into two components: cytosol and organelles.

Cytosol

Cytosol is the watery fluid of the cytoplasm in which various organelles are suspended. It is composed of 75–90% water and various dissolved and suspended substances such as various ions, glucose, amino acids, lipids, ATP and waste products.

Organelles

The organelles (meaning small organs) are highly specialized subcellular structures having a characteristic shape and specific functions. The various organelles include cytoskeleton, ribosomes, the endoplasmic reticulum (ER), the Golgi apparatus, lysosomes and the mitochondria. Each organelle performs a specific function and cooperates with each other to maintain homeostasis.

The organelles present in the cytoplasm are of two types: nonmembranous and membranous.

❑ **Nonmembranous organelles**: These organelles lack the membrane and are in direct contact with the cytosol, for example, ribosomes and cytoskeleton.

❑ **Membranous organelles**: These organelles are surrounded by the lipid bilayer membrane, for example, the endoplasmic reticulum, the Golgi apparatus, the mitochondria and lysosomes.

The sections that follow provide a detailed description about various organelles.

Mitochondria

The mitochondria (singular: *mitochondrion*) are small oblong-shaped structures enclosed by two membranes. The outer mitochondrial membrane is smooth and gives the mitochondria its characteristic shape; however, the inner mitochondrial membrane is arranged in a series of folds called *cristae* that provides large surface area for the energy-producing chemical reactions that occur on it. Enclosed by the inner membrane and cristae is the central fluid-filled cavity of the mitochondria called the *matrix* (Fig. 1.13a).

The major function of the mitochondria is production of energy in the form of ATP by chemical reactions of aerobic respiration, that is, the citric acid cycle and the electron transport system that occur in the matrix and cristae of the mitochondria. The matrix also contains various enzymes that catalyse these reactions. Because of their functions in ATP generation, the mitochondria are also called the *power house of the cell*.

A cell may have as few as a hundred or as many as several thousand mitochondria. Physiologically active cells that have high energy requirement such as in muscles, liver and kidneys have a larger number of mitochondria because they use ATP at a higher rate.

Lysosomes

Lysosomes are the membrane-enclosed vesicles that are formed by the Golgi apparatus. They contain powerful digestive or hydrolytic enzymes that are capable of breaking down a wide variety of molecules (e.g. DNA, RNA, proteins and carbohydrates) (Fig. 1.13b).

Function of lysosomes

The lysosomal enzymes, also called *lysozymes,* are involved in the following processes:

❏ Digestion of proteins, carbohydrates, lipids and nucleic acids and release of their final breakdown products into cytosol.
❏ *Autophagy* (*auto*: self; *phagy*: eating), i.e. the digestion of worn-out organelles and release of the digested components in the cytosol for reuse. In this way, the lysosomal enzymes recycle the own structures of the cell.
❏ *Autolysis,* i.e. the digestion of the entire cell that may occur in certain pathological conditions and immediately after death. In this process, the lysosomes expel all of their enzymes directly into the cytosol to destroy the cell and its organelles.
❏ Lysosomes in WBCs digest the foreign bodies such as microbes.

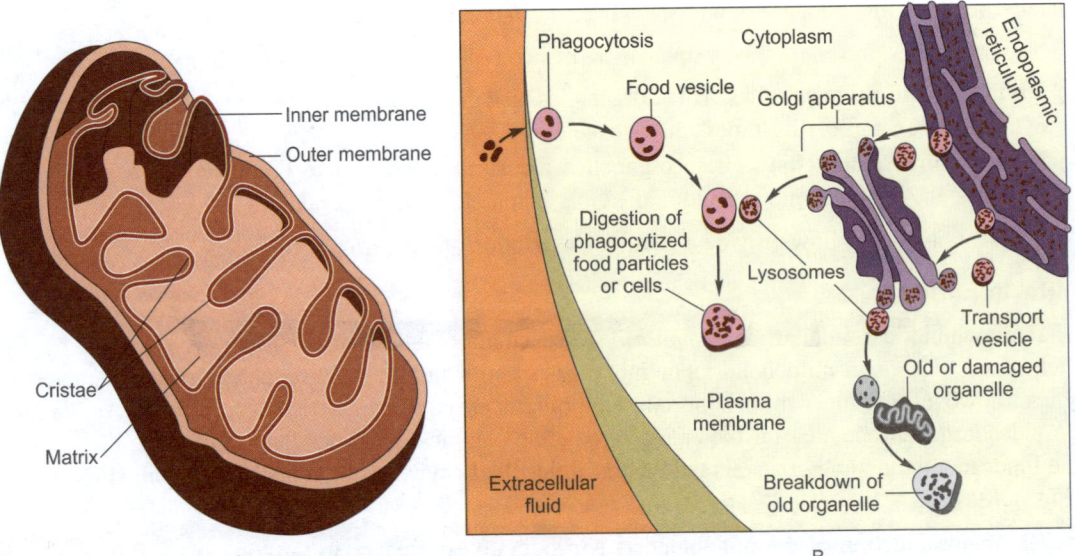

Figure 1.13 (a) Mitochondria; (b) Lysosomes.

Peroxisomes

These are small membrane-enclosed vesicles that are similar in structure to lysosomes. They contain some oxidative enzymes that are capable of oxidizing various organic substances such as amino acids, fatty acids and toxic substances such as alcohol. These oxidation reactions generate hydrogen peroxide (H_2O_2) as a by-product, which is a very toxic compound. The peroxisomes also decompose H_2O_2 and protect the other parts of the cell from the toxic effects of H_2O_2.

Endoplasmic reticulum

Endoplasmic reticulum is a series of interconnecting membranous canals in the cytoplasm. The membranous canals form flattened sacs or tubules called *cisternae* that extend from the nuclear membrane to the plasma membrane, and thus form a link between the nucleus and the plasma membrane (Fig. 1.14).

The endoplasmic reticulum is of two types: rough endoplasmic reticulum and smooth endoplasmic reticulum.

Rough endoplasmic reticulum: The outer surface of the rough endoplasmic reticulum is studded with ribosomes, hence the name rough. The ribosomes are the sites of protein synthesis. The proteins synthesized by ribosomes are processed within the endoplasmic reticulum and then released from cells, for example, hormones and enzymes. In addition, the rough endoplasmic reticulum is involved in the synthesis of glycoproteins and phospholipids that are incorporated in the plasma membrane.

Smooth endoplasmic reticulum: Smooth endoplasmic reticulum extends from the rough endoplasmic reticulum to form a network of membranous tubules. Unlike the rough endoplasmic reticulum, the smooth endoplasmic reticulum does not have ribosomes on the outer surface of its membrane. Smooth endoplasmic reticulum synthesizes lipids and steroid hormones such as estrogen and testosterone and is also associated with the detoxification of certain toxic substances such as drugs and carcinogens.

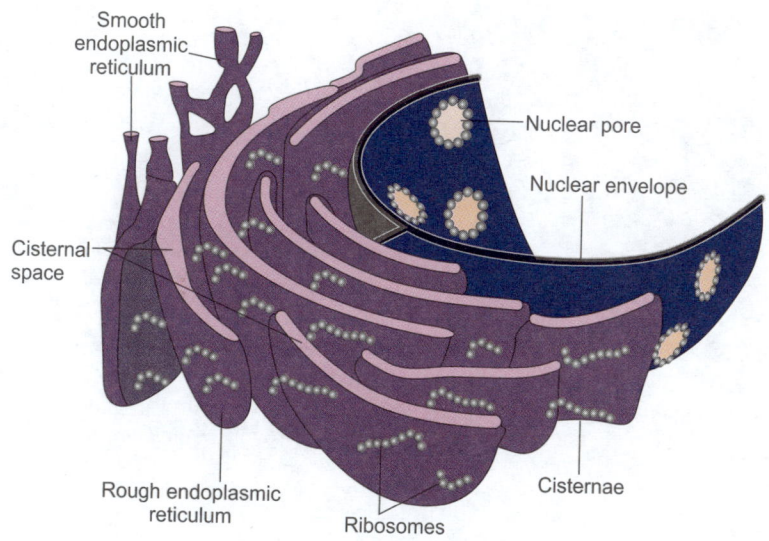

Figure 1.14 Endoplasmic reticulum.

Ribosomes

Ribosomes are tiny granules composed of ribosomal RNA (rRNA) and proteins. They are the sites for protein synthesis; hence, they are also called *protein factories*.

Some ribosomes are present as 'free ribosomes' in the cytoplasm and are involved in the synthesis of proteins for use within the cell, for example, enzymes required for metabolism and the protein part of haemoglobin. The remaining ribosomes are attached to the outer surface of the nuclear membrane and endoplasmic reticulum and are called *membrane-bound ribosomes*. These ribosomes synthesize proteins for insertion in the plasma membrane or for release outside the cell, for example, phospholipids, hormones and enzymes.

Golgi apparatus

The Golgi apparatus or Golgi body or Golgi complex consists of 3–20 flattened membranous sacs called *cisternae* (Fig. 1.15). It is present in all cells except RBCs. Most cells have only one Golgi apparatus and it is larger in cells that synthesise and secrete proteins in the extracellular fluid.

The major function of the Golgi apparatus is processing, packaging and delivering protein molecules to different parts of the cell. The proteins synthesized by ribosomes in the endoplasmic reticulum are transported to the Golgi apparatus in the form of membrane-bound vesicles. In the Golgi apparatus, the vesicles are processed, sorted out and packed in the form of secretory granules, secretory vesicles, lysosomes, etc., and stored. When needed, these vesicles and granules move to the plasma membrane where the proteins are released by exocytosis into the extracellular fluid.

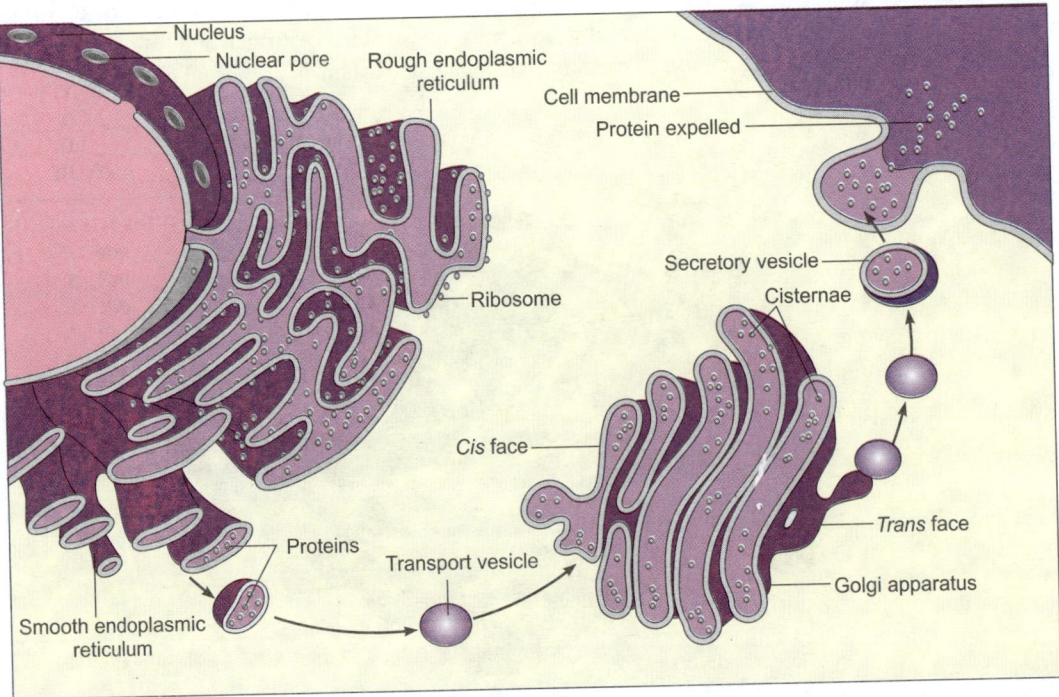

Figure 1.15 Golgi apparatus.

Cytoskeleton

The *cytoskeleton* is a complex network of tiny strands of proteins that extend throughout the cytosol. It provides a structural framework for the cell and determines its shape. It is also responsible for cellular movements including the movement of chromosomes during cell division and the movement of whole cells such as phagocytes.

The cytoskeleton is composed of three types of protein fibres: microfilaments, intermediate filaments and microtubules (Fig. 1.16).

Microfilaments: They are the thinnest fibres of the cytoskeleton. Most of the microfilaments are composed of the protein *actin* and are concentrated at the cell periphery. The microfilaments provide structural support, maintain the characteristic shape of the cell and are responsible for cellular movements, for example, contraction in muscle cells and migration of skin during wound healing.

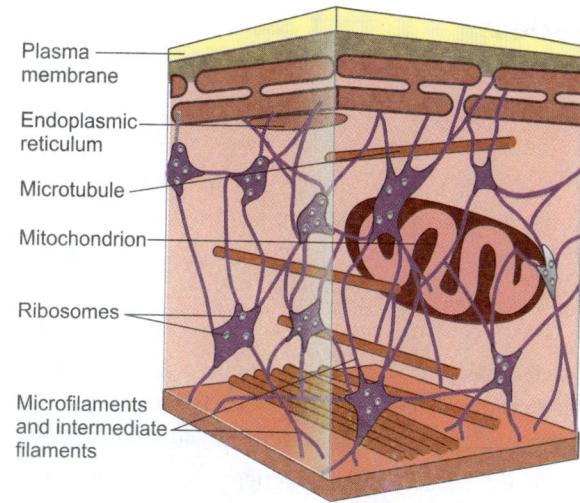

Plasma membrane

Endoplasmic reticulum

Microtubule

Mitochondrion

Ribosomes

Microfilaments and intermediate filaments

Figure 1.16 Cytoskeleton.

Intermediate filaments: They are thicker than microtubules. These protein fibres form a network around the nucleus and extend to the cell periphery. They maintain the shape of the cell and also help hold the organelles firmly.

Microtubules: They are the largest of the cytoskeletal components and are mainly composed of a protein called *tubulin*. They give the structural strength to the cell and are responsible for the movement of the organelles within the cell, chromosomes during cell division and cell extensions, that is, cilia and flagella.

Centrosome

The centrosome is located near the nucleus and consists of two components: pericentriolar area and centrioles. The pericentriolar area is responsible for the formation of mitotic spindle during cell division and for the organization of microtubules in the cell. Within the pericentriolar area is a pair of centrioles, present at right angles to each other near the nuclear membrane. The centrioles consist of small clusters of microtubules that are responsible for the movement of cell extensions and the movement of chromosomes during cell division (discussed in detail in the Cell Division section).

Cell extensions

The *cell extensions* are the motile projections of the plasma membrane that consists of microtubules as their major component. They include:

Cilia: These are small, hair-like projections that extend from the cell surface. Many cilia move together in coordination and result in the movement of substances along the cell surface, for example, the movement of hundreds of cilia in the respiratory tract moves the foreign particles trapped in the mucus upwards away from the lungs.

Flagella: These are long, whip-like projections that can move an entire cell, for example, tail of spermatozoa.

Nucleus

The nucleus is the most prominent, spherical- or oval-shaped structure in the cell. Every cell in the body has a nucleus except mature RBCs. Most of the body cells have a single nucleus, whereas few cell types such as skeletal muscle cells contain several nuclei.

The nucleus is covered by a double-layered membrane called *nuclear membrane*, which is similar to the plasma membrane but has tiny perforations called *nuclear pores* that regulate the movement of substances between the nucleus and the cytoplasm. The outer layer of the nuclear membrane is continuous with the endoplasmic reticulum.

The nuclear membrane encloses various structures of the nucleus including:

Nucleoplasm: It is the fluid medium of the nucleus that contains large amount of the genetic material in the form of deoxyribonucleic acid (DNA). This genetic material forms the cell's hereditary units called *genes*, which control the cellular structure and regulate most of the cellular activities.

Nucleoli: These are the spherical bodies present inside the nucleus and are composed of clusters of DNA, RNA and proteins that are not enclosed by a membrane. They serve as the sites of the assembly of ribosomes, which play a key role in protein synthesis (Fig. 1.17).

Genetic information is stored in the form of DNA that contains the cell's hereditary units called *genes*. To simplify, gene is a portion of DNA molecule that contains the message or code for the synthesis of a specific protein. Many genes make up a DNA, and many DNA make up a chromosome. Thus, a

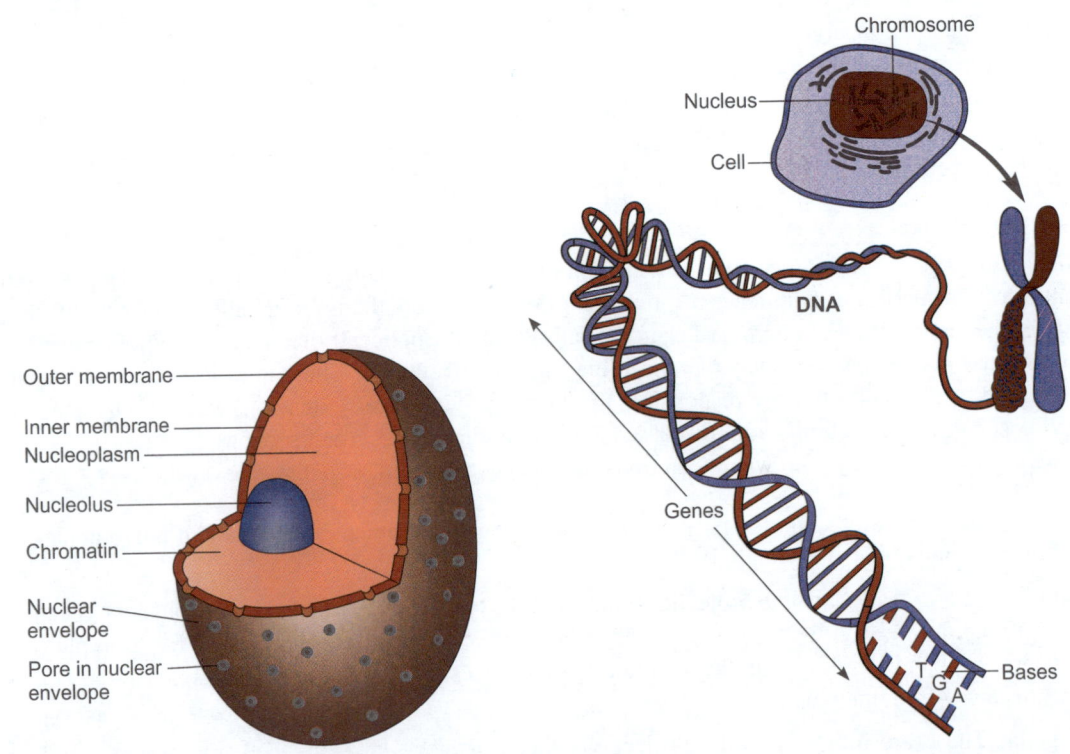

Figure 1.17 Nucleus.

chromosome is a thread-like linear strand of DNA that carries the genes and plays an important role in the transmission of hereditary information. The cells of the human body contain 46 chromosomes, 23 inherited from each parent. When the cell is not dividing, the chromosomes resemble a fine network of threads called *chromatin*.

The nucleus forms the control centre of all the activities of the cell and contains hereditary material in the genes that is passed from one generation to the next. In addition, the DNA molecule in the nucleus contains instructions or codes to make a particular protein.

❑ To synthesize proteins, the information encoded in a region of DNA is first transcribed (copied) to a specific molecule of RNA (mRNA). This process is called *transcription*, and it occurs in the nucleus with the assistance of an enzyme called RNA polymerase.

❑ The mRNA then leaves the nucleus through a nuclear pore and enters ribosomes in the cytoplasm where the information contained in it is *translated* into a corresponding sequence of amino acids that form a protein molecule (Fig. 1.18).

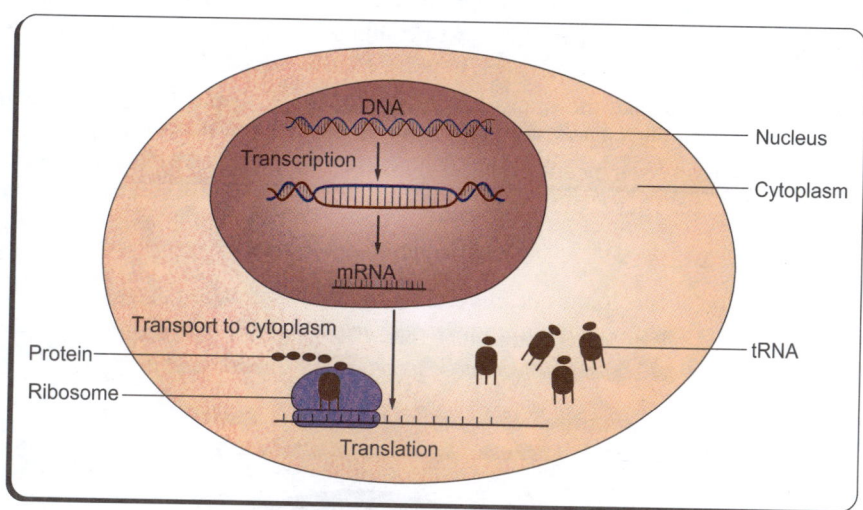

Figure 1.18 Transcription and translation.

CELL DIVISION

Cell division can be defined as the process by which a cell divides into two and duplicates its genetic material. The frequency with which cell division occurs varies with different types of cells.

There are two types of cell divisions: *somatic cell division* and *reproductive cell division*.

❑ **Somatic cell division**: In this process, a cell undergoes a nuclear division called *mitosis* and a cytoplasmic division called *cytokinesis* to produce two genetically identical daughter cells. Most of the body cells divide by mitosis to replace the damaged, diseased or worn-out cells.

❑ **Reproductive cell division**: It is a special kind of two-step division called *meiosis* that occurs only in the gonads for the formation of gametes (sex cells, i.e. ova and spermatozoa). In this process, the genetic material must not only be duplicated but also reduced to half in the daughter cells so that the female egg and sperm carries half of the genetic material (i.e. 23 chromosomes each).

Somatic cell division

There are three main stages in somatic cell division: interphase, mitosis and cytokinesis (Fig. 1.19).

Interphase

❑ Interphase is the longest and most dynamic phase during which the cell undergoes certain changes in anticipation of the cell division. Interphase has three subphases: G_1, S and G_2.

➤ G_1 *phase*: It is the primary growth phase of the cell in which the cell duplicates its organelles and cytosolic components.

➤ *S Phase* or *synthetic phase*: It is the interval between the G_1 and the G_2 phase during which the DNA strands duplicate themselves. The chromosomes resemble a fine network of dark threads called *chromatin*. The chromatin becomes tightly coiled and replicates, thereby forming identical double chromosomes called *sister chromatids* that attach to each other at a central region called the *centromere*. Replication of the centrosome also begins at this phase.

➤ G_2 *phase*: It is the final phase for the preparation of cell division during which the enzymes and other proteins are synthesized and cell growth continues. The centrosome finishes its replication in this phase.

❑ Towards the end of interphase, the microscopic view of a cell displays a clearly defined nuclear membrane, nucleolus and chromatin. The mitotic phase begins after the cell completes its activities in the G_1, S and G_2 phases. Some cells however remain in the G_1 phase for a very long time and are said to be in the G_0 phase. These cells never divide again (e.g. most of the nerve cells).

Mitosis or the mitotic phase

This phase of cell division occurs in the nucleus and results in the formation of two identical nuclei. It is a continuous process that is subdivided into four stages: *prophase*, *metaphase*, *anaphase* and *telophase* (Fig. 1.20).

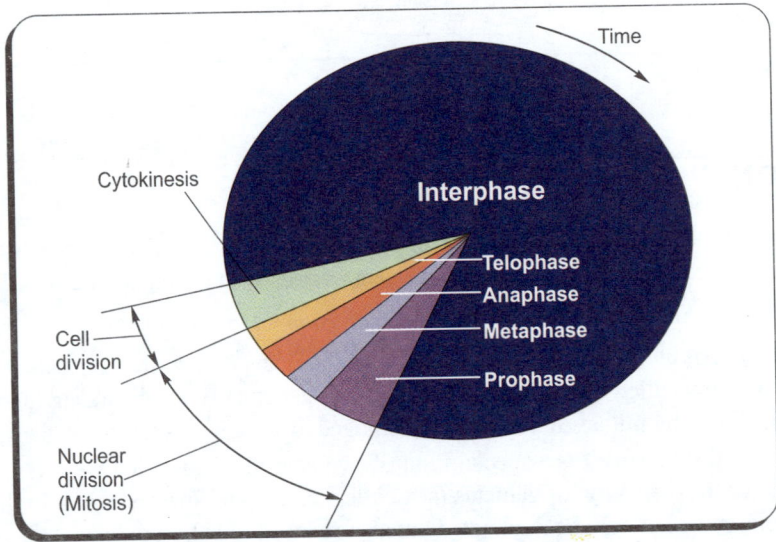

Figure 1.19 Phases of somatic cell division.

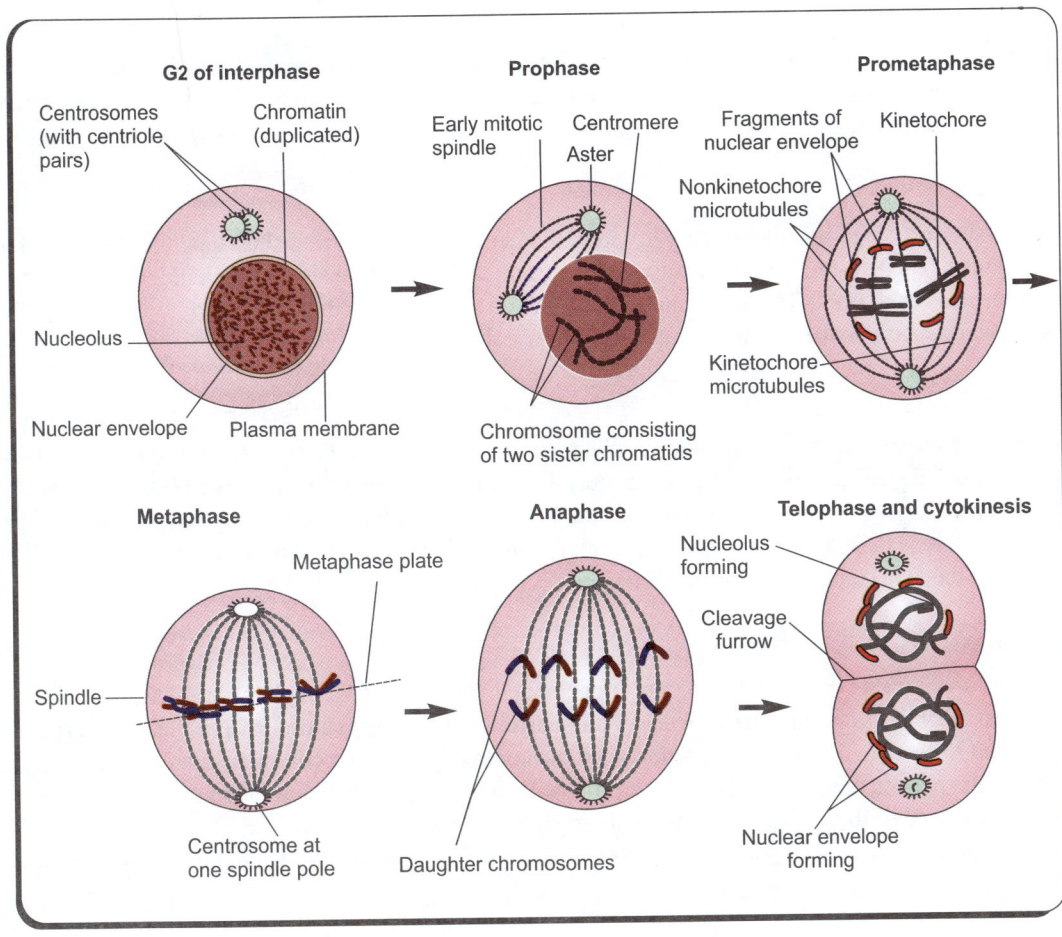

Figure 1.20 Somatic cell division.

Prophase

❏ During early prophase, the sister chromatids that are attached to one another at the centromere become visible within the nucleus.

❏ Each centrosome moves to an opposite pole (end) of the cell, where the pericentriolar area of the centrosome starts to form the *mitotic spindle*, a football-shaped assembly of microtubules. The lengthening of microtubules between the centrosomes pushes the centrioles present within the pericentriolar area to the ends of the cell. At this time, the nuclear membrane breaks down and the nucleolus disappears.

❏ As prophase continues, microtubules of the mitotic spindle extend from the poles (ends) towards the centromeres of the chromosomes. The microtubules coming from two poles (ends) attach to the opposite sides of the centromere in such a way that each of the two sister chromatids are attached to microtubules from different poles. This alignment ensures the separation of the sister chromatids to the opposite poles of the cell.

Metaphase

It is the second stage of mitosis. During metaphase, the microtubules align the centromeres of the sister chromatids at the exact centre of the mitotic spindle. This midpoint region is called the *metaphase plate* or *equatorial plane region*.

Anaphase

It is the shortest stage of mitosis during which the centromeres split and thus separate the two sister chromatids of each chromosome. The divided centromere, each with a sister chromatid, moves towards opposite poles of the cell. The sister chromatids take on a V shape as they are drawn to their respective poles. Once separated, the sister chromatids are now called *daughter chromatids*.

Telophase

The sister chromatids, which can now be called chromosomes reach the opposite poles of the cell and begin to uncondense and uncoil. The uncondensed chromosomes revert back to threadlike chromatin. A nuclear membrane forms around each chromatin mass and nucleoli reappear in the daughter nuclei. The mitotic spindle is disassembled as the microtubules are broken down into units of tubulin that are used to develop the cytoskeleton of new daughter cells.

Cytokinesis

❑ During cytokinesis, the actual separation of the cell into two new daughter cells takes place. This process begins in late anaphase or early telophase, with the indentation of the plasma membrane referred to as a *cleavage furrow* produced by the contraction of the actin microfilaments that lie just inside the plasma membrane. These microfilaments pull the plasma membrane progressively inward into the centre of the cell and eventually divide the cell into two.

❑ Each new daughter cell now enters the interphase stage of the cell division and continues to grow until it is ready to divide once again.

Reproductive cell division

Reproductive cell division by meiosis occurs only in special organs of the body (i.e. in the female gonads or ovaries and in the male gonads or testes) and results in the production of gametes that contain half of the genetic material (i.e. 23 chromosomes). This reduced number is called the *haploid* (n), and thus gametes are *haploid cells*. The fertilization of male gametes (sperm) and female gametes (ova) restores the genetic material to its full complement of 46, and thus the zygote becomes a diploid cell (2n).

Thus, somatic cells such as brain cells, stomach cells and kidney cells contain 23 pairs of chromosomes, or a total of 46 chromosomes in which one member of each pair is inherited from each parent. The chromosomes that make up each pair are called *homologous chromosomes* as they contain similar genes arranged in the same order. An exception to the homologous chromosomes is a pair of chromosomes called the *sex hormones*, designated X and Y. In females, the homologous pair of sex chromosomes consists of two X chromosomes, whereas in males, it consists of one X and one Y chromosome. The other 22 pairs of chromosomes are called *autosomes*.

Meiosis occurs in two successive stages: *meiosis I* and *meiosis II*. The interphase stage precedes meiosis I; in this stage, the chromosomes replicate in the manner similar to that in the interphase before mitosis in somatic cell division.

Meiosis I

Meiosis I consists of four phases: prophase I, metaphase I, anaphase I and telophase I (Fig. 1.21).

Prophase I

❑ In prophase I, the replicated chromosomes shorten, coil, thicken and become visible. The nuclear membrane and nucleoli disappear and the mitotic spindle develops. At this time, the chromosomes pair up with their homologue and are brought so close together by a process called *synapsis* wherein they are lined side by side. The resulting pair of homologous chromosomes, each with two sister chromatids, is called a *tetrad*.

❑ The sister chromatids are so close together that they may exchange genetic material in a process called *crossing over*, which occurs only in meiosis. This crossing over results in genetic recombination (i.e. the formation of new combinations of genes and may be responsible for the genetic variation among humans).

Metaphase I

The centromeres of the two homologous chromosomes attach to the microtubules extending from the opposite poles (ends) of the cell. This alignment ensures that the homologous chromosomes will be pulled to the opposite poles of the cell. The homologous pairs of chromosomes now line along the metaphase plate or the equatorial plate of the cell.

Anaphase I

The microtubules of the spindle shorten and pull the homologous chromosomes in such a manner that one member of each pair separate and move to the opposite pole of the cell. (Unlike mitosis, the centromere does not split in this phase.)

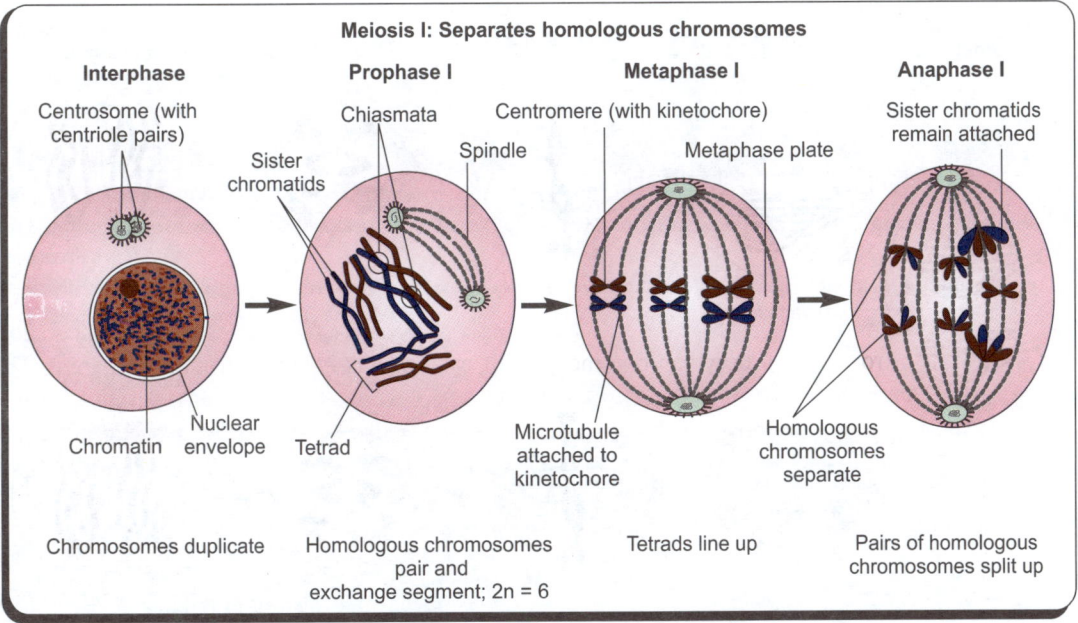

Figure 1.21 Reproductive cell division (meiosis I).

Telophase I

One member of each pair reaches the opposite poles of the cell and each pole now contains haploid (n) (i.e. 23) chromosomes. Now, the spindle disappears and a new nuclear membrane forms around each cluster of chromosomes at the opposite poles. Cytokinesis occurs similar to that in somatic cell division.

The net effect of meiosis I is two daughter cells that contain the haploid number of chromosomes. However, each chromosome still consists of two sister chromatids attached by a common centromere.

Meiosis II

❏ Meiosis II also consists of four phases: prophase II, metaphase II, anaphase II and telophase II (Fig. 1.22). These phases are very similar to those occuring in mitosis.
  ➤ **Prophase II**: In each of the two daughter cells formed in meiosis I, a spindle develops and the chromosomes shorten, coil and thicken. The nuclear membrane disappears but no duplication of DNA occurs.
  ➤ **Metaphase II**: The chromosomes line up on the equatorial plate and microtubules bind to the opposite sides of the centromere.
  ➤ **Anaphase II**: The centromeres split and the sister chromatids separate and move towards the opposite poles of the cell. Now, each chromosome is haploid, consisting of one chromatid and one centromere.
  ➤ **Telophase II**: The spindle disappears and a new nuclear membrane forms around the separated chromatids. The result is four haploid daughter cells, each containing half the genetic material compared with the original parent cell (i.e. 23 chromosomes).

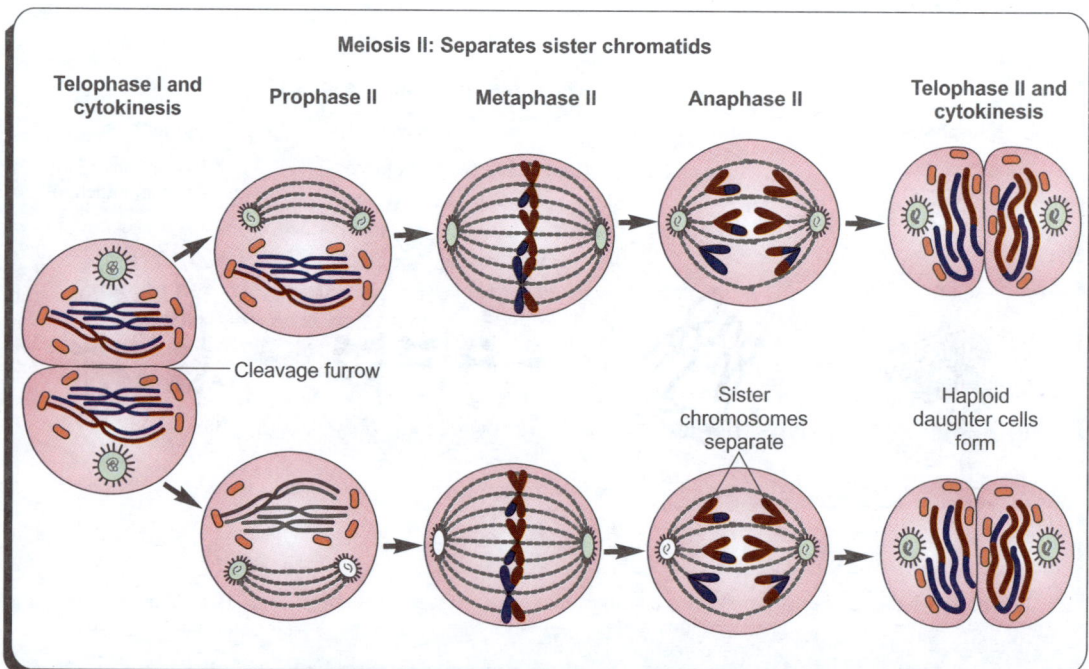

Figure 1.22 Reproductive cell division (meiosis II).

❑ In summary, meiosis I results in two daughter cells, each with the haploid number of chromosomes, and meiosis II results in the division of each haploid cell and the formation of four haploid cells.

THE TISSUE LEVEL OF ORGANIZATION

A *tissue* is a group of similar cells that work together to perform a specialized function. The science that deals with the study of tissues is called *histology*.

Body tissues can be classified into four basic types (Fig. 1.23):

1. **Epithelial tissue or the epithelium**: It covers the body surface and lines the body cavities, hollow organs and ducts.
2. **Connective tissue**: It is the most abundant tissue in the body. It protects and supports the body and its organs.
3. **Muscle tissue**: It is responsible for the movement of the various body structures and of the body as a whole.
4. **Nervous tissue**: It detects the changes in the internal and external environment and responds by generating nerve impulses.

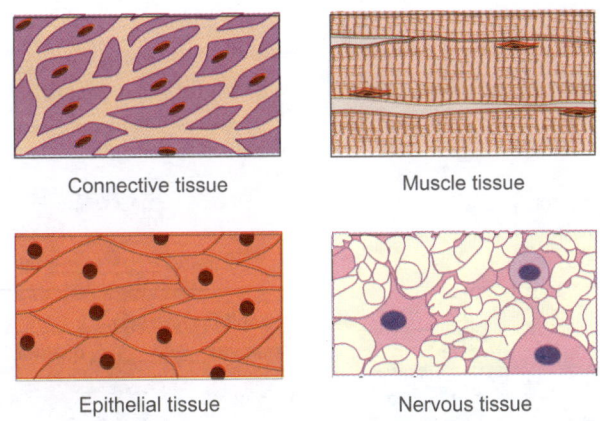

Figure 1.23 Four types of tissues.

EPITHELIAL TISSUE

The epithelial tissue consists of cells arranged in continuous sheets, in either single or multiple layers.

Epithelial tissue performs various functions, which include:

1. **Protection of underlying tissues**: For example, our skin is the epithelial tissue that protects the underlying tissues from dehydration and any mechanical or chemical damage.
2. **Secretion**: All glands involved in secretion are made of epithelial tissue (e.g. endocrine glands secrete hormones and mucous glands secrete mucus).
3. **Absorption**: The epithelial tissue lining the small intestine absorbs nutrients from the digested food.

The cells in the epithelial tissue are very tightly packed together, and the intercellular substance called the *matrix* is minimal. The epithelial cells are separated from the underlying tissues by a specialized membrane called the *basement membrane*. This membrane provides protection to the underlying tissues such as the connective tissue. The epithelial tissue lacks its own blood supply; hence, the absorption of nutrients and the removal of wastes take place from blood vessels located in the underlying connective tissue.

Epithelial tissue can be divided into two types:

1. **Covering and lining epithelium**: It covers the body surface and lines the body cavities, hollow organs and ducts.
2. **Glandular epithelium**: It is a group of epithelial cells that produce specialized secretions (e.g. sweat glands and thyroid gland).

Covering and lining epithelium (Fig. 1.24)

The covering and lining epithelium can be classified based on:
❑ Arrangement of cells
❑ Shape of cells

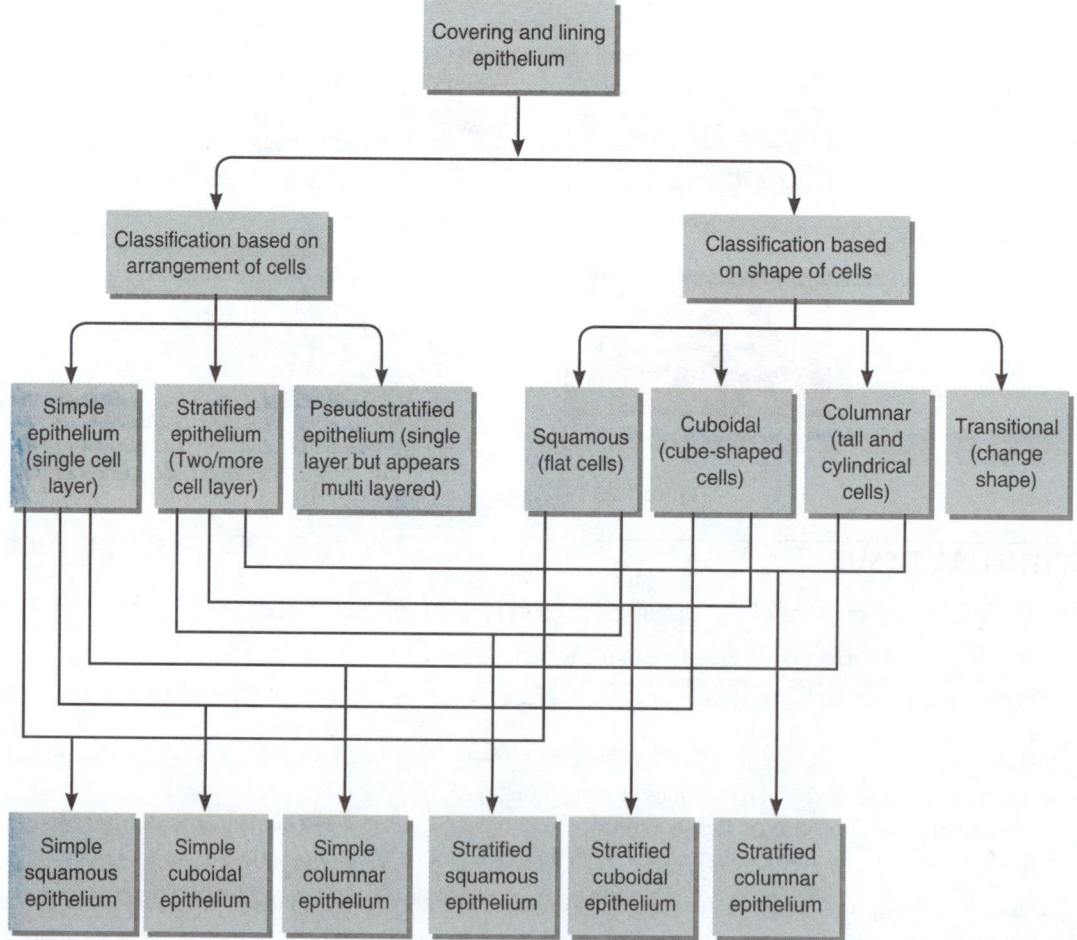

Figure 1.24 Covering and lining epithelium.

Classification based on arrangement of cells

1. **Simple epithelium** consists of a *single layer of cells* and is usually found on absorptive or secretory surfaces.
2. **Stratified epithelium** consists of *two or more layers of cells* and is usually found on surfaces subjected to stress. It protects the underlying structures from mechanical wear and tear.
3. **Pseudostratified epithelium** contains only a single layer of cells, but it appears to have multiple layers due to the position of cell nuclei at different levels.

Classification based on shape of cells

1. **Squamous cells**: These are *flattened cells* that fit closely together to form a thin and smooth membrane.
2. **Cuboidal cells**: These are *cube-shaped cells* lying on a basement membrane.
3. **Columnar cells**: These are *tall and cylindrical cells* that protect the underlying tissues.
4. **Transitional cells**: These cells *change shape* from cuboidal to flat, and back, as the body parts expand or stretch.

The combination of the two bases of classification provides the different types of covering and lining epithelium present in the body. Thus, the classification scheme of covering and lining epithelial tissues is as follows (Fig. 1.25):

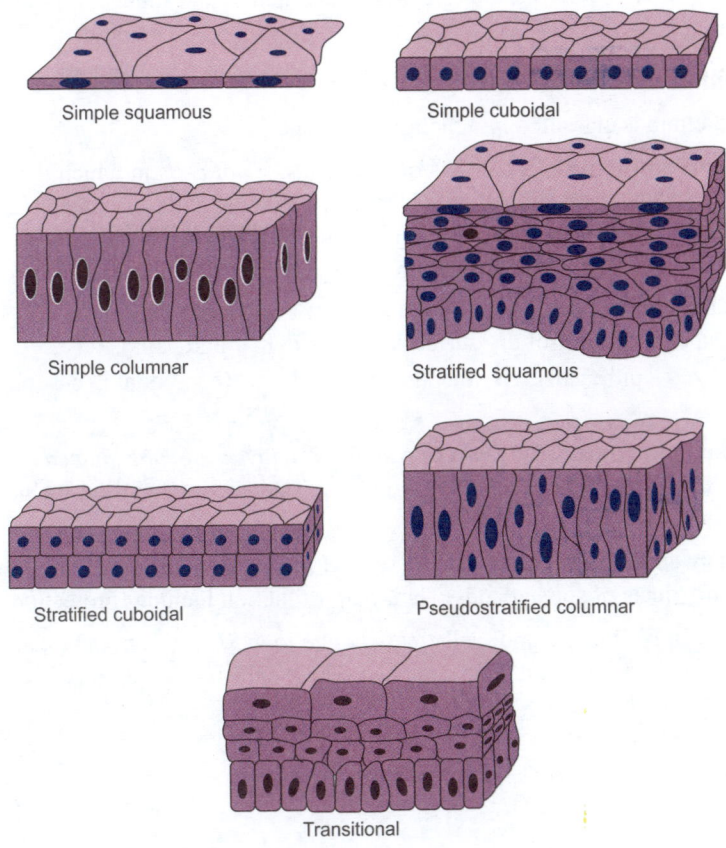

Simple squamous

Simple cuboidal

Simple columnar

Stratified squamous

Stratified cuboidal

Pseudostratified columnar

Transitional

Figure 1.25 Simple and stratified epithelial tissue.

1. Simple epithelium

The simple epithelium is classified into the following:

Simple squamous epithelium: It consists of a *single layer of flattened cells*. These cells line the heart, blood vessels and lymphatic vessels where this layer is also known as the *endothelium*. These cells also line the alveoli (air sacs) of lungs and glomerular (Bowman's) capsule of kidneys. The major functions of these cells include secretion, diffusion and absorption.

Simple cuboidal epithelium: It consists of a *single layer of cube-shaped cells*. These cells line the kidney tubules, smaller ducts of many glands and the surface of the ovary. Their major function includes secretion, absorption and excretion.

Simple columnar epithelium: It consists of a *single layer of cylindrical cells*. These cells exist in two forms: nonciliated and ciliated.

- ❑ The nonciliated simple columnar epithelium consists of cells with microvilli (finger-like projections) and goblet cells (secrete mucus). These cells line the organs of the gastrointestinal tract and are involved in absorption and secretion.
- ❑ The ciliated simple columnar epithelium contains cells with cilia (hairlike projections on the free surface), which line a few portions of the upper respiratory tract, uterine tubes and the uterus. The wavelike motion of cilia propels the mucus and other substances in one-way direction. For example, cilia propel ova present in uterine tubes towards the uterus, and mucus in the respiratory passage towards the throat.

2. Stratified epithelium

The stratified epithelium is classified into the following subtypes:

Stratified squamous epithelium: It consists of *several layers of cells* in which the superficial layer is of flattened cells, whereas the deepest layer is of mainly columnar cells. The major function of stratified squamous epithelial cells is protecting the underlying structures. These cells exist in two forms: keratinized and nonkeratinized.

- ❑ The keratinized epithelial cells have a tough layer of keratin protein on the cell surface, and these cells form the superficial layer of dry surfaces (e.g. skin, hair and nails).
- ❑ The nonkeratinized epithelial cells line the wet surfaces (e.g. mouth, oesophagus, tongue and vagina).

Stratified cuboidal epithelium: It consists of *two or more layers of cube-shaped cells*. These cells are present in the male urethra and ducts of sweat glands. Their major function includes protection and secretion.

Stratified columnar epithelium: It consists of *several layers of cylindrical cells*. These cells line the urethra and excretory ducts of some glands. Their major function includes protection and secretion.

Transitional epithelium: It consists of cells that *change their shape* from cuboidal to squamous, and back as the body parts are relaxed and then stretched. These cells line the urinary bladder and permit the stretching of bladder as it fills.

3. Pseudostratified columnar epithelium

This kind of epithelium contains only a single layer of cells but appears to be multilayered when viewed from the side, hence the name pseudostratified (*pseudo*: false). These cells line most of the upper respiratory tract and ducts of many glands. Their main functions are secretion and movement of mucus by ciliary action.

Glandular epithelium

The glandular epithelium consists of a group of highly specialized epithelial cells that secrete substances into ducts, into blood or on the surface. These highly specialized epithelial cells are referred to as *glands* and they are of two types: endocrine glands and exocrine glands.

Endocrine glands

The secretions from these cells, called *hormones,* directly enter the blood stream without passing through ducts; hence, they are also called *ductless glands,* e.g. pituitary gland, thyroid gland, adrenal gland, etc. (discussed in detail in Endocrine System).

Exocrine glands

❑ The secretions from these cells enter the ducts (tubes that release these secretions) at the surface of covering and lining epithelium or into the lumen (cavity) of a hollow organ (e.g. sweat glands [secrete sweat] and salivary glands [secrete saliva]).

❑ Exocrine glands can be either *unicellular glands*, which are single celled (e.g. goblet cell), or *multicellular glands*, which contain several cells (e.g. sweat and salivary glands).

❑ The multicellular exocrine glands can be classified structurally (Fig. 1.26):
  ➤ Based on the branching of ducts:
    — Unbranched ducts (e.g. simple glands); branched ducts (e.g. compound glands)
  ➤ Based on the shape of the secretory portion:
    – Tubular shape (e.g. tubular gland), flask-like shape (e.g. acinar [or alveolar] gland) and both flask-like and tubular shape (e.g. tubuloacinar gland)

❑ Thus, the structural classification scheme of exocrine gland is as follows:
  ➤ *Simple gland*: Single, unbranched duct
    – Simple tubular (e.g. intestinal glands); simple acinar (e.g. urethra)
  ➤ *Compound gland*: Branched duct
    – Compound tubular (e.g. Cowper's glands); compound acinar or alveolar (e.g. mammary glands); compound tubuloacinar or tubuloalveolar (e.g. pancreatic glands)

❑ The multicellular exocrine glands can be functionally classified into three types (Fig. 1.27):
  1. **Merocrine glands**: These glands form the secretion and release it from the cell (e.g. salivary glands, pancreas).

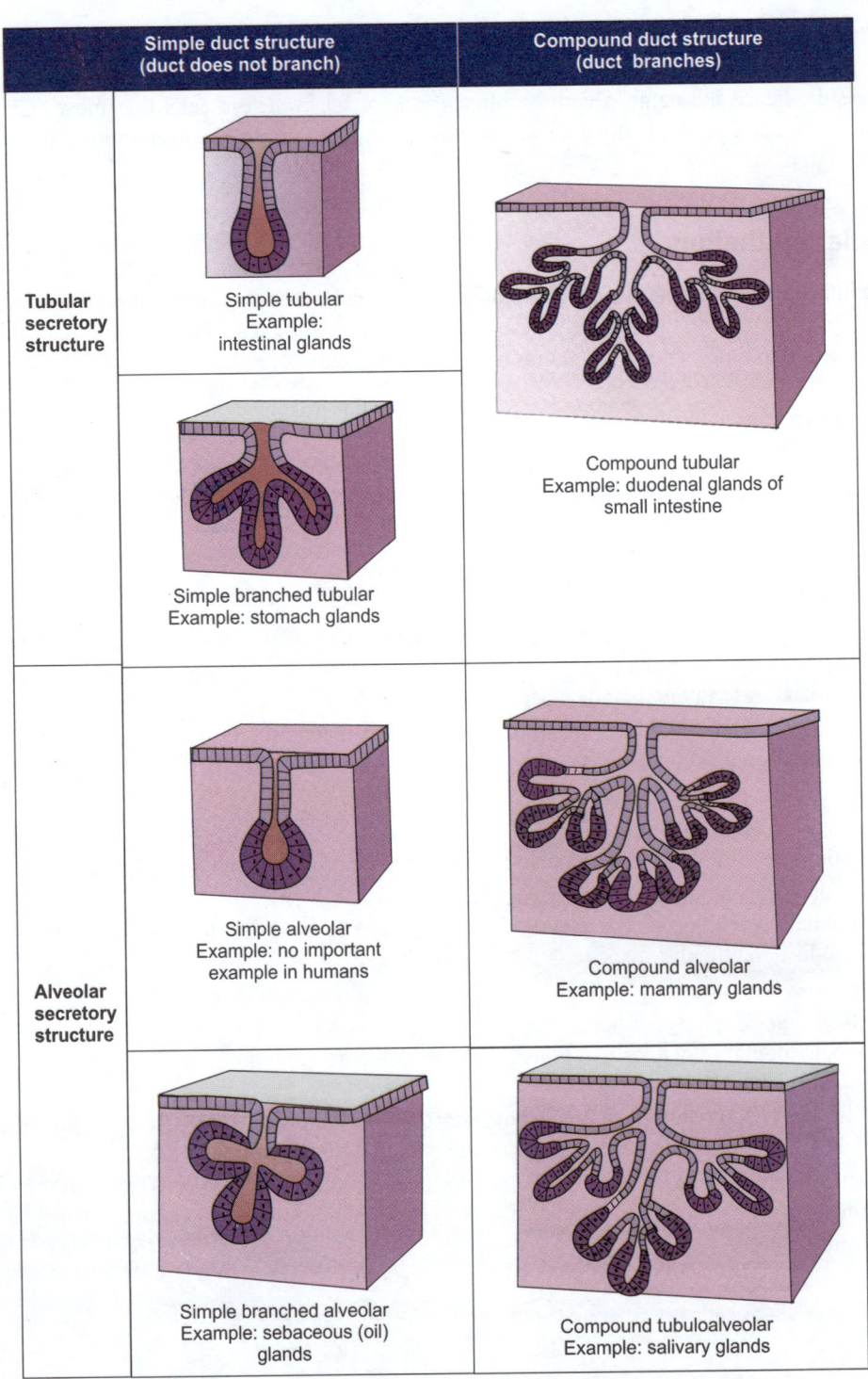

Figure 1.26 Structural classification of exocrine gland.

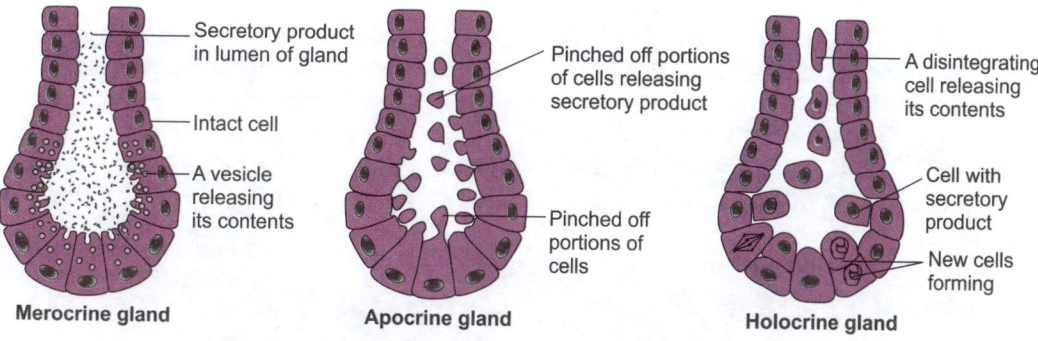

Figure 1.27 Functional classification of exocrine gland.

2. **Apocrine glands**: These glands accumulate the secretion at the apical surface of the cell, and this apical portion separates from the rest of the cell to form the secretion.
3. **Holocrine glands**: These glands accumulate the secretion in the cytosol of the cell. As the cell matures, it dies and becomes the secretion (e.g. sebaceous (oil) gland of skin).

CONNECTIVE TISSUE

Connective tissue is the most abundant and widely distributed tissue in the body. Unlike epithelial tissue, it has a rich blood supply.

Connective tissue performs various functions, which include the following:

1. **Structural support**: The connective tissue binds together the other body tissues and supports them (e.g. bones provide support to muscles, nerves, blood vessels and the skin).
2. **Protection**: It protects and insulates internal organs (e.g. bones protect the vital organs of the body such as the heart, lungs, brain and spinal cord).
3. **Transport**: It serves as the major transport system within the body (e.g. blood, a fluid connective tissue transports gases, nutrients and hormones to the cells).
4. **Storage**: It is the major site of stored energy reserves (e.g. adipose tissue stores the high-energy fat molecules, which are converted to ATP when required).

The components of connective tissue

The connective tissue comprises:

❏ Cells of connective tissue
❏ Intercellular substance called *matrix* (Fig. 1.28)

Cells of Connective Tissue

The different types of cells present in various connective tissues include the following:

1. **Fibroblasts** (*fibro*: fibres; *blasts*: immature cells that can undergo cell division): These cells are the most numerous large, flat cells with irregular processes. These cells secrete collagen and elastic

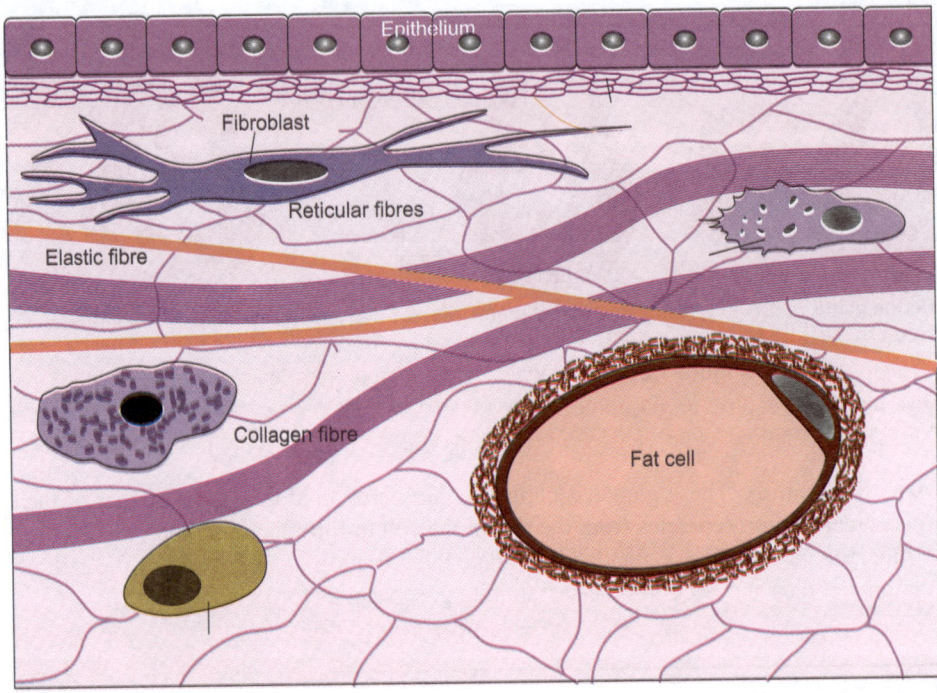

Figure 1.28 Components of connective tissue.

fibres and the connective tissue's extracellular matrix, i.e. the material present between its widely spread cells.

2. **Fat cells or adipocytes**: These cells store triglycerides (fats) and are abundant in the adipose connective tissue.

3. **Macrophages** (*macro*: large; *phages*: eaters): Macrophages are irregular-shaped cells that are capable of engulfing cell debris, bacteria and other foreign bodies by phagocytosis. Some macrophages are fixed (i.e. attached to connective tissue fibres), whereas others are wandering or motile (i.e. they have the ability to move throughout the tissue).

4. **Leukocytes or white blood cells**: These cells are found in small numbers in normal healthy connective tissue but migrate from blood into the connective tissues in response to infections or allergy (e.g. neutrophils, a type of WBC migrates from blood and gather at the site of infection as the body's defence response).

5. **Plasma cells**: They are small cells that develop from B-lymphocytes, a type of white blood cell. They secrete specific proteins called *antibodies* that attack and neutralize the foreign substances in the body.

6. **Mast cells**: Mast cells are mainly found in loose connective tissue and around blood vessels. They produce granules that contain heparin and histamine, which are released when there is cell injury. *Histamine* is a chemical that dilates small blood vessels and is involved in inflammatory response. Heparin prevents blood coagulation and helps in the passage of protective substances from blood to the affected tissue.

Intercellular substance—the matrix

The matrix is the intercellular material present in large amounts between the cells of connective tissue. The matrix is usually secreted by the cells themselves and varies in different connective tissues.

The matrix consists of two major components: ground substance and fibres.

❑ **Ground substance**: This is present between the cells of connective tissue and fibres. It may be of a semisolid jelly-like consistency (like in cartilage) or hard and inflexible (like in bones). The ground substance is responsible for binding the cells together and supporting them. It also provides a medium through which materials are exchanged between the blood and cells.

❑ **Fibres**: The fibres are usually embedded in the matrix and they support the connective tissue. There are three types of fibres, which include:

➤ *Collagen fibres*: They consist of collagen protein and provide strength to the connective tissue. These fibres are mainly found in bones and cartilages.

➤ *Elastic fibres*: They consist of elastin protein and provide strength as well as elasticity. These are found in skin and walls of blood vessels.

➤ *Reticular fibres*: They consist of collagen with a coating of glycoprotein. They provide support and strength to the cells. They are mainly present in reticular connective tissue.

Classification of connective tissue

The connective tissue can be classified into three subgroups: loose connective tissue, dense connective tissue and specialized connective tissue.

Loose connective tissue

As the name implies, loose connective tissue consists of a large number of cells and fibres that are loosely woven among them. There are three types of loose connective tissue: areolar, adipose and reticular.

Areolar connective tissue

This is the most widely distributed connective tissue. The matrix is semisolid and consists of several types of cells including fibroblasts, mast cells and macrophages widely separated by elastic and collagen fibres (Fig. 1.29).

The areolar connective tissue is mainly found in the epidermis of the skin and in the subcutaneous layer along with adipose tissue where it attaches the skin to its underlying tissues and organs. It provides elasticity and strength to the other tissues and serves as the basic support tissue around organs, muscles, blood vessels and nerves.

Adipose tissue

Adipose tissue consists of fat cells called *adipocytes*, which are specialized for storage of fats. The fats are stored in a large central area of adipocytes, which pushes the nuclei and cytoplasm to the periphery of the cell (Fig. 1.29). The adipose tissue is mainly found around organs such as the heart, kidneys and eyes and between muscle fibres where it supports and protects these organs. It is also present in the subcutaneous layer, where it acts as a thermal insulator and energy store.

There are two types of adipose tissue: *white adipose tissue* found mainly in adults and *brown adipose tissue* present in the fetus and infant. The brown adipose tissue generates more heat on metabolism and thus maintains the body temperature in the newborn.

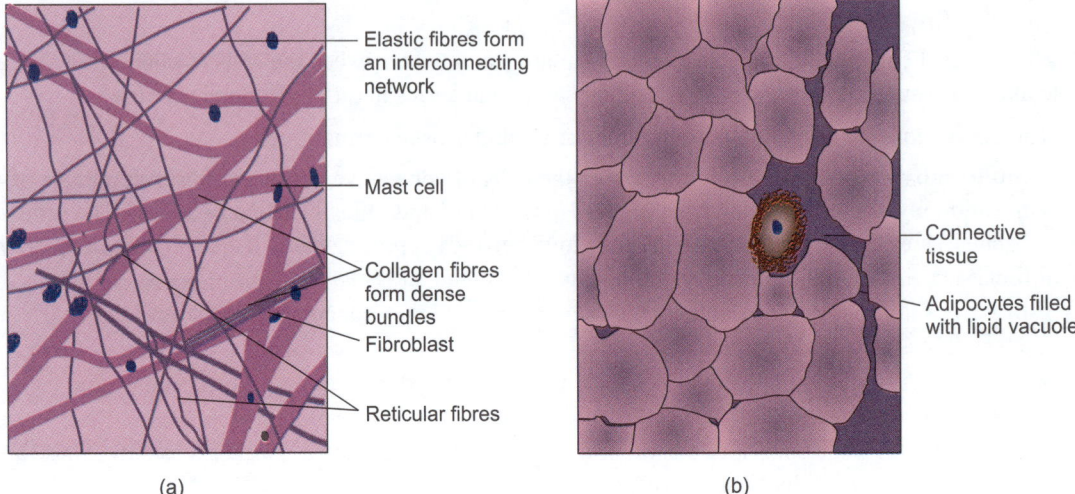

- Elastic fibres form an interconnecting network
- Mast cell
- Collagen fibres form dense bundles
- Fibroblast
- Reticular fibres
- Connective tissue
- Adipocytes filled with lipid vacuole

(a)   (b)

Figure 1.29 (a) Areolar tissue; (b) Adipose tissue.

Reticular connective tissue

It consists of a fine network of reticular fibres and reticular cells (Fig. 1.30). The reticular connective tissue supports the organs such as liver, bone marrow, spleen and lymph nodes and also helps in binding smooth muscle tissue cells.

Dense connective tissue

As the name implies, dense connective tissue consists of more numerous, tightly packed fibres and fewer cells. There are two types of dense connective tissue: fibrous and elastic.

Fibrous connective tissue: It consists of mainly collagen fibres that are tightly packed with very little matrix. Between bundles of collagen fibres, are few fibroblasts present in rows (Fig. 1.30a). The fibrous connective tissue is found in tendons (attach muscle to bone), ligaments (attach bone to

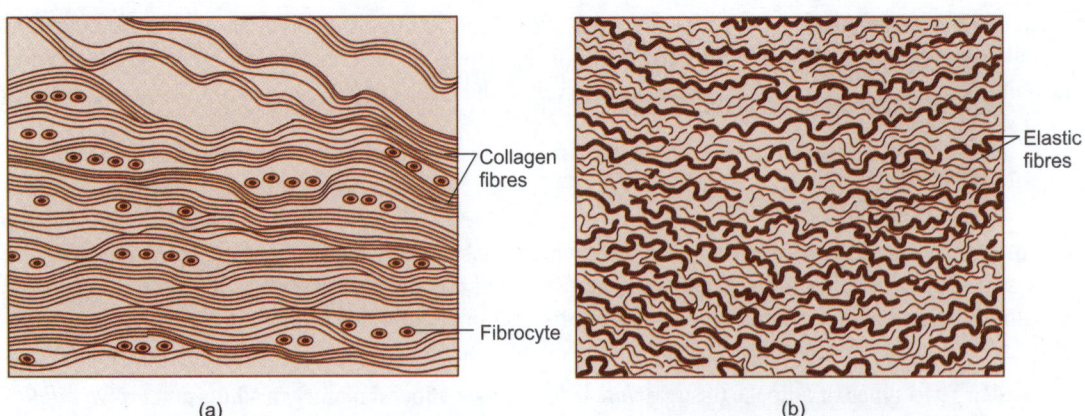

- Collagen fibres
- Fibrocyte
- Elastic fibres

(a)   (b)

Figure 1.30 (a) Fibrous connective tissue; (b) Elastic connective tissue.

bone), periosteum of bone, around some organs like kidneys, lymph nodes and muscle fasciae (covers whole muscle). The collagen fibres in this tissue are responsible for its strength and help it to attach various structures strongly.

Elastic connective tissue: It consists of mainly elastic fibres with a few fibroblasts present in the spaces between fibres (Fig. 1.30b). Elastic connective tissue is quite strong and is capable of considerable extension that can be recoiled to its original shape. Thus, this tissue is mainly found in organs where stretching is required, for example, large blood vessels, bronchi and lungs.

Specialized connective tissue

This subtype of connective tissue includes a number of connective tissues that have specialized functions such as cartilage, bone, blood and lymphoid tissue.

❑ **Cartilage**: Cartilage consists of small cavities called *lacunae* that contain cells of cartilage called *chondrocytes* embedded in the matrix consisting of a dense network of collagen and elastic fibres. The cartilages have more strength as compared to the loose or dense connective tissue. There are three types of cartilages: hyaline cartilage, fibrocartilage and elastic cartilage.

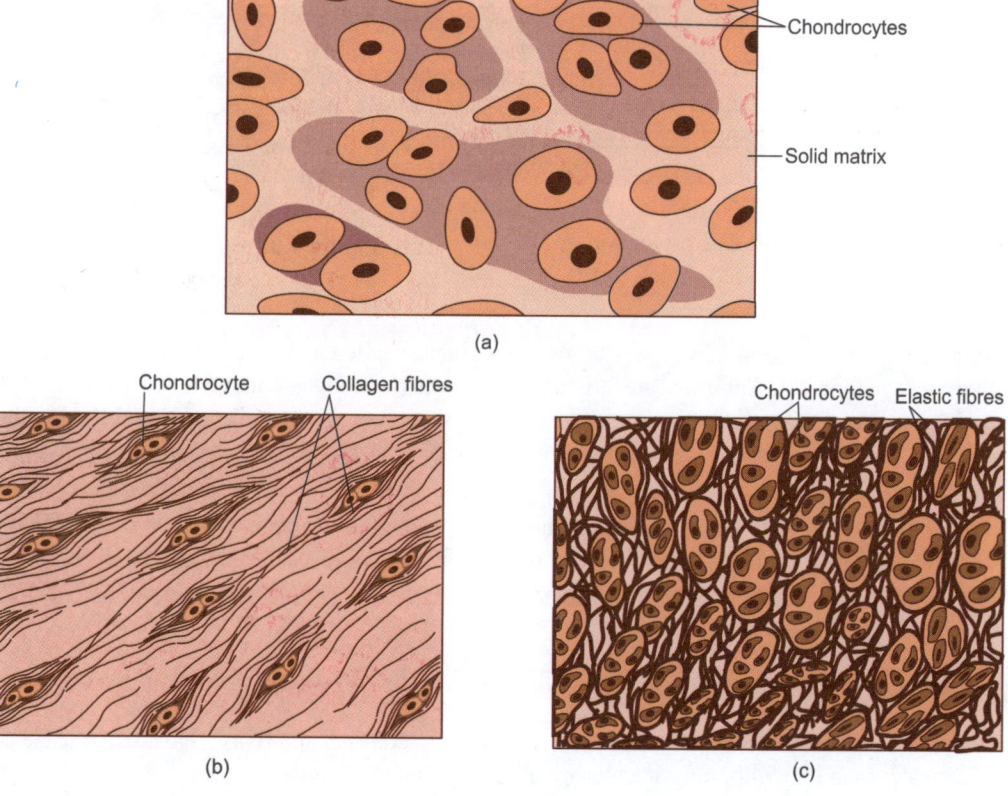

Figure 1.31 (a) Hyaline cartilage; (b) Fibrocartilage; (c) Elastic cartilage.

➤ *Hyaline cartilage*: It is the most abundant cartilage in the body. It consists of small groups of chondrocytes within lacunae embedded in the matrix with fine collagen fibres (Fig. 1.31a). The fine collagen fibres in this tissue permit movement and provide firm and flexible support for the movement at joints. It is mainly found at the ends of long bones, anterior ends of ribs, part of larynx, trachea and bronchi and embryonic skeleton.

➤ *Fibrocartilage*: It consists of a dense mass of collagen fibres embedded in the matrix with chondrocytes widely dispersed in it (Fig. 1.31b). The dense collagen fibres act as a shock absorber and permit limited movement at the joints. It is a tough, flexible and supporting tissue found in the intervertebral discs and pubic symphysis (joint between pelvic bones).

➤ *Elastic cartilage*: It consists of chondrocytes embedded in the matrix consisting of elastic fibres (Fig. 1.31c). These fibres permit the elastic cartilage to be easily stretched and allow the tissue to be flexible. It is located at the lobe of the ear, epiglottis and auditory (Eustachian) tubes.

❑ **Bone**: It consists of bone cells called *osteocytes* embedded in the matrix of collagen fibres and strengthened by inorganic salts, especially calcium and phosphorus (Fig. 1.32). The inorganic salts and collagen fibres make this tissue rigid and strong. There are two types of bones:

➤ *Compact bone*: It has dense appearance and forms the outer layer of bone.

➤ *Spongy bone*: It has spongy or 'honey comb'-like appearance.

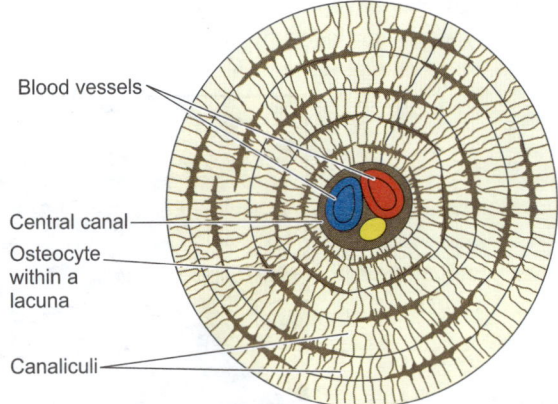

Figure 1.32 Bone tissue.

The bone tissue makes up the skeletal system and provides support and protection to the internal organs (discussed in detail in the Skeletal System section).

❑ **Blood**: Blood is a fluid connective tissue composed of matrix called plasma and formed elements (cells) including red blood cells (erythrocytes), white blood cells (leukocytes) and platelets (thrombocytes). Blood transports oxygen, carbon dioxide, nutrients and waste products. The white blood cells are involved in defence response and the platelets participate in blood clotting (discussed in detail in Haemopoietic System).

❑ **Lymphoid tissue**: It is found in the lymph nodes, thymus gland, spleen, tonsils and adenoids. It is involved in antibody production and helps in protecting us from disease and foreign microorganisms (discussed in detail in the section Lymphatic System).

MUSCLE TISSUE

Muscle tissue consists of fibres (cells) that have the ability to contract and relax. Because a muscle cell's length is greater than its width, muscle cells are often referred to as muscle fibres. There are three types of muscle tissues: skeletal or striated muscle tissue, smooth or visceral muscle tissue and cardiac muscle tissue (Fig. 1.33).

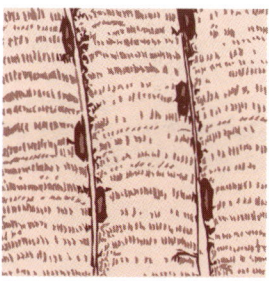
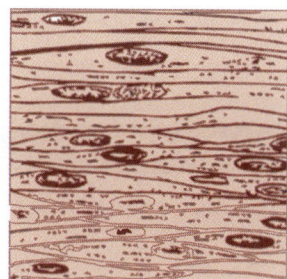
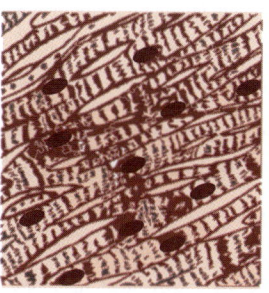

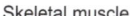

Skeletal muscle   Smooth muscle   Cardiac muscle

Figure 1.33 Muscle tissue.

Skeletal (striated) muscle tissue: These muscles are attached to the bones of the skeleton and have alternate light and dark bands called *striations*, hence named *striated muscle tissue*. Skeletal muscle is voluntary because it is under conscious control. The skeletal muscle fibre is very long, cylindrical in shape and contains several nuclei located at the periphery of the cell. Its major functions include maintenance of posture and movement of bones.

Smooth (visceral) muscle tissue: Smooth muscle is nonstriated and involuntary because it lacks the striations and is not under conscious control. The smooth muscle fibre is small, spindle shaped with only one central nucleus. It is found in the walls of hollow organs such as blood vessels, stomach, intestine, gallbladder and urinary bladder. The contraction of smooth muscle helps regulate the diameter of blood vessels, propel the contents of ureters and gastrointestinal tract, and expel the contents of the urinary bladder and uterus.

Cardiac muscle tissue: This tissue is found only in the heart wall and is striated like the skeletal muscle and involuntary like the smooth muscle. The cardiac muscle fibres are cylindrical, branched and usually have only one nucleus. They attach to one another by *intercalated discs* that can be seen as lines that are thicker and darker than the ordinary cross stripes. This end-to-end continuity of cardiac muscle cells has significance in the coordinated pumping action of the heart.

NERVOUS TISSUE

The nervous tissue consists of two types of cells: neurons and neuroglia (Fig. 1.34).

❏ The *neurons* or *nerve cell* converts stimuli into nerve impulses and then conducts these impulses to other neurons, muscles or glands. Most neurons have three basic parts: *cell body* that contains nucleus and other organelles; *dendrites,* that is, short processes that receive stimuli and conduct them to cell body; and *axons,* that is, long processes that transmit the impulses towards another neuron or some other tissue.

❏ *Neuroglia* does not generate or conduct nerve impulses; these cells support the neurons.

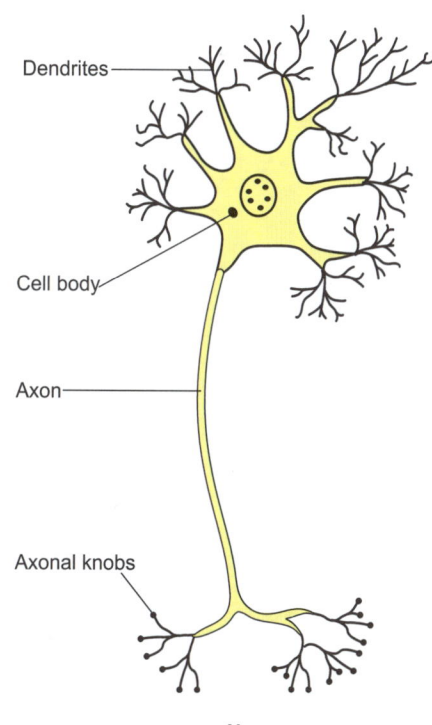

Dendrites

Cell body

Axon

Axonal knobs

Nerve

Figure 1.34 Nerve tissue.

The nervous tissue makes up the brain, spinal cord and various nerves of the body. It allows us to perceive the stimuli and helps adapt to the changing situations. It also controls and coordinates various body activities.

THE SYSTEM LEVEL OF ORGANIZATION

A *system* is an organization of two or more organs and associated structures working as a unit to perform a common function or set of functions.

The basic structure and function of the major body systems is presented below:

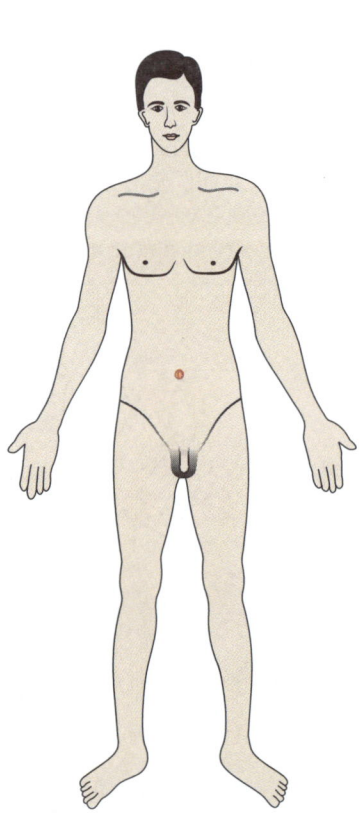

Figure 1.35 Integumentary system.

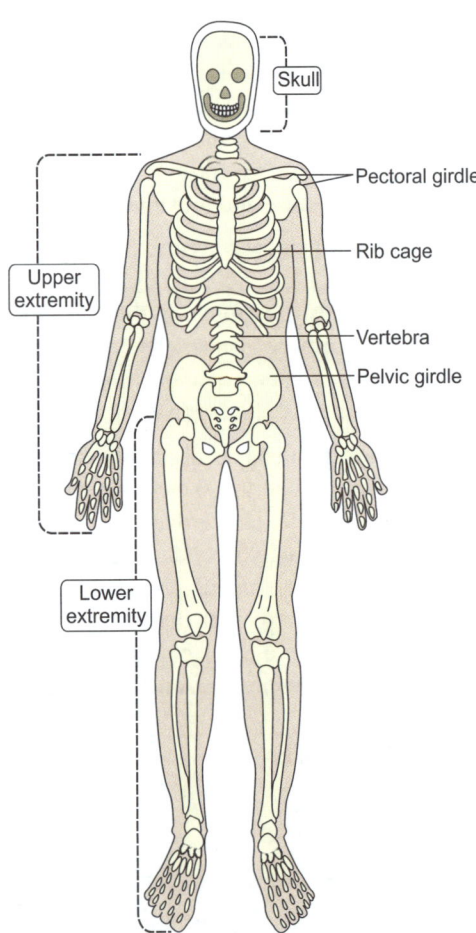

Figure 1.36 Skeletal system.

Definition: The integumentary system includes skin and structures derived from it (hair, nails and oil and sweat glands) (Fig. 1.35).

Functions: Protects the body, regulates body temperature, eliminates wastes and receives certain stimuli (tactile, temperature and pain).

Definition: The skeletal system includes bones, cartilage and ligaments (Fig. 1.36).

Functions: Provides body support and protection, permits movement and leverage, produces blood cells (haematopoiesis) and stores minerals.

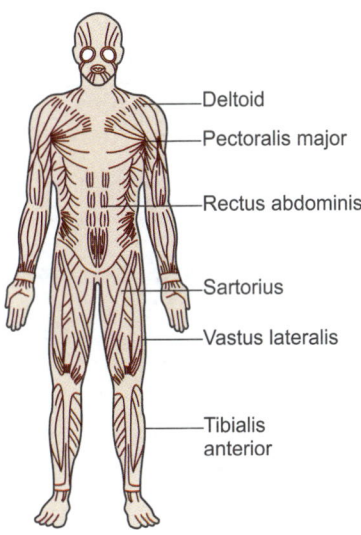

Figure 1.37 Muscular system.

Definition: The muscular system includes skeletal muscles of the body and their tendinous attachments (Fig. 1.37).

Functions: Role in body movements, maintains posture and produces body heat.

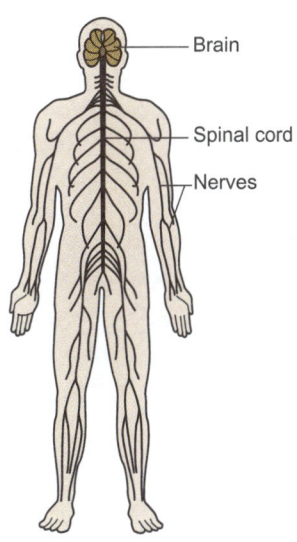

Figure 1.38 Nervous system.

Definition: The nervous system includes the brain, spinal cord and nerves (Fig. 1.38).

Functions: Detects and responds to changes in the internal and external environment, enables reasoning and memory and regulates body activities.

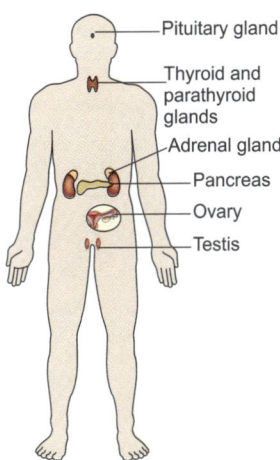

Figure 1.39 Endocrine system.

Definition: The endocrine system includes the hormone-producing glands (Fig. 1.39).

Functions: Controls and integrates body functions via hormones secreted into the bloodstream.

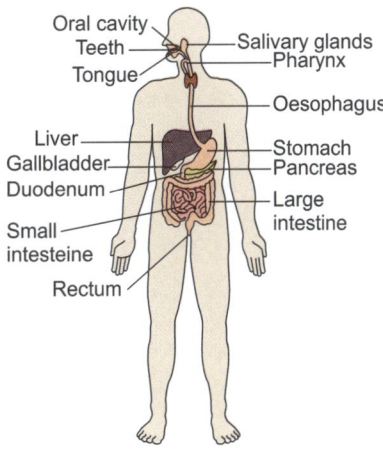

Figure 1.40 Digestive system.

Definition: The digestive system includes the various body organs that render ingested foods absorbable (Fig. 1.40).

Functions: Mechanically and chemically breaks down foods for cellular use and eliminates undigested wastes.

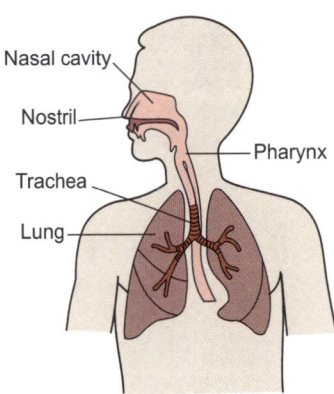

Figure 1.41 Respiratory system.

Definition: The respiratory system includes the body organs concerned with the movement of respiratory gases (O_2 and CO_2) to and from the pulmonary blood (the blood within the lungs) (Fig. 1.41).

Functions: Supplies oxygen to the blood and eliminates carbon dioxide; also helps regulate the acid–base balance.

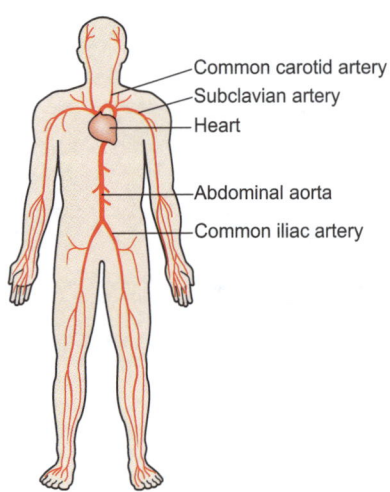

Figure 1.42 Cardiovascular system.

Definition: The cardiovascular system includes heart and the vessels that carry blood or blood constituents (lymph) through the body (Fig. 1.42).

Functions: Transports respiratory gases, nutrients, wastes and hormones; protects against disease and fluid loss; helps regulate body temperature and the acid–base balance.

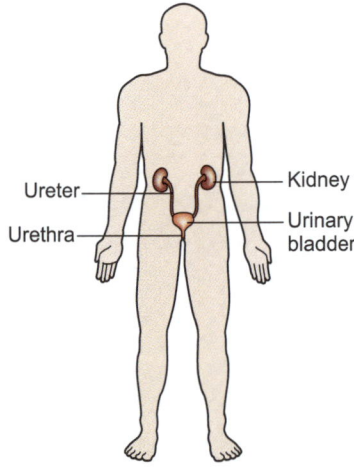

Figure 1.43 Urinary system.

Definition: The urinary system includes the organs that operate to remove wastes from the blood and to eliminate urine from the body (Fig. 1.43).

Functions: Removes various wastes from the blood; regulates the chemical composition, volume and electrolyte balance of the blood; helps maintain the acid–base balance of the body.

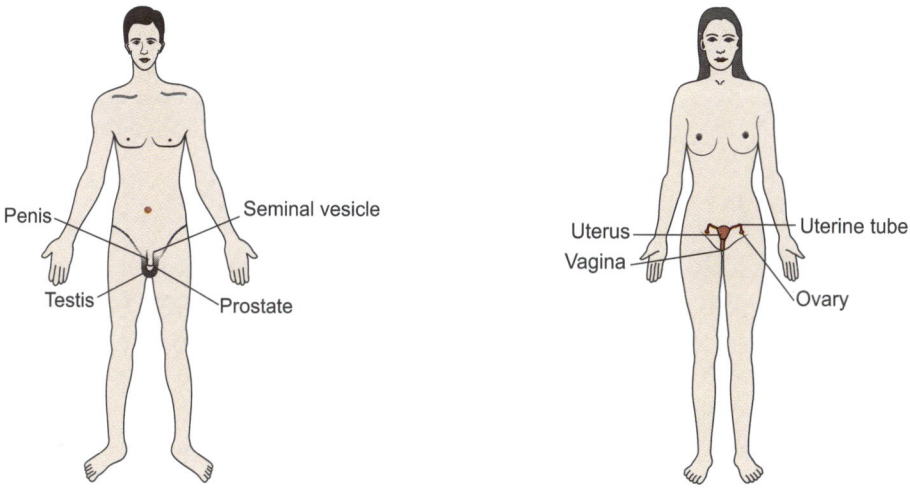

Figure 1.44 Male and female reproductive systems.

Definition: The reproductive system includes the body organs that produce, store and transport reproductive cells (gametes, or sperm and ova) (Fig. 1.44).
Functions: Reproduce the organism; produce sex hormones.

Summary of Various Systems of Human Body

S. no.	System	Components	Functions
1.	Integumentary system	Skin, hair, nails, sebaceous glands and sweat glands.	Protects the body; regulates body temperature and water content; detects sensations such as warmth, cold and touch
2..	Skeletal system	Bones, cartilage and joints	Supports and protects the body; helps in body movement; manufactures blood cells in red bone marrow
3.	Muscular system	**Muscles** Skeletal muscles Smooth muscles Cardiac muscles	Allows movement; pushes food through the GI tract and blood through blood vessels; Causes contraction of heart.
4.	Nervous system	Brain, spinal cord and nerves	Controls and regulates other systems of the body; detects changes in the internal and external environment; gives appropriate response
5.	Endocrine system	Endocrine glands	Produce hormones that regulate the body's functions

S. no.	System	Components	Functions
6.	Cardiovascular system	Heart, blood vessels and blood	Heart pumps blood through blood vessels. Blood carries oxygen and nutrients to cells, and carbon dioxide and wastes away from the body cells.
7.	Lymphatic system	Lymph, lymph vessels, lymph nodes, spleen and thymus	Protects body from disease-causing microorganisms; absorbs fats from the intestine and carries it to the blood; returns proteins and fluid to the blood.
8.	Respiratory system	Lungs, pharynx, larynx, trachea and bronchi	Transfers oxygen from inhaled air to blood and carbon dioxide from blood to exhaled air
9.	Digestive system	Alimentary canal (mouth, oesophagus, stomach, small and large intestine, anus) and glands (salivary, liver, pancreas)	Carries out physical and chemical breakdown of food and produces nutrients that can be absorbed by body cells; eliminates undigestible wastes
10.	Urinary system	Kidney, ureters, urinary bladder, urethra	Produces, stores and eliminates urine and regulates the acid–base balance and homeostasis
11.	Reproductive system	**Male**: Testes, vas deferens, seminal vesicles, prostate gland, penis **Female**: Ovaries, uterine tubes, uterus, vagina.	Maintains sexual characteristics and the continuation of a species

DISEASES ASSOCIATED WITH CELLS AND TISSUES

CANCER

Cancer is a group of diseases characterized by uncontrolled cell proliferation, which is faster than normal and in an uncoordinated manner. The mass of tissue that develops due to this excess growth is called *tumour*. Tumours may be cancerous, referred to as *malignant tumour*, or non-cancerous (harmless), referred to as *benign tumour*. This process of uncontrolled cell multiplication is termed *carcinogenesis*, and the agents precipitating this condition are *carcinogens*.

Causes

❏ Chemical carcinogens (e.g. aniline dyes, asbestos, cigarette smoke)
❏ Radiation carcinogens (e.g. X-rays, ultraviolet rays in sunlight, radioactive isotopes)
❏ Viruses (Some viruses incorporate their DNA or RNA into the host's genetic material and cause malignant changes in the cells.)
❏ Miscellaneous (e.g. inherited factors, age, race and diet)

SYSTEMIC LUPUS ERYTHEMATOSUS

It is a chronic inflammatory disease of connective tissue that results in tissue damage in almost every body system.

Symptoms are Painful joints, fatigue, weight loss, mouth ulcers and anorexia.

In severe conditions, it may cause inflammation of the kidneys, liver, spleen, lungs, brain and gastrointestinal tract.

Effect of Ageing on Cells

❑ Ageing is a normal process that produces observable changes in the structure and function and makes us more vulnerable to disease and environmental conditions. As we age, cellular repair and cell division to replace old cells become slower, causing delay in wound healing and gradually ceases to occur, thereby leading to cellular deterioration and death.

❑ Collagen fibres become structurally irregular, lose their strength and extensibility and thus become more fragile. Elastic fibres thicken, fragment and thus lead to changes that may be associated with the development of atherosclerosis. The muscle cells and neurons decrease with age, causing decline in memory, reduced brain capacity and decreased muscle contraction in the elderly.

Review Questions

Long Answer Questions

1. Describe the basic characteristics of living organisms.
2. Describe the levels of organization of the human body.
3. List the four principal types of tissues and describe the functions of each.
4. What is a negative feedback, and how is it used to help maintain homeostasis?
5. Describe the anatomical position of the human body.
6. Describe the composition of cell (plasma) membrane.
7. Discuss the various processes by which substances are transferred across cell membranes.
8. Describe the structure and function of various organelles in the cell.
9. Describe the processes of mitosis and meiosis.
10. Discuss the various types of epithelial tissues.
11. Describe the characteristics, locations and functions of the connective tissue.
12. Describe muscle tissue and distinguish between the three types.

Multiple Choice Questions

1. A person in the anatomical position would be
   - (a) Lying face down
   - (b) Lying face up
   - (c) Standing erect facing forward
   - (d) In a fetal position

2. Which is *not* one of the four principal tissue types?
   - (a) Nervous tissue
   - (b) Bone tissue
   - (c) Epithelial tissue
   - (d) Muscle tissue
   - (e) Connective tissue

3. The abdominal cavity contains
   - (a) The heart
   - (b) The lungs
   - (c) The spleen
   - (d) The trachea

4. The thoracic cavity is separated from the abdominopelvic cavity by
   - (a) The mediastinum
   - (b) The abdominal wall
   - (c) The abdominal septum
   - (d) The diaphragm

5. The cell membrane
   - (a) Encloses components of the cell
   - (b) Regulates absorption
   - (c) Gives shape to the cell
   - (d) Does all of the preceding

6. Which organelle contains hydrolytic enzymes?
   - (a) Lysosome
   - (b) Ribosome
   - (c) Mitochondrion
   - (d) The Golgi apparatus

7. Endoplasmic reticulum (ER) with attached ribosomes is called
   - (a) Smooth ER
   - (b) A Golgi apparatus
   - (c) Nodular ER
   - (d) Rough ER

8. Engulfing of solid material by cells is called
   - (a) Pinocytosis
   - (b) Phagocytosis
   - (c) Active transport
   - (d) Diffusion.

9. The function of the Golgi apparatus is
   - (a) Packaging of material in membranes for transport out of the cell
   - (b) Production of mitotic and meiotic spindles
   - (c) Excretion of excess water
   - (d) Production of ATP by oxidative phosphorylation

10. The function of the mitochondria is
    - (a) Packaging of materials in membranes for transport out of the cell
    - (b) Conversion of light energy to chemical energy in the form of ATP
    - (c) Excretion of excess water from the cell
    - (d) Synthesis of ATP by oxidative phosphorylation

11. The flow of genetic information in most organisms may be indicated as
    (a) Protein–DNA–mRNA
    (b) Protein–tRNA–DNA
    (c) DNA–mRNA–protein
    (d) Four nucleotides

12. The two daughter cells formed by mitosis have
    (a) Identical genetic constitutions
    (b) Exactly half as many genes as the parent cell
    (c) The same amount of cytoplasm as the parent cell
    (d) None of the preceding

13. Which of the following is *not* a specialized type of cell found in connective tissues?
    (a) Lymphocyte
    (b) Macrophage
    (c) Goblet cell
    (d) Mast cell

14. Intercalated discs are found in
    (a) Cardiac muscle tissue
    (b) Movable joints
    (c) The vertebral column
    (d) Bone tissue

15. Which of the following is *not* a type of epithelium?
    (a) Simple squamous
    (b) Transitional
    (c) Simple ciliated columnar
    (d) Complex stratified

State True or False

1. Histology is the microscopic examination of tissues.

2. A group of cells cooperating in a particular function is called a tissue.

3. In the anatomical position, the subject is standing erect, the feet are together and the arms are relaxed to the side of the body with the thumbs forward.

4. A sagittal plane divides the body into right and left halves.

5. The term *parietal* refers to the body wall, and the term *visceral* refers to internal body organs.

6. Active transport does not require energy and is the mechanism by which O_2 enters a cell.

7. Meiosis is the process of gamete (sex cell) formation.

8. Skeletal and cardiac muscle fibres are striated.

9. Neuroglia are specialized cells of nervous tissue that react to stimuli.

10. Cells of epithelia are tightly packed, mostly avascular, and without significant matrix.

Fill in the Blanks

1. The _____ system includes the skin, hair, nails and oil and sweat glands.

2. _____ is the dynamic maintenance of a nearly stable internal environment in the body so that metabolism can occur.

3. _____ feedback mechanisms provide input to controlling organs in the process of maintaining homeostasis.

4. The _____ plane divides the body into equal right and left portions.

5. _____ is a directional term meaning 'away from the head' or 'towards the lower portion of the body'.

6. _____ is the scientific study of tissues.

7. Epithelium consisting of two or more layers is classified as _____.

8. The _____ of a neuron receive a stimulus and conduct the nerve impulse to the cell body.

Careers Related to Cells and Tissues

✓ Cell biologists are trained in the study of structure and functions of cellular organelles.

✓ Histologists are medical professionals who specialize in the study of structure and functions of tissues.

✓ Forensic scientists are medical professionals who specialize in analysing tissue samples and help in solving the criminal cases.

The Integumentary System

STUDY OBJECTIVES

✓ To describe the structure and principal functions of skin.

✓ Discuss about the accessory structures of skin, i.e. hair, nails and skin glands.

The integumentary system (*inte*: whole; *gument*: body covering) includes the skin and its accessory structures: hair and nails, along with various glands, muscles and nerves.

The skin is the largest organ of the body, with a surface area of about 1.5–2 m² in adults. It protects the underlying structures from injury and microbial invasion, thus guarding the body's integrity. It contains sensory nerve endings of pain, temperature and touch and is also involved in the regulation of body temperature. The branch of medicine specialized for diagnosis and the treatment of skin disorders is called *dermatology* (*derma*: skin; *logy*: study).

STRUCTURE OF THE SKIN

The skin consists of two main layers: the outer *epidermis* and the inner *dermis*. A subcutaneous layer or hypodermis (*hypo*: below) lies beneath the dermis, consisting of areolar and adipose tissues. This layer anchors the skin to the underlying tissues and organs (Fig. 2.1).

THE EPIDERMIS

The outermost or epidermal layer of skin is composed of stratified squamous keratinized epithelial cells. The epidermal layer varies in thickness in different parts of the body. It is thickest where it receives the most abrasion and weight—on the palms of hands and soles of feet, whereas it is much thinner over the ventral surface of the trunk. Although it does not have blood vessels or nerves, it receives nutrition from capillaries of the dermis.

The epidermis is made up of the following five layers (Fig. 2.2):

1. Stratum corneum (horny layer)
2. Stratum lucidum (clear layer)
3. Stratum granulosum (granular layer)
4. Stratum spinosum (spiny layer)
5. Stratum germinativum or stratum basale (regenerative layer)

The cells in the lowermost layer divide by mitosis, and the new cells formed push the older cells upwards toward the surface. Thus, the old cells at the surface are continuously replaced by new cells.

DO YOU KNOW

❑ The attachment of the human skin to muscles is what causes dimples.
❑ Human hair and fingernails continue to grow after death.
❑ Globally, dead skin accounts for about a billion tons of dust in the atmosphere. Your skin sheds 50,000 cells every minute.
❑ An average adult's skin spans 21 sq ft, weighs 9 pounds and contains more than 11 miles of blood vessels.
❑ Intelligent people have more zinc and copper in their hair.
❑ There are 3000 sweat glands per square inch on the palms of our hands.
❑ Hair is the second fastest growing tissue in the body.
❑ Hair grows faster in warm and sunny weather.
❑ About 100 hair fall out of the scalp (normally) every day.
❑ The fastest growing nail is on the middle finger. The slowest growing nail is on the thumbnail.

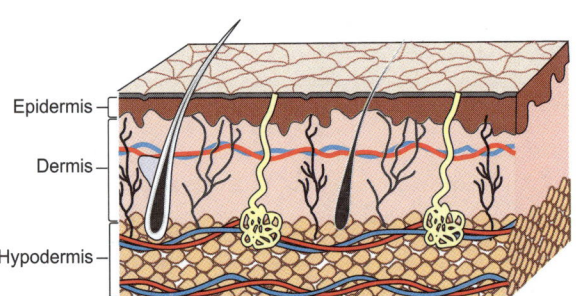

Epidermis —
Dermis —
Hypodermis —

Figure 2.1 Structure of skin.

MEDICAL TERMINOLOGY

❑ **Albinism**: Inherited inability of an individual to produce melanin due to gene mutation.
❑ **Alopecia**: Baldness, especially in men, and is regulated by ageing and genetic factors.
❑ **Desmosomes**: They are highly convoluted, interlocking cellular links that connect one cell to another.
❑ **Elasticity**: It is the ability to return to its original shape after stretching.
❑ **Extensibility**: It is the ability to stretch.
❑ **Mole**: Localized overgrowth of melanocytes in childhood/adolescence.
❑ **Tonofilaments**: The scattered intermediate filaments present in cells that consist of a protein that forms keratin.
❑ **Vitiligo**: Partial or complete loss of melanocytes from patches of skin that results in irregular white spots on the skin.

1. **Stratum corneum**

   (a) It is the outermost layer that consists of 25–30 layers of dead keratinized cells that are nonnucleated and are filled with keratin (protein), which is responsible for its structural strength.

   (b) The keratinized cells are also covered with lipids, which make this layer an effective barrier, abrasion resistant and protect the deeper layers from injury and microbial invasion. These cells are constantly shed and replaced by the cells from the stratum germinativum.

   Note: Constant exposure of skin to abrasion or friction results in abnormal thickening of the stratum corneum called *callus*.

2. **Stratum lucidum (*lucid*: clear)**: It lies directly beneath the stratum corneum and consists of 3–5 layers of flattened, transparent, dead keratinized cells. These cells exhibit a shiny character; hence, this layer is named *lucidum*.

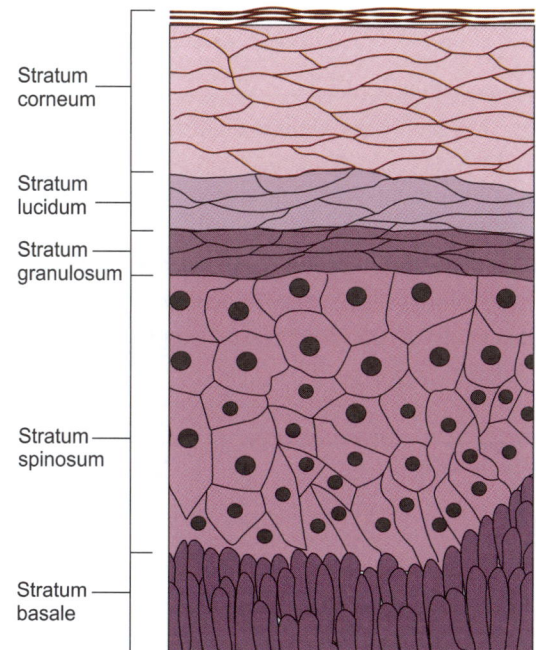

Figure 2.2 Layers of the epidermis.

3. **Stratum granulosum**

   (a) It is a thin layer that consists of 2–5 layers of flattened keratinocytes (cells containing keratin). The cytoplasm of these cells contains keratohyalin granules, which convert tonofilaments into keratin and lamellar granules, which release a lipid-rich, water-repellent secretion.

   (b) The cells in this layer undergo apoptosis because of which they lose nuclei and die. Thus, this layer marks the transition between dead, keratinized cells in the upper layers and deep, alive cells of the lower strata.

4. **Stratum spinosum**: It lies above the stratum germinativum and consists of 8–10 layers of spiny keratinocytes. These cells have spine (thorn)-like projections, which connect one cell to another and provide both strength and flexibility to the skin.

5. **Stratum germinativum or stratum basale**

   (a) It is the deepest and most important layer of the skin because it is responsible for the formation of all other upper epidermal layers. It consists of a single row of cuboidal or columnar keratinocytes, out of which some are stem cells that have the ability to divide by mitosis and thus continually produce new cells known as *keratinocytes*. When new cells are formed, they undergo morphological and nuclear changes as they get pushed upwards by the dividing cells beneath them.

   (b) These cells contain tonofilaments that attach to desmosomes and bind the cells of the stratum germinativum to each other and to the cells between the epidermis and the dermis, thus providing anchor and nutrition to the epidermal cells.

(c) The stratum germinativum also contain cells called *melanocytes*, which are responsible for producing skin colour (discussed later in detail).

The epidermis is maintained by the synchronization of three processes:

1. Shedding of the keratinized cells from the surface.
2. Movement of the cells from the stratum germinativum towards the surface. (As the cells move upwards, they tend to accumulate increased keratin, a process called *keratinization,* after which they undergo apoptosis.)
3. Continuous cell division in the stratum germinativum to form new cells.

These three processes take about 4 weeks in an average epidermis of about 0.1 mm thickness, but the rate of cell division increases in skin injury.

The excessive amount of keratinized cells that are shed from skin of the scalp is called *dandruff.*

THE DERMIS

The second, deeper part of the skin, the dermis, lies directly beneath the epidermis and is composed of dense connective tissues with white collagen fibres and yellow elastin fibres. Blood vessels, nerves, lymph vessels, smooth muscles (arrector pili around hair follicles), glands and hair follicles are all embedded in the dermis (Fig. 2.3).

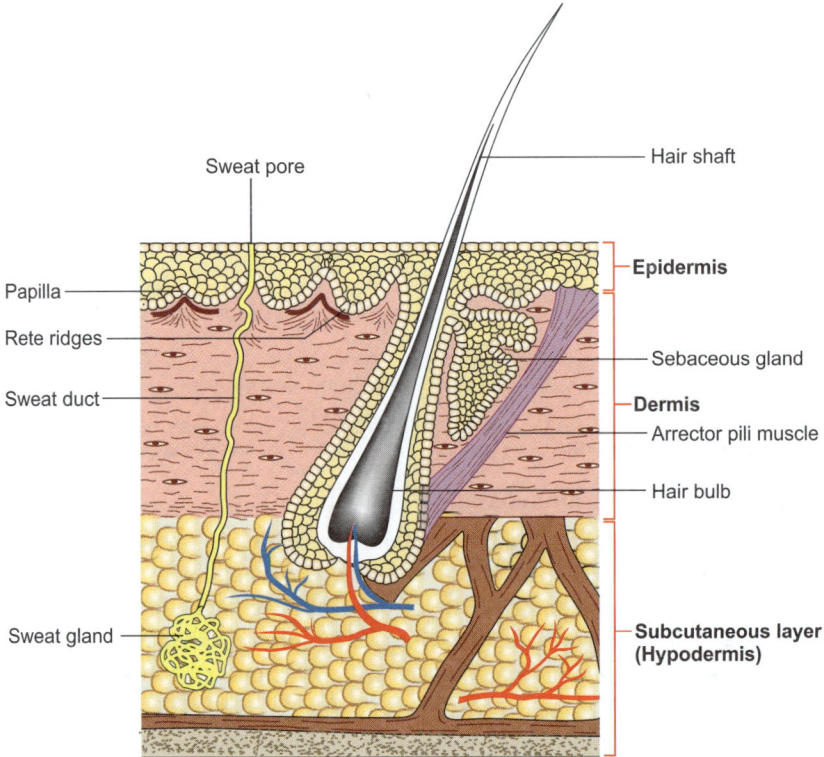

Figure 2.3 Detailed structure of the skin.

The specialized nerve endings (sensory receptors) sensitive to touch (Meissner's corpuscles), temperature, pressure (Pacinian corpuscles) and pain are also widely distributed in the dermis.

The dermis is made up of two layers: papillary layer and reticular layer.

1. **Papillary layer**
   (a) It is the layer adjacent to the epidermis and consists of fine elastic fibres.
   (b) The cells in this layer, called *papillae*, extend their projections towards the surface of the epidermis. These projections from the dermis to the epidermis are called *epidermal ridges*, and these are unique for each individual. The impression made by them forms *fingerprints*, which serves as the basis for identification.

2. **Reticular layer**
   (a) It lies between the papillary layer and the fatty subcutaneous (hypodermis) layer and consists of bundles of tough collagen fibres, fibroblasts and some elastic fibres.
   (b) The collagen and elastic fibres in the reticular layer are responsible for extensibility, elasticity and strength of skin.
   (c) The overstretching of skin causes rupture of elastic fibres, resulting in permanent *striae* or *stretch marks* (red or silvery white streaks on the skin surface) as found in pregnancy and obesity.

COLOUR OF THE SKIN

The colour of the skin depends on two important factors: pigmentation of the skin and haemoglobin (Hb) in the blood.

1. **Pigmentation of the skin**
   (a) The stratum germinativum contains cells called *melanocytes* that synthesize a brown pigment called *melanin*, which is responsible for skin pigmentation. Melanin is synthesized from the amino acid tyrosine in the presence of tyrosinase enzyme by melanocytes. Most of the melanocytes are present in the epidermis of penis, nipples of breast, area just around nipples and face (moles).
   (b) The number of melanocytes in all races is fairly constant, but the difference in colour depends on the genes that determine the amount of melanin produced by melanocytes. Dark-skinned individuals have more active melanocytes that produce more melanin and vice versa.
   (c) Exposure to sunlight promotes the synthesis of melanin that absorbs ultraviolet (UV) radiation, prevents DNA damage in epidermal cells and thus protects the skin from harmful UV radiation.

2. **Hb in blood**: The amount and nature of blood pigment, Hb, circulating in the cutaneous blood vessels play an important role in skin coloration. Light-skinned individuals exhibit pink to red skin colour because of Hb in red blood cells.

Decreased Hb $\longrightarrow$ Anaemia $\longrightarrow$ Paleness of skin

Reduced Hb due to CO_2 in blood $\longrightarrow$ Cyanosis or bluish discoloration of the skin

ACCESSORY STRUCTURES OF THE SKIN

The structures associated with the skin include hair, nails and various glands of skin.

HAIR

Hair or pili is the main characteristic feature of all the mammals. It covers most of the body surface except the palms of hands, soles of feet and certain portions of external genitalia (e.g. the head of penis). In adults, it is most heavily distributed on the head, in the eyebrows, in the axillae (armpits) and around the external genitalia. The thickness and pattern of hair distribution depend on genetic and hormonal factors.

The hair on the head provides protection from injury and sun rays, whereas the hair on eyebrows protects the eyes from foreign particles.

Anatomy of hair

Each hair is composed of columns of dead keratinocytes bonded together by extracellular proteins. The *shaft* is the visible portion of the hair present above the skin surface. The *root* is the portion of hair deep to the shaft that penetrates into the dermis. The root of the hair is surrounded by an epidermal tube called the *hair follicle*, which is made up of epidermal cells and contains a cluster of cells called *bulb* at the base of the hair follicle. The bulb is the site of mitotic cell division and is responsible for the growth of existing hair and production of new hair.

The shaft and root of the hair both consist of three concentric layers of cells: cuticle, cortex and medulla. The cuticle is the outermost portion and consists of a highly keratinized single layer of thin, flat cells. The middle cortex forms the major part of the shaft and consists of the elongated cells. The inner medulla is composed of two or three rows of irregularly shaped cells (Fig. 2.4).

A bundle of smooth muscle fibres, called *arrector pili,* is attached to the hair follicle. The contraction of this muscle in response to fear or cold pulls on the hair follicle and makes the hair stand erect and also raises the skin around the hair, causing 'goose flesh' appearance on skin.

Hair growth

Each hair follicle grows in cycles, which consists of a growth stage and a resting stage. During the growth stage, the epithelial cells in the bulb of the hair follicle divide by mitosis and get pushed upwards due to which hair grows longer. As the new cells move upwards, they die and become keratinized. At this time, the resting stage begins where the hair follicle rests and the growth of hair stops.

Hair loss means that hair is being replaced as the old hair falls out of the hair follicle and a new hair begins to grow in its place. Normally, hair grows for 2–6 years and rests for about 3 months.

Normal hair loss in an adult is about 70–100 hair per day. Some men suffer a permanent loss of hair due to the loss of hair along with its hair follicles. In this case, the male sex hormone testosterone affects the hair follicles and men become bald. Pathological conditions such as radiation therapy, chemotherapy, illness or severe emotional stress also affect the growth and resting stages.

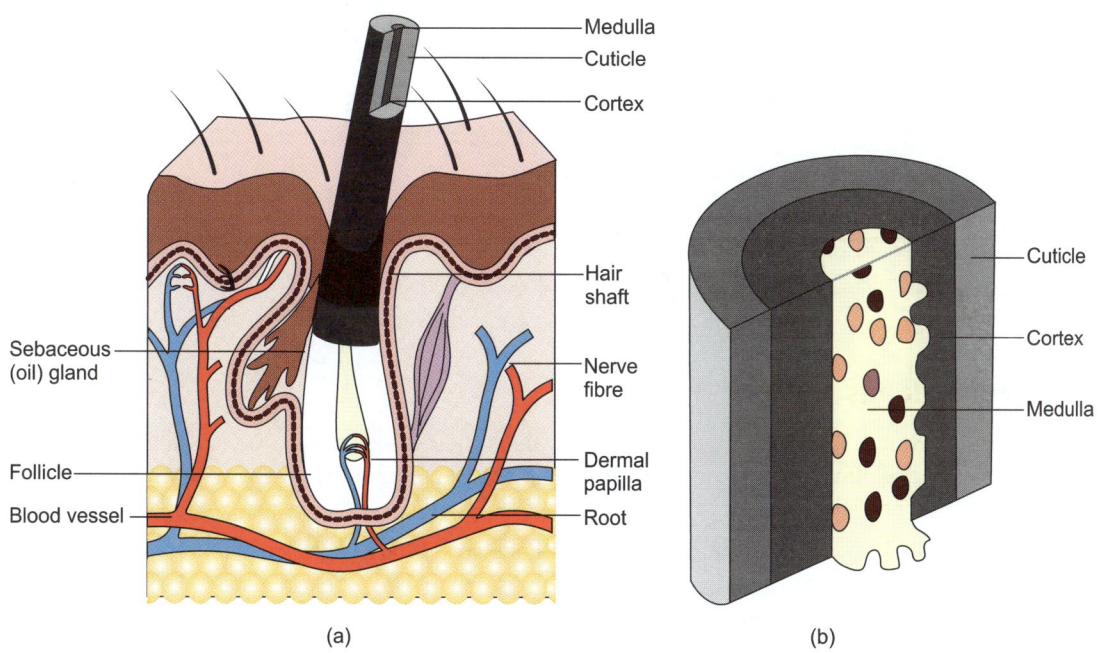

Figure 2.4 (a) Structure of the hair; (b) Layers of cells in the hair.

Note: Hair is straight, curled or tightly curled due to genetic factors that control the cross-linking and polymerization of the keratin in the cortex of the hair. This characteristic configuration of keratin makes the fibres elastic and produces different hair textures.

Hair colour

Hair colour is determined by genetic factors that control the amount of melanin present in its keratinized cells. Hair becomes grey due to progressive decline in melanin production, whereas white hair results from the lack of melanin and accumulation of air bubbles in the shaft.

NAILS

The nails are the plates of tightly packed, hard, dead keratinized epidermal cells. They protect the tips of the fingers and toes.

Each nail consists of a nail body, a free edge and a nail root. The *nail body* is the visible part of the nail and appears pinkish because of blood flowing through capillaries in the underlying dermis. The *free edge* forms the hemispherical pale area called the *lanula* or the proximal end of the nail body. The *nail root* is the part of the nail body attached to the nail bed, where the cells divide by mitosis to produce growth of nails.

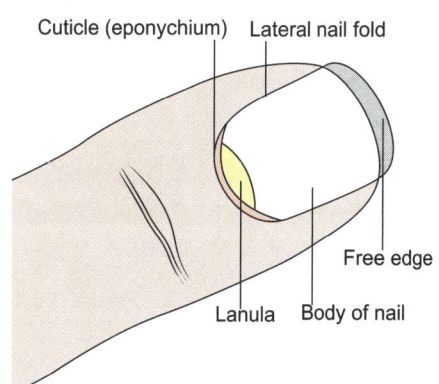

Figure 2.5 Structure of the nail.

The root of nail is embedded in the skin and is covered by the cuticle or eponychium (stratum corneum) (Fig. 2.5).

The finger nails grow at an average rate of 1 mm/week, whereas it is somewhat slower in the toe nails. The growth rate varies according to the environmental temperature (increases at high temperature), season and pathological conditions (decreases in illness).

SKIN GLANDS

The skin contains two types of glands: *sebaceous glands* and *sweat glands* (Fig. 2.6).

Sebaceous glands

Sebaceous glands or oil glands develop along the walls of hair follicles and produce an oily substance called *sebum*. The sebum is secreted into the hair follicles and on the skin of all parts of the body, except the palms of hand and soles of feet.

Sebum lubricates the surface of the skin and hair and also acts as a bactericidal and fungicidal agent, thus preventing infections. It also prevents the drying of skin and hair when exposed to heat and sunlight and gives them a shiny appearance.

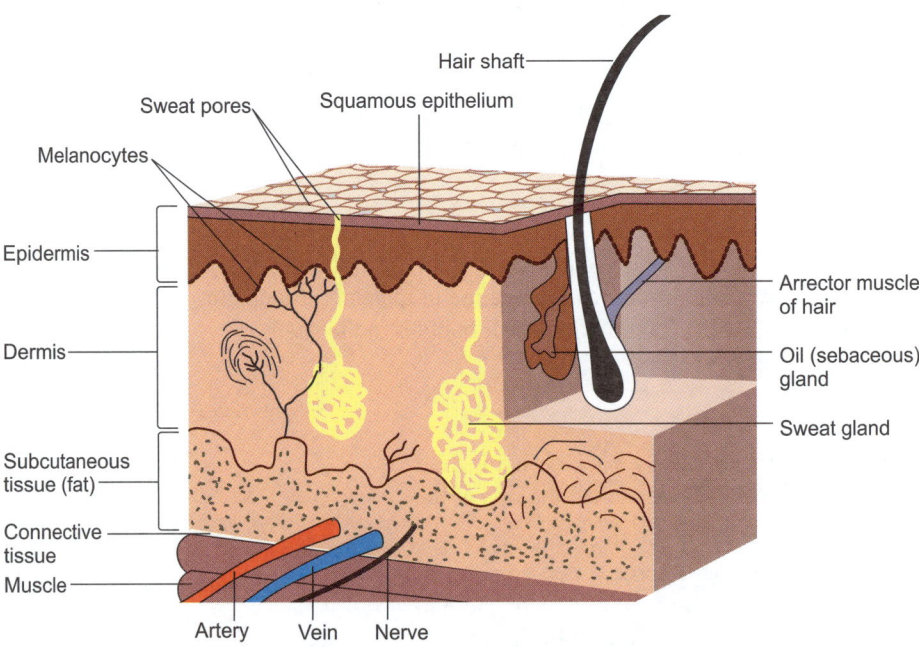

Figure 2.6 Sebaceous gland and sweat gland.

Sweat glands

Sweat glands or sudoriferous glands (*sudori*: sweat; *ferrous*: bearing) are simple tubular glands widely distributed throughout the skin and are most numerous in the palms of hand, soles of feet, axillae and groins. It has been estimated that there are 300 sweat glands per square inch on the palms of our hands.

Each sweat gland consists of a secretory portion (coiled in deep dermis) that releases its secretion by exocytosis and an excretory duct that empties the secretions on the skin surface or hair follicles. Glands that open into the hair follicles do not become active until puberty. These glands produce an odourless milky fluid, which, if decomposed by surface microbes, produces an unpleasant odour.

The most important function of sweat glands is the regulation of body temperature. Sweating leads to loss of heat from the body and helps lower body temperature.

FUNCTIONS OF THE INTEGUMENTARY SYSTEM

The various functions of the integumentary system are as follows:

1. **Protective function**: Skin covers all the organs of the body and protects these organs from:
   (a) **Microbial invasion:** The tightly interlocked keratinocytes in the skin resist the microbial invasion on skin surface. Moreover, the epidermis contains specialized immune cells called *Langerhans cells* and macrophages that phagocytize bacteria and viruses, which manage to penetrate the skin surface.
   (b) **Toxic chemicals:** The skin offers resistance against toxic chemicals such as acids and alkalis by acting as a chemical barrier.
   (c) **UV rays:** The melanin pigment in skin provides protection against damaging effects of UV rays in sunlight.
   (d) **Dehydration:** The lipid content of the skin inhibits the excessive loss of water and electrolytes through the skin.
2. **Regulation of body temperature**: The skin plays an important role in the regulation of body temperature, which is maintained at 98.6°F (37°C) approximately by two ways: liberating sweat and adjusting the flow of blood in the dermis.
   (a) **Sweat evaporation**
       (i) High environmental temperature increases sweat production and helps lower body temperature
       (ii) Low environmental temperature decreases sweat production and helps conserve heat
   (b) **Blood flow in the dermis**
       (i) High environmental temperature or increased heat production in the body leads to vasodilation in the dermis and causes more blood flow at the body surface. This increases the amount of heat loss and lowers body temperature.

Chapter 2

(ii) Low environmental temperature or decreased heat production in the body causes vasoconstriction and decreases the blood flow near skin surface and conserves heat balance

3. **Excretory function**: Skin is a minor excretory organ for some substances like small amounts of salts (sodium chloride), ammonia and urea (breakdown products of protein).

4. **Absorptive function**: The substances that can be absorbed through skin include fat-soluble substances (vitamin A, D, E and K), oxygen and carbon dioxide gases and toxic chemicals (e.g. mercury and acetone).

5. **Sensory function**: Skin has many sensory nerve endings, which are specialized to form cutaneous receptors. The sensations of touch, pain, pressure or temperature stimulates the cutaneous receptors, which then convey these sensations to the brain and the spinal cord, where these different sensations are interpreted and perceived.

6. **Synthesis of vitamin D**: 7-Dehydrocholesterol is a lipid-based substance in the skin, which is converted to vitamin D by the action of UV rays. Vitamin D is necessary for our body because it stimulates the intake of calcium and phosphorus in our intestine.

DISORDERS OF THE INTEGUMENTARY SYSTEM

1. **Dermatitis**
   (a) It is an inflammatory condition that is accompanied by redness, swelling, exudation of serous fluid and pruritus (itching).
   (b) It may be caused by allergens or irritants (e.g. strong acids or alkalis, industrial chemicals and hypersensitivity reactions to drugs and other chemicals).

2. **Pressure ulcers**
   (a) Pressure ulcers is also known as decubitus ulcers or bedsores.
   (b) They are caused by a constant deficiency of blood flow to tissues when the skin is compressed for long periods between bony projections and a hard surface, for example, bed or chair.
   (c) Blistering of the affected area may indicate superficial damage, but reddish blue discoloration indicates deep tissue damage. It occurs mostly in bedridden patients, but can be prevented with proper care.

3. **Skin cancer**
   (a) Skin cancer usually develops due to excessive exposure to the UV rays of the sun.
   (b) It is of three types:
      (i) *Basal cell carcinoma:* It is the most common cancer that produces an open ulcer and can be easily treated with radiation therapy or surgical removal.
      (ii) *Squamous cell carcinoma:* It produces nodular tumours and can spread to dermis, metastasize and may cause death.
      (iii) *Malignant carcinoma:* It is the most dangerous and rare type of cancer that is associated with a mole on skin. It appears as a dark nodule or a spreading lesion. Unless treated early, this cancer is fatal.

4. **Moles**: They are common disorders produced by grouping of melanocytes that develop during the first years of life. If the moles darken and enlarge later around 30 years, they may be a first indication of skin cancer.

OVERVIEW OF THE INTEGUMENTARY SYSTEM

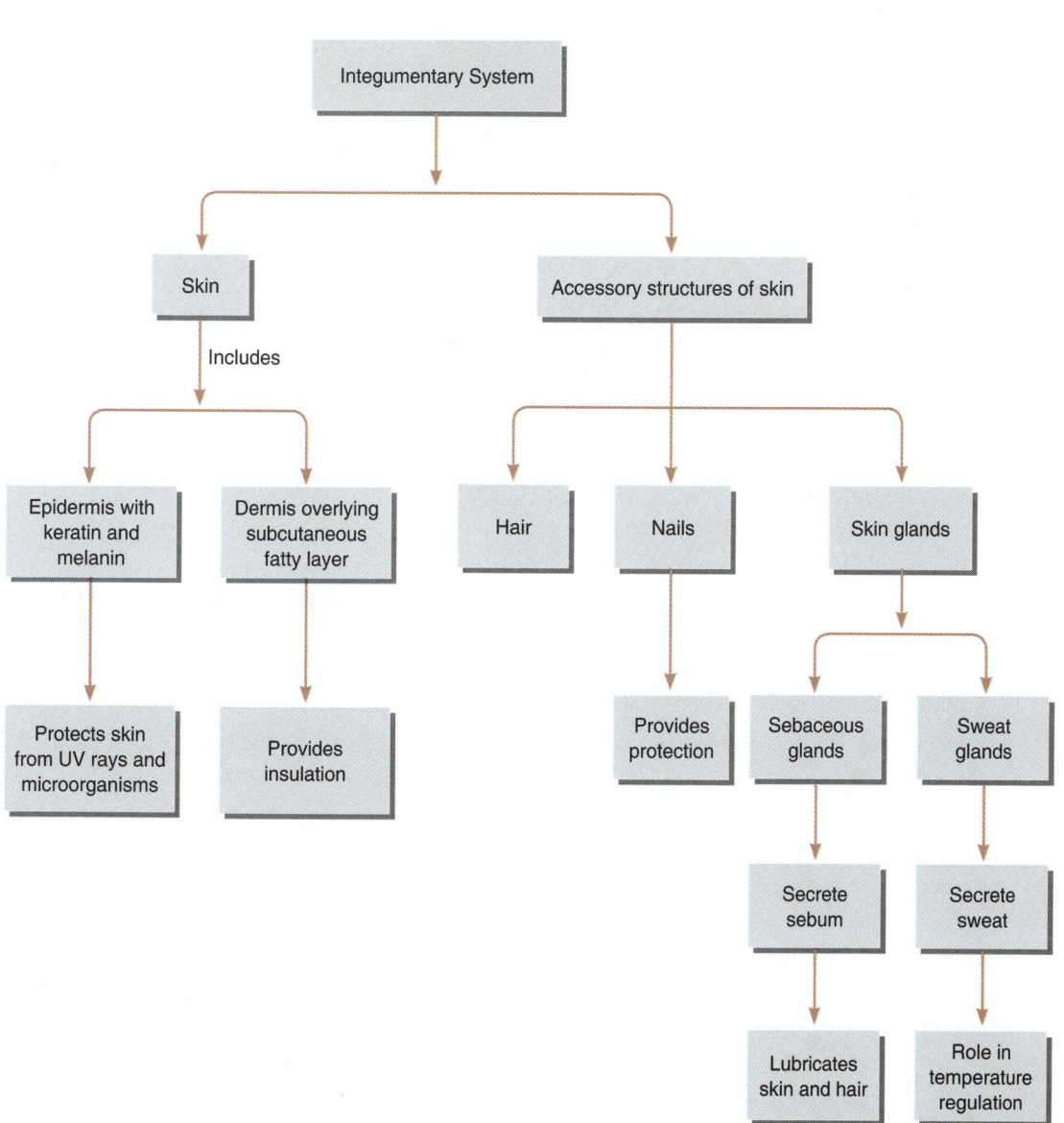

Wound Healing

❏ Damage to the skin stimulates a sequence of events that repairs the skin to its normal structure and function.

❏ There are two types of wound healing depending on the injury:

1. **Epidermal wound healing**—when only the epidermis is wounded.

2. **Deep wound healing**—when the wound penetrates the dermis.

❏ Epidermal wound healing: In small wounds such as abrasions or burns, only the superficial epidermal cells get damaged. In response, the basal cells of the epidermis enlarge and migrate across the wound. Migration stops when each cell is in contact with all epidermal cells on all sides, thus repairing the wound.

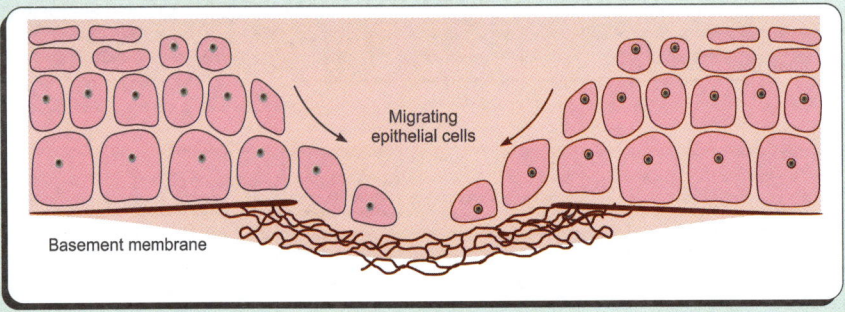

❏ Deep wound healing: In deep wounds, healing is more complex and occurs in four phases:

1. **Inflammation**: The cut surfaces become inflamed and blood clot and cell debris fill the gap between the cuts in the first few hours.

2. **Migration**: Phagocytes and fibroblasts migrate to the blood clot. Phagocytes begin to phagocytize microbes, clot and cell debris, whereas fibroblasts secrete collagen fibres that bind the damaged surface.

3. **Proliferation**: Epithelial cells proliferate across the wound and the clot becomes the scab. Collagen fibres deposit randomly and the growth of blood vessels continues.

4. **Maturation**: Collagen fibres rearrange and become more organized. The scab sloughs off after the epidermis is restored to normal thickness and blood vessels are restored to normal.

Wound Healing Phases

Inflammatory

1. Immediate to 2–5 days

2. Bleeding stops (haemostasis)
   (a) Constriction of the blood supply
   (b) Platelets start to clot
   (c) Formation of a scab

3. Inflammation
   (a) Opening of the blood supply
   (b) Cleansing of the wound

Proliferative

1. 5 days to 3 weeks

2. Granulation
   (a) New collagen tissue is laid down
   (b) New capillaries fill in defect

3. Contraction
   (a) Wound edges pull together

4. Epithelialization
   (a) Cells cross over the moist surface
   (b) Cells travel about 3 cm from point of origin

Maturation

1. Collagen forms, which increases tensile strength to wounds

2. Scar tissue is only 80 percent as strong as original tissue

3. 3 weeks to 2 years

Chapter 2

Burns

❑ Burn is tissue damage caused by excessive heat, cold, electricity, ionizing radiation and corrosive chemicals that destroy the proteins in the skin cells.

❑ Burns are classified into three major categories:

1. **First-degree burns**: They involve only the epidermis. Symptoms include redness, pain, slight swelling or oedema. These burns can heal in about 7 days.

2. **Second-degree burns**: They involve both the epidermis and the dermis. Symptoms include redness, pain, swelling and blisters. Healing can take up to 2 weeks or may extend up to several months in case of severe burns.
   First-degree and second-degree burns are also called *partial thickness burns.*

3. **Third-degree burns**: They are also called *full-thickness burns* as the epidermis and the dermis are completely destroyed. These burns are usually painless because the sensory receptors in the skin are also destroyed. The treatment usually requires skin grafts as burns take a long time to heal.

Complications of Burns

❑ Extensive burns can be life threatening or fatal. The major complications include:

1. **Dehydration and hypovolaemia**: Due to excessive loss of water and plasma proteins from the surface of the damaged skin.

2. **Hypothermia**: Due to loss of excessive heat.

3. **Infection**

4. **Kidney failure**: Due to hypovolaemia.

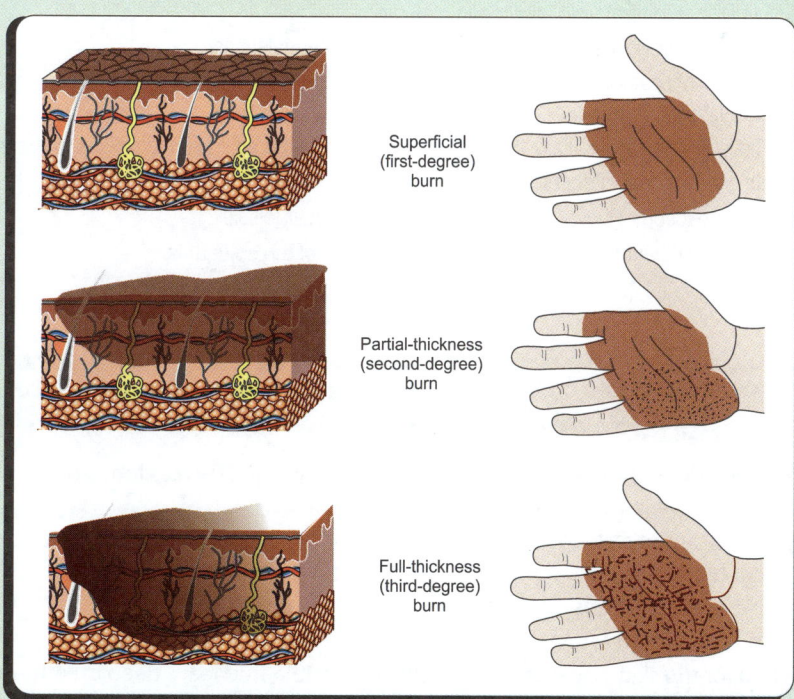

Superficial (first-degree) burn

Partial-thickness (second-degree) burn

Full-thickness (third-degree) burn

Ageing and Integumentary System

❑ With advancing age, many visible changes occur in the skin that includes dry skin, wrinkles, sagging skin, greying of hair and brittle nails.

❑ Collagen fibres in the dermis begin to decrease in number, stiffen and disorganize into a shapeless, matted tangle. Elastic fibres lose some of their elasticity and began to decrease in number. The loss of collagen and elastic fibres results in skin sagging and wrinkles.

❑ The number of melanocytes decreases in some areas that result in greying and whitening of hair with advancing age. Moreover, growth of nails and hair slows during the second and third decades of life. The toenails become brittle and break easily and become more susceptible to fungal infections.

❑ The skin glands reduce in size which leads to dry and broken skin that is more susceptible to infections.

❑ These all age related factors along with poor healing of skin makes the elderly people much more susceptible to skin infections and pathological conditions like skin cancer, itching and pressure sores.

Embryonic Development of the Integumentary System

❑ As the fertilized egg develops, a portion of the developing embryo develops into three layers of tissue called as *primary germ layers*: ectoderm, mesoderm and endoderm.

❑ During the 4th week of development, the ectoderm forms epidermal layers.

❑ During the 11th week of development, the mesoderm differentiates into the dermis and the underlying connective tissue and blood vessels.

❑ At 10 weeks, nails develop that initially consist of a thick layer of the epithelium called as *primary nail field*.

❑ During the 12th week of development, hair follicles develop.

➤ At 16 weeks, sebaceous glands develop from the sides of hair follicles.

➤ At 20 weeks, sweat glands develop from the downgrowths of the epidermis.

TIPS TO MAINTAIN HEALTHY SKIN

1. One of the top tips for healthy skin care is to eat healthy foods such as foods containing omega-3 fatty acids, vitamin A, zinc and fresh fruits and vegetables.

2. Getting a good night's sleep is important for healthy skin care because when we sleep, skin rejuvenation takes place and the cells undergo a process of repair.

3. Drinking lots of water keeps our skin healthy.

4. Avoid taking tea or coffee; instead replace it with green tea or buttermilk.

5. Stress is bad for the skin. Avoid stress as much as possible, and learn deep breathing exercises, or other stress-reducing techniques, for those times when you are stressed.

Review Questions

Long Answer Questions

1. Describe the basic functions of the integumentary system.
2. List the layers of the skin and describe their structure.
3. What accounts for the variation in normal skin colour?
4. What is the functional relationship among melanocytes, melanin and tanning?
5. Describe the innervation of the skin.
6. Describe the hair, nails, sebaceous glands, sudoriferous glands, and ceruminous glands.
7. What are the functions of human hair?
8. Describe the structure and function of nails.
9. Describe the structure and function of sebaceous glands. Why are they of clinical significance?
10. Write notes on (a) dermis (b) sebaceous glands (c) hair.

Multiple Choice Questions

1. Which of the following word pairs is appropriately matched?
   - (a) Skin–gland
   - (b) Skin–tissue
   - (c) Skin–organ
   - (d) Skin–body system
2. The skin is derived from
   - (a) Ectoderm and endoderm
   - (b) Ectoderm and mesoderm
   - (c) Mesoderm and endoderm
   - (d) Ectoderm, mesoderm and endoderm
3. What percentage of the body weight does the skin account for?
   - (a) 2%
   - (b) 10%
   - (c) Less than 2%
   - (d) 7%
4. Which of the following is *not* a function of the skin?
   - (a) Prevention of body dehydration
   - (b) Synthesis of vitamin A
   - (c) Prevention of pathogen entry
   - (d) Regulation of body temperature
5. Loss of body fluids through the integument is restricted by
   - (a) Keratin
   - (b) The stratum basale
   - (c) Melanocytes
   - (d) The thickness of the dermis
6. Which of the following pairings is appropriate?
   - (a) Stratum corneum–melanocytes
   - (b) Stratum granulosum–keratin
   - (c) Stratum lucidum–blood vessels
   - (d) Stratum spinosum–cornified

7. Fingerprint patterns are established prenatally during the development of

   (a) The stratum corneum

   (b) The dermal papillary layer

   (c) The stratum basale

   (d) The dermal reticular layer

   (e) The hypodermis

8. It is *false* that the dermis

   (a) Is highly vascular

   (b) Gives rise to sebaceous and sweat glands

   (c) Contains reticular, elastic and smooth muscle fibres

   (d) Contains numerous nerve endings

9. It is *false* that the epidermis

   (a) Is highly vascular

   (b) Contains melanin and keratin

   (c) Is distinctly stratified

   (d) Gives rise to sebaceous and sweat glands

10. What is the proper sequence of epidermal strata (layers) pierced as a sliver penetrates the epidermis on the palm of the hand?

   (a) Spinosum, basale, granulosum, lucidum, corneum, disjunction

   (b) Basale, spinosum, granulosum, disjunction, lucidum, corneum

   (c) Disjunction, corneum, lucidum, granulosum, spinosum, basale

   (d) Corneum, disjunction, lucidum, spinosum, granulosum, basale

11. Cells from the stratum basale reach the stratum disjunction in approximately

   (a) 15–20 days   (b) 6–8 weeks

   (c) 8–10 days   (d) 12–15 weeks

   (e) 4–6 months

12. Produced in the epidermis of the skin, melanin

   (a) Protects against ultraviolet light   (b) Prevents infections

   (c) Helps regulate body temperature   (d) Reduces water loss

13. The most probable cause of alopecia is

   (a) Protein deficiencies   (b) Dermal viral infection

   (c) Genetic inheritance   (d) Stress

14. Which of the following statements about sebaceous glands is *true*?

   (a) They secrete sebum directly to the skin surface

   (b) They derive from specialized mesoderm

   (c) They are a type of oil-secreting gland

   (d) They are a compound saccular type

15. Which of the following is *not* a function of the integument?
    (a) Elimination of certain body salts, urea and uric acid
    (b) Absorption of fat-soluble vitamins, steroid hormones and certain toxic chemicals
    (c) Storage of lipids
    (d) Thermoregulation
    (e) Synthesis of proteins and carbohydrates
    (f) Prevention of desiccation and blood loss

State True or False

1. Skin is the largest tissue of the body, accounting for approximately 7% of the body weight.
2. Hair, nails and integumentary glands are specializations of the epidermis and are derived from the embryonic ectodermal germ layer.
3. A burn that damaged both the epidermis and dermis so that regeneration could occur only from the edges of the wound would be classified as a second-degree burn.
4. People of African descent have more melanocytes in their skin than do lighter complexioned people.
5. Mammary glands are modified sebaceous glands that are hormonally prepared to lactate in association with the birth of a baby.
6. Stimulation of the free nerve endings within the skin would cause the perception of cold and may autonomically induce shivering.
7. Water-soluble substances would be more readily absorbed through the skin than fat-soluble substances.
8. The principal danger of a third-degree burn is excessive body fluid loss and disruption of homeostasis.
9. Alopecia is a disease that results in excessive loss of hair.
10. Warts, shingles and acne are all viral infections of the integument.

Fill in the Blanks

1. The term _____ is synonymous with skin.
2. The epidermis of the skin consists of _____ epithelial tissue.
3. The outermost layer of the epidermis of the skin is the stratum _____, and the deepest layer is the stratum _____.
4. Normal skin coloration reflects a combination of three pigments: haemoglobin, _____, and _____.
5. The dermis of the skin consists of an upper _____ layer and a deeper _____ layer.
6. _____ is a protein in the skin that strengthens the stratified squamous epithelium of the epidermis.
7. _____ glands secrete sebum into the hair follicles of the skin.

Careers in Integumentary System

✓ Cosmetologists are trained professionals who develop career as makeup artists and hair stylists and occupy various positions in television, cinema and local hair salons.

✓ Dermatologists are physicians who specialize in the diseases and disorders of the skin.

✓ Plastic surgeons are the physicians who specialize in cosmetic surgery to counteract the effects of ageing and to correct birth defects.

✓ Allergists are the physicians specialized in the inflammatory responses of the skin.

3 The Skeletal System

CHAPTER OUTLINE

STUDY OBJECTIVES

- ✓ To describe the basic functions of the skeletal system
- ✓ To discuss the general structure and types of bones
- ✓ To explain the structure of compact and spongy bone tissue
- ✓ To describe the process of bone development and bone healing
- ✓ To identify the bones of the skull (face and cranium)
- ✓ To discuss the various regions in the vertebral column
- ✓ To describe the bones that form the thoracic cage and the appendicular skeleton
- ✓ To discuss the various bones in the upper and lower limbs
- ✓ To discuss joints and their various types
- ✓ To explain the characteristics of fibrous and cartilaginous joints
- ✓ To describe the structure and various types of synovial joints

INTRODUCTION

The entire framework of bones and their cartilages constitutes the skeletal system. The skeletal system is the supporting structure of the body that enables us to stand erect and move in our environment and gives us the ability to perform stressful efforts such as running and jumping. The scientific study of bone structure and the treatment of bone disorders is called *osteology* or *skeletology*. The branch of science concerned with the prevention or correction of disorders of the musculoskeletal system is called *orthopaedics*.

The skeletal system includes all the bones of the body and their associated cartilages, tendons and ligaments. The hard, 'dead' stone-like appearance of bones is due to mineral salts such as calcium phosphate embedded in the inorganic matrix of the bone tissue. Leonardo da Vinci (1452–1519), the famous Italian Renaissance artist and scientist, is credited as the first anatomist to correctly illustrate the skeleton with its 206 bones.

FUNCTIONS OF THE SKELETAL SYSTEM

The various functions of the skeletal system include:

1. **Support**: The skeleton serves as the structural framework of the body. It gives attachment to muscles and tendons and supports and stabilizes surrounding tissues such as muscles, blood vessels, nerves, fat and skin.

2. **Protection**: The skeleton encloses the vital organs of the body, such as the brain, spinal cord, heart and lungs, and protects them from injury.

3. **Assists in movement**: The skeleton allows the movement of the body as a whole and of parts of the body, by forming joints.

4. **Haemopoiesis**: A connective tissue called *red bone marrow* is present within certain bones that produce red blood cells, white bloods cells and platelets, and this process is called *haemopoiesis*.

5. **Mineral homeostasis**: Bone tissue serves as the storage area for mineral salts, especially phosphorus and calcium, which strengthen the bone. The homeostasis of minerals in the body is maintained by releasing the minerals into the blood when required.

DO YOU KNOW

- The pelvis or hip bone is the largest bone in the body.
- The 'femur' in the thigh is the longest bone in the body. It makes up almost one quarter of the body's total height.
- The ears and end of the nose do not have bones inside them. Their inner supports are cartilage, which is lighter and more flexible than bone. This is why the nose and ears can be bent.
- After death, cartilage rots faster than bone. This is why the skulls of skeletons have no nose or ears.
- Humans and giraffes have the same number of bones in their necks. Giraffe's neck vertebrae are just much, much longer!
- There are over 230 moveable and semimoveable joints in the body.

STRUCTURE OF THE BONE

At the macroscopic level, the structure of bone can be analysed by studying the parts of a long bone.

A typical long bone consists of the following parts (Fig. 3.1):

1. **Diaphysis** (*dia*: growing between): It is the long cylindrical main portion of the bone that constitutes bone's shaft or body.

2. **Epiphyses**: These are the extremities, i.e. the distal and proximal ends of the bone.

3. **Metaphyses**
   - These are the regions in mature bone where the diaphysis joins the epiphysis.
   - In a growing bone, each metaphysis includes a layer of hyaline cartilage called *epiphyseal plate* that allows the diaphysis of the bone to grow in length. When the bone stops to grow in length at

MEDICAL TERMINOLOGY

- **Blasts**: They are cells that secrete the extracellular matrix.
- **Cartilage**: It is a connective tissue that is present at the ends of certain bones and joints and provides a smooth surface for adjacent bones to move against each other.
- **Cytes**: These are cells in any tissue that maintain the tissue.
- **Ligaments**: These are tough connective tissue structures that attach bones to bones.
- **Tendons**: These are structures that attach muscle to bone.

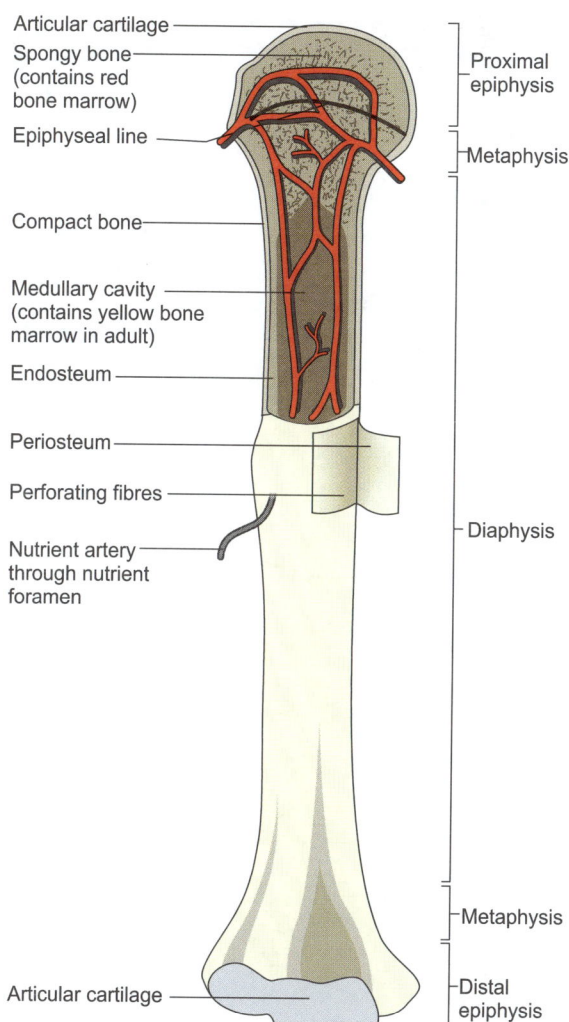

Articular cartilage

Spongy bone (contains red bone marrow)

Epiphyseal line

Compact bone

Medullary cavity (contains yellow bone marrow in adult)

Endosteum

Periosteum

Perforating fibres

Nutrient artery through nutrient foramen

Articular cartilage

Proximal epiphysis

Metaphysis

Diaphysis

Metaphysis

Distal epiphysis

Figure 3.1 Structure of a long bone.

puberty, the cartilage in the epiphyseal plate is replaced by bone and the resulting bone structure is called the *epiphyseal line*.

4. **Articular cartilage**: It is a thin layer of hyaline cartilage that covers the part of epiphyses, forming articulation (joint) with another bone. Articular cartilage reduces friction at freely movable joints.

5. **Periosteum**: It is a tough sheath of dense irregular tissue that surrounds the surface of bone wherever it is not covered by articular cartilage. The periosteum protects the bone, helps nourish bone tissue, helps in fracture repair and serves as an attachment point for ligaments and tendons. The periosteum also contains bone-forming cells that enable bones to grow in thickness.

6. **Medullary cavity**: It is a space within diaphysis in adults that contains the fatty yellow bone marrow.

7. **Endosteum**: It is a thin membrane of bone-forming cells and connective tissue that lines the medullary cavity.

TYPES OF BONES

Bones can be classified into five categories based on their shape: long, short, flat, irregular and sesamoid (Fig. 3.2).

1. **Long bones**
   - ❏ These are bones whose length exceed their width and consist of a shaft, or diaphysis, and two extremities, or epiphysis. The epiphysis consists of an outer thin covering of compact bone with spongy (cancellous) bone inside that usually contains red marrow.
   - ❏ Examples include the femur, tibia, fibula and humerus.

2. **Short bones**
   - ❏ They have no shafts or extremities, have a nearly cubic shape and are almost equal in length and width.
   - ❏ Examples include carpals (wrist) and tarsals (foot).

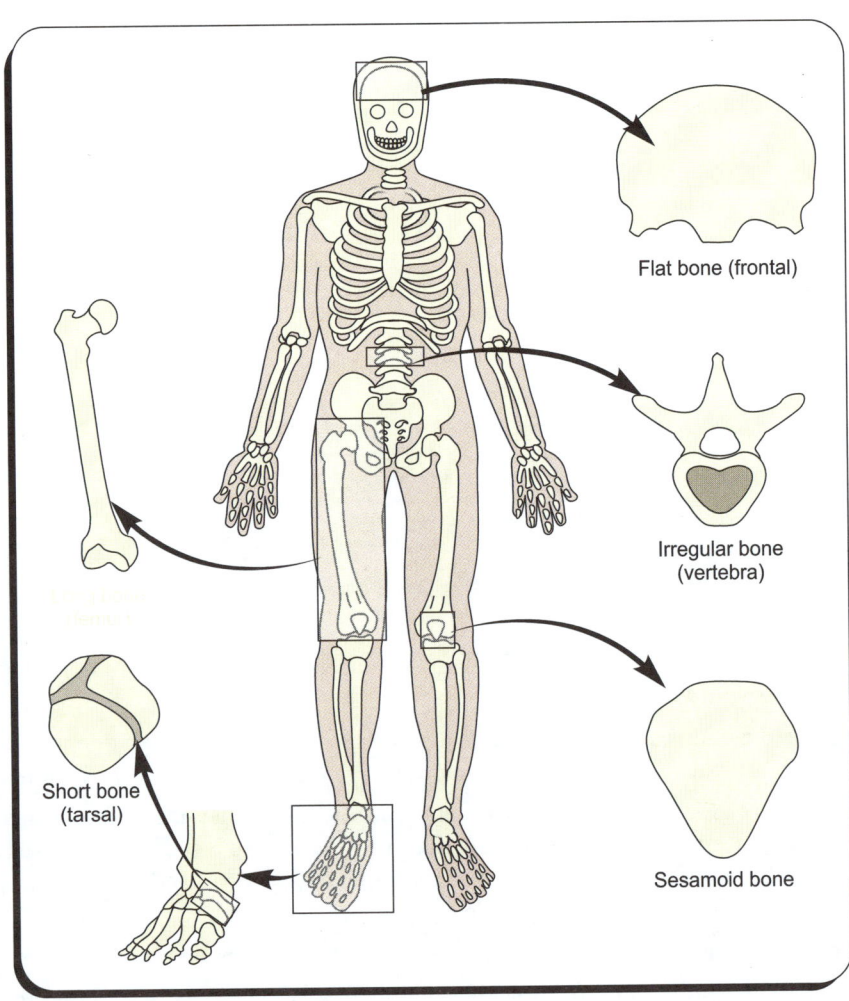

Figure 3.2 Types of bones.

3. **Flat bones**
   - ❏ Flat bones are thin bones present in areas that need extensive muscle attachment or that protect the soft or vital parts of the body. These bones are usually curved and consist of two flat plates of compact bone tissues enclosing a layer of cancellous (spongy) bone.
   - ❏ Examples include sternum, ribs and most skull bones.
4. **Irregular bones**
   - ❏ These are irregularly shaped bones that consist of spongy (cancellous) bone enclosed by relatively thin layers of compact bone.
   - ❏ Examples include vertebrae, ossicles (ears) and some skull bones.
5. **Sesamoid bones**
   - ❏ These are small rounded bones that assist in the functioning of muscles. They are located adjacent to joints.
   - ❏ Examples include patella (knee cap).

HISTOLOGY OF BONE TISSUE

Bone is a strong and durable connective tissue that consists of *the extracellular matrix* and *the bone cells*.

The extracellular matrix includes 25% water, 25% collagen fibres and 50% crystallized mineral salts (mainly calcium phosphate, calcium hydroxide and calcium carbonate). The mineral salts undergo calcification (i.e. they crystallize in the spaces between collagen fibres and are responsible for the hardness of the bone). The collagen fibres in the extracellular matrix give slight flexibility to the bone.

The bone tissue contains four types of cells: osteogenic cells, osteoblasts, osteocytes and osteoclasts (Fig. 3.3).

1. **Osteogenic cells**
   - ❏ These are the unspecialized stem cells that undergo cell division and the resulting cells develop into osteoblasts.
   - ❏ Osteogenic cells are found in the periosteum and endosteum of bones.

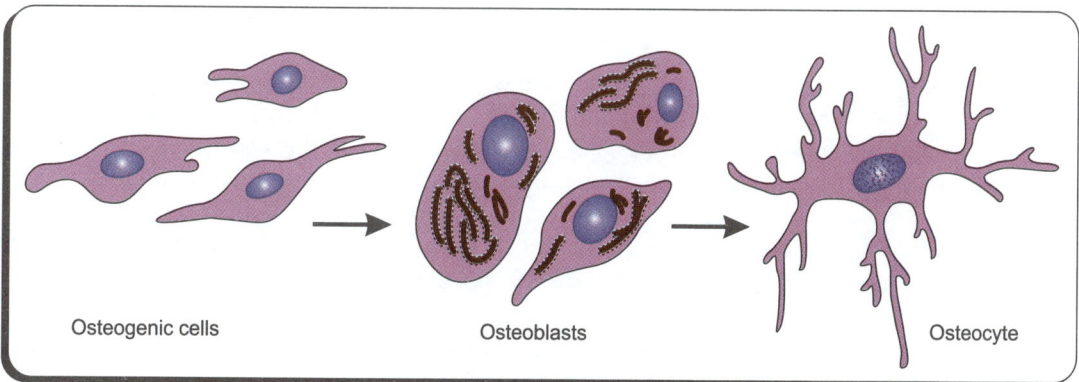

Osteogenic cells   Osteoblasts   Osteocyte

Figure 3.3 Cells of bone tissue.

Chapter 3

2. **Osteoblasts**
   - ❏ These are bone-forming cells that secrete collagen and other organic components required to build the extracellular matrix of bone tissues.
   - ❏ Osteoblasts are present in the deeper layers of periosteum, ends of diaphysis and at the fracture site.
3. **Osteocytes:** As the bone develops, osteoblasts become trapped within the newly formed bone and develop into osteocytes, which are the mature bone cells that maintain the bone tissue.
4. **Osteoclasts**
   - ❏ These are huge cells mainly concentrated in the endosteum of bones. The plasma membrane of osteoclasts is deeply folded into a ruffled border.
   - ❏ The main function of these cells is resorption of bone to maintain the optimum shape. These cells contain powerful lysosomal enzymes and acids that digest the protein and mineral components of the bone matrix and cause bone resorption.

A fine balance between osteoblasts and osteoclasts maintains the structure and functions of normal bone.

TYPES OF BONE TISSUES

There are two types of bone tissues: *compact or dense bone* and *cancellous or spongy bone*. In both types of tissue, the osteocytes are the same, but the arrangement of blood supply to the bone cells is different.

Compact bone tissue

- ❏ Compact bone tissue makes up about 80% of the body bone mass. It is found mainly beneath the periosteum of all bones and in the diaphysis of long bones.
- ❏ It is made up of a large number of repeating units called *osteons* or *Haversian systems*; each osteon is made up of a central canal or Haversian canal (Fig. 3.4).
  - ➤ The osteons are aligned in the same direction along the lines of stress (e.g. in the long bones, osteons are parallel to the long axis of the bone, which gives the bone strength and resists it from bend or fracture even when considerable force is applied from either end).
  - ➤ The central canal runs parallel to the surface of bone and contains blood vessels (capillaries, arterioles, venules) that bring in oxygen and nutrients and remove waste products and carbon dioxide.
- ❏ The central canals are surrounded by concentric rings of the calcified extracellular matrix, each layer of which is called a *lamella*. Between the two lamellae are small cavities called *lacunae* (singular is lacuna), which contain osteocytes. The lacunae are connected to each other and to the larger haversian (central) canals by small canals or channels called *canaliculi*, filled with extracellular fluid. The areas between osteons are *interstitial lamellae* that contain fragments of older osteons that have been partially destroyed during bone remodelling or growth. Each central canal is linked with neighbouring canals through perforating or *Volkmann's canals* that run horizontally to the central canal.
- ❏ The Volkmann's canal, central canal and the canaliculi that connect the lacunae with one another and with the central canal form an intricate system of interconnected canals throughout the bone. This system provides many routes for providing oxygen and nutrients and for the removal of wastes and keeps the osteocytes alive and healthy.

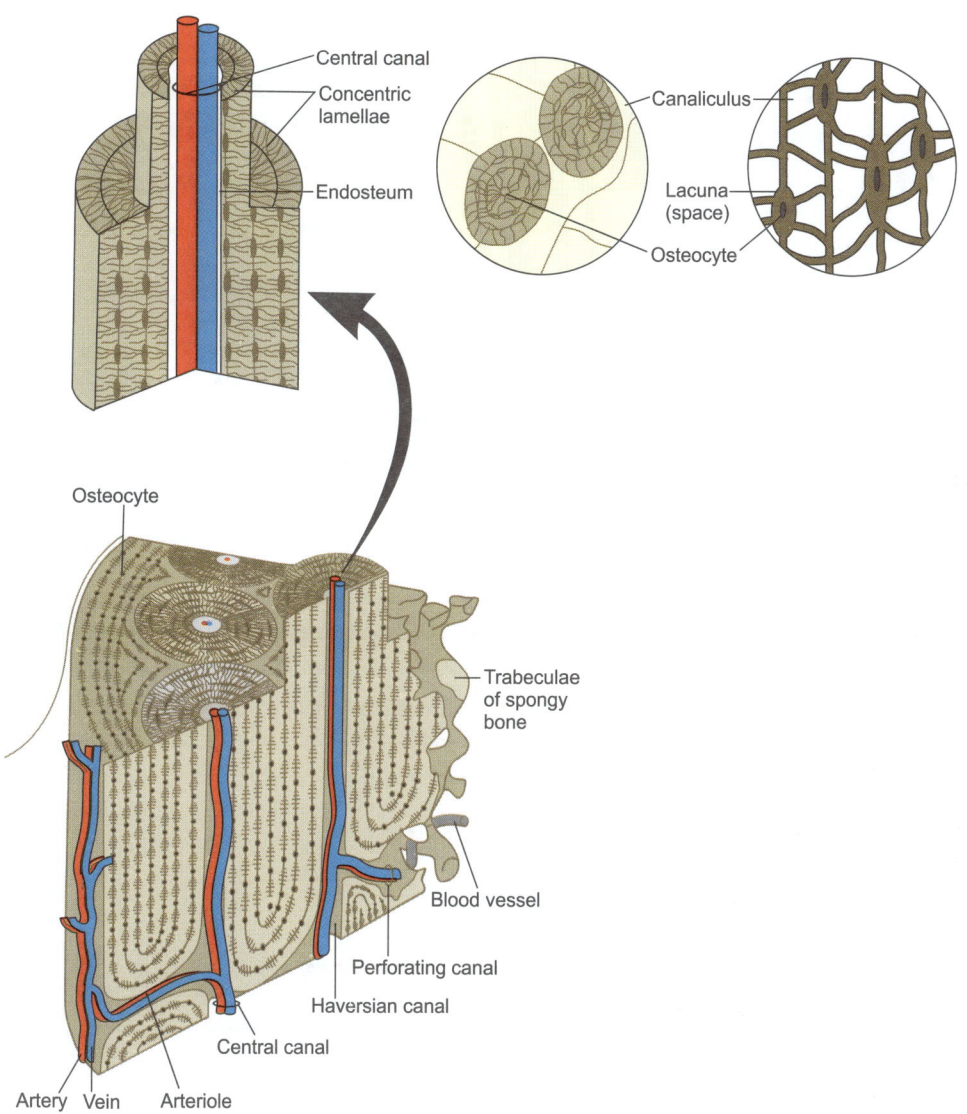

Figure 3.4 Compact bone tissue.

Spongy (trabecular) bone tissue

❑ Spongy bone tissue is located at the ends of long bones and forms the centre of all other bones. It consists of a framework of interconnecting sections called *trabeculae*, creating the sponge-like appearance of the bone tissue. Each trabecula consists of several lamellae with osteocytes, interconnected by canaliculi just as in compact bone (Fig. 3.5). The trabecula gives strength to the bone without adding weight to the bone, which makes it light weight compared with the compact bone tissue.

❑ The spaces between the trabeculae are filled with red bone marrow, where haematopoiesis (blood cell production) occurs in adults.

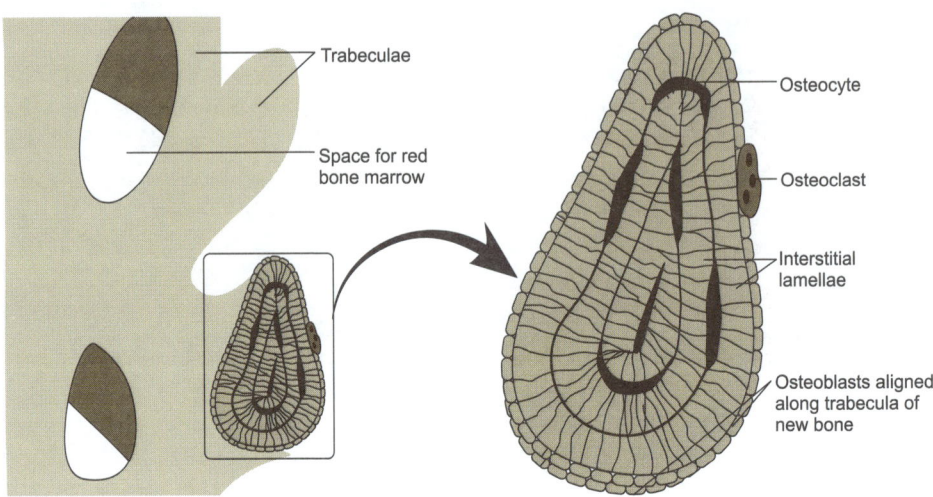

Figure 3.5 Spongy bone tissue.

DEVELOPMENT OF BONE TISSUE OR FORMATION OF BONE

The process of bone formation is called *ossification* or *osteogenesis*. The skeleton of a developing fetus is completely formed by the end of the third month of pregnancy. However, at this time, the skeleton is predominantly made of cartilage. Ossification occurs only during the subsequent months of pregnancy.

There are two types of ossification (bone formation) (Fig. 3.6):

1. Intramembranous ossification
2. Endochondral ossification

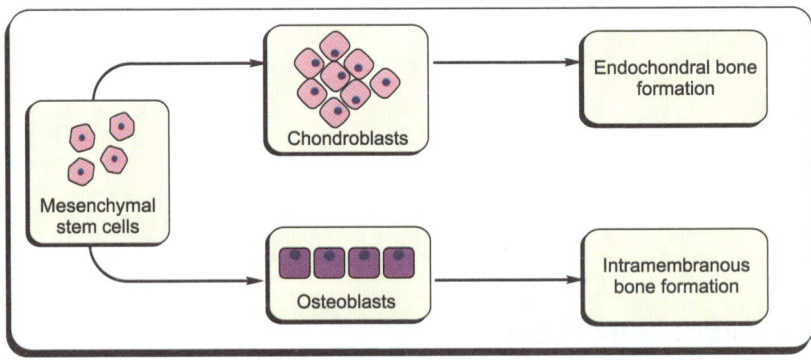

Figure 3.6 Differentiation of mesenchymal cells.

1. Intramembranous ossification (*intra*: within; *membranous*: membrane): This method of bone formation results in the formation of flat bones as in the skull and mandible (lower jaw bone). Bone formation by this process continues for a few months after birth, which is why the membranes can still be felt on the top of a baby's skull, at the *soft spots* or *fontanelle*. These soft spots help the fetal skull pass through the birth canal. After birth, it undergoes intramembranous ossification and thus hardens.

The various steps by which intramembranous ossification occurs are as follows (Fig. 3.7):

Development of the ossification centre

- ❑ The mesenchymal cells cluster together at the site of bone development called as the *ossification centre*. (*Mesenchyme* is the tissue from which all other connective tissues arise.)
- ❑ At the ossification centre, the mesenchymal cells differentiate into osteogenic cells and then further into osteoblasts that secrete the extracellular matrix of the bone.

Calcification and trabeculae formation

- ❑ The osteoblasts get surrounded by the extracellular matrix and develop into mature bone cells or osteocytes. Eventually, calcification commences and the matrix begins to harden.
- ❑ The extracellular matrix develops into trabeculae to form spongy bone, while some of the connective tissue in the trabecula differentiates into red bone marrow.

Development of mature bone: The mesenchyme at the bone periphery condenses and develops into periosteum. Underneath the periosteum, the surface layer of spongy bone is replaced by compact bone, but the spongy bone remains at the centre. Most of the newly formed bone is remodelled to develop it into mature bone (adult size and shape).

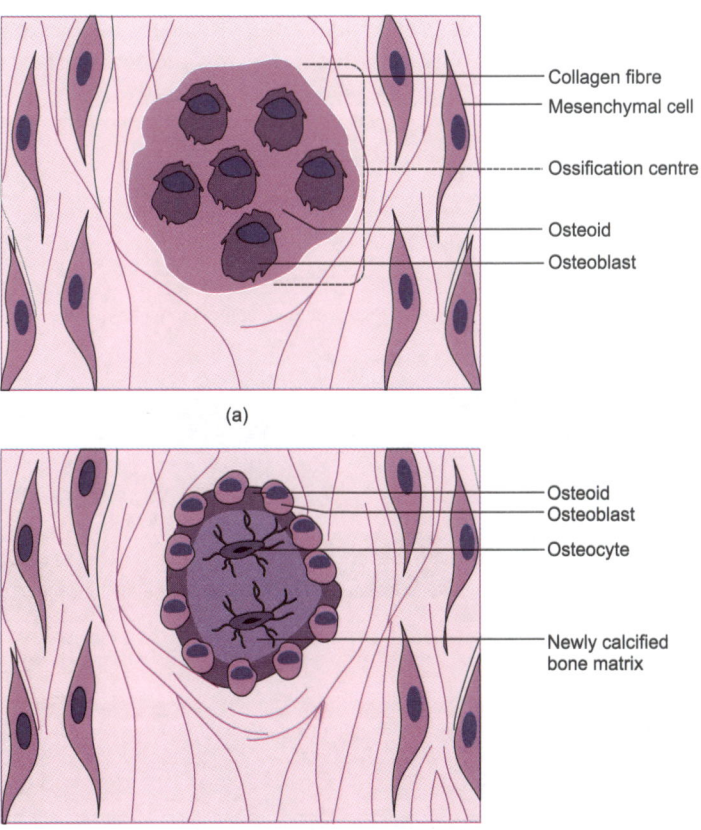

(a)

(b)

Figure 3.7 Intramembranous ossification: (a) Ossification centres from within thickened regions of mesenchyme; (b) Bone matrix (osteoid) undergoes calcification.

2. Endochondral ossification (*endo*: within; *chondral*: cartilage): This is the process in which bone formation occurs by the replacement of cartilage with the bone. Most of the bones of the body are formed by this method.

The following are the steps of endochondral ossification (Fig. 3.8):

Development of the cartilage model: At the site of bone development, the mesenchymal cells cluster together and differentiate into chondroblasts. The chondroblasts secrete the cartilage extracellular matrix and develop into a *cartilage model* that consists of hyaline cartilage.

Development of the primary ossification centre: The chondroblasts develop into mature cells or chondrocytes that undergo cell division continuously along with the secretion of extracellular matrix. Later, with the development of the blood supply, the bone tissue replaces most of the cartilages at a site close to the middle of the model called the *primary ossification centre*. Primary ossification proceeds inwards from the external surface of the bone, forming spongy trabeculae at the centre. Later, the bone lengthens as ossification continues and extends to the epiphyses.

Formation of medullary cavity: The osteoclasts break down some of the newly formed spongy trabeculae in the centre and form a medullary canal. However, most of the walls of diaphysis are replaced by compact bone.

Development of secondary ossification centre: Around birth, secondary ossification centres develop in the epiphyses and ossification proceeds outwards, that is, towards the outer surface of the bone.

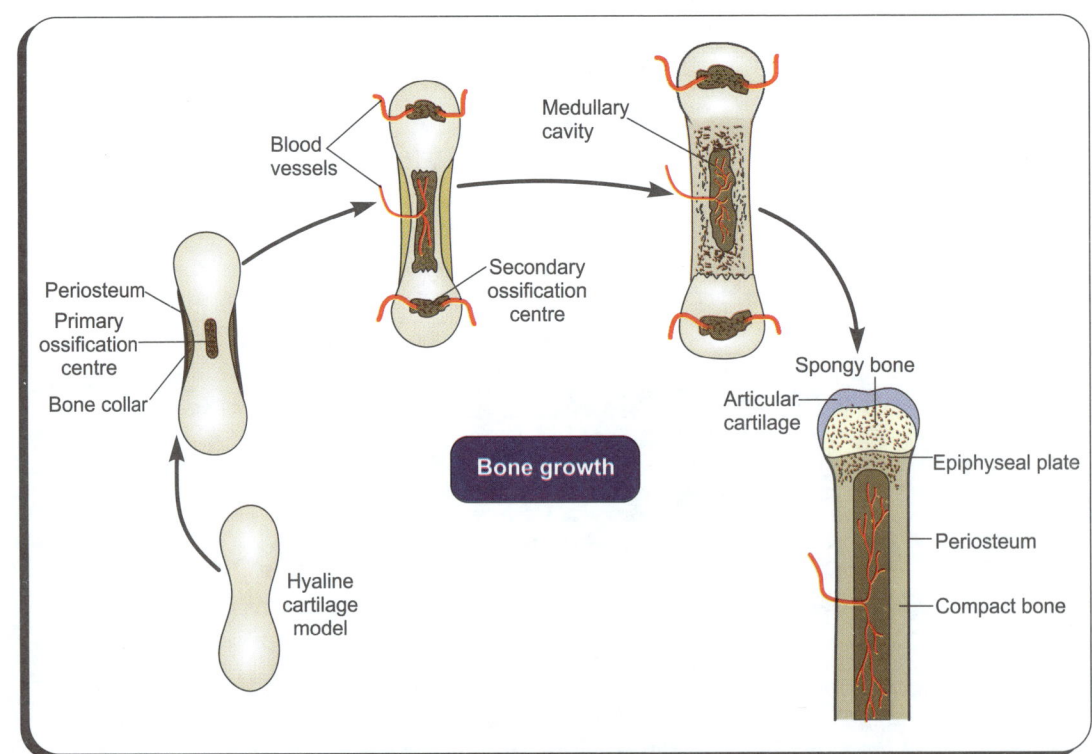

Figure 3.8 Endochondral ossification.

Formation of articular cartilage and epiphyseal plate

❏ The hyaline cartilage develops into the articular cartilage, which covers the bone. Prior to adulthood, the hyaline cartilage remains between the diaphysis and the epiphysis as the *epiphyseal plate* where the epiphyseal cartilage cells continue to divide and are responsible for the lengthwise growth of long bones.

❏ At puberty (around 18 years in females and 21 years in males), the epiphyseal plate closes, the epiphyseal cartilage cells stop dividing, the bone replaces all the cartilage and the epiphyseal plate transforms into the *epiphyseal line*. The epiphyseal line signifies that the bone has stopped growing in length.

REMODELLING OF BONE

Bone remodelling is the ongoing replacement of old bone tissues by new bone tissues. It involves bone resorption by osteoclasts and bone deposition by osteoblasts. The osteoblasts and osteoclasts work in accord to maintain the shape, size and integrity of the bone.

❏ **Bone resorption**: It is the process of removal of minerals and collagen fibres from bone, which destroys the bone extracellular matrix.

❏ **Bone deposition**: It is the addition of minerals and collagen fibres to the bone, resulting in the formation of the bone extracellular matrix.

FACTORS AFFECTING BONE GROWTH AND BONE REMODELLING

The various factors that regulate the growth, size and shape of bones are as follows:

1. Minerals

The growing bones need a large amount of calcium and phosphorus and comparatively smaller amounts of fluoride, magnesium, iron and manganese. These minerals are necessary for bone growth as well as during bone remodelling.

2. Vitamins

❏ **Vitamin A**: It stimulates osteoblast activity.
❏ **Vitamin C**: It is required for collagen synthesis and for activity of osteoblasts.
❏ **Vitamin K and B$_{12}$**: It is required for protein synthesis.
❏ **Vitamin D**: It is necessary for normal growth of bone.

3. Hormones

The following are the hormones that regulate the growth and remodelling of bones:

1. **Growth hormone (GH) and the thyroid hormones** (Thyroxine [T$_4$] and tri-iodothyronine [T$_3$])
   These hormones are especially important during infancy and childhood as they stimulate osteoblasts and promote bone growth.

Chapter 3

2. **Sex hormones (testosterone and oestrogen)**

   (a) The secretion of these hormones at puberty dramatically affects the growth of bones. These hormones cause increased osteoblast activity and synthesis of the bone extracellular matrix and thus are responsible for the sudden *growth spurt* of puberty.

   (b) They influence the physical changes that occur at puberty such as the widening of pelvis in females and also help maintain the bone structures throughout life.

   (c) In later stages, these sex hormones, especially oestrogen in both sexes, stimulate closure of the epiphyseal plates, causing the bone elongation to cease.

   (d) During adulthood, sex hormones contribute to bone remodelling by slowing resorption of old bone and promoting deposition of new bone.

3. **Parathyroid hormone and calcitonin**

   (a) Parathyroid hormone (PTH) and calcitonin control the blood levels of calcium and maintain calcium between 9 and 11 mg per 100 mL.

   (b) The decrease in blood Ca^{2+} levels stimulate parathyroid gland to release PTH into the blood.

   (c) PTH maintains the blood Ca^{2+} level by the following ways:

      (i) PTH increases the number and activity of osteoclasts and speeds up bone resorption that causes release of Ca^{2+} from the bone into blood.

      (ii) PTH acts on kidneys and decreases loss of Ca^{2+} from the urine.

      (iii) PTH stimulates calcitriol formation that promotes the absorption of calcium from foods in the gastrointestinal tract into blood.

   (d) PTH elevates and maintains Ca^{2+} level whenever the Ca^{2+} level in blood is decreased (discussed in detail in the Endocrine System).

   (e) The increase in blood Ca^{2+} level stimulates the thyroid gland to secrete calcitonin. Calcitonin inhibits osteoclasts activity and increases the calcium uptake into bones. This leads to deposition of calcium in bones and decreased blood Ca^{2+} level.

FRACTURE AND HEALING OF BONE

A fracture can be defined as any break in a bone. The common types of fractures are as follows (Fig. 3.9):

1. **Open (compound) fracture**: The broken end of the bone protrudes through the skin.
2. **Closed (simple) fracture**: The broken bone ends do not protrude through the skin.
3. **Comminuted fracture**: The bone breaks into small fragments at the impact site and the smaller bone fragments lie between the two main fragments.
4. **Impacted fracture**: One end of the fractured bone is forcefully pushed into the interior of the other.

The repair of a bone fracture involves the following steps (Fig. 3.10):

1. Formation of fracture haematoma: As the blood vessels break at the fracture site, the blood leaks out and forms a clot called *fracture haematoma*. It is followed by the development of acute inflammation and accumulation of inflammatory exudates, containing phagocytes (neutrophils and macrophages) that begin to remove the dead and damaged tissues in and around the fracture haematoma. This stage may last up to 1–2 weeks.

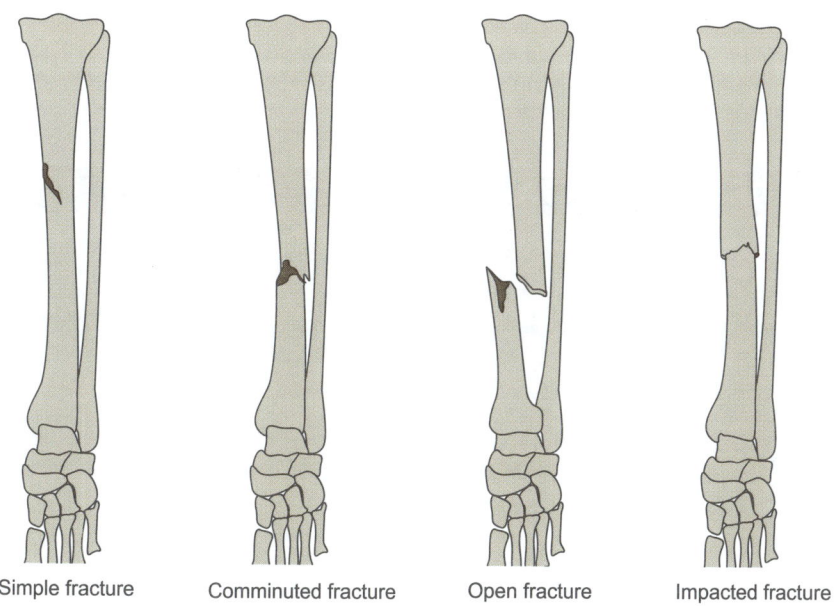

Simple fracture Comminuted fracture Open fracture Impacted fracture

Figure 3.9 Common types of fractures.

2. Formation of callus: Fibroblasts and cells of periosteum invade the fracture site and begin to produce collagen fibres and fibrocartilage, which lead to the development of a mass of repair tissue called *fibrocartilaginous callus*. This callus mainly consists of collagen fibres and cartilage, which forms a bridge and unites the broken ends of the bone. Eventually, osteoblasts convert the fibrocartilage into spongy bone and the callus is then referred to as *bony callus*. This stage may last up to 2–16 weeks.

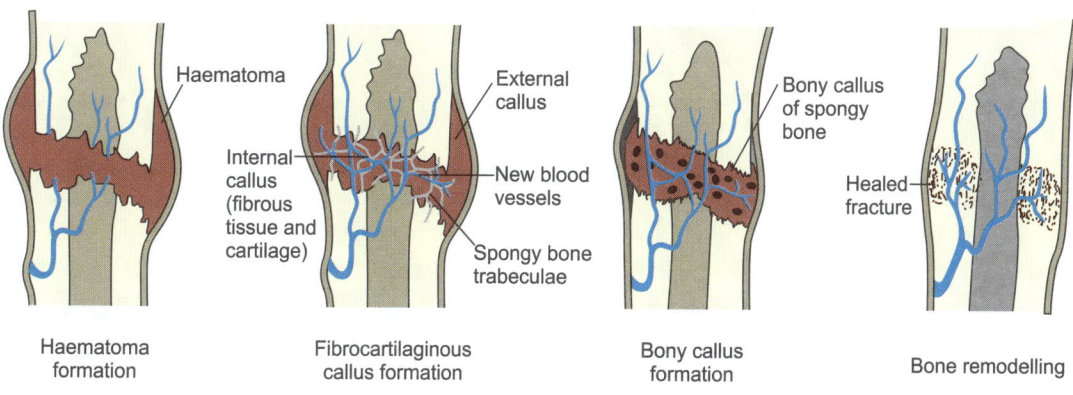

Haematoma formation   Fibrocartilaginous callus formation   Bony callus formation   Bone remodelling

Figure 3.10 Various events in fracture repair.

3. Bone remodelling: This is the final phase of fracture repair in which dead portions of the broken bone are gradually resorbed by osteoclasts and reshaping of the bone continues. The compact bone replaces the spongy bone at the bone periphery, and often the repaired bone is thicker and stronger than the original bone.

DIVISIONS OF THE SKELETAL SYSTEM

The adult human skeleton consists of 206 bones, most of which are paired and present on the right and left sides of the body.

The bones of the skeleton are divided into two main divisions: the *axial skeleton* and the *appendicular skeleton* (Fig. 3.11).

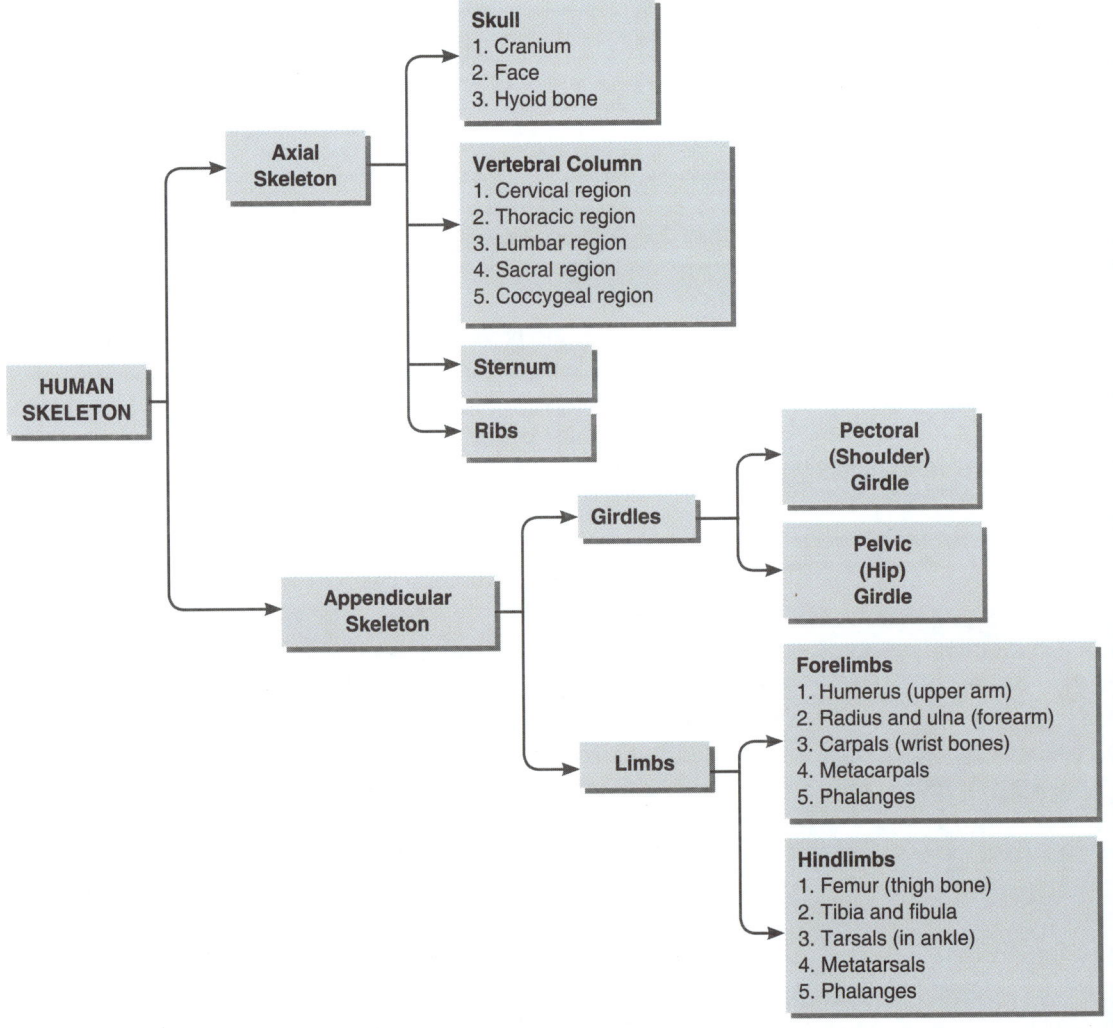

Figure 3.11 Divisions of the skeletal system.

The axial skeleton consists of the skull, vertebral column, ribs and sternum. The bones of the axial skeleton lie around the longitudinal axis of the human body and constitute the central bony core of the body.

The appendicular skeleton consists of the shoulder girdle with the upper limbs and the pelvic girdle with the lower limbs (Fig. 3.12).

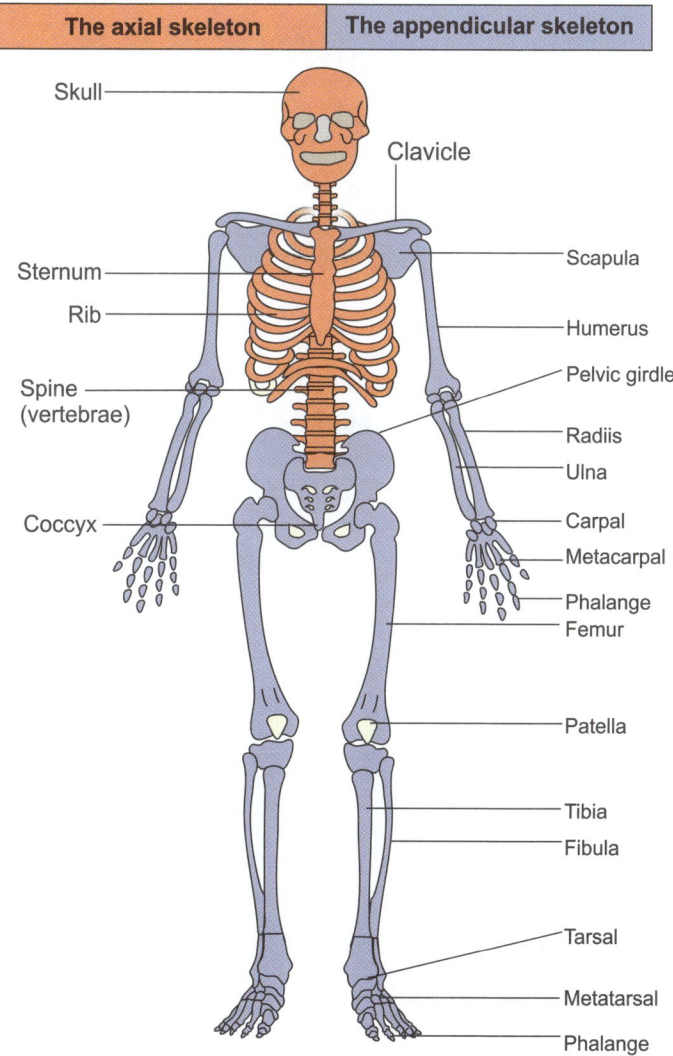

Figure 3.12 Axial and appendicular skeleton.

BONE MARKINGS

The surfaces of the bones have characteristic marking features that are adapted for specific functions. These markings are either processes, i.e. projections (outgrowths)) or fossae (depressions). The various bone markings and their terminology are described in Table 3.1.

Table 3.1 The various bone markings and their terminology

Terms	Bone markings
Articulating surface	The part of the bone that enters into the formation of a joint
Bony sinus	A hollow cavity within a bone
Condyle	A smooth rounded projection of bone that forms part of a joint
Fissure	A narrow slit
Foramen	A hole
Fossa	A hollow or depression
Styloid process	A sharp downward projection of bone that gives attachment to muscles and ligaments
Spinous process	A sharp ridge of bone

THE AXIAL SKELETON

The axial skeleton consists of the skull (cranium and face), vertebral column and thoracic cage (ribs and sternum).

SKULL

The skull rests on the upper end of the vertebral column.

The bones of the skull are divided into two parts: *the cranium (cranial bones)* and the *face (facial bones)*.

Cranial bones

There are eight cranial bones (*crani*: brain case) that enclose and protect the brain. These bones are united or joined by immovable (fibrous) joints called *sutures*. The sutures help dissipate the shock of a blow to the head.

Cranial bones have numerous perforations (e.g. foramina, fissures) for the passage of blood vessels, lymph vessels and nerves.

The eight cranial bones (Fig. 3.13) are as follows:
- ❏ 1 Frontal bone
- ❏ 2 Parietal bones
- ❏ 2 Temporal bones
- ❏ 1 Occipital bone
- ❏ 1 Sphenoid bone
- ❏ 1 Ethmoid bone

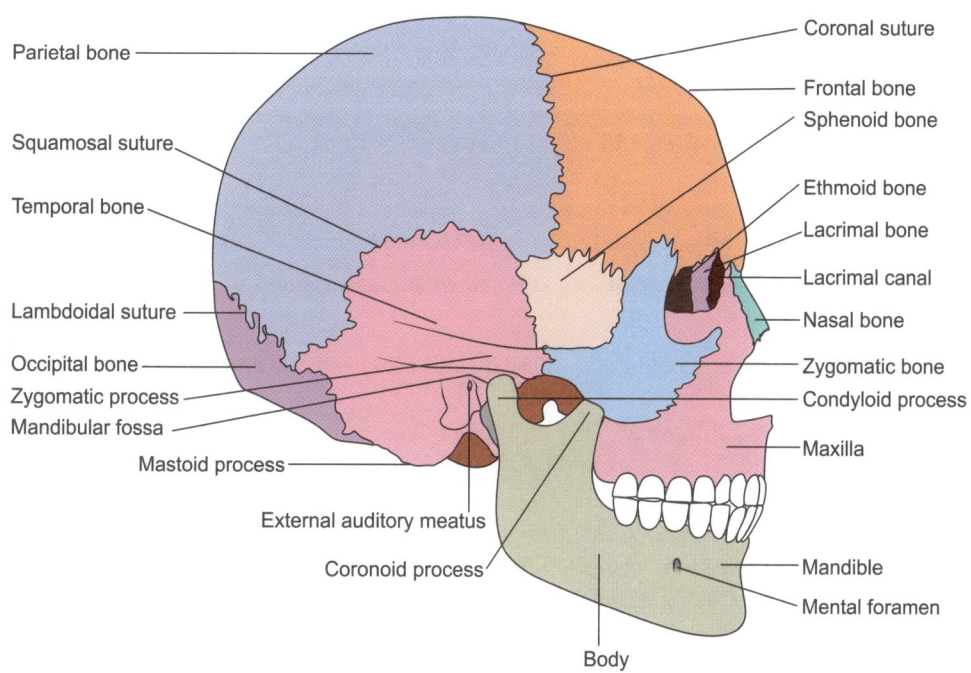

Parietal bone

Squamosal suture

Temporal bone

Lambdoidal suture

Occipital bone

Zygomatic process

Mandibular fossa

Mastoid process

External auditory meatus

Coronoid process

Coronal suture

Frontal bone
Sphenoid bone

Ethmoid bone

Lacrimal bone

Lacrimal canal

Nasal bone

Zygomatic bone
Condyloid process

Maxilla

Mandible

Mental foramen

Body

Figure 3.13 Cranial bones.

Frontal bone

The frontal bone forms the forehead and the roof of the orbits (eye sockets) and the nasal cavity.

The bone markings on the frontal bone are as follows:

- ❑ **Orbital margin**: Ridge above each orbit; located where eyebrows are found.
- ❑ **Supraorbital margin**: Prominent ridges above the eyes.

Just above the supraorbital margin are the two air-filled cavities or sinuses lined with the ciliated mucous membrane that open into the nasal cavity.

The frontal and parietal bones are joined by a suture called the *coronal suture*.

Parietal bones

These bones form the sides and roof of the skull. They are joined with each other at the sagittal suture, with the frontal bone at the coronal suture, with the occipital bone at the lambdoidal suture and with temporal bones at the squamous suture.

Temporal bones

These bones lie one on each side of the head and form fibrous immovable joints with the parietal, occipital, sphenoid and zygomatic bones. Each temporal bone encloses an ear and bears a fossa for articulation with the lower jaw or mandible.

The temporal bones are irregular in shape, with each bone consisting of the following three parts (Fig. 3.14):

1. **Squamous**
   (a) It is the largest and most superior of the three parts.
   (b) It is a thin fan-shaped area that articulates with the parietal bone. The zygomatic process projects from the lower part of the squamous portion of the temporal bone and articulates with the zygomatic bone (cheek bone) to form the zygomatic arch.

2. **Petrous**: It forms part of the base of the skull and contains the organs of hearing and balance.

3. **Mastoid**
   (a) It is located behind and below the external auditory meatus (meatus: passage way) or the ear canal.
   (b) It contains the mastoid process that provides attachment to several neck muscles and assists in moving the head. The mastoid process contains a large number of air sinuses lined with the squamous epithelium.

The temporal bones articulate with the mandible (lower jaw) at the temporomandibular joint, the only movable joint of the skull.

The styloid process projects from the inferior surface of the temporal bone and serves as a point of attachment for muscles and ligaments of the tongue and neck.

Note: Processes are named according to the bones they go to; thus the zygomatic process of the temporal bone goes towards the zygomatic bone and forms the zygomatic arch.

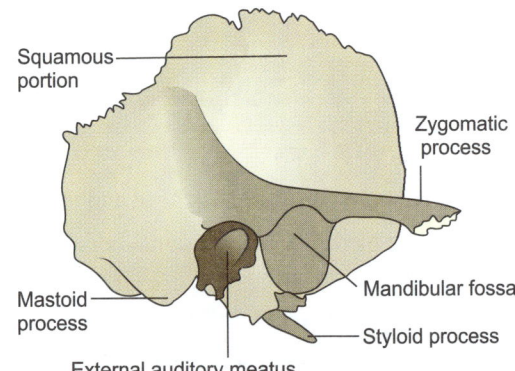

Figure 3.14 Temporal bone.

Occipital bone

Occipital bone forms the back of the head and part of the base of the skull. It joins the parietal bones superiorly at the lambdoid suture (Fig. 3.15).

The inferior portion of this bone has a large opening called the foramen magnum through which the spinal cord connects with the brain. On each lower side of the occipital bone, there are articular condyles that form condyloid joints or atlanto-occipital joints with the first bone of the vertebral column, the atlas. This joint allows the nodding movements of the head.

Sphenoid bone

Sphenoid bone occupies the middle portion of the base of the skull. It acts as an anchor binding all the cranial bones together.

The shape of the sphenoid bone resembles a bat with outstretched wings. The body of the bone contains sphenoidal sinuses (air sinuses) that open into the nasal cavity. The middle portion of the bone has a little saddle-shaped depression on the superior surface called as *hypophyseal fossa*, in which the

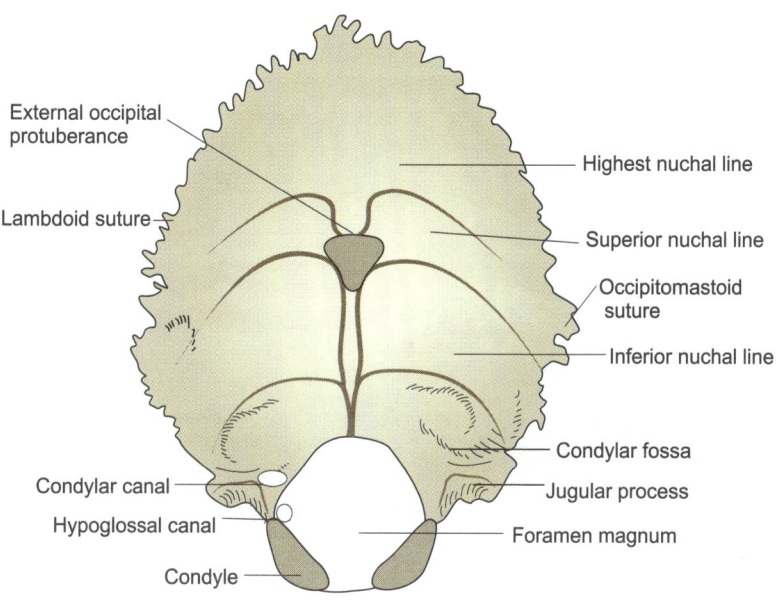

Figure 3.15 Occipital bone.

pituitary gland rests. It also contains the optic foramen, for the passage of the optic (II) nerve and the ophthalmic artery.

Ethmoid bone

It is the lightest of the cranial bones and occupies the anterior part of the base of the skull. It helps form the orbital cavity, the nasal septum and the lateral walls of the nasal cavity.

The horizontal part, called the *cribriform plate*, lies in the anterior portion of the cranium and forms the roof of the nasal cavity. The cribriform plate contains numerous olfactory foramina through which the olfactory nerves pass upwards from the nasal cavity to the brain (Fig. 3.16).

On each side of the ethmoid bone are two projections into the nasal cavity, the superior conchae and the middle conchae; they contain many air sinuses with openings into the nasal cavity. There is also a very fine perpendicular plate of the bone that forms the upper part of the nasal septum.

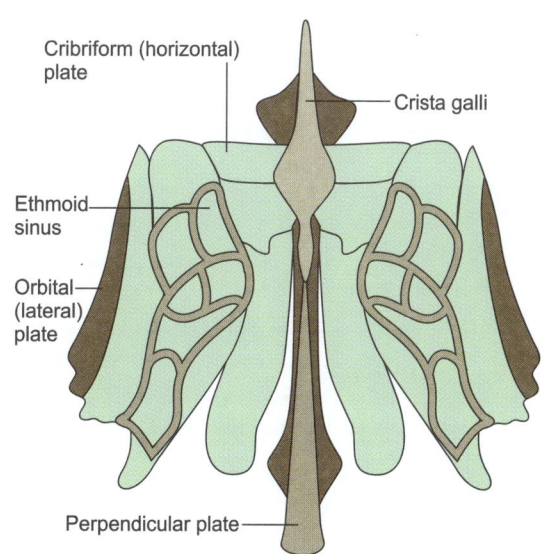

Figure 3.16 Ethmoid bone.

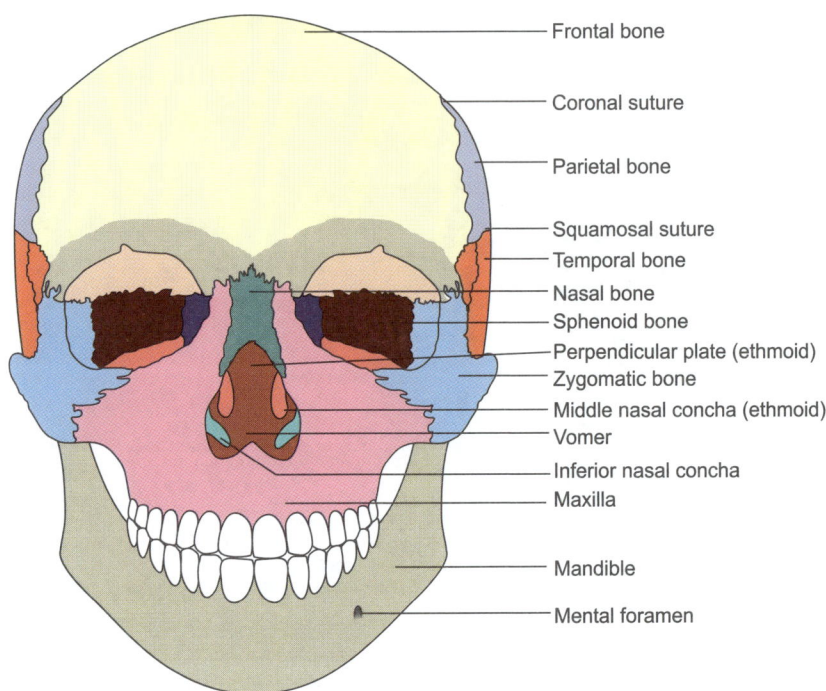

Figure 3.17 Facial bones.

Facial bones

The skeleton of the face is formed by the following 13 bones (Fig. 3.17):

❑ 2 Zygomatic (cheek) bones
❑ 1 Maxilla (originated as 2)
❑ 2 Nasal bones
❑ 2 Lacrimal bones
❑ 1 Vomer
❑ 2 Palatine bones
❑ 2 Inferior conchae
❑ 1 Mandible (originated as 2)

Zygomatic bones

The two zygomatic bones, commonly called cheek bones, form the prominences of the cheeks and part of the floor and lateral walls of orbital cavities. They articulate with the frontal, maxilla, sphenoid and temporal bones.

It forms the zygomatic arch by articulation with the temporal bone (refer to *temporal bones*).

Maxilla (upper jaw bone)

Maxilla originates as two bones, but fusion takes place before birth. It articulates with every bone of the face except the mandible (lower jaw) bone.

The maxilla forms the upper jaw, part of the floor of orbital cavities, part of the lateral walls and the floor of nasal cavity, and the anterior part of the roof of the mouth.

Each maxilla contains a large air sinus or the maxillary sinus that opens into the nasal cavity. The alveolar process (*alveola*: small cavity) of the maxilla is an arch that contains the alveoli (sockets) for the upper teeth.

Nasal bones

These are two small and delicate bones that meet at the midline of the face and form the bridge of the nose. The rest of the supporting tissues of the nose consist of cartilage.

Lacrimal bones

These two bones, the smallest bones of the face, are posterior and lateral to the nasal bones and form part of the medial walls of the orbital cavities.

Their lateral surface has a depression or fossa that houses the lacrimal sac or tear sac and a foramen for the passage of nasolacrimal duct that carries the tears from the eyes towards the nasal cavity.

Vomer bone

Vomer is a thin flat bone on the floor of the nasal cavity that articulates superiorly with the perpendicular plate of the ethmoid bone. It forms the inferior portion of the nasal septum.

Palatine bones

The two L-shaped palatine bones form the posterior portion of hard palate (roof of mouth), part of the floor and lateral walls of the nasal cavity, and a small portion of the floor of the orbital cavities.

Inferior conchae

These bones are very thin and fragile and present on the lateral side of each nostril. These are inferior to the middle nasal conchae of the ethmoid bone and project into the nasal cavity.

All the three pairs of nasal conchae (superior, middle and inferior) increase the surface area in the nasal cavity, allowing the inspired air to be swirled, warmed and filtered before it passes into the lungs.

Mandible

The mandible or the lower jaw bone is the largest and strongest facial bone. It is the only movable bone of the skull. It originates as two parts that unite at the midline.

Each half of the bone consists of two main parts: a *curved body* with the alveolar ridge to hold the teeth of lower jaw and a *ramus* that extends perpendicularly upwards.

At the upper end, the ramus divides into the condylar process that articulates with the temporal bone to form the temporomandibular

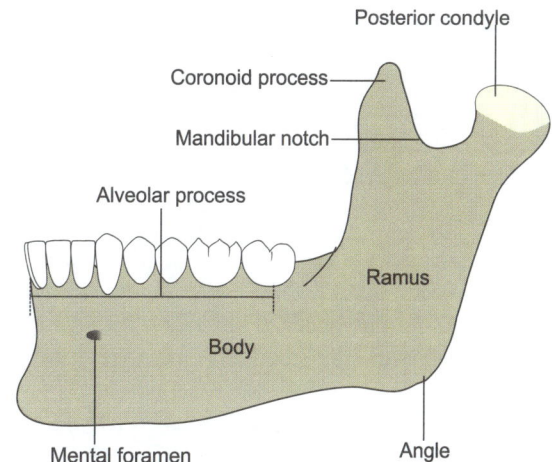

Figure 3.18 Mandible.

Posterior condyle

Coronoid process

Mandibular notch

Alveolar process

Ramus

Body

Mental foramen

Angle

Chapter 3

joint and the coronoid process that attaches to the muscle and ligaments which close the jaw. The point where the ramus joins the body is the angle of the jaw (Fig. 3.18).

Important terms regarding the bones of the skull

1. **Nasal Septum**
   - ❏ Nasal septum is the vertical partition that divides the inside of the nose into the right and left sides. The three components of the nasal septum are vomer, septal cartilage (hyaline cartilage) and the perpendicular plate of the ethmoid bone.
   - ❏ The term *broken nose* often refers to the damage to the septal cartilage.

2. **Hyoid Bone**
   - ❏ It is a single horse-shoe-shaped bone located in the anterior neck between the mandible and the larynx (Fig. 3.19). It does not articulate with any other bone but is attached to the styloid process of the temporal bone by ligaments.
   - ❏ The hyoid bone acts as a support for the tongue and its associated muscles. It also helps elevate the larynx during swallowing and speech.

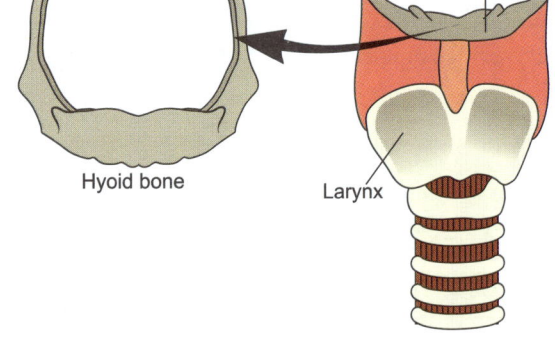

Figure 3.19 Hyoid bone.

3. **Fontanelles**
   - ❏ The skeleton of newly formed embryo mainly consists of cartilage. Gradually, ossification occurs and most of the cartilage is replaced by bones. Thus, at birth, spaces called *fontanelles* or soft spots are present between the cranial bones, which help the fetal skull pass though the birth canal.
   - ❏ The major fontanelles (Fig. 3.20) present in the skull at birth are as follows:
     - ➤ *Anterior fontanelle*: It is the largest fontanelle and is located between the parietal bones and the cranial bone. It usually closes 18–24 months after birth.
     - ➤ *Posterior fontanelle*: It is located at the midline between the parietal bones and occipital bone. It generally closes 2 months after birth.

4. **Sinuses**
   - ❏ The sinuses are the air-filled cavities present in sphenoid, ethmoid, maxillary and frontal bones (Fig. 3.21). They are lined with ciliated mucous membrane and are continuous with the nasal cavity.
   - ❏ Their major function involves providing resonance to the voice and reducing the weight of the skull.

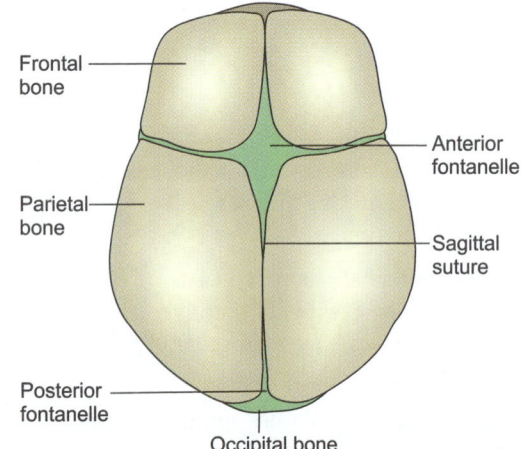

Figure 3.20 Anterior and posterior fontanelles.

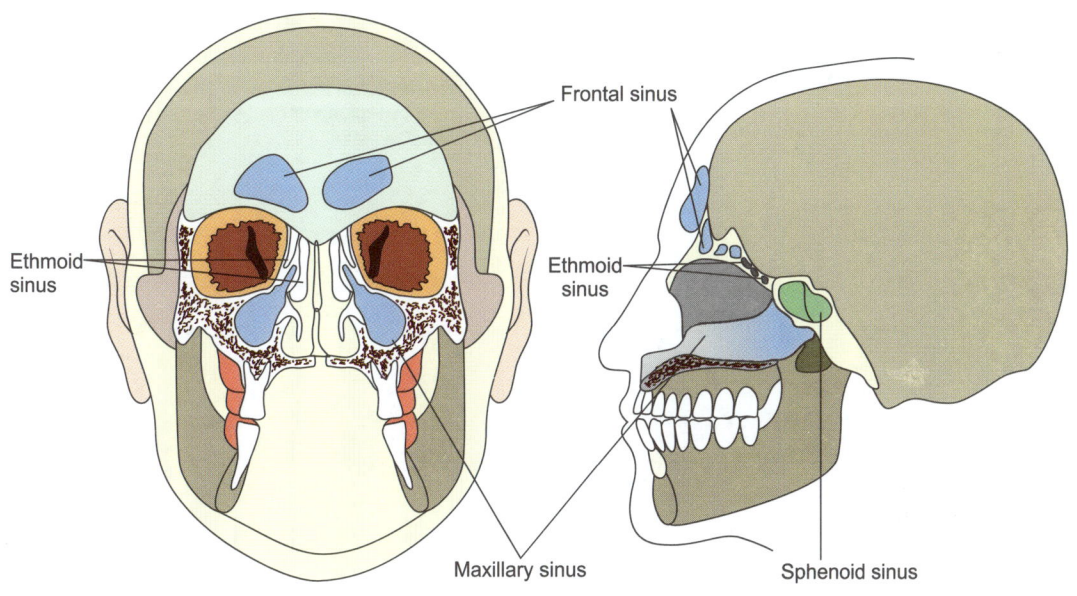

Figure 3.21 Sinuses.

Functions of the skull

The various parts of the skull serve different and specific functions (Fig. 3.13):

1. The cranium houses and protects the delicate tissues of the brain.
2. The bony eye sockets protect the eyes against injury and provide attachment to the muscles that move the eyes.
3. The temporal bone protects the delicate structures of the ear.
4. Some skull bones contain air-filled cavities called *sinuses* that give resonance to the voice and open into the nasal cavity.
5. The maxilla and mandible provide the alveolar ridges in which the teeth are embedded.
6. The cranial and facial bones serve as attachment sites for the muscles involved in mastication, facial expression and movement of the head.

VERTEBRAL COLUMN

The vertebral column, also called the spine or backbone, encloses and protects the spinal cord, supports the head and serves as a point of attachment for the ribs, pelvic girdle and muscles of the back.

The vertebral column is composed of a series of 26 irregular bones called *vertebrae* (singular: *vertebra*) divided into 5 regions (Fig. 3.22):

1. The **cervical region** (*cervic*: neck) contains 7 cervical vertebrae.
2. The **thoracic region** (*thorac*: chest) contains 12 thoracic vertebrae.
3. The **lumbar region** contains 5 lumbar vertebrae.

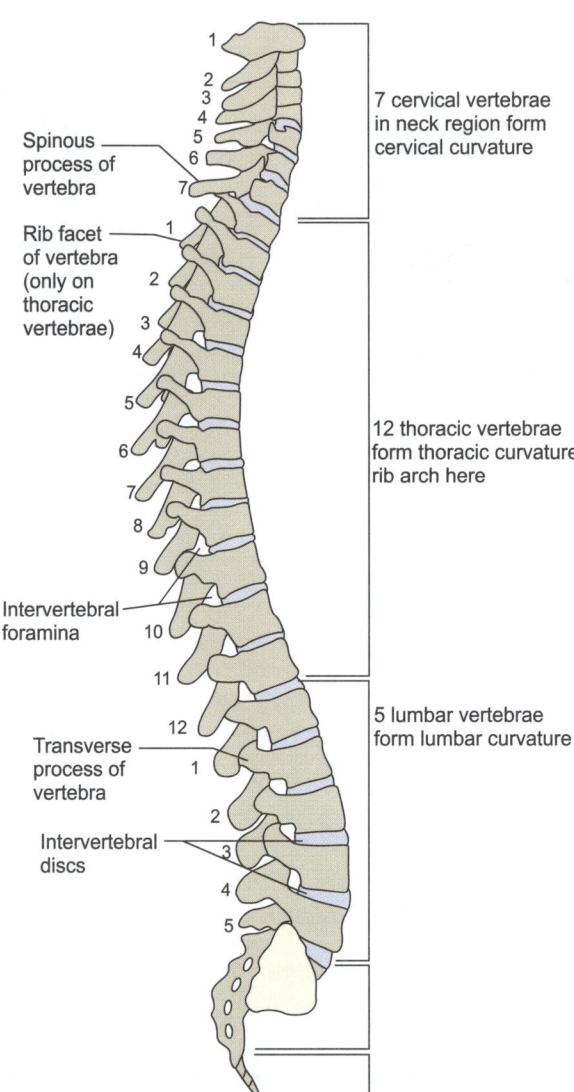

Spinous process of vertebra

Rib facet of vertebra (only on thoracic vertebrae)

Intervertebral foramina

Transverse process of vertebra

Intervertebral discs

7 cervical vertebrae in neck region form cervical curvature

12 thoracic vertebrae form thoracic curvature rib arch here

5 lumbar vertebrae form lumbar curvature

Figure 3.22 Vertebral column.

4. The **sacral region** contains 5 sacral vertebrae that are fused to form a single sacrum.
5. The **coccygeal region** contains 4 coccygeal vertebrae that are fused to form the single coccyx or tailbone.

The total number of vertebrae is 33 before the fusion of the sacral and coccygeal regions to form a single sacrum and coccyx, respectively.

The cervical, thoracic and lumbar vertebrae are movable, whereas the sacrum and coccyx are fixed.

Each vertebra is identified by the first letter of its region followed by a number indicating its position (e.g. the top most vertebrae are called C_1, and the third thoracic vertebrae are called T_3.

A typical vertebra has the following parts (Fig. 3.23):

1. **The body**: The body of each vertebra is a thick disc-shaped anterior portion that varies in size in different regions. They are the smallest in the cervical region and become larger towards the lumbar region.

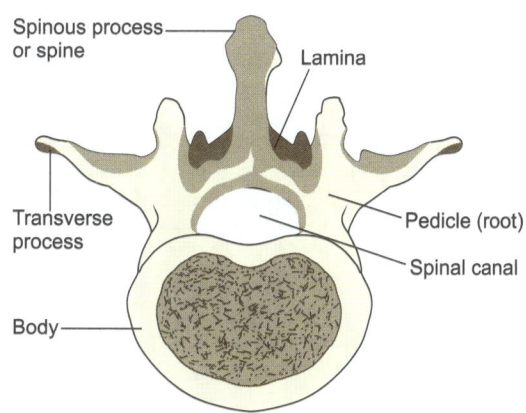

Figure 3.23 Parts of a typical vertebra.

2. **The vertebral (neural) arch**
   (a) The vertebral arch is the area behind the body and forms the posterior and lateral walls of the vertebral foramen. The lateral walls are formed from plates of bone called *pedicles* and the posterior walls are formed from laminae. The vertebral foramen is a large space present between the vertebral arch and the body.
   (b) Collectively, the vertebral foramina of all vertebrae form the vertebral (spinal) canal that encloses the spinal cord.

3. **Processes**: The vertebral arch has seven processes:
   (a) The transverse processes, on each side of the vertebra, and present at the point where the pedicle joins the lamina.
   (b) A single spinous process is at the back where the two laminae meet. These three processes serve as the point for muscle attachment.

The remaining four processes form the joints with the vertebra immediately above and the vertebra immediately below by the two superior and the two inferior articular processes, respectively.

Regions of the vertebral column

Cervical region

These are the smallest vertebrae present in the neck. All cervical vertebrae have three foramina: *one vertebral foramen* for the passage of the spinal cord and two *transverse foramina* in the transverse processes through which a vertebral artery passes upwards to the brain.

The first two cervical vertebrae differ considerably from the others. The first cervical vertebra (C_1) is called the *atlas*, and it supports the head by articulation with the condyles of the occipital bone. The articulation of the occipital bone and atlas forms the atlanto-occipital joint, which allows the nodding movement of the head.

The second cervical vertebra (C_2) is the *axis* and has a small body with a small superior projection called the *odontoid process* (also called the *dens*, meaning tooth). The dens acts as a pivot on which the atlas and head rotate, and it allows the side-to-side rotation of the head.

The third to sixth cervical vertebrae (C_3–C_6) are as per the structural pattern of the typical vertebra. The seventh cervical vertebra (C_7), also known as the *vertebra prominens*, has a single large spinous process; it can be easily felt at the base of the neck.

Thoracic region

The thoracic vertebrae are larger and stronger than the cervical vertebrae and are present in the upper back. The bodies and transverse processes of thoracic vertebrae have facets (articulating surfaces) for articulation with the ribs.

Lumbar region

The lumbar vertebrae are the largest and strongest in the vertebral column as they have to support the weight of the upper body. They have broad and thick spinous processes for the attachment of powerful back muscles.

Sacrum

The sacrum is a triangular and slightly curved bone formed by the union of five sacral vertebrae. The female sacrum is shorter, wider and more curved between S_2 and S_3 compared with males.

The upper part articulates with the fifth lumbar vertebra to form the lumbosacral joint. On both lateral surfaces, sacrum articulates with the ilium of each hip bone to form the sacroiliac joint; at its inferior tip, sacrum articulates with the coccyx. The anterior edge of the base, the promontary, protrudes into the pelvic cavity. There is a series of foramina on each side of the bone for the passage of nerves and blood vessels.

Coccyx

Coccyx is also triangular in shape formed by the fusion of four coccygeal vertebrae. It has a broad base that articulates with the tip of the sacrum.

Features of the vertebral column

Intervertebral discs

❑ The bodies of the adjacent vertebra are separated by intervertebral discs, consisting of an outer fibrous ring of fibrocartilage (annulus fibrosus) and a central core of elastic substance (nucleus pulposus). The discs form strong joints, permit various movements of the vertebral column and absorb shock.
❑ Displacement of an intervertebral disc, called *slip disc*, is harmful.

Intervertebral foramina

When viewed from the side, a foramen formed by a gap between pedicles is seen on each side between every pair of vertebra. This gap forms a passage for the spinal nerves, blood vessels and lymph vessels.

Curves of the vertebral column

❑ The side view of the vertebral column shows four curves: two primary and two secondary.

❏ The fetus in the uterus shows only a single anterior curve called the *primary curve*. The thoracic and sacral curves are called the *primary curves* because they form first during fetal development. The secondary cervical curve develops when the infant begins to hold its head erect (after about 3 months after birth) and the secondary lumbar curve develops when the child sits up, stands and walks (after 12–15 months after birth).

Functions of the vertebral column

The following are the various functions of the vertebral column:

1. The vertebral canal provides a strong bony protection for the delicate spinal cord.
2. The intervertebral discs act as shock absorbers and enable various movements of the vertebral column.
3. The vertebral column provides support to the body.
4. It forms the axis of the trunk and provides attachment to the ribs, pelvic girdle, shoulder girdle, limbs and muscles of the back.

THORACIC CAGE

The thoracic cage (thorax) is formed by the sternum, 12 pairs of ribs and the 12 thoracic vertebrae (Fig. 3.24).

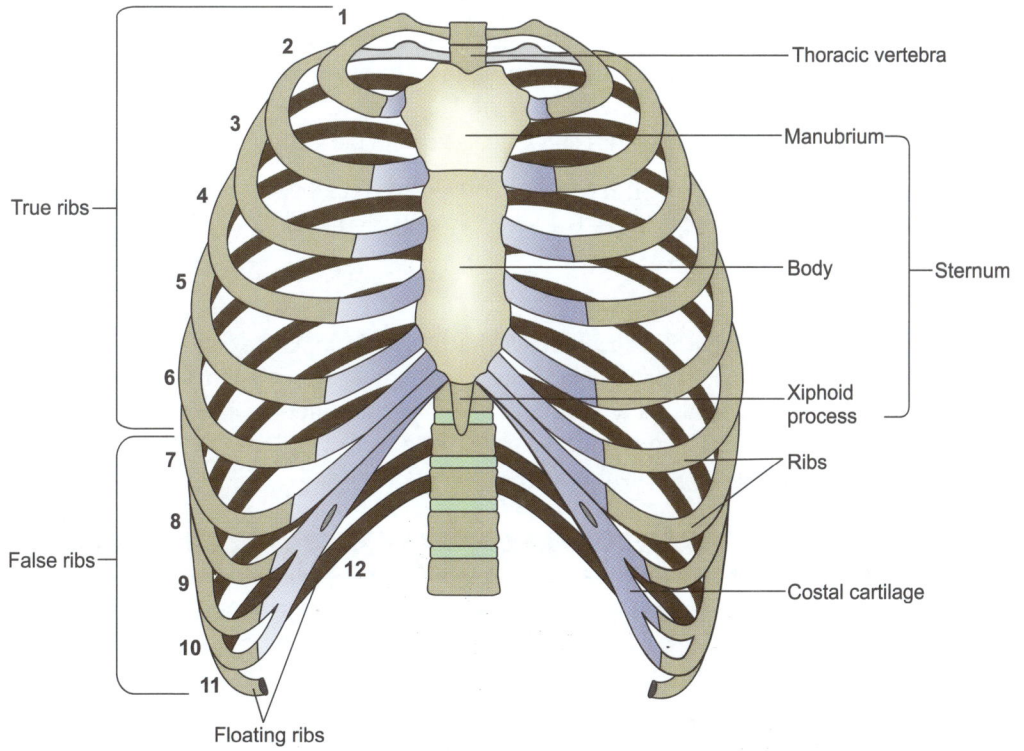

Figure 3.24 Thoracic cage.

Sternum (breast bone)

The sternum is a long narrow, flat vertical bone located in the middle of the front of the chest. It is about 15 cm long and consists of the following three parts:

❏ The manubrium is the uppermost part and articulates with the clavicles at sternoclavicular joints and with the first two pairs of ribs.

❏ The body or middle part articulates with the 2nd to 10th ribs. The junction of the manubrium and the body forms the sternal angle.

❏ The xiphoid process is the tip of the bone. It provides attachment to the diaphragm and some abdominal muscles.

Ribs

The ribs are the curved bones that articulate posteriorly with the thoracic vertebrae and attach anteriorly with the sternum through costal cartilages (*costae*: rib). There are 12 pairs of ribs.

❏ The upper 7 pairs of ribs attach directly to the sternum and are called *true ribs*. The lower 5 pairs of ribs are called *false ribs*.

❏ The 8th, 9th and 10th pairs of ribs attach indirectly to the sternum (attach to the rib above each), and the 11th and 12th pairs do not attach to the sternum at all, and thus these false ribs are called *floating ribs*.

A typical rib consists of two parts: *vertebral* and *sternal*.

❏ The vertebral part is long and bony. It articulates with the thoracic vertebrae by two facets, the *capitulum* and *tubercle,* in the first nine ribs and by a single facet, the head in the remaining vertebrae. (Head is the projection at the posterior end of the rib.)

❏ The sternal part is short and cartilaginous and articulates with the sternum or the upper rib.

The inner surface of the rib is deeply grooved, which protects the blood vessels and intercostal nerves. The spaces between ribs, called intercostal spaces, are occupied by intercostal muscles, blood vessels and nerves.

Functions of ribs

1. Ribs protect the internal organs (i.e. heart, lungs, trachea, bronchi, kidney and blood vessels).
2. Ribs play a vital role in the respiratory mechanism as the first rib is fixed to the sternum and to the first thoracic vertebrae, and thus the ribs do not move during inspiration. Thus, when the intercostal muscles contract, they pull the entire ribcage upwards towards the first rib to increase the surface area for inspiration (discussed in detail in the Respiratory System).

THE APPENDICULAR SKELETON

The appendicular skeleton consists of the shoulder girdle with the upper limbs and the pelvic girdle with the lower limbs.

SHOULDER (PECTORAL) GIRDLE

The human body has two shoulder girdles that attach the bones of the upper limbs to the axial skeleton. Each of the two shoulder girdle consist of the following (Fig. 3.25):

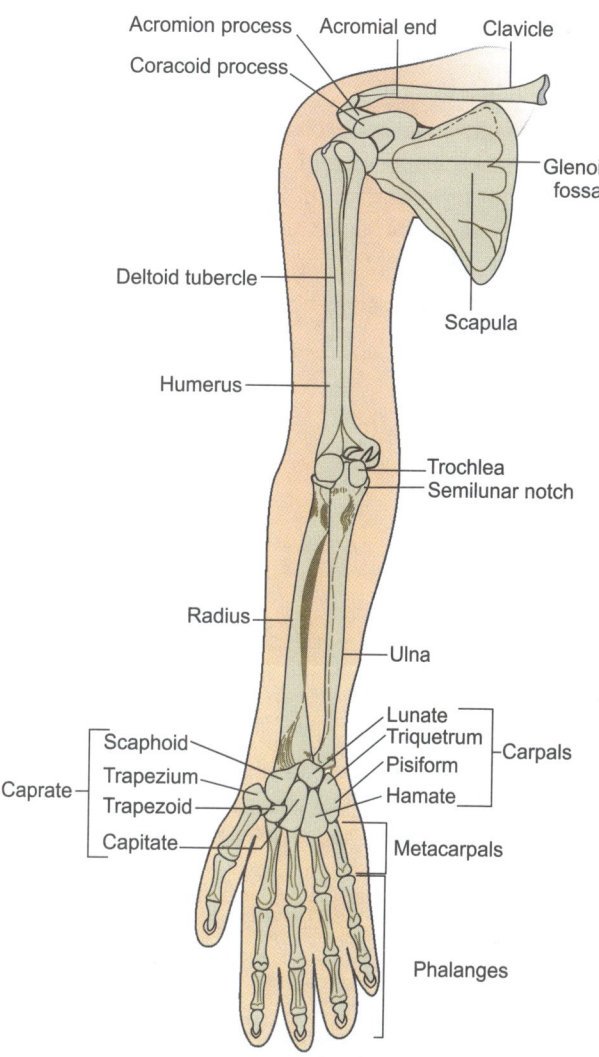

Figure 3.25 Shoulder girdle and upper limbs.

□ 2 Clavicle (collar bone)
□ 2 Scapulae (singular: scapula)

Clavicle (collar bone)

The clavicle is an S-shaped long bone located horizontally across the anterior part of the thorax superior to the first rib. The medial (sternal) end articulates with the manubrium of the sternum to form the sternoclavicular joint, and the lateral end articulates with the acromion of the scapula to form the acromioclavicular joint.

Scapula (shoulder blade)

The scapula is a large, flat, triangular bone located in the superior part of the posterior thorax.

It has, at its lateral angle, a shallow concavity, *the glenoid cavity*, which articulates with the head of the humerus (arm bone) to form the glenohumeral joint (shoulder joint). A prominent ridge called the *spine* runs diagonally across the posterior surface of the scapula and overhangs the glenoid cavity. This prominent overhang, which can be easily felt as the highest point of the shoulder, is called the *acromion process* and forms a joint with the clavicle, the acromioclavicular joint. A projection from the upper border of the bone, the coracoid process, provides attachment to muscles that move the shoulder joint.

UPPER LIMBS

Each upper limb has 30 bones, which are as follows:

1. Humerus in the upper arm
2. Radius and ulna in the forearm
3. 8 Carpals in the wrist
4. 5 Metacarpals in the palm
5. 14 Phalanges in the fingers

Humerus

Humerus is the longest and largest bone of the upper limb.

The proximal end of the humerus has a rounded head that articulates with the glenoid cavity of the scapula to form the shoulder joint. Distal to the scapula are two roughened projections, the greater and lesser tubercles, for muscle attachment, and between them there is a groove called *bicipital* or *intertubercular sulcus*.

The distal end has two surfaces, *capitulum* and *trochlea*, that articulate with the head of the radius and ulna, respectively, to form the elbow joint.

Ulna and radius

Ulna is the longer, medial bone of the forearm, whereas radius is the shorter and lateral bone of the forearm.

Ulna and radius articulate with the humerus at the elbow joint, with the carpal bones at the wrist joint and with each other at the proximal and distal radioulnar joint. In addition, the shafts of the two bones are also joined by a broad, flat and fibrous connective tissue called the *interosseous membrane*.

Carpal (wrist) bones

The bones of the wrist are called *carpals*. There are eight carpals joined to one another by ligaments to form the intercarpal joints.

Carpals are arranged in two rows of four bones each. From outside inward they are as follows:

❑ **Proximal row**: Scaphoid (boat like), lunate (moon shaped), triquetrum (three cornered) and pisiform (pea shaped)
❑ **Distal row**: Trapezium (four sided), trapezoid, capitate (head shaped) and hamate (hooked)

The bones of the proximal row are associated with the wrist joint, whereas those of the distal row articulate with the metacarpal bones.

Metacarpal bones

The metacarpal bones are the five bones that form the palm of the hand. They are numbered I to V, starting from the thumb. The proximal ends of these bones articulate with the carpal bones to form the carpometacarpal joints, whereas the distal end articulates with the proximal phalanges to form the metacarpophalangeal joints.

Phalanges

There are 14 phalanges, 3 in each finger and 2 in the thumb. The phalanges are joined to each other by *interphalangeal joints*.

PELVIC GIRDLE

The pelvic girdle consists of two hip bones that attach the lower limbs to the axial skeleton (Fig. 3.26). The hip bones are joined anteriorly to one another at the pubic symphysis and are joined posteriorly with the sacrum at the sacroiliac joints. The complete ring composed of the hip bones, pubic symphysis and sacrum forms a deep, basin-like structure called *pelvis*. The pelvis provides a strong and stable support for the vertebral column and pelvic organs.

Each hip bone consists of three fused bones: the *ilium*, the *ischium* and the *pubis*.

Ilium

Ilium is the uppermost and largest portion of the hipbone. The superior border of the ilium, the iliac crest, is projected into the anterior superior iliac spine and the anterior inferior iliac spine.

The ilium articulates with the sacrum to form the sacroiliac joint.

Ischium

Ischium is the inferior, posterior portion of the hip bone. The rough, thickened projection of the ischia, the ischial tuberosity, bears the weight of the body in the sitting position.

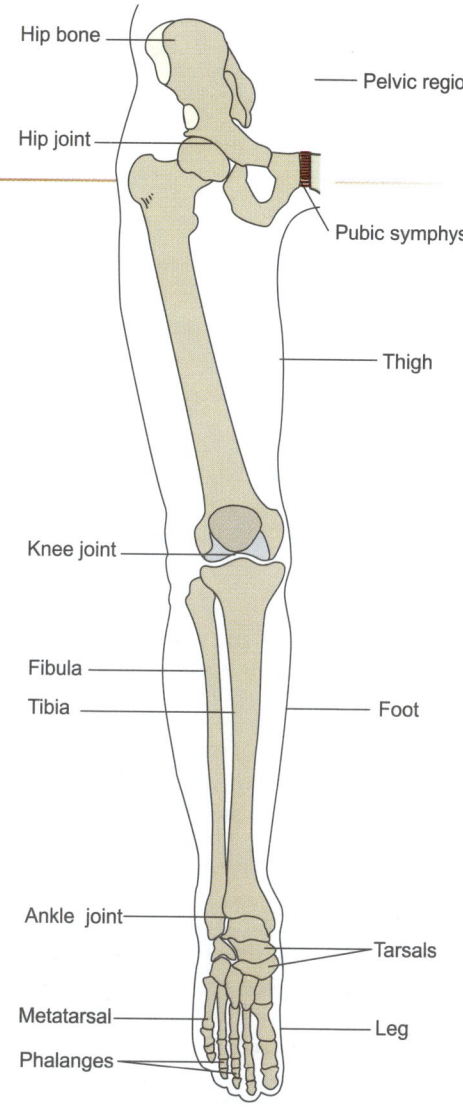

Figure 3.26 Pelvic girdle and lower limb.

Chapter 3

Pubis

Pubis is superior and slightly anterior to the ischium. Between the pubis and ischium is the obturator foramen. This is the largest foramen in the body and serves as the passage for nerves, blood vessels and tendons.

On the lateral surface of the hip bone just above the obturator foramen is a deep depression called *acetabulum,* which is formed by the fusion of the ilium, ischium and pubis. It forms the hip joint with the rounded head of the femur.

False and true pelvis

The pelvis is divided into upper and lower parts by the pelvic brim (brim of the pelvis). The portion of the pelvis superior to pelvic brim is referred to as *false (greater) pelvis* as it does not contain pelvic organs, whereas the portion of pelvis inferior to the pelvic brim is called the *true (lesser) pelvis* and it surrounds the pelvic cavity.

The female pelvis differs structurally from the male pelvis as an adaption for requirements of pregnancy and childbirth. The female pelvis has lighter bones and is wider and shallower than the male pelvis.

LOWER LIMBS

Each lower limb has 30 bones, which are as follows:

1. 1 Femur in the thigh
2. 1 Patella (kneecap)
3. 1 Tibia and 1 fibula in the lower leg
4. 7 Tarsals in the ankle
5. 5 Metatarsals in the sole
6. 14 Phalanges in the toes

Femur

Femur is the longest and heaviest bone of the body. The body (shaft) of the femur is positioned at an angle that slants downwards and inwards. This unique design allows it to bear and distribute the weight of the body.

The proximal end of the femur consists of a rounded head that articulates with the acetabulum of the hip bone to form the hip joint. The distal end of the femur is widened into a medial condyle and a lateral condyle, which articulate with the tibia.

Patella

Patella or kneecap is a small, triangular bone located anterior to the knee joint. It is enveloped within the tendons of the quadriceps femoris muscle. Patella's posterior surface articulates with the femur in the knee joint and protects the knee joint.

Tibia and fibula

Tibia is the larger, medial bone of the leg. The proximal end of the tibia is expanded into a lateral condyle and a medial condyle that articulate with the condyles of the femur to form the tibiofemoral (knee) joint. The distal end articulates with the talus of the ankle and the fibula.

The fibula is lateral to the tibia, but it is considerably smaller. The head of the fibula articulates with the lateral condyle of the tibia to form the proximal tibiofibular joint. The distal end articulates with the talus of the ankle and the tibia.

Tarsal bones

The bones of the ankle are known as the *tarsal bones*. The seven tarsal bones include calcaneous (heel), the talus or ankle bone, navicular (little boat), cuboid (cube shaped), and medial (I), intermediate (II) and lateral (III) cuneiforms.

The calcaneous is the strongest and largest tarsal bone. The talus is the only bone of the foot that articulates with the fibula and tibia to form the ankle joint. The other bones articulate with each other and with the metatarsal bones.

Metatarsal bones

There are five metatarsal bones, numbered I to V. The proximal ends articulate with the tarsals, whereas the distal ends articulate with the phalanges.

Phalanges

There are 14 phalanges in a similar manner as those in the fingers (i.e. 2 in the thumb and 3 in each of the other toes). The phalanges are joined with each other at interphalangeal joints.

Arches of the foot

The bones of the foot are arranged in a series of arches that are held in position by ligaments and tendons and give a curved shape to the sole of the foot. The arches enable the foot to bear the weight of the body and provide leverage while walking.

There are two longitudinal arches and one transverse arch (Fig. 3.27). The medial longitudinal arch is formed by calcaneous, talus, navicular, three cuneiforms and three metatarsals. This is the highest arch of the foot. The lateral longitudinal arch is much lower and is formed by the calcaneous, cuboid and 2 metatarsals. The longitudinal arch is so high that only calcaneous and metatarsals should touch the ground while walking on a hard surface.

The transverse arch is perpendicular to the longitudinal arches and is formed by 1 navicular, 3 cuneiforms and 5 metatarsals.

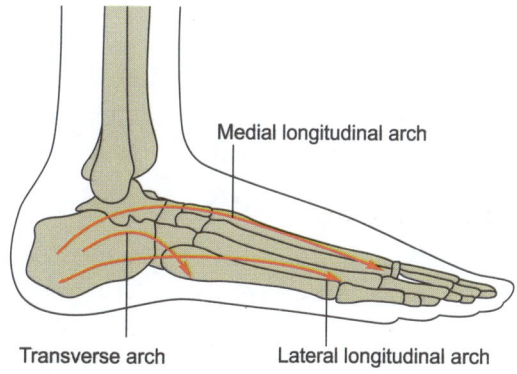

Figure 3.27 Arches of the foot.

Flat foot

It is the condition when the height of the longitudinal arch decreases due to the weakening of ligaments and tendons. This results in uneven distribution of body weight and may cause sore feet when standing, walking or running for long periods.

Causes may be genetic, excessive weight, weakened muscles in the foot or postural abnormalities.

JOINTS

Joint, also called as an *articulation* or *arthrosis*, is a place of union or junction between two or more bones. Joints allow flexibility and movement of the skeleton and allow attachment between bones. The scientific study of joints is called *arthrology* (*arthros*: joint; *logos*: study).

CLASSIFICATION (TYPES) OF JOINTS

Joints can be classified into three major groups based on the degree of movement they allow and based on the connective tissue that holds the bones of the joint together.

The three main types of joints are:

1. Fibrous or immovable joints
2. Cartilaginous or slightly movable joints
3. Synovial or freely movable joints

Fibrous joint

The bones forming fibrous joints are held together by fibrous connective tissues and such an arrangement permits little or no movement.

Examples of fibrous joint include the following:

1. The joints between skull bones formed by dense fibrous connective tissues are called *sutures*.
2. Joint between the tibia and the fibula formed by a sheet of fibrous tissue is called *intraosseous membrane*.
3. Joint between the tooth and the mandible formed by dense fibrous connective tissues called *periodontal ligament*.

Cartilaginous joint

The bones forming cartilaginous joints are held together by fibrocartilage or hyaline cartilage that acts as a shock absorber and permits little movement.

Examples include the following:

1. Pubic symphysis, which is the joint between two pelvic bones
2. Joint between the vertebra

Synovial joint

Synovial joints are characterized by the presence of a space called *synovial cavity* between the articulating bones. These joints allow a great deal of movement.

Structure of the synovial joint

All synovial joints have certain common characteristics, which are as follows (Fig. 3.28):

1. **Articular cartilage**: The ends of bones at the joint are covered by a layer of hyaline cartilage called *articular cartilage*. This layer of cartilage provides a smooth and somewhat elastic surface and reduces friction.
2. **Articular capsule**
   (a) This joint is surrounded and enclosed by a sleeve-like articular capsule that holds the bones together and encloses the synovial cavity.

(b) The articular capsule is composed of the following two layers:

   (i) Outer fibrous capsule: It consists of dense, fibrous tissue that attaches to the periosteum of the articulating bones. The flexibility of the fibrous capsule allows sufficient movement, whereas the tensile strength of the fibrous capsule prevents bones from dislocating. The fibres of some fibrous capsules are arranged in bundles called *ligaments* that hold the bones together.

   (ii) Inner synovial membrane: It is composed of areolar connective tissue and elastic fibres. This membrane contains secretory cells that secrete a thick, sticky synovial fluid.

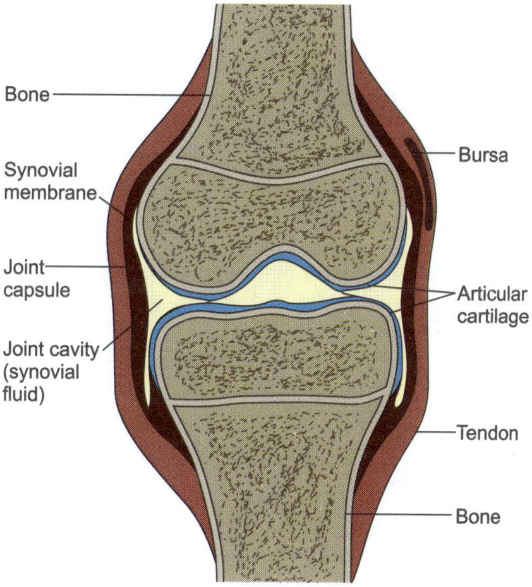

Figure 3.28 Synovial joint.

3. **Synovial fluid**

   (a) Synovial fluid is secreted by the synovial membrane into the synovial cavity. This fluid lubricates the joint to allow frictionless movement of bones and provides nutrition for the structures within the cavity.

   (b) It also serves to hold the bones together similar to the activity of a film of water between two glass plates.

   (c) Small membrane-bound packets, called *bursae*, are present in some joints, e.g. knee. These bursae store synovial fluid and reduce friction between bones and other nearby structures such as muscles and skin where the joint is close to the surface.

4. **Accessory ligaments**: Many synovial joints also contain accessory ligaments called *extracapsular ligaments* and *intracapsular ligaments*.

   (a) *Extracapsular ligaments* lie outside the articular capsule and provide additional stability (e.g. fibular collateral ligaments at the knee joint).

   (b) *Intracapsular ligaments* occur within the articular capsule, but outside the synovial membrane. They assist in the maintenance of stability (e.g. cruciate ligaments at the knee joint).

Some synovial joints also contain pads of fibrocartilage that are attached to the fibrous capsule. These pads are called *menisci* and they help maintain the stability of the joint.

Types of synovial joint

Synovial joints can be divided into the following six types (Fig. 3.29):

1. **Ball and socket joint**

   ❏ It consists of a ball-like head of one bone fitted into a socket or cuplike depression of another bone. This joint allows a wide range of movement including flexion, extension, adduction, abduction, rotation and circumduction.

   ❏ Examples are the shoulder joint and hip joint.

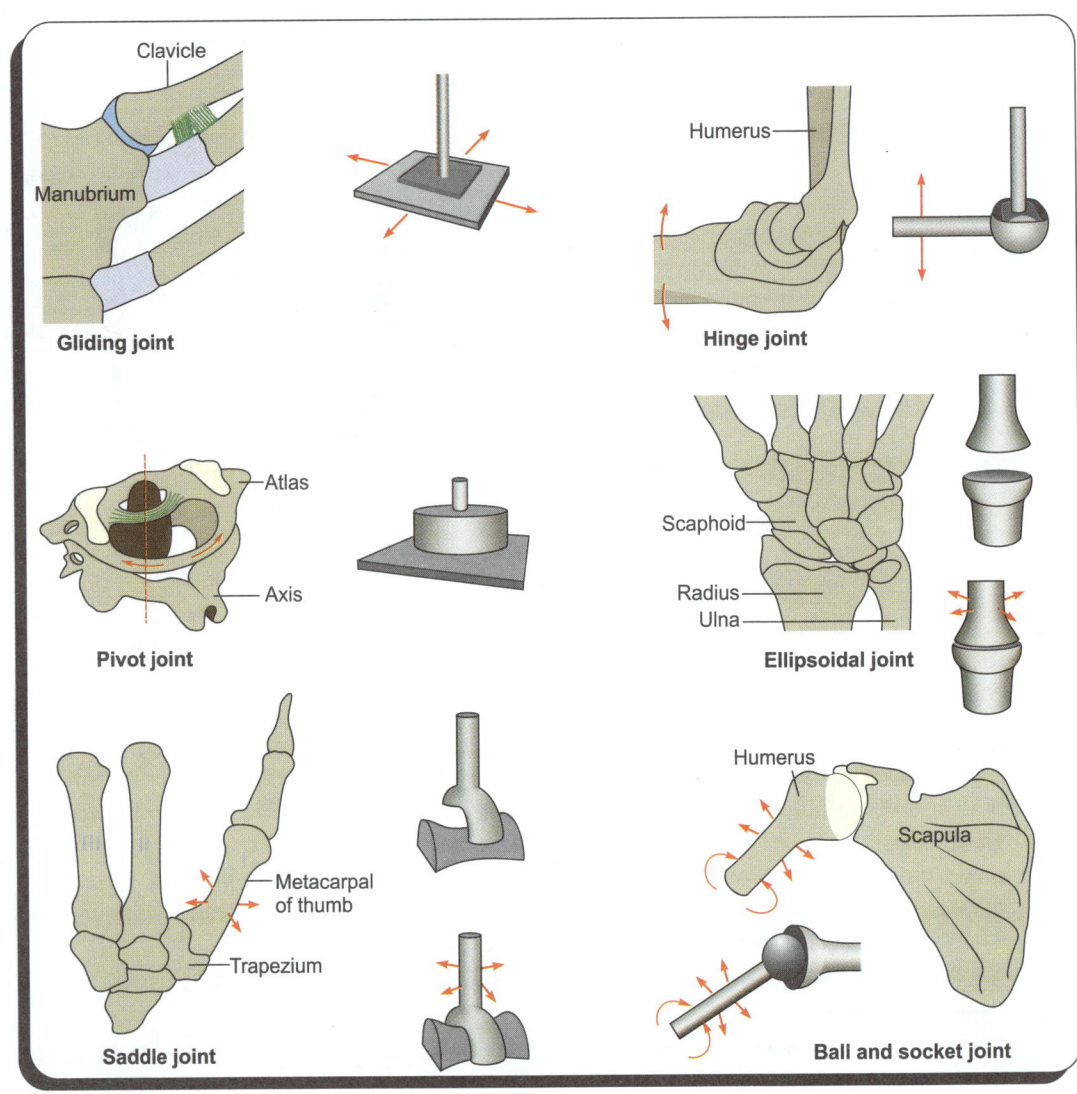

Figure 3.29 Types of synovial joints.

2. **Hinge joint**
   - ❏ In the hinge joint, the convex surface of one bone fits into the concave surface of another bone. The movement is restricted to only flexion and extension.
   - ❏ Examples include the knee joint, elbow joint, ankle joint and joints between phalanges.
3. **Condyloid joint or ellipsoidal joint**
   - ❏ In this joint, the convex oval-shaped projection of one bone fits into the cup-shaped depression of another bone. This joint permits flexion, extension, adduction, abduction and circumduction.
   - ❏ Examples include the wrist joint and metacarpophalangeal joint.

4. **Gliding joint**
   - ❏ This joint permits sliding movement of two bones over each other. The articular surfaces are usually flat or slightly curved.
   - ❏ Examples include joints between carpals in wrist, tarsals in foot and between the sternum and the clavicle.

5. **Pivot joint**
   - ❏ In this joint, the rounded end of one bone fits into a shallow pit of another bone. This joint allows only a rotary movement of one bone on the other.
   - ❏ Examples include joints between the atlas and the axis.

6. **Saddle joint**
   - ❏ In the saddle joint, the articular surface of one bone is saddle shaped and the articular surface of another bone fits into the saddle.
   - ❏ Example includes the carpometacarpal joint of the thumb.

Movements at synovial joints

The following movements can occur at synovial joints (Fig. 3.30):

S. no.	Movement	Description
1.	Flexion	Bending or decreasing angle between bones
2.	Extension	Opposite to flexion (i.e., increasing angle between bones)
3.	Hyperextension	Continuation of extension beyond the anatomical position
4.	Abduction	Movement away from the midline of the body
5.	Adduction	Movement towards the midline of the body
6.	Circumduction	Moving the bone in such a way that body parts move in a circle
7.	Rotation	Movement around the central axis
8.	Pronation	Turning the palm of the hand down
9.	Supination	Turning the palm of the hand up
10.	Inversion	Turning the sole of the feet inwards
11.	Eversion	Turning the sole of the feet outwards
12.	Protraction	Movement forward on a plane parallel to ground
13.	Retraction	Movement backward on a plane parallel to ground
14.	Elevation	Upward movement of a body part
15.	Depression	Downward movement of a body part
16.	Dorsiflexion	Bending the foot in the direction of dorsum (superior surface)
17.	Plantar flexion	Bending the foot in the direction of plantar surface

Chapter 3

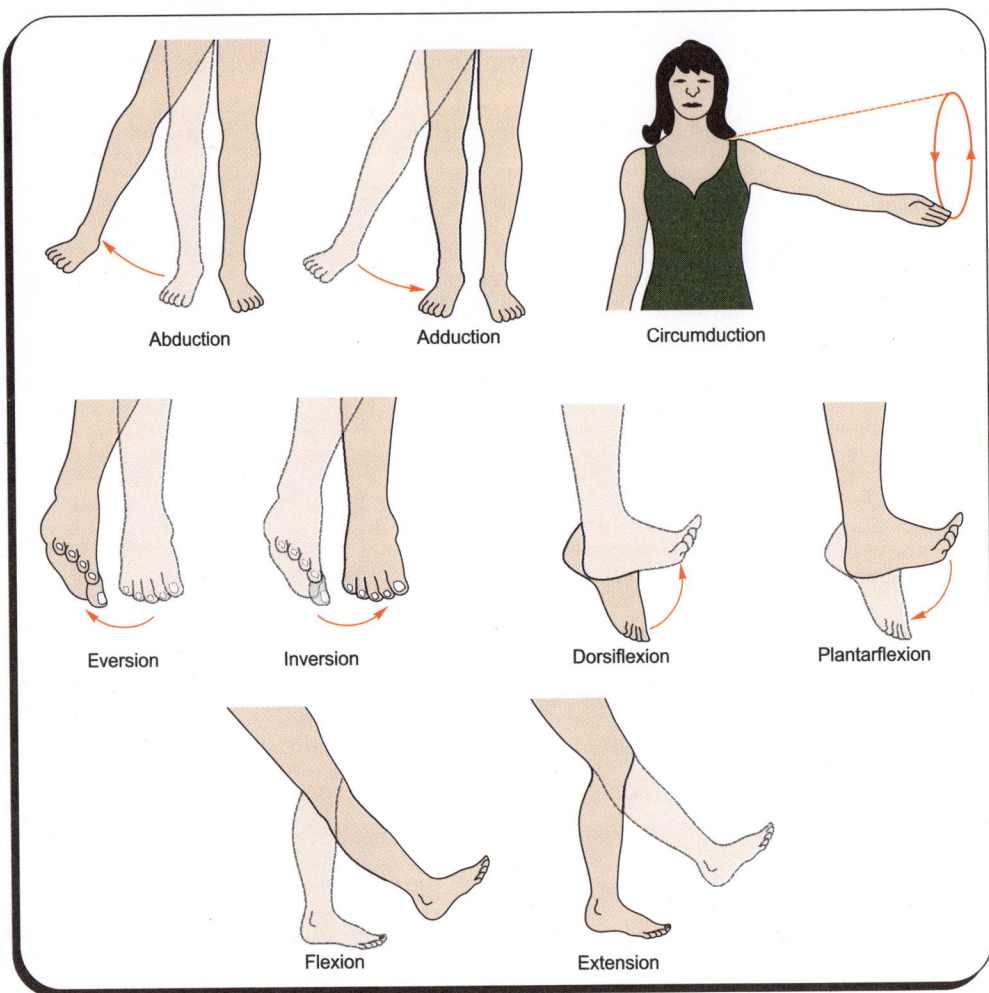

Figure 3.30 Movements at synovial joints.

DISORDERS ASSOCIATED WITH THE SKELETAL SYSTEM

OSTEOPOROSIS

It is a condition in which bone density decreases or bone tissue mass reduces, resulting in weakening of skeletal strength and increased susceptibility to bone fractures. It occurs due to excessive resorption of calcium and phosphorus from the bone than is absorbed from the diet. More loss occurs to the trabecular bone than to the compact bone.

This disorder mainly affects middle-aged and elderly people, and it is more common in women after menopause.

Osteoporosis results in fractures, shrinkage of vertebrae, height loss, hunched backs and bone pain.

Preventive measures include adequate calcium intake, weight-bearing exercise and oestrogen replacement therapy (for postmenopausal women).

RICKETS

It is a condition in which the bones fail to calcify, resulting in the softening of the bones in children, thereby leading to fractures and deformity of bones.

Rickets mainly affects the growing bones of children and leads to characteristic bowing and deformity of the lower limbs.

The common cause includes deficiency of vitamin D or defective vitamin D metabolism (due to limited exposure to sunlight).

OSTEOMALACIA

It is a condition caused by the deficiency of vitamin D in adults, which leads to failure of bone calcification during the normal turnover of bone (also called *adult rickets*). This disorder causes bone pain and tenderness of bones, especially in the hip and leg, resulting in increased risk of fracture.

OSTEOMYELITIS

It is the bacterial infection of bone characterized by high fever, pain, pus formation and oedema in the affected bone. The bacteria may reach the bone from outside the body (through open fracture or surgical procedures) or from blood-borne infections in the body (due to urinary tract infections or upper respiratory tract infections).

PAGET'S DISEASE

It is a condition characterized by excessive bone destruction and unorganized bone repair, resulting in irregular thickening and softening of bones. This predisposes to deformities and fractures, especially of the skull, pelvis and limbs.

Treatment includes a high-protein and high-calcium diet with regular mild exercise.

RHEUMATOID ARTHRITIS

It is a chronic progressive inflammatory autoimmune disease mainly affecting the peripheral synovial joints. It usually starts in small joints in the hand and may eventually result in crippling deformities in severe cases.

It is more common in females than in males. Symptoms include inflammation of the synovial membrane, joint pain and stiffness, particularly in the morning and after rest.

Chapter 3

OSTEOARTHRITIS

It is degenerative progressive noninflammatory disease of the synovial joints, particularly the weight-bearing joints, resulting in pain and restricted movement of the affected joints. It mainly occurs in overweight people in their late middle age and mainly affects the larger joints (i.e. knees and hips).

Joint deterioration can be arrested by mild exercise, which increases the ability to maintain movement at joints.

ARTHRITIS

It is an inflammation of the whole joint and usually involves all the tissues of the joint: cartilage, bone, muscles, tendons and ligaments. In this condition, the joints become swollen, stiff and painful.

Joint deterioration can be kept at bay by mild exercise, which increases the ability to maintain movement at joints, and pain can be relieved using analgesics.

GOUT

It is the accumulation of uric acid crystals in the joints and tendons that usually result in an acute inflammatory response. This usually occurs in the joints of the feet and legs and is more common in men than in women.

The risk factors of gout include obesity, hyperuricaemia, high alcoholic intake and heredity.

BURSITIS

It is an inflammation of the synovial bursa that is caused by excessive stress on the bursa. It can also be caused by local or systemic inflammatory response. The elbow and the shoulder are the common sites of bursitis.

OVERVIEW OF THE SKELETAL SYSTEM

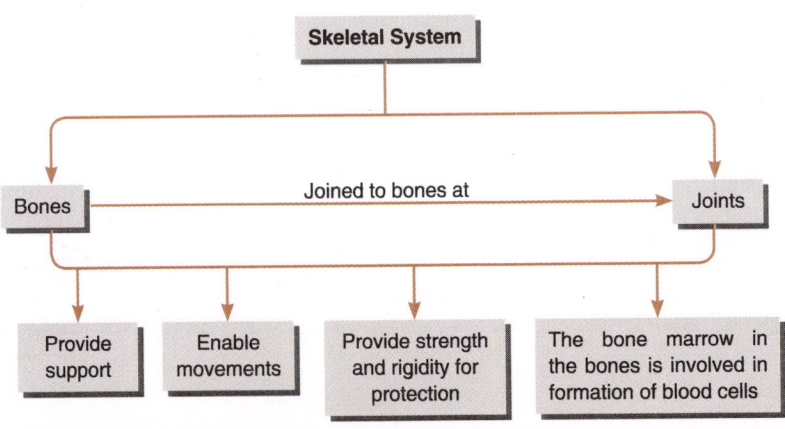

Ageing and Bone Tissue

❏ From birth till adolescence the rate of bone deposition is more than the rate of resorption.

❏ At puberty, the rates of deposition and resorption are almost similar.

❏ With advancing age, the rate of resorption greatly increases, leading to a decrease in the bone mass, especially in women after menopause. Thus, there is a higher incidence of osteoporosis in females, which may also be due to the smaller and less-massive bones in females compared with males.

❏ With ageing, demineralization, that is, loss of calcium and other minerals, occurs and the rate of protein synthesis also decreases. Furthermore, the amount of collagen protein in ligaments and tendons decreases, thereby decreasing the flexibility of the bone. These make the bone very brittle and susceptible to fractures.

❏ Also with ageing, the production of synovial fluid in joints decreases and the articular cartilage becomes thinner. By age 80 years, some type of degeneration in the knees, elbows, hips and shoulders develops in almost all adults.

Embryonic Development of Skeletal System

❏ All skeletal tissues develop from mesenchymal cells that are derived from the *mesoderm*.

❏ 4th week of fertilization: Mesenchyme around the developing brain gives rise to the skull. The mesenchyme consists of two major portions:
   1. *Neurocranium*: Forms bones of the skull
   2. *Viscerocranium*: Forms bones of the face

❏ Portions of cube-shaped mesodermal cells form the vertebrae.

❏ The processes from the vertebrae in the thoracic region develop into ribs.

❏ During the middle of the 4th week, the sides of the trunk develop small elevations called as upper limb buds, which form the upper limbs, and subsequently, after two days the lower limb buds appear, which give rise to the lower limbs.

Exercise and Bone Tissue

❏ When stress is applied within limits, the bone tissue becomes stronger through increased deposition of the extracellular matrix by osteoblasts. Without stress or weight-bearing exercises, bone resorption is quicker than bone formation.

❏ Owing to immobility or fracture, the strength of unstressed bones greatly diminishes due to loss of bone minerals and decreased collagen fibres.

❏ Weight-bearing activities such as walking and moderate weightlifting help build and retain bone mass; thus, adolescents and young adults should engage in exercises before closure of the epiphyseal plates to build their bone mass.

TIPS TO MAINTAIN STRONG BONES

1. Diet rich in calcium and vitamin D such as dark green leafy vegetables, broccoli, sardines, salmon, kelp, oysters and dairy products should be included in the diet.
2. Avoid eating whole grains and calcium-rich foods at the same time as whole grains contain a substance that binds with calcium and prevents proper absorption.
3. Avoid taking phosphate-containing foods such as soft drinks as phosphorus causes calcium excretion from the body.
4. Include garlic and onions in the diet as they contain sulphur.
5. Limit or avoid a high-protein diet as protein causes calcium excretion.
6. Reduce caffeine intake.
7. Exercise regularly.
8. Additional supplements of calcium, magnesium and vitamin D may be taken if not provided enough through diet.
9. Bone-building herbs such as alfalfa, barley grass, dandelion root, nettle, parsley and rose hips may be taken as tea, tincture or tablets.

Review Questions

Long Answer Questions

1. Describe the principal functions of the skeletal system.
2. What is the composition of bones? Categorize bones according to shape.
3. Distinguish between the axial and appendicular portions of the skeletal system.
4. Distinguish between endochondral and intramembranous bone formation.
5. Describe the gross structure of a typical long bone.
6. List the cranial and facial bones of the skull along with their locations and structural characteristics.
7. Where is the hyoid bone located and what are its functions?
8. Describe the structure and functions of the vertebral column.
9. List the bones of the upper extremity.
10. Describe the structure and functions of the pelvic girdle.
11. Describe the kinds of articulations or joints in the body and the range of movement permitted by each.
12. Describe the structure of a synovial joint.

Multiple Choice Questions

1. Which of the following is *not* a function of the skeletal system?
   - (a) Production of blood cells
   - (b) Storage of minerals
   - (c) Storage of carbohydrates
   - (d) Protection of vital organs

2. Mitosis resulting in elongation of bone occurs at
   - (a) The articular cartilage
   - (b) The periosteum
   - (c) The epiphyseal plate
   - (d) The diploe

3. Synovial fluid that lubricates a synovial joint is produced by
   - (a) A meniscus
   - (b) The synovial membrane
   - (c) A bursa
   - (d) The articular cartilage
   - (e) The mucous membrane.

4. A flattened or shallow articulating surface of a bone is called
   - (a) A tubercle
   - (b) A fossa
   - (c) A fovea
   - (d) A facet

5. Which of the following bones is *not* part of the axial skeleton?
   - (a) Hyoid bone
   - (b) Sacrum
   - (c) Sphenoid bone
   - (d) Clavicle
   - (e) Manubrium

6. The optic foramen is located within
   - (a) The ethmoid bone
   - (b) The occipital bone
   - (c) The palatine bone
   - (d) The sphenoid bone

7. An example of a gliding joint is
   - (a) The intercarpal joint
   - (b) The radiocarpal joint
   - (c) The intervertebral joint
   - (d) The phalangeal joint

8. Teeth are supported by
   - (a) The maxillae and mandible
   - (b) The mandible and palatine bones
   - (c) The maxillae and palatine bones
   - (d) The maxillae, mandible and palatine bones

9. Remodelling of bone is a function of
   - (a) Osteoclasts and osteoblasts
   - (b) Osteoblasts and osteocytes
   - (c) Chondrocytes and osteocytes
   - (d) Chondroblasts and osteoblasts

10. The sagittal suture is positioned between
    - (a) The sphenoid and temporal bones
    - (b) The temporal and parietal bones
    - (c) The occipital and parietal bones
    - (d) The occipital and frontal bones
    - (e) The right and left parietal bones

Match the Following

1.	Flexion	(a)	Movement away from the midline of the body
2.	Extension	(b)	Turning the sole of the feet outwards
3.	Hyperextension	(c)	Upward movement of a body part
4.	Abduction	(d)	Bending the foot in the direction of dorsum (superior surface)
5.	Adduction	(e)	Turning the palm of the hand down
6.	Circumduction	(f)	Downward movement of a body part
7.	Rotation	(g)	Movement backward on a plane parallel to ground
8.	Pronation	(h)	Bending the foot in the direction of plantar surface down
9.	Supination	(i)	Movement towards the midline of the body
10.	Inversion	(j)	Moving the bone in such a way that body parts move in a circle
11.	Eversion	(k)	Movement around the central axis
12.	Protraction	(l)	Turning the sole of the feet inwards
13.	Retraction	(m)	Continuation of extension beyond the anatomical position
14.	Elevation	(n)	Turning the palm of the hand up
15.	Depression	(o)	Bending or decreasing angle between bones
16.	Dorsifl exion	(p)	Opposite to flexion (i.e., increasing angle between bones)
17.	Plantar flexion	(q)	Movement forward on a plane parallel to ground

State True or False

1. The tibia and fibula articulate with the femur at the knee joint.
2. The proximal and distal ends of a long bone are referred to as diaphyses.
3. Supination and pronation are specific kinds of circumductional movements.
4. Yellow bone marrow in certain long bones of an adult produces red blood cells, white blood cells and platelets.
5. Bone matrix is composed primarily of calcium and magnesium, which may be withdrawn in small amounts as needed elsewhere in the body.
6. Most of the bones of the skeleton form through intramembranous ossification.
7. Articular cartilage and synovial membranes are found only in synovial joints.
8. All joints or articulations in the body permit some degree of movement.
9. Osteoblasts actually destroy bone tissue in the process of demineralization.
10. A person has seven pairs of true ribs and five pairs of false ribs, the last two pairs of which are designated as floating ribs.

Fill in the Blanks

1. Red bone marrow produces blood cells in a process called _____ .

2. The _____ skeleton consists of the skull, vertebral column, and rib cage; the _____ skeleton consists of the girdles and the appendages.

3. The _____ is a diamond-shaped soft spot on the top of a newborn's skull that facilitates childbirth and permits brain growth.

4. Separating the diaphysis and epiphysis of a child's long bone is a_____, which permits linear bone growth.

5. The _____ foramen is an opening in the mandible on the lateral side below the second premolar tooth.

6. The _____ and the perpendicular plate of the _____ bone compose the bony framework of the nasal septum.

9. In an adult, the ilium, ischium and pubis are fused to form the _____ or hipbone.

10. The foot contains _____ tarsal bones, _____ metatarsal bones and _____ phalanges.

Careers in the Skeletal System

✓ Orthopaedists specialize in prevention and correction of disorders of the skeleton, joints and muscles.

✓ Prosthetists specialize in creating artificial limbs.

✓ Athletic trainers are individuals who develop bones and muscles for agility and sports training.

The Muscular System

STUDY OBJECTIVES

- ✓ To describe the structure and basic functions of skeletal muscles.
- ✓ To discuss the anatomy of smooth and cardiac muscles.
- ✓ To discuss the physiology of muscle contraction.
- ✓ To explain the location of skeletal muscles in different parts of the body.

INTRODUCTION

The bones form the framework of the body but they cannot move body parts without the muscle tissue. Movement is brought about by the alternating contraction and relaxation of muscles. In addition, the muscle tissues stabilize body position, generate heat and push the fluids and food through various systems of the body. They also allow us to perform stressful effort (like running and playing sports) for a prolonged period. The scientific study of muscles is called *myology* (*myo*: muscle; *logy*: study).

The muscular system comprises the specialized contractile tissue called the *muscle tissue*. This is the most abundant tissue in most animals, accounting for 40–50% of the adult body weight. Human body has about 639 separate muscles that bring about movement of the body as a whole and allow proper function of our internal organs.

FUNCTIONS OF MUSCLE TISSUE

The various functions of muscle tissue are as follows:

1. **Body movement**: The integrated functioning of bones and skeletal muscles brings about movement of the body as a whole. The contractions of smooth muscles in the internal organs propel

fluid and food through various body tracts and the contraction of cardiac muscles in the heart pumps the blood through the blood vessels of the body.

2. **Body posture**: The contraction of skeletal muscle stabilizes the joints and helps maintain the body posture while standing and sitting.

3. **Heat generation**: The muscles help maintain normal body temperature by generating heat during muscle contraction.

DO YOU KNOW

- ❏ The human body contains more than 600 voluntary muscles.
- ❏ Masseter muscle, which is used for chewing, is the strongest muscle of the body.
- ❏ Our hand contains 20 different muscles.
- ❏ If all the muscles of the body could pull in one direction, it could create a force of 25 tons
- ❏ Muscles contribute ~40% of our body weight.
- ❏ It takes 17 muscles in our face to smile, but it takes 43 muscles to frown.
- ❏ We use our leg muscles to take approximately 5 million steps per year.

PROPERTIES OF MUSCLE TISSUE

The muscle tissue possesses four special properties that enable them to function properly.

The four properties of muscle tissues are as follows:

1. **Excitability**: It is defined as the ability of a tissue to respond to certain stimuli by producing electrical signals called *action potential*. The action potential can be triggered by the muscular tissue itself (e.g. heart pacemaker) or by chemical stimuli (e.g. neurotransmitters or hormones).

2. **Contractility**: It is the ability of a muscle tissue to contract forcefully in response to an action potential. The contraction in the muscle tissue is manifested by change in either the length or the tension of the muscle fibres.

3. **Extensibility**: It is the ability of muscle tissue to stretch without being damaged, for example stretching of smooth muscles in the stomach when filled with food or stretching of cardiac muscles in the heart when filled with blood.

4. **Elasticity**: It is the ability of muscle tissue to return to its original shape and length after contraction or extension.

TYPES OF MUSCLE TISSUE

The following are the three types of muscle tissue (Fig. 4.1):

1. Skeletal or striated muscle tissue
2. Smooth or visceral muscle tissue
3. Cardiac muscle tissue

MEDICAL TERMINOLOGY

- ❏ **Cartilage**: It is a connective tissue present at the ends of certain bones and joints and provides a smooth surface for adjacent bones to move against each other.
- ❏ **Ligaments**: They are tough connective tissue structures that attach bones to bones.
- ❏ **Tendons**: They are structures that attach muscle to bone.

Chapter 4

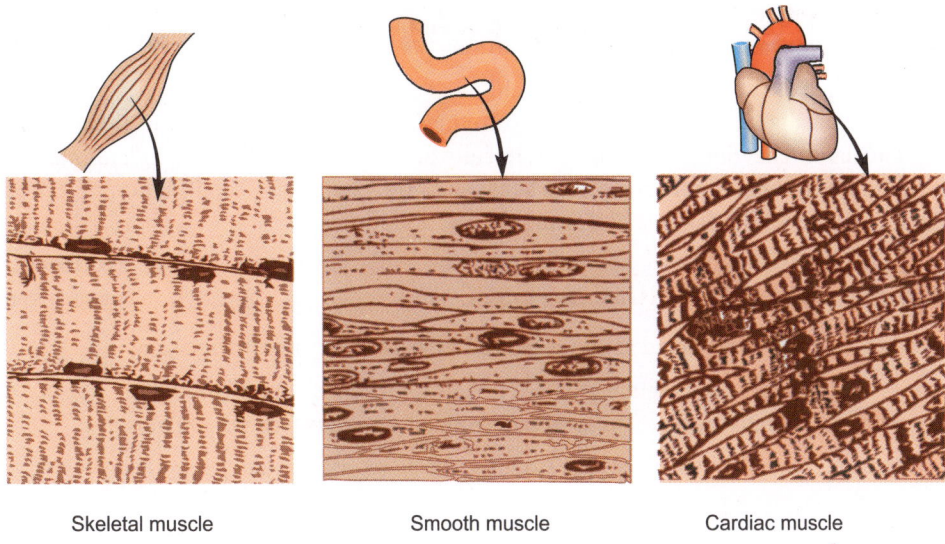

Skeletal muscle   Smooth muscle   Cardiac muscle

Figure 4.1 Types of muscle tissue.

1. **Skeletal muscle tissue**

   (a) Skeletal muscle tissue is named so because these muscles are attached to the bone and are used to move the bones of the skeleton. It is also referred to as *striated muscle* because of the characteristic alternating light and dark bands (striations) of tissue when it is examined under the microscope.

   (b) It is also called *voluntary muscle* because the activities of these muscles can be controlled voluntarily (at will) due to the innervation of somatic (voluntary) nerves.

2. **Smooth muscle tissue**

   (a) Smooth muscle tissue is named so because it does not have the striated appearance under the microscope. It is also referred to as *visceral muscle* as it is situated in association with viscera, i.e. in the walls of hollow internal organs of the digestive tract, respiratory tract, excretory system, reproductive system and blood vessels.

   (b) These muscles are involuntary (cannot be consciously controlled).

3. **Cardiac muscle tissue**

   (a) Cardiac muscle tissue is found exclusively in the wall of the heart. It is also striated (has characteristic light and dark bands when seen under a microscope) but its actions are involuntary (not controlled consciously).

   (b) Both smooth muscle tissue and cardiac muscle tissue are regulated by neurons of the autonomic (involuntary) nervous system and by hormones released from endocrine glands.

Note: This chapter mainly focuses on the structure and functions of skeletal muscle tissue. Cardiac muscle and smooth muscle are discussed in detail later, in Chapters 11 and 12, respectively.

Chapter 4

SKELETAL MUSCLE TISSUE

Mature skeletal muscle cells are the longest and most slender cells in the range 1–50 mm in length and 10–100 μm in diameter. Because of this unique structure of the cell, i.e. their length being much greater than their width, skeletal muscle cells are often referred to as *skeletal muscle fibres*. The contraction of a skeletal muscle occurs because of the coordinated contraction of its individual fibres.

ANATOMY OF SKELETAL MUSCLE TISSUE

The skeletal muscle cell is surrounded and protected by layers of connective tissues.

A thick layer of fibrous connective tissue termed as *fascia* surrounds the whole muscle trunk. It provides a pathway for nerves, blood vessels and lymphatic vessels through the muscles.

Three layers of connective tissue extend from the fascia to support and strengthen skeletal muscles, which are as follows:

1. **Epimysium**: It is the outermost layer of connective tissue present beneath the fascia and it encircles the entire muscle.
2. **Perimysium**: Within the muscle, the cells are collected into separate bundles called fascicles, and each fascicle is covered in a connective tissue sheath called *perimysium*.
3. **Endomysium**: The individual muscle cells lie within the fascicles, each wrapped in a fine areolar connective tissue layer called *endomysium* (Fig. 4.2).

These three layers of connective tissue act like cement holding all of the muscle cells and their bundles together. These connective tissue layers may extend beyond the muscle fibres to form a tendon, i.e. a cord of dense connective tissue composed of collagen fibres that attach a muscle to the bone.

Microscopic anatomy of skeletal muscle fibre

When the skeletal muscle is examined under a microscope, the cells are seen to be roughly cylindrical in shape, lying parallel to one another with characteristic alternate light and dark bands.

Each skeletal muscle cell is multinucleated and is surrounded by sarcolemma, the plasma membrane of the muscle cell. Thousands of tiny invaginations of sarcolemma, called *transverse (T) tubules*, tunnel in from the surface towards the centre of each muscle fibre. These T tubules help in rapid transmission of the nerve impulse along the muscle fibre.

Within the sarcolemma is the sarcoplasm, the cytoplasm of the muscle fibre. The sarcoplasm contains a substantial amount of glycogen (used for ATP synthesis), many mitochondria (produce ATP) and a red-coloured protein called *myoglobin*. Myoglobin is a specialized oxygen-binding protein, found only in muscle cell that stores oxygen within the muscle cell and releases it when it is required by mitochondria for ATP production.

At high magnification, the sarcoplasm appears to be stuffed with thousands of smaller units called *myofibrils* (*myo*: muscle; *fibril*: little fibre). Myofibrils are about 2 μm in diameter and are present through the entire length of a muscle fibre. Each myofibril is made up of two types of contractile filaments: thick (dark) filaments and thin (light) filaments arranged in a repeating pattern.

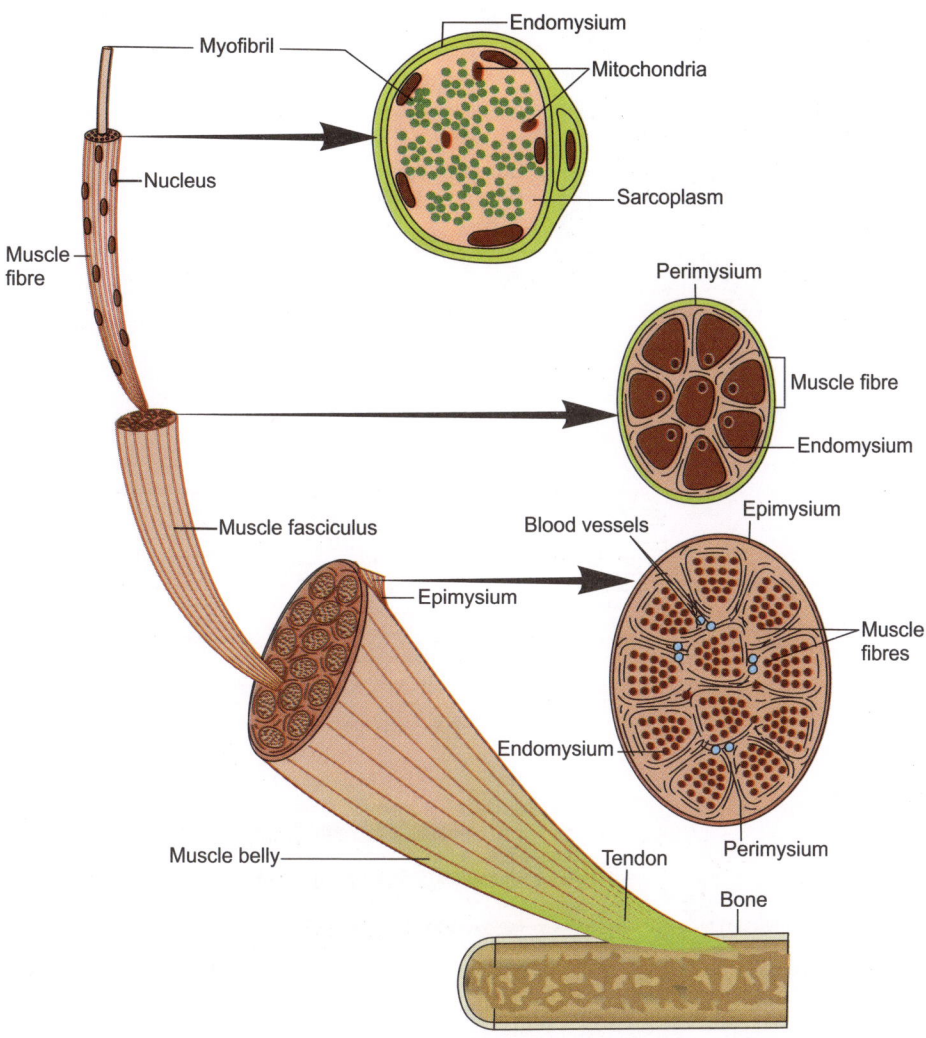

Figure 4.2 Anatomy of skeletal muscle tissue.

The characteristic striated appearance (alternate light and dark bands) of the muscle is due to the overlapping of the thick (dark) and thin (light) filaments on the myofibrils.

The dark bands are made up of thick filaments made up of the protein myosin. They appear dark because of their thickness and are called as *A bands* (clue to remember: the second letter in the word *dark* is A). The light bands are made up of thin filaments made up of the protein actin. They appear light as they are thin and are referred to as *I bands* (clue to remember: the second letter in the word *light* is I).

The I band is crossed through its centre by a dark narrow band called *Z line*. The area between two adjacent Z lines is called a *sarcomere*, the basic functional unit of a myofibril. The dark A band has a

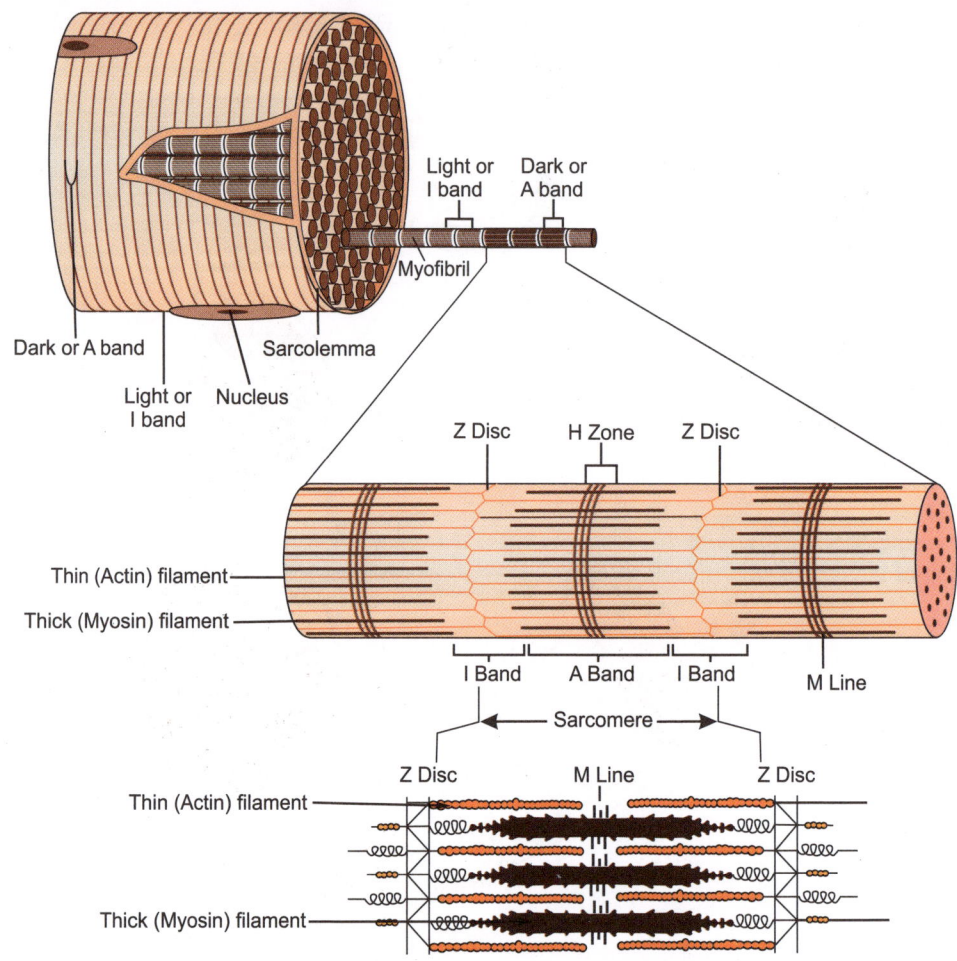

Figure 4.3 Microscopic anatomy of skeletal muscle fibre.

middle light zone called the *H zone* or *H band*. In the middle of the H zone lies the middle part of the myosin filament called the *M line* (named so as it is at the middle of the sarcomere) (Fig. 4.3).

Electron microscopy has revealed that muscle fibrils are surrounded by a fluid-filled system of membranous sacs called *sarcoplasmic reticulum (SR)*. The SR is similar to the smooth endoplasmic reticulum in nonmuscular cells and is specialized for calcium storage. Release of calcium from SR triggers muscle contraction.

PHYSIOLOGY OF SKELETAL MUSCLE CONTRACTION

The muscle fibres in the skeletal muscle are arranged in groups. Each group is under the control of a single motor neuron. A group of muscle fibres innovated by one motor neuron is called a *motor unit* because these muscle fibres are always excited simultaneously and therefore contract together. The number of muscle fibres in a unit is variable and depends on the fineness of the control exercised by a motor unit.

For example, an eyeball muscle has about 10 muscle fibres and a finger muscle has 3–6 muscle fibres.

Mechanism of muscle contraction

The contractile proteins, myosin and actin present in the thick and thin filaments of the sarcomere generate the force during muscle contraction. The actin molecule contains a site on which a myosin head can attach; this site is called the *myosin-binding site.* The interaction between myosin and actin causes contraction.

The theory about the contraction of skeletal muscle is called the *sliding filament theory*, which states that muscle contraction results from the sliding of thin actin filaments over the thick myosin filaments. According to this theory, during muscle contraction, the myosin heads attach to and slide along the thin actin filaments at both ends of a sarcomere. As a result, the thin filaments are pulled towards the M line, the Z lines come closer together and the sarcomere shortens. Shortening of the sarcomeres causes shortening of the whole muscle fibre and thereby of the entire muscle (Fig. 4.4).

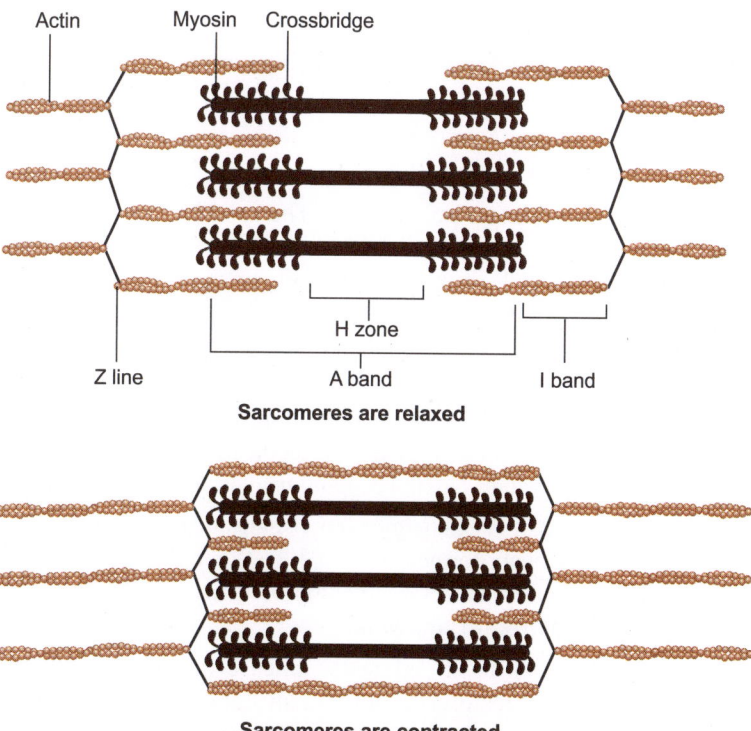

Figure 4.4 Sliding filament mechanism of muscle contraction.

Chapter 4

Electrical and biochemical events in muscle contraction

Muscle contraction involves the following complex electrical and biochemical events:

❑ The sarcolemma of the membrane of the muscle fibre is surrounded by ions. In a resting muscle fibre, the outer region of the sarcolemma is positively charged with respect to the inside. This potential difference across a membrane is called *resting potential* (−60 mV) and the membrane with such a resting potential is said to be *polarized*. The resting potential is maintained by the following mechanism:

  1. Sodium (Na^+) ions predominate outside the sarcolemma, whereas potassium (K^+) ions predominate inside the cell.
  2. Sarcolemma is more permeable to potassium (K^+) ions than to sodium (Na^+) ions and because of the uneven distribution of the ions, potassium (K^+) ions tend to leave the muscle fibre faster than sodium (Na^+) ions can enter and this builds up a positive charge on the outside.

❑ When a muscle fibre is stimulated, the sarcolemma suddenly becomes more permeable to sodium (Na^+) ions, causing the sodium (Na^+) ions to rush inside the muscle cell. This rapid influx of sodium (Na^+) ions creates an electrical potential and makes the inside of sarcolemma positive with respect to the outside and generates an *action potential*. The sarcolemma is now said to be *depolarized*, and this is the signal for contraction of the muscle fibres.

❑ Depolarization of sarcolemma, i.e. action potential, passes into the muscle fibre by way of T tubules and Z lines and increases the permeability of the SR membrane for calcium. This causes the release of calcium ions stored in SR into the sarcoplasm surrounding the thick and thin filaments. The released calcium then triggers a series of biochemical events, resulting in the contraction of muscle fibres.

The various biochemical events are as follows (Fig. 4.5):

1. **Uncovering of the myosin-binding sites on actin**: The calcium ions released from SR binds to troponin and causes the troponin–tropomyosin molecules to move away from the myosin-binding sites on actin. (In relaxed muscle, the myosin-binding site on the actin is occupied by two inhibitor proteins: tropomyosin and troponin.)

2. **ATP hydrolysis**: The myosin head contains an ATP-binding site and an ATPase [an enzyme that hydrolyses ATP (adenosine triphosphate) into ADP (adenosine diphosphate) and a phosphate group (Pi)]. Now, an ATP molecule joins the ATP-binding site on the myosin head and hydrolyzes to ADP and Pi, which remain temporarily bound to the head. The energy released by hydrolysis reaction reorients and energizes the myosin head and triggers the power stroke of contraction.

3. **Attachment of myosin and actin**: The energized myosin head attaches to the myosin-binding site on actin and releases the previously formed ADP and Pi. When the myosin heads attach to actin, the crossbridges are formed, and it causes contraction by generating the force that slides the thin filament over the thick filament towards the M line.

When the action potential ceases to stimulate the release of calcium ions from the SR, the sodium–potassium pump begins to restore the ionic distribution to its normal resting potential. As a result, Na^+ ions are pumped out and K^+ ions enter the cell, and the resting potential is again maintained.

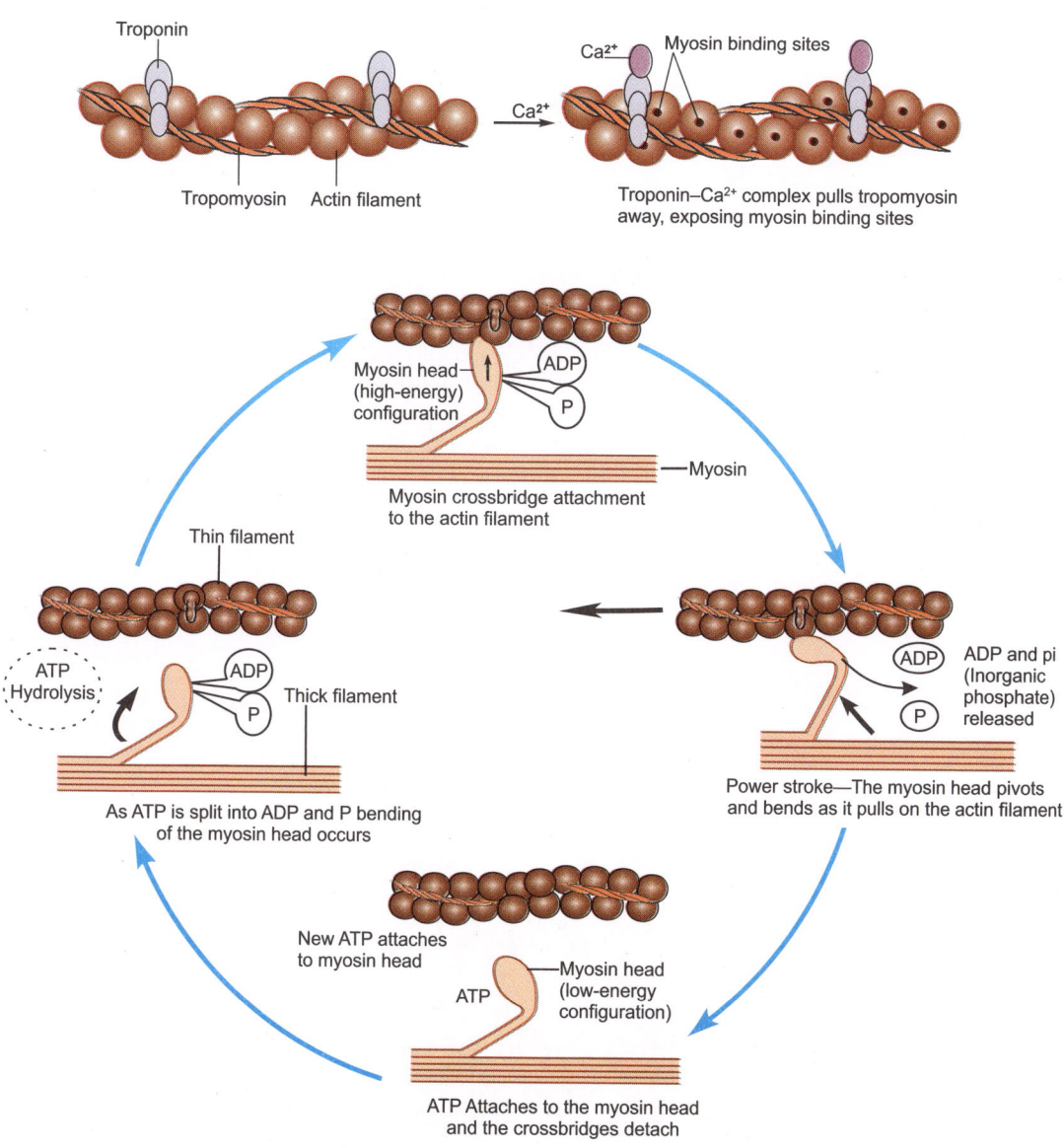

Figure 4.5 Skeletal muscle contraction.

Now, the contraction ceases and the binding of fresh ATP causes the myosin head to return to its resting position. It leads to the detachment of the myosin head from actin filaments and the Z lines move further apart. Troponin and tropomyosin molecules move back and again block the myosin-binding site on actin filaments.

Contraction occurs in a few thousand of a second and once the sodium–potassium pump restores ionic distribution, contraction ceases and all the calcium ions are once again bound to SR. A continued series of action potentials is necessary to provide enough calcium ions to maintain a continued contraction.

The neuromuscular junction

The skeletal muscle cell contracts in response to stimulation from a nerve fibre. The region where the nerve and muscle come into the closest proximity and the transmission of the action potential takes place is called the *neuromuscular junction*.

The axon (ends) of motor neurons widens to form a motor end plate at the site where it meets the skeletal muscle fibre. At this site, the axon loses its myelin sheath and divides into a cluster of synaptic end bulbs that contain hundreds of membrane-enclosed sacs called *synaptic vesicles*. Each synaptic vesicle contains thousands of neurotransmitters, that is acetylcholine (ACh) molecules (Fig. 4.6).

Thus, a neuromuscular junction includes synaptic end bulbs on one side and the motor end plate of the muscle fibre on the other side. The gap between these two is called the *synaptic cleft*. The motor end plate has many ACh receptors that bind specifically to ACh.

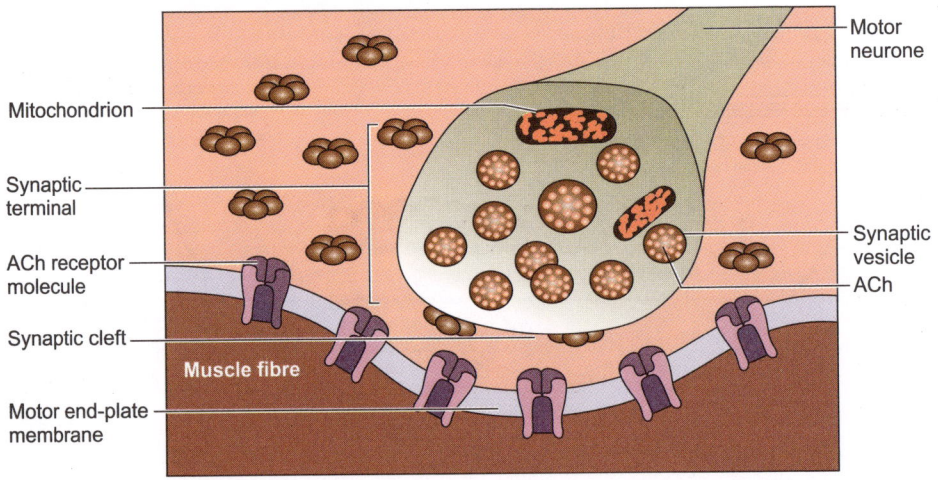

Figure 4.6 The neuromuscular junction (ACh = acetylcholine).

A nerve impulse results in muscle contraction in the following ways:

1. **Release of ACh**: Arrival of the nerve impulse at the neuromuscular junction causes many synaptic vesicles to release ACh into the synaptic cleft.

2. **Activation of ACh receptors**: Binding of ACh to the receptors on the motor end plate depolarizes the muscle cell's sarcolemma and generates an action potential.

3. **Contraction of skeletal muscle fibre**: The action potential spreads into the interior of muscle fibres via T tubules and Z lines, resulting in the contraction of muscle fibre (discussed in detail in the section Electrical and Biochemical Events in Muscle Contraction).

4. **Termination of ACh activity**: The effect of acetylcholine ACh binding lasts only for a short time because ACh is rapidly broken down by an enzyme called acetyl cholinesterase present in the synaptic cleft.

If another nerve impulse releases more ACh, steps 2 and 3 are repeated and the contraction of the muscle fibre continues.

Steps of muscle contraction

Nerve impulse arrives at the neuromuscular junction, triggering the release of Ach

↓

ACh binds to its receptors and depolarizes the sarcolemma, thus triggering an action potential

↓

SR releases calcium (Ca^{2+}) into the sarcoplasm

↓

Increased calcium (Ca^{2+}) results in the attachment of myosin and actin, leading to muscle contraction

↓

Acetylcholinesterase breaks down ACh and the action potential ceases

↓

Release of calcium (Ca^{2+}) is stopped and the resting potential is again maintained by Na^+/K^+ pump

↓

Muscle relaxes

Rigor Mortis: After death, the cellular membranes become leaky, due to which calcium ions leak out of SR into the sarcoplasm, allowing the myosin to bind with actin. ATP synthesis ceases shortly after breathing stops, which does not allow the detachment of the crossbridges between the myosin and the actin. The resulting condition of rigid muscles is called rigor mortis (rigidity of death).

Energy source for muscle contraction

The muscle cells convert chemical energy (ATP and ADP) into mechanical energy (contraction). The energy for muscle contraction is obtained by the hydrolysis of ATP into ADP and Pi by the ATPase enzyme.

Chapter 4

Muscle fibres produce ATP by the following three ways:

1. Glycolysis
2. Krebs citric acid cycle and electron transport
3. From phosphocreatine (unique to muscle fibres)

In glycolysis, glucose present in the blood enters cells, where it is broken down through a series of chemical reactions to pyruvic acid. These reactions use 2 ATP molecules and produce 4 ATP molecules, resulting in a net gain of 2 ATP molecules.

In the Krebs citric acid cycle and electron transport, pyruvic acid is further broken down into CO_2 and H_2O, with a net gain of 36 more ATP molecules from each glucose molecule in the presence of oxygen. But if oxygen is not available to the muscle cell, the pyruvic acid changes to lactic acid and builds up in the muscle cell with only 2 ATP molecules produced in glycolysis. A small portion of lactic acid diffuses out into blood and enters the liver, where it is converted back to glucose.

Muscle cells have an additional source of ATP. When muscles are at rest, excess ATP is not needed for contraction, so the ATP produced by muscle is used to synthesize phosphocreatine, an energy-rich molecule found only in muscle fibres. During strenuous exercise, phosphocreatine takes up ADP to release ATP and creatine, thus supplying the muscle with an additional supply of ATP.

To summarize:

1. In muscle contraction,

$$ATP + H_2O \xrightarrow{ATPase} ADP + Pi + Energy$$

2. Glycolysis: $\text{Glucose} \xrightarrow{Glycolysis} \text{Pyruvic acid} + 2\ ATP$
3. Krebs cycle and electron transport
   Aerobic condition: $\text{Pyruvic acid} \longrightarrow CO_2 + H_2O + 36\ ATP$
   Anaerobic condition: $\text{Pyruvic acid} \longrightarrow \text{Lactic acid}$
4. $\text{Phosphocreatine} + ADP \longrightarrow \text{Creatine} + ATP$

Muscle fatigue

The inability of a muscle to maintain force of contraction after prolonged activity is called *muscle fatigue*. The factors that contribute to muscle fatigue include insufficient oxygen, depletion of glucose and other nutrients, deposition of lactic acid and depletion of phosphocreatine in muscles.

A muscle gets fatigued sooner by strenuous exercise than by mild exercise. During vigorous exercise, the supply of oxygen to the muscle fibres becomes insufficient in spite of faster breathing and quicker heart beat. After muscle contraction has stopped, heavy breathing continues for a while and oxygen consumption is more than that in the resting condition. This added oxygen, over and above the oxygen consumption in the resting state, which is taken into the body after exercise is termed as *oxygen debt*. This oxygen is used to convert lactic acid back to glucose, synthesize phosphocreatine and ATP in muscle fibres, and replace the oxygen removed from myoglobin.

Muscle tone

Muscle tone is defined as a property of muscle in which a sustained state of partial contraction is maintained in a muscle. The tone is maintained by a constant flow of nerve impulses to the muscle fibres. To sustain muscle tone, small groups of motor units are alternately active and inactive in a constantly shifting pattern, i.e. some muscle cells in a muscle will always be contracting while others are at rest.

Muscle tone keeps skeletal muscles firm, but it does not generate strong force to produce movement, for example maintenance of upright posture of the head requires constant activity of muscles of the neck and shoulders.

Tone also maintains pressure on abdominal contents, maintains blood pressure in the arteries and veins and helps in digestion in the stomach and intestine.

Muscle twitch

Muscle twitch or twitch contraction is the brief contraction of all the muscle fibres in a motor unit in response to a single action potential in its motor neurons. In the laboratory, twitch can be produced by direct stimulation of a motor neuron or its muscle fibres to record the muscle contraction.

The strength of the contraction of a muscle fibre depends on a number of factors, which are as follows:

1. Strength of stimulus (weak stimulus cannot cause contraction).
2. Duration of stimulus (even if a strong stimulus is applied for a millisecond, it would not be effective).
3. Speed of stimulus (a strong stimulus applied quickly and immediately pulled away will not be effective).
4. Temperature (muscles operate best at normal body temperature, i.e. 37°C or 98.6°F in humans).

When each muscle fibre contracts, it obeys the *all or none principle*, i.e. the whole fibre either contracts completely or not at all.

Isotonic and isometric contractions

Muscle contractions are classified as either isotonic or isometric.

In an isotonic contraction, the tension (force of contraction) developed by the muscle remains almost constant while the muscle changes its length, for example during body movements and for moving objects.

In an isometric contraction, the tension in the muscle increases while the muscles involved remain at a constant length. These contractions are important for maintaining posture and for supporting objects in a fixed position, for example holding a book steady using an outstretched arm.

TYPES OF SKELETAL MUSCLE FIBRES

All skeletal muscle fibres are not alike in composition and function. The following are the two types of skeletal muscle fibres (Fig. 4.7):

1. Tonic/red/slow muscle fibres
2. Twitch/white/fast muscle fibres

1. **Tonic/red/slow muscle fibres**
   - ❑ These are thin, dark red and slow-contracting muscle fibres. They contain a high amount of myoglobin, abundant mitochondria and poorly formed SR. High myoglobin content imparts them a dark red colour and hence are termed *red muscle fibres*.
   - ❑ They carry on slow and sustained contractions for long time periods without fatigue and hence the body muscles meant for sustained work at a slow rate for a prolonged duration are composed

Chapter 4

mostly or entirely of red muscle fibres, for example extensor muscles in the back, to maintain erect posture against gravity and long-distance running.

2. **Twitch/white/fast muscle fibres**
   - ❏ These are much thicker, lighter in colour and fast-constricting muscle fibres. They have low myoglobin content, few mitochondria and well-formed SR.
   - ❏ The body muscles meant for fast and strenuous work for short durations are composed mostly or entirely of white muscle fibres, for example intense movements such as weightlifting or throwing a ball.

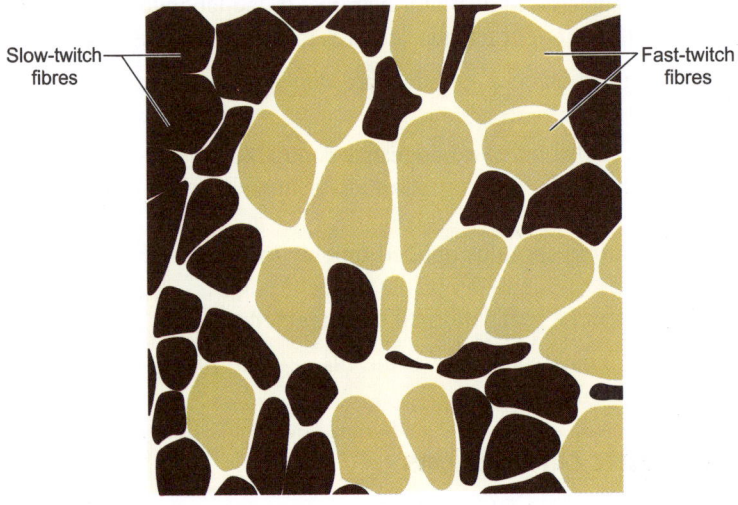

Figure 4.7 Fast and slow muscle fibres.

CARDIAC MUSCLE TISSUE

Cardiac muscle tissue is found exclusively in the wall of heart. They have the same arrangement of actin and myosin and the same bands and zones as the skeletal muscle fibres. However, the microscopic

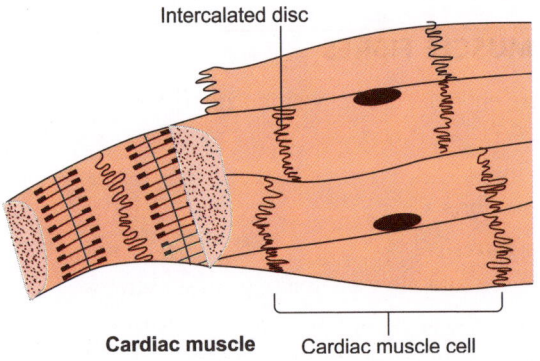

Figure 4.8 Cardiac muscle tissue.

structure called as *intercalated discs* are unique to cardiac muscle fibres. These intercalated discs connect the ends of cardiac muscle fibres to one another (Fig. 4.8).

The cardiac muscle tissue remains contracted 10–15 times longer than the skeletal muscle fibres in response to an action potential (discussed in detail in the chapter Cardiovascular System) and it has a unique property of autorhythmicity.

SMOOTH MUSCLE TISSUE

Smooth muscle tissue is nonstriated, involuntary and is of the following two types:

1. Single-unit smooth muscle tissue
2. Multiunit smooth muscle tissue

1. **Single-unit smooth muscle tissue**
   - ❏ It is found in the walls of small arteries, veins and hollow organs such as the stomach, intestine, uterus and urinary bladder.
   - ❏ The muscle fibres are connected to one another by gap junctions that form a network through which action potential spreads and contracts the whole muscle as a unit.
2. **Multiunit smooth muscle tissue**
   - ❏ It consists of individual fibres with very few gap functions between neighbouring fibres. The stimulation of a multiunit fibre contracts that particular fibre only.
   - ❏ It is found in the walls of large arteries, ciliary body, iris muscle and arrector pili.

MICROSCOPIC ANATOMY OF SMOOTH MUSCLE TISSUE

A single relaxed smooth muscle fibre is 30–200 µm long. It is thickest in the middle and tapers at each end. The sarcoplasm contains both thick and thin filaments but they are not arranged in sarcomeres as in the skeletal muscle.

Smooth muscle fibres contain thin filaments called *dense bodies*, which are functionally similar to Z discs in skeletal muscle fibres. During contraction, the sliding filament mechanism is involved in the sliding of thick and thin filaments, which in turn pulls the dense bodies and causes shortening of muscle fibre.

PHYSIOLOGY OF SMOOTH MUSCLE TISSUE

Contraction in the smooth muscle fibre starts slowly and lasts much longer as compared to skeletal muscle fibres. Also, the smooth muscle fibres can both shorten and stretch to a greater extent than the other muscle types.

Smooth muscle tissues have very little SR (as compared to skeletal muscle) to store Ca^{2+}, which results in longer time for Ca^{2+} to trigger the contractile process, resulting in slow onset of contraction. Moreover, the smooth muscle tissue contains a protein called *calmodulin* that binds to Ca^{2+} and activates an enzyme, myosin light chain kinase *(MLCK)*. This enzyme binds ATP to the myosin head and results in the interaction between myosin and actin, which causes contraction. The MLCK also works slowly, contributing to the slow contraction of smooth muscle tissue (Fig. 4.9).

Chapter 4

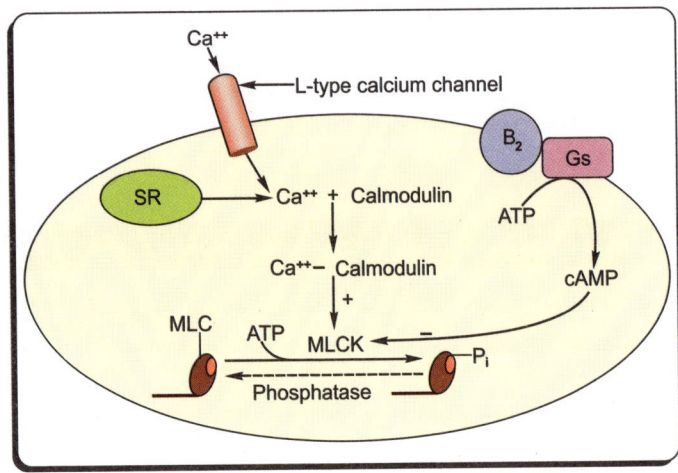

Figure 4.9 Contraction in smooth muscle tissue.

Moreover, the Ca^{2+} that enters the smooth muscle fibre moves out slowly from the muscle fibre, which delays relaxation. Thus, the prolonged presence of Ca^{2+} in the cytosol is responsible for the smooth muscle tone, i.e. a state of continued partial contraction.

SKELETAL MUSCLES IN THE HUMAN BODY

Skeletal muscles produce movements by exerting force on tendons, which in turn pull on bones or other structures (such as the skin). Generally, the attachment of a muscle's tendon to the stationary bone is called *origin*. It is usually the proximal attachment that remains still while the muscle contracts. The attachment of the muscle's other tendon to the movable bone is called *insertion* and it is the distal attachment site (Fig. 4.10).

The fleshy portion of the muscle between the tendons is called *belly*, and the actions of a muscle include the major movements that occur when the muscle contracts.

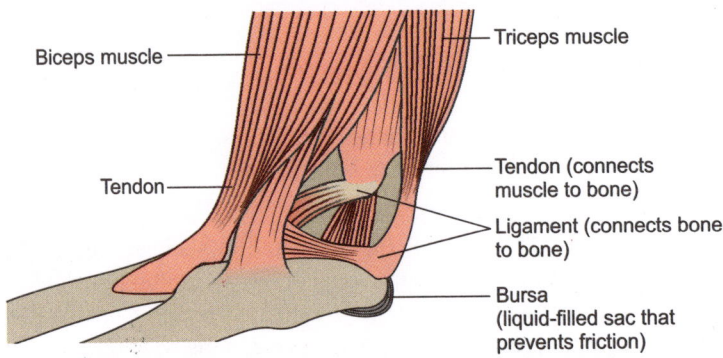

Figure 4.10 Pictorial representation of tendon, ligament and muscles.

The body movements are often the result of several skeletal muscles acting as a group. Most skeletal muscles are arranged in opposing (antagonistic) pairs at joints and in performing any movement, such as bending the leg at the knee joint, the muscles performing the actual movement (i.e. contracting to cause action) are called *prime movers* or *agonists*, whereas the muscles that strengthen the knee are the *antagonists*. The antagonists and prime movers are usually located on the opposite sides of the bone or joint. The muscles that assist the prime movers are called the *synergists* (Fig. 4.11).

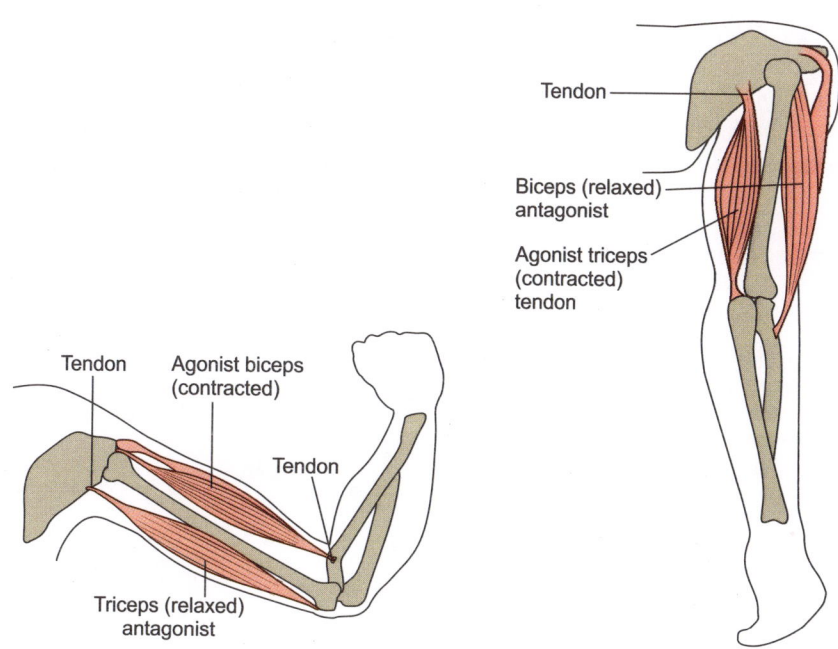

Figure 4.11 Agonists and antagonists in body movements.

MUSCLE TERMINOLOGY: NAMING OF SKELETAL MUSCLES

Muscles can be named according to their action (adductor, flexor, extensor), shape (quadratus, trapezius), location (tibialis, radialis), number of divisions (biceps, triceps) and the directions their fibres run into (transverse, oblique).

Functional classification of skeletal muscles

Based on the type of motion they cause, the skeletal muscles can be classified into the following types:

1. **Flexors**: They bend one part of a limb on another at a joint, for example biceps → bring forearm towards the upper arm.
2. **Extensors**: They extend or strengthen a limb at a joint, for example triceps → extends forearm.
3. **Abductors**: They pull a limb away from the midline of the body, for example deltoideus.

4. **Adductors**: They bring a limb towards the midline of the body
5. **Depressors**: They lower a part of the body
6. **Elevators**: They raise a part of the body
7. **Rotators**: They rotate a part of the body
8. **Pronators**: They rotate the forearm to turn the palms downward or backward
9. **Supinators**: They rotate the forearms to turn the arm upward or forward

LOCATION AND FUNCTION OF SKELETAL MUSCLES

The sections that follow covers the major muscles that move the limbs as well as the major muscles of the face and neck, back, chest, pelvic floor and abdominal wall. The muscles are present in pairs, one on each side (except where indicated).

Muscles of face and neck

Muscles of facial expression

These are the muscles of face involved in changing facial expression (Fig. 4.12).

Table 4.1 Muscles of facial expression

S. no.	Muscle	Location	Function
1.	Occipitalis (unpaired)	Present over occipital bone	Draws scalp backwards
2.	Frontalis (unpaired)	Present over frontal bone	Raises eyebrows and wrinkles skin of forehead
3.	Zygomaticus	Zygomatic bone	Involved in smiling and laughing
4.	Levator labii superioris	Maxilla	Raises the upper lip
5.	Levator palpebrae superioris	Extends from orbital cavity to upper eyelid	Raises the eyelid
6.	Orbicularis oculi	Surrounds the eye, eyelid and orbital cavity	Closes the eyes
7.	Orbicularis oris (unpaired)	Surrounds the opening of mouth	Closes the lips and when strongly contracted, shapes the mouth for whistling
8.	Buccinator	Cheeks	Compresses cheek and assists in mastication

Occiput: back of head; *zygomatic*: cheek bone; *levator*: raises/elevator; *bucc*: cheek; *oculi*: of the eye; *palpebrae*: eyelids; *labii*: lip.

Note: The two muscles orbicularis oris and buccinators are involved in puckering up to kiss.

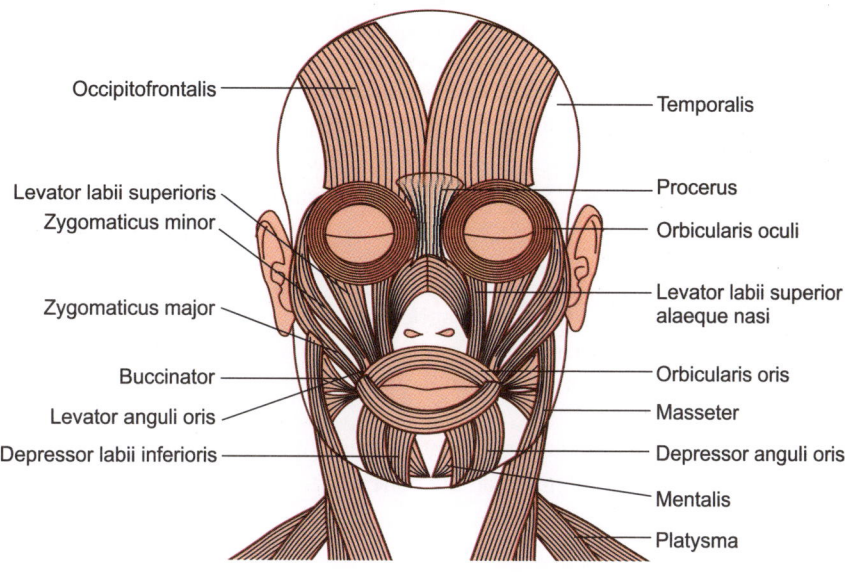

Occipitofrontalis

Temporalis

Levator labii superioris
Zygomaticus minor

Procerus

Orbicularis oculi

Zygomaticus major

Levator labii superior
alaeque nasi

Buccinator

Orbicularis oris

Levator anguli oris

Masseter

Depressor labii inferioris

Depressor anguli oris

Mentalis

Platysma

Figure 4.12 Muscles of facial expression.

Muscles of mastication

These are the muscles of face involved in moving the mandible (lower jaw bone) and are known as the *muscles of mastication* (chewing) (Fig. 4.13).

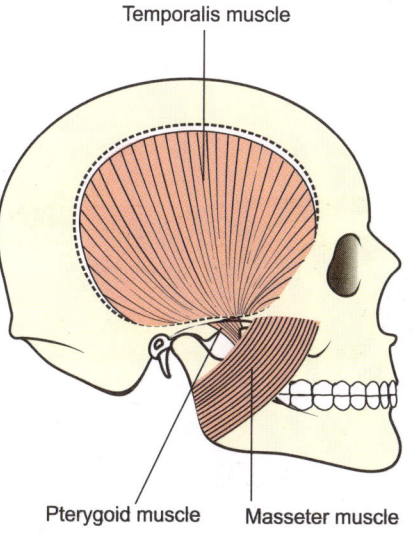

Temporalis muscle

Pterygoid muscle   Masseter muscle

Figure 4.13 Muscles of mastication.

Chapter 4

Table 4.2 Muscles of mastication

S.no.	Muscle	Location	Function
1.	Masseter (chewer)	Maxilla and zygomatic arch	Closes the jaw and exerts considerable pressure on the food
2.	Temporalis	Temporal bone	Elevates and retracts the mandible, closes the mouth and assists in chewing
3.	Pterygoid	Extends from sphenoid bone to mandible	Closes the mouth and pulls the lower jaw forward

Muscles of eyes

- ❏ These are the muscles involved in the movement of eyes (Fig. 4.14).
- ❏ They are unique in that they do not insert on the bone, but insert on the eyeball.

Table 4.3 Muscles of eyes

S.no.	Muscle	Location	Function
1.	Superior rectus	Superior and central part of eyeball	Moves eyeball upwards
2.	Inferior rectus	Inferior and central part of eyeball	Moves eyeball downwards
3.	Medial rectus	Medial side of eyeball	Moves eyeball medially (adduction)
4.	Lateral rectus	Lateral side of eyeball	Moves eyeball laterally (abduction)
5.	Superior oblique	Between superior and lateral recti	Rotates the eyeball on axis
6.	Inferior oblique	Between inferior and lateral recti	Rotates the eyeball on axis

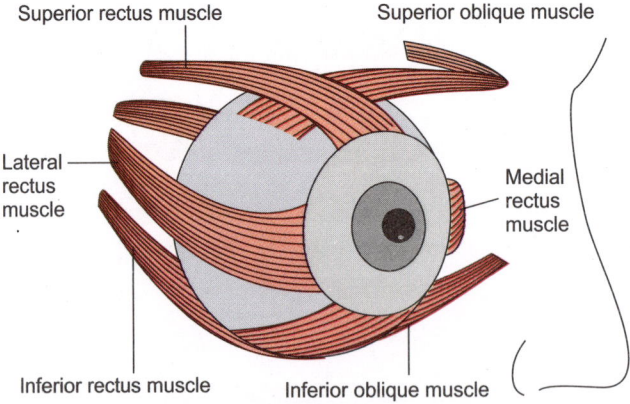

Figure 4.14 Muscles of eyes.

Muscles that move the head

The major muscle that moves the head is the sternocleidomastoid muscle. It arises from the sternum and clavicle and extends upwards to the mastoid process of the temporal bone. It helps in turning the head from side to side. When the muscle contracts on one side, it draws the head towards the shoulder. When both (pair) contracts at the same time, the head is maintained in a fixed position (Fig. 4.15).

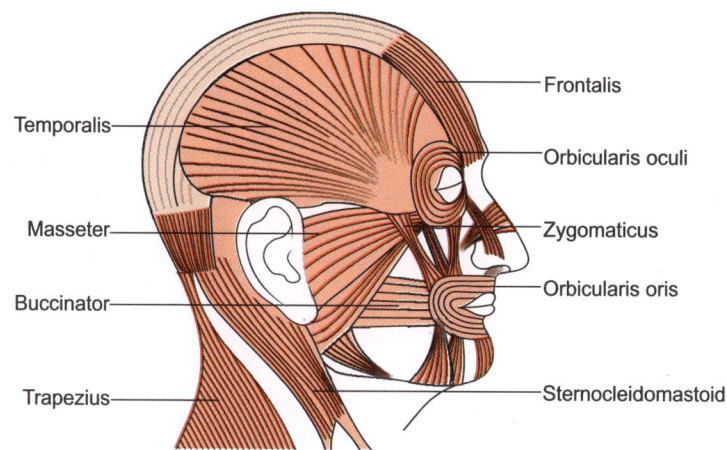

Figure 4.15 Muscles of the head and neck.

Muscles of the shoulder and upper limbs

Muscles that move the shoulder (pectoral) girdle

The main action of the muscles that move the shoulder girdle is to stabilize scapula (Fig. 4.16)

Table 4.4 Muscles that move the shoulder (pectoral) girdle

S. no.	Muscle	Origin	Insertion	Function
1.	Levator scapulae	Cervical vertebrae	Scapula	Elevates scapula
2.	Rhomboid	Thoracic verte-brae	Scapula	Elevates and retracts scapula
3.	Pectoralis minor	Ribs	Scapula	Abducts scapula and rotates it downwards
4.	Trapezius	Occipital bone	Clavicle	Pulls head backwards and rotates scapula
5.	Serratus anterior	Ribs	Scapula	Abducts scapula and rotates it upwards

Levator: raises; *rhomboid*: diamond shaped; *trapezius*: trapezoid shaped; *serratus*: saw shaped.

Chapter 4

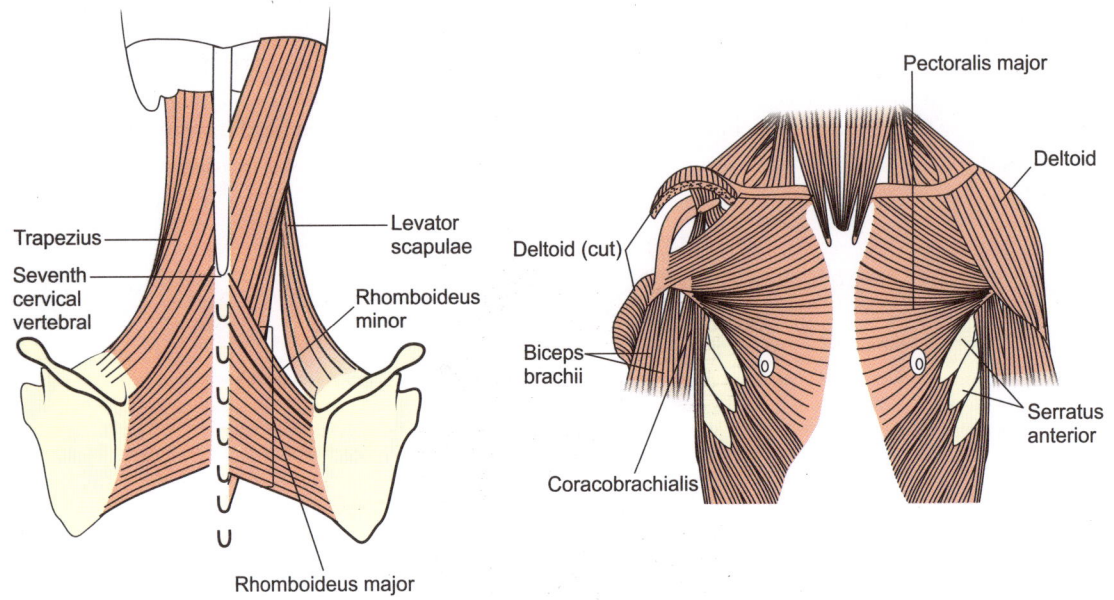

Figure 4.16 Muscles of the shoulder (pectoral) girdle and humerus.

Muscles that move the humerus (arm bone)

Most of these muscles originate on the bones of the shoulder girdle (Fig. 4.16). Table 4.5 describes the major muscles involved in the movement of humerus.

Table 4.5 Muscles that move the humerus (arm bone)

S. no.	Muscle	Origin	Insertion	Function
1.	Pectoralis major	Clavicle; sternum	Humerus	Flexes and adducts (i.e. draws the arm forward and towards the body)
2.	Coracobrachialis	Scapula	Humerus	Flexes the shoulder joint
3.	Deltoid	Clavicle; scapula	Humerus	Abducts and rotates the arm
4.	Latissimus dorsi *swimmer muscle*	Thoracic and lumbar vertebrae	Humerus	Extends, adducts and rotates the arm medially

Major: larger; *brachi*: arm; *deltoid*: triangle shaped; *latissimus*: widest

Muscles that move the radius and ulna (forearm bones or elbow)

Table 4.6 describes the major muscles involved in the movement of radius and ulna (Fig. 4.17).

Table 4.6 Muscles that move the radius and ulna (forearm bones)

S. no.	Muscle	Origin	Insertion	Function
1.	Brachialis	Humerus	Ulna	Main flexor of the elbow joint
2.	Biceps brachii	Scapula	Humerus	Stabilizes and flexes the shoulder joint and assists in supination and flexion at the elbow joint
3.	Triceps brachii	Scapula, humerus	Ulna	Adduction of the arm and extends the elbow joint
4.	Brachioradialis	Humerus	Radius	Flexes the elbow joint
5.	Anconeus	Humerus	Ulna	Extends the forearm

brachii: arm; *ancon*: elbow; *biceps*: two heads; *triceps*: three heads.

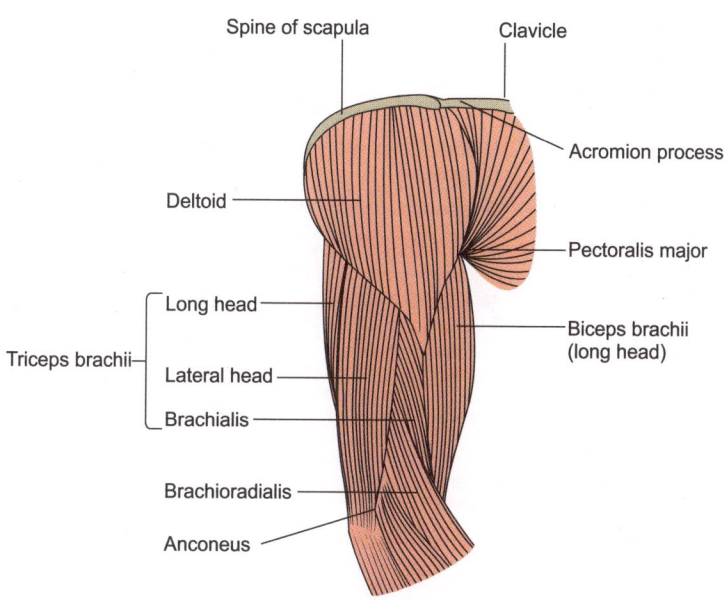

Figure 4.17 Muscles that move the forearm or elbow.

Muscles that move the wrist

Table 4.7 describes the major muscles involved in the movement of wrist (Fig. 4.18).

Table 4.7 Muscles that move the wrist

S. no.	Muscle	Origin	Insertion	Function
1.	Flexor carpi radialis	Humerus	Metacarpal bones	Flexes and abducts the wrist
2.	Flexor carpi ulnaris	Humerus; ulna	Metacarpal bones	Flexes and adducts the wrist
3.	Extensor carpi radialis longus and extensor carpi radialis brevis	Humerus	Metacarpal bones	Extends and abducts the wrist
4.	Extensor carpi ulnaris	Humerus	Metacarpal bones	Extends and adducts the wrist
5.	Palmarus longus	Humerus	Palm of hand	Flexes the wrist joint
6.	Extensor digitorum communis	Humerus	Phalanges of each finger	Extends the wrist joint

Carpi: wrist; *brevis*: short.

Muscles that move the hand and digits

Table 4.8 describes the major muscles involved in the movement of hand and digits (Fig. 4.18).

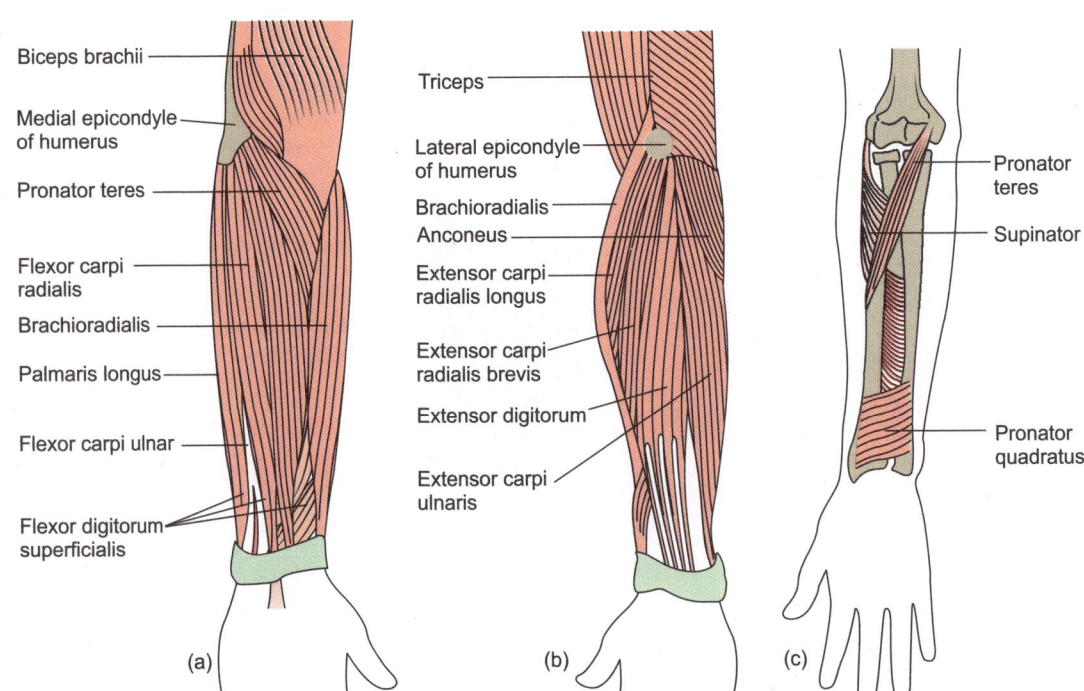

Figure 4.18 Muscles that move the wrist and hand: (a) Anterior view (flexors and pronators); (b) Posterior view (flexors and pronators); (c) Internal view.

The thumb is capable of moving in many directions, which gives the hand a unique capability of grasping, thus distinguishing humans from all other animals. Table 4.9 describes the major muscles involved in the movement of thumb (Fig. 4.19).

Table 4.10 describes the major muscles involved in the movement of fingers.

Table 4.8 Muscles that move the hand

S. no.	Muscle	Origin	Insertion	Function
1.	Supinator	Humerus; ulna	Radius	Supinates the forearm
2.	Pronator teres	Humerus; Ulna	Radius	Pronates the forearm
3.	Pronator quadratus	Ulna	Radius	Pronates forearm

Pronator: turns palm posteriorly; *supinator*: turns palm anteriorly.

Table 4.9 Muscles that move the thumb

S. no.	Muscle	Origin	Insertion	Function
1.	Flexor pollicis longus	Radius	Thumb	Flexes the distal phalanx of the thumb
2.	Extensor pollicis longus	Ulna	Thumb	Abducts and extends the thumb
3.	Extensor pollicis brevis	Radius	Thumb	Extends thumb
4.	Abductor pollicis longus	Radius; ulna	Thumb	Abducts and extends the thumb
5.	Abductor pollicis brevis	Radius; ulna	Thumb	Abducts the thumb
6.	Opponens pollicis	Radius; ulna	Thumb	Flexes and moves the thumb across the palm to meet the little finger
7.	Flexor pollicis brevis	Radius; ulna	Thumb	Flexes the thumb
8.	Adductor pollicis	3rd metacarpal	Thumb	Adducts the thumb

Pollic: thumb; *abductor*: moves away from midline; *adductor*: moves towards midline; *longus*: long.

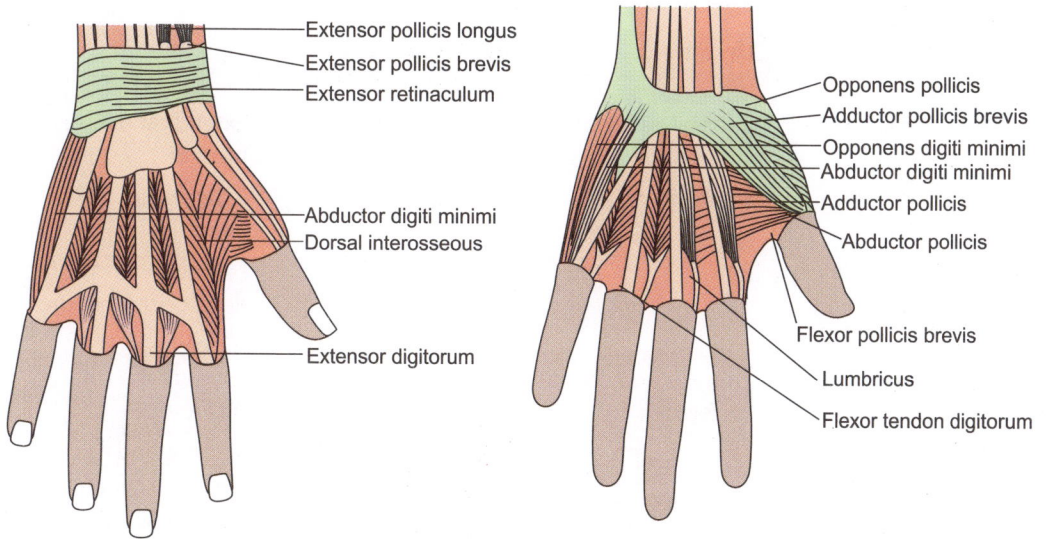

Figure 4.19 Muscles that move the thumb and fingers.

Table 4.10 Muscles that move the fingers

S. no.	Muscle	Origin	Insertion	Function
1.	Flexor digitorum profundus	Ulna	Phalanx of each finger	Flexes the phalanges of each finger
2.	Flexor digiti minimi brevis	Ulna	Little finger	Flexes the little finger
3.	Dorsal interossei	Metacarpals	Phalanx of each finger	Abducts and extends the fingers
4.	Flexor digitorum superficialis	Humerus, ulna, radius	Phalanx of each finger	Flexes the middle phalanges
5.	Extensor indicis	Ulna	Index finger	Extends the index fingers
6.	Palmar interossei	Metacarpal of all fingers	Phalanges of all fingers	Adducts and flexes each finger
7.	Abductor digiti minimi	Ulna	Little finger	Abducts the little finger
8.	Opponens digiti minimi	Ulna	Little finger	Rotates and abducts the little finger
9.	Extensor digitorum	Humerus	Phalanges of each finger	Extends the fingers

Digit: finger; *minimi*: little; *superficialis*: closer to surface; *palmer*: palm; *dorsal*: back surface; *interossei*: between bones; *indicis*: index.

Muscles that move the vertebral column (backbone)

Table 4.11 describes the major muscles involved in the movement of vertebral column (Fig. 4.20).

Table 4.11 Muscles that move the vertebral column (backbone)

S. no.	Muscle	Origin	Insertion	Function
1.	Splenius capitis	Cervical and thoracic vertebrae	Occipital and temporal bone	Extends and flexes the head
2.	Splenius cervicis	Thoracic vertebrae	Cervical vertebrae	Extends and flexes the head
3.	Iliocostalis cervicis; thoracis and lumborum	Ribs	Cervical vertebrae	Extends and maintain erect posture of the vertebral column
4.	Longissimus capitis	Thoracic and cervical vertebrae	Temporal bone	Extends and rotates the head
5.	Longissimus cervicis	Thoracic vertebrae	Cervical vertebrae	Extends and flexes the vertebral column
6.	Longissimus thoracis	Lumbar vertebrae	Ribs	Extends and flexes the vertebral column

7.	Spinalis capitis; cervicis; thoracis	Cervical; thoracic vertebrae	Occipital bone; thoracic vertebrae	Extends the vertebral column
8.	Scalene	Cervical vertebrae	Ribs	Flexes and rotates the head
9.	Interspinales and intertransversarii	All vertebrae	Spinous process of vertebrae	Extends the vertebral column and stabilizes it during movement
10.	Semispinalis capitis; cervicis; thoracis	Cervical, thoracic vertebrae	Occipital bone; Cervical vertebrae	Extends and rotates the head

Capit: head; *cervic*: neck; *longissimus*: longest; *costa*: ribs; *thorac*: chest.

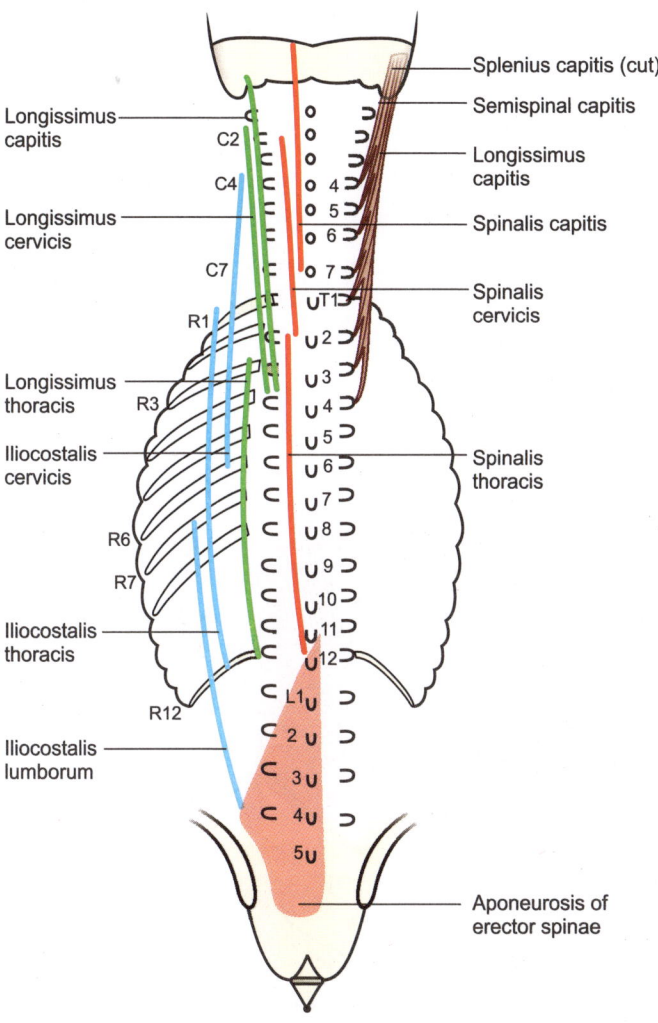

Figure 4.20 Muscles that move the vertebral column.

Muscles of the abdominal wall

Three layers of muscles along the sides of the abdomen constrict and hold the abdominal contents in place (Fig. 4.21).

Table 4.12 Muscles of the abdominal wall

S. no.	Muscle	Origin	Insertion	Function
1.	External oblique	Lower eight ribs	Iliac crest	Compress the abdominal organs and their contents
2.	Internal oblique	Iliac crest	Costal cartilage lower three or four ribs	Compress the abdominal organs and their contents
3.	Transversus abdominis (abdomen)	Iliac crest cartilage of the lower six ribs	Xiphoid cartilage	Compress the abdominal organs and their contents
4.	Rectus abdominis	Crest of pubis, pubic symphysis	Cartilage of 5th, 6th and 7th rib	Flexes the vertebral column, assists in compressing the abdominal wall
5.	Quadratus lumborum	Iliac crest	Last rib and upper four lumbar vertebrae	Flexes the trunk laterally

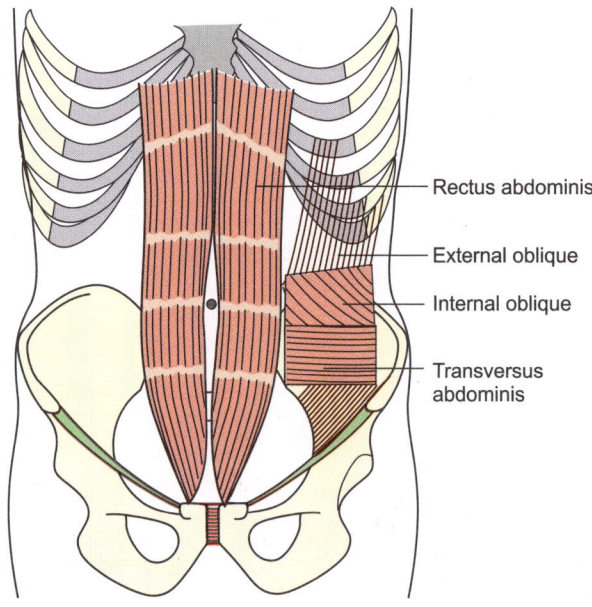

Rectus abdominis

External oblique

Internal oblique

Transversus abdominis

Figure 4.21 Muscles of the abdominal wall.

Muscles of breathing or respiration

The main muscle used in breathing is the diaphragm (Fig. 4.22), as its contraction causes air to enter lungs while relaxation expels air from lungs.

Table 4.13 Muscles of respiration

S. no.	Muscle	Origin	Insertion	Function
1.	Diaphragm	Xiphoid process, costal cartilages, lumbar vertebrae	Central tendon	Increases vertical dimension of the thorax
2.	External intercostals	Lower border of the rib	Upper border of the rib below	Draws adjacent ribs together
3.	Internal Intercostals	Ridge on inner surface of the rib	Upper border of the rib below	Draws adjacent ribs together

Dia: across; *phragm*: wall.

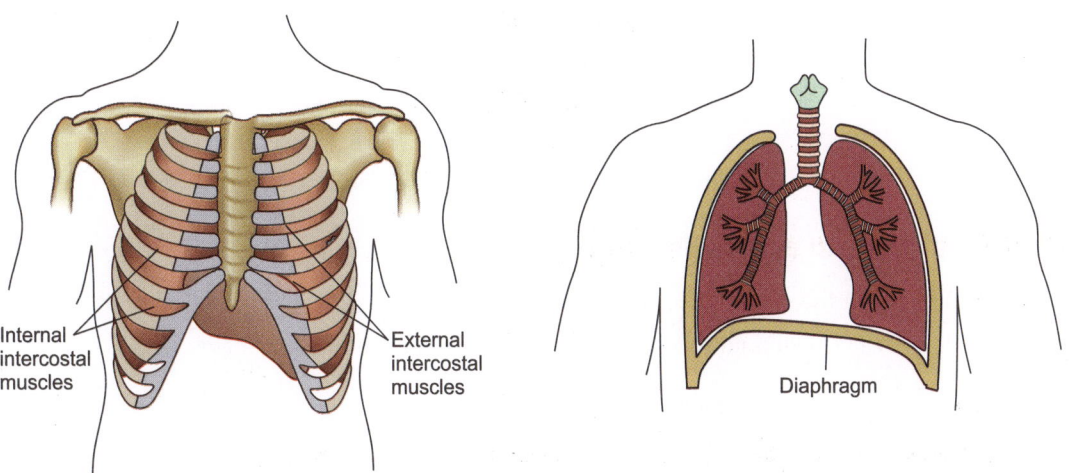

Internal intercostal muscles

External intercostal muscles

Diaphragm

Figure 4.22 Muscles of respiration or breathing.

Muscles of the pelvic floor

Table 4.14 describes the major muscles of the pelvic floor (Fig. 4.23).

Table 4.14 Muscles of the pelvic floor

S. no.	Muscle	Origin	Insertion	Function
1.	Levator ani (divided in two parts)			
	(a) Pubococcygeus	Pubis	coccyx, urethra and anal canal	Supports the pelvic organs
	(b) Iliococcygeus	Ischial spine	coccyx	Supports the pelvic organs
2.	Coccygeus	Ischial spine	sacrum and coccyx	Supports the pelvic organs and maintains continence (i.e. resists raised intrapelvic pressure during micturition and defecation)

Levator: raises; *ani*: anus; *pubo*: pubis; *coccygeus*: coccyx; *ilio*: ilium.

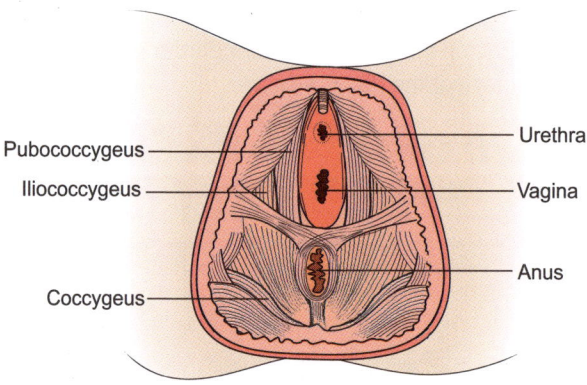

Figure 4.23 Muscles of the pelvic floor.

Muscles of the hip and lower limb

Muscles that move the femur (thigh bone)

Table 4.15 describes the major muscles involved in the movement of the femur (Fig. 4.24).

Table 4.15 Muscles that move the femur

S. no.	Muscle	Origin	Insertion	Function
1.	Psoas major	Transverse process of lumbar vertebrae	Femur	Flexes, rotates the hip joint
2.	Iliacus	Last thoracic and lumbar vertebrae	Junction of ilium and pubis	Flexes, rotates the hip joint
3.	Gluteus maximus	Ilium, sacrum and coccyx	Fascia lata, gluteal ridge	Extends, rotates the thigh laterally
4.	Gluteus medius	Ilium	Tendon on femur	Extends, abducts, rotates the thigh at hip joint

S. no.	Muscle	Origin	Insertion	Function
5.	Gluteus minimus	Ilium	Femur	Extends, abducts, rotates the thigh at hip joint
6.	Tensor fascia lata	Ilium	Femur	Flexes and abducts the thigh at hip joint
7.	Abductor brevis	Pubis	Femur	Abducts, rotates the thigh at hip joint
8.	Adductor magnus	Ischium, ischiopubic ramus	Femur	Adducts, extends the thigh at hip joint
9.	Obturator externus	Ischium, ischiopubic ramus	Femur	Rotates the thigh laterally
10.	Pectineus	Pubis	Femur	Flexes, adducts the thigh at hip joint
11.	Adductor longus	Crest and symphysis of pubis	Femur	Adducts, rotates, flexes the thigh at hip joint

Muscles that move the knee joint

Table 4.16 describes the major muscles involved in the movement of the knee joint (Fig. 4.24).

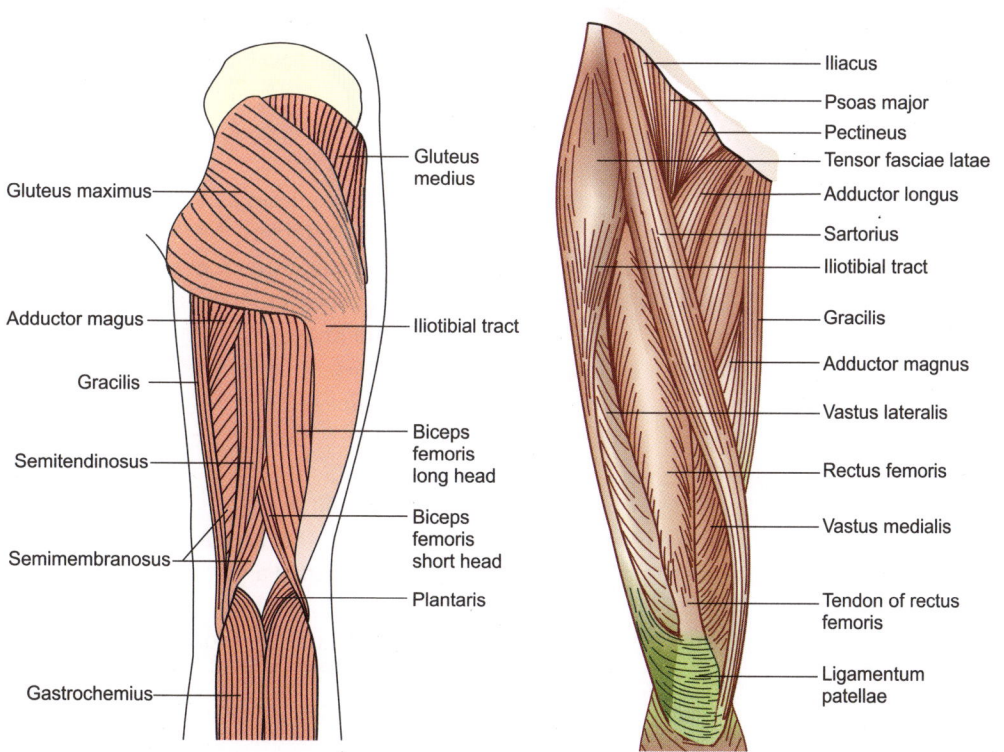

Figure 4.24 Muscles that move the femur and knee joint.

Table 4.16 Muscles that move the knee joint

S. no.	Muscle	Origin	Insertion	Function
1.	Biceps femoris (two heads)	Ischium	Tibia, Fibula	Flexes the leg at knee joint and extends the thigh at hip joint
2.	Semitendinosus	Ischial tuberosity	Tibia	Flexes the leg at knee joint and extends the thigh at hip joint
3.	Semimembranosus	Ischial tuberosity	Tibia	Flexes the leg at knee joint and extends the thigh at hip joint
4.	Sartorius (longest muscle in the body)	Iliac spine	Tibia	Flexes the thigh, abducts and rotates the thigh at hip joint
5.	Quadriceps femoris (four heads) Rectus femoris Vastus lateralis Vastus medialis Vastus intermedius	Femur	Tibia	Extends the leg and flexes the thigh at hip joint

Muscles that move the foot

Table 4.17 describes the major muscles involved in the movement of the foot (Fig. 4.25).

Table 4.17 Muscles that move the foot

S. no.	Muscle	Origin	Insertion	Function
1.	Gastrocnemius	Femur	Calcaneous by way of calcaneous tendon	Plantar flexes foot, flexes leg, supinates foot
2.	Soleus	Tibia, Fibula	Calcaneous by way of calcaneous tendon	Plantar flexes foot at ankle joint and helps stabilize the joint while standing
3.	Tibialis posterior	Tibia, Fibula	Metatarsals	Plantar flexes foot at ankle joint and helps stabilize the joint while standing
4.	Tibialis anterior	Tibia, Fibula	Metatarsals	Dorsally flexes foot at ankle joint and helps to stabilize the joint while standing
5.	Peroneus tertius	Fibula	Metatarsals	Dorsally flexes foot at ankle joint and helps stabilize the joint while standing
6.	Peroneus longus	Tibia, Fibula	Metatarsals	Everts foot and plantar flexes at ankle joint and helps stabilize the joint while standing
7.	Peroneus brevis	Fibula	Metatarsals	Everts foot and plantar flexes foot at ankle joint and helps stabilize the joint while standing
8.	Plantaris	Femur	Calcaneous by way of calcaneous tendon	Plantar flexes foot at ankle joint and flexes leg at knee joint
9.	Popliteus	Femur	Tibia	Flexes leg at knee joint and rotates tibia

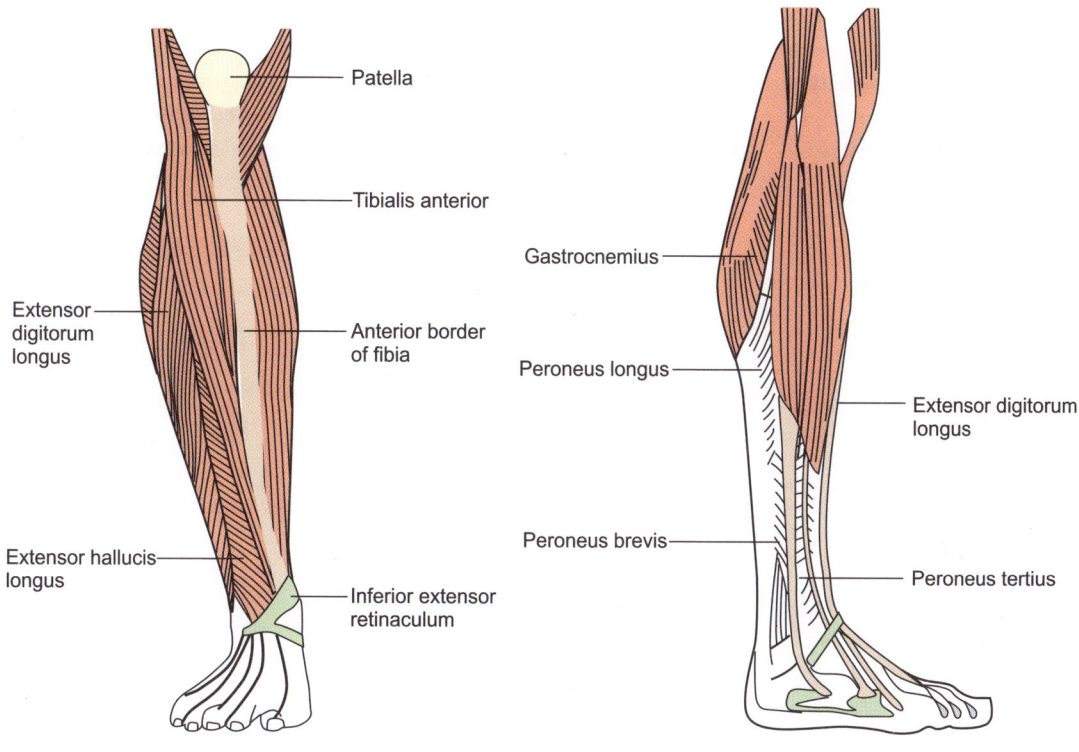

Figure 4.25 Muscles that move the foot.

Muscles that move the toes

Table 4.18 describes the major muscles involved in the movement of the toes (Fig. 4.26).

Table 4.18 Muscles that move the toes

S. no.	Muscle	Origin	Insertion	Function
1.	Flexor hallucis brevis	Metatarsal	Phalanx of great toe	Flexes the great toe at the metatarsophalangeal joint
2.	Flexor hallucis longus	Fibula	Phalanx of great toe	Flexes the great toe at the metatarsophalangeal joint
3.	Extensor hallucis longus	Fibula	Phalanx of great toe	Extends the great toe, dorsiflexes the ankle at the metatarsophalangeal joint
4.	Interossei dorsales	Metatarsal	Phalanges	Abduct, flex toes at the metatarsophalangeal joint
5.	Flexor digitorum longus	Tibia	Phalanges	Flexes toes, extends foot at the metatarsophalangeal joint

6.	Extensor digitorum longus	Tibia and fibula	Phalanges	Extends toes and dorsiflexes foot at the ankle joint
7.	Abductor hallucis	Metatarsal	Great toe	Abducts, flexes the great toe at the metatarsophalangeal joint
8.	Abductor digiti minimi	Metatarsal	Little toe	Abducts and flexes the little toe at the metatarsophalangeal joint

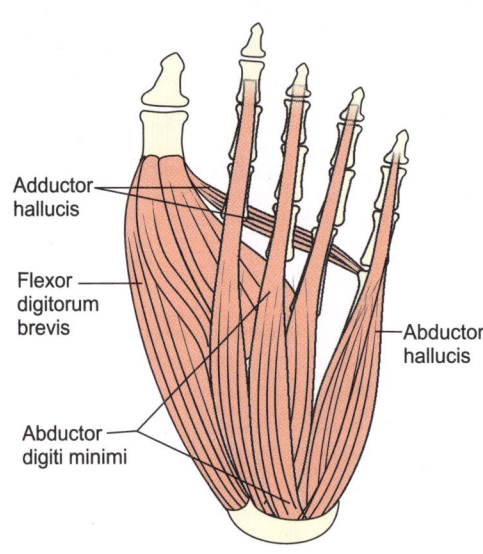

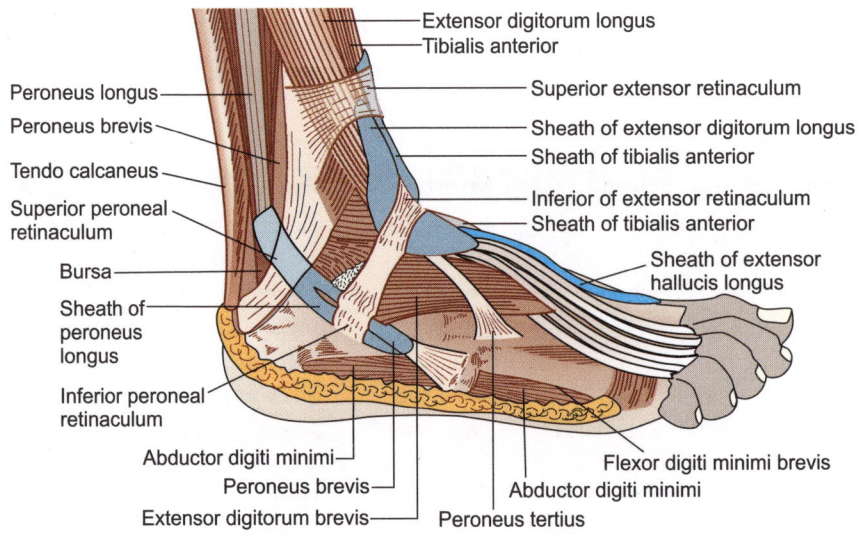

Figure 4.26 Muscles that move the toes.

DISORDERS ASSOCIATED WITH THE MUSCULAR SYSTEM

MYASTHENIA GRAVIS

Myasthenia gravis is an autoimmune disorder that causes chronic, progressive damage to the neuromuscular junction. The antibodies produced by the immune system bind to and block some ACh receptors, thereby decreasing the number of functional acetylcholine receptors at the motor end plate of skeletal muscles.

Symptoms include progressive and extensive muscle weakness that initially affects eye muscles causing diplopia (double vision), followed by affecting muscles of the neck leading to difficulty in chewing, swallowing and speech and eventually affecting the limbs. Death may result from paralysis of respiratory muscles.

Treatment involves mainly the use of anticholinesterase drugs such as pyridostigmine and neostigmine.

MUSCULAR DYSTROPHY

It refers to a group of inherited diseases that cause progressive degeneration of skeletal muscles. The most common form of muscular dystrophy is Duchenne muscular dystrophy or DMD. In this condition, the gene that codes for the dystrophin protein is mutated on the X chromosome of female carriers. The disorder is present before birth but usually becomes apparent between the ages of 2 and 5 years.

Symptoms include weakness of the muscles of the lower and upper limbs, which leads to difficulty in running, walking and jumping. Death may occur due to respiratory failure, cardiac arrhythmia or cardiomyopathy.

Treatment involves gene therapy by inducing the protein utrophin, which is similar to dystrophin.

CRUSH SYNDROME

It is characterized by massive muscle necrosis due to sustained pressure on the trunk or limbs. When circulation is restored after pressure is relieved, the damaged muscle releases myoglobin and other necrotic products that are highly toxic to the kidneys and may eventually cause acute renal failure.

ABNORMAL CONTRACTIONS OF SKELETAL MUSCLES

1. **Spasm:** It is a sudden involuntary contraction of a single muscle in a large group of muscles.
2. **Cramp**: It is a painful spasmodic contraction due to inadequate blood flow to muscles, dehydration or injury.
3. **Tremor**: It is rhythmic, involuntary contractions that produce shaking movements.

MYOSITIS

It is the inflammation of muscular tissue.

Chapter 4

MYALGIA

It is the pain associated with muscles. In this condition there is pain, tenderness and stiffness of muscles, tendons and the surrounding soft tissues.

Treatment consists of regular exercise, application of heat, gentle massage and medication for pain relief.

MUSCLE ATROPHY AND HYPERTROPHY

Atrophy is the decrease in the size of muscles due to the lack of exercise or immobility for prolonged periods. In severe cases, the muscle fibres are lost and replaced with connective tissues.

Hypertrophy (opposite of atrophy) is the increase in the size of muscles due to exercises like weightlifting.

OVERVIEW OF THE MUSCULAR SYSTEM

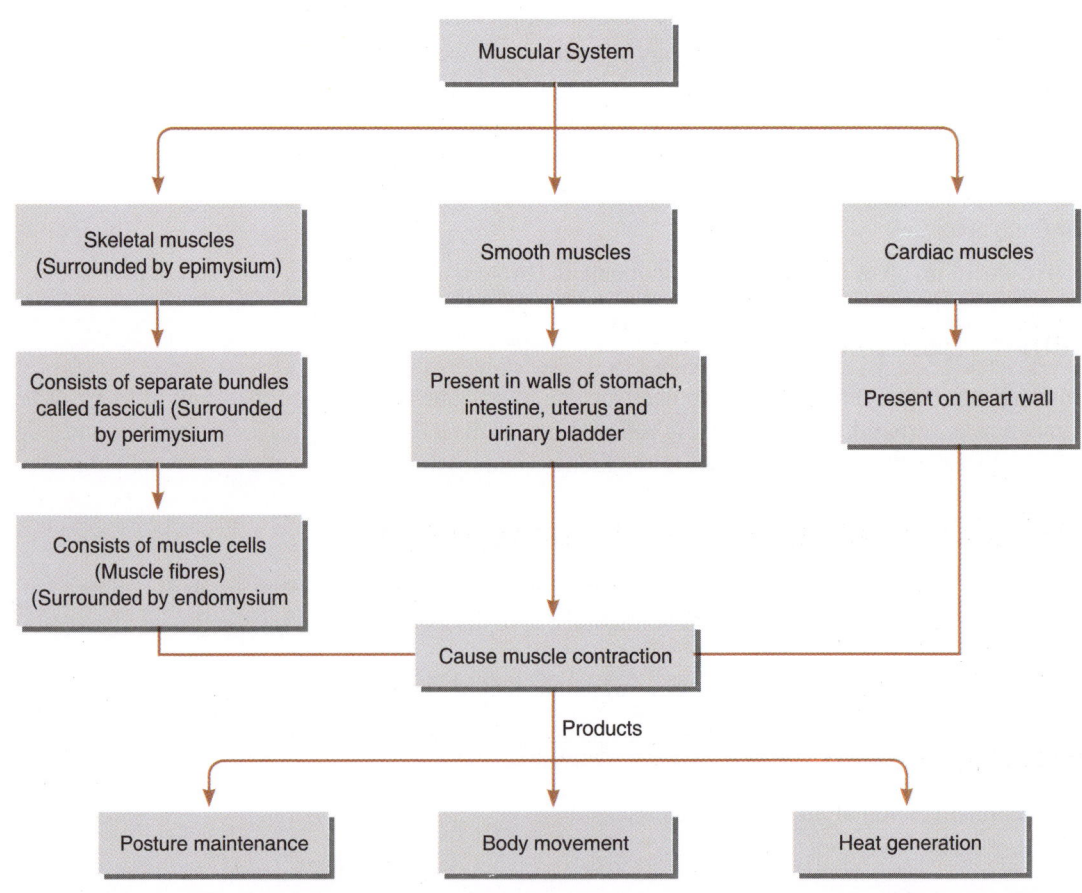

Ageing and the Muscular System

❏ With age, the skeletal muscle mass is progressively and slowly replaced by fibrous connective tissue and adipose tissue, which leads to decrease in muscle strength, slowing of muscle reflexes and loss of flexibility.

❏ In addition, with ageing, the slow red muscle fibres begin to increase. This could be due to either atrophy of other type of muscles fibres or limited physical activity.

❏ Thus, elderly are encouraged to include certain aerobic activities in their daily routine, which can slow down or even reverse the age-associated decline in muscular performance.

Embryonic Development of the Muscular System

❏ All muscles in the body (except iris of the eyes and arrector pili attached to the hair) develop from *mesoderm*.

❏ A part of the developing mesoderm arranges in dense columns on either side of the nervous system and forms cube-shaped structures called *somites*.

❏ End of 5th week: Somites → Give rise to skeletal muscles

Cells of somites differentiate into the following three regions:

1. Myotome → Forms skeletal muscles of the head, neck and limbs
2. Dermatome → Forms connective tissue
3. Sclerotome → Forms vertebrae

❏ Mesodermal cells that migrate towards developing heart → Form cardiac muscle

❏ Mesodermal cells that migrate towards developing GIT and viscera → Form smooth muscle

Exercise and Skeletal Muscle Tissue

❏ Various types of exercises induce different changes in skeletal muscle fibres.

❏ Aerobic exercises like running or swimming increase the diameter, strength, number of mitochondria and blood supply in the fast muscle fibres. These exercises also result in cardiovascular (increase heart beat) and respiratory changes (increase breathing) that adapt the skeletal muscles to receive more oxygen and nutrients but does not increase muscle mass.

❏ Regular exercise improves the speed of muscle contraction and relaxation, improving muscle performance.

❏ Exercises that require greater strength for short periods produce an increase in size of muscles by increasing the synthesis of thick and thin filaments. This results in muscle enlargement, as evident in the bulging muscles of body builders.

Chapter 4

TIPS TO MAINTAIN THE MUSCULAR SYSTEM

Keep Your Muscles Healthy with Proper Nutrition

1. Have lots of whole grains (whole-grain bread, oatmeal and brown rice) to keep muscles healthy.
2. Include dairy products such as milk, cheese and yoghurt in diet as they are rich in calcium and aid in healthy bones.
3. Drink more water to keep your muscles strong and avoid soft drinks.
4. Eat plenty of fruits and vegetables as they are full of vitamins and minerals, including iron, calcium and vitamin D.

Keep Your Muscles Healthy with Exercise

1. Warming up before exercise by stretching increases flexibility and reduces the risk of muscle pulls and other injuries.
2. Cardiovascular exercises like running, walking, swimming and sports keep the heart active and healthy.
3. Exercises should be changed often and should include all muscle groups in different combinations as the same exercise routine decreases effectiveness dramatically.
4. It is very essential to cool down after exercise as it helps bring the heart down to its resting rate and avoids muscle cramping.

Review Questions

Long Answer Questions

1. Describe the classification and functions of muscle tissue.
2. Why do skeletal and cardiac muscle fibres appear striated?
3. Describe the fine structure (electron micrograph) of a skeletal muscle fibre.
4. Explain the sequence of events in muscle contraction.
5. Describe the neuromuscular junction.
6. List the sequence of events occurring at the neuromuscular junction.
7. Distinguish between isotonic and isometric contractions.
8. List the muscles of facial expression, eyes and head.
9. List the muscles that move the vertebral column.
10. Discuss the muscles present in femur.

Multiple Choice Questions

1. Muscle fibres characterized by lack of striations, a single centrally located nucleus in each cell and involuntary contractions are referred to as
   - (a) Skeletal muscle fibres
   - (b) Smooth muscle fibres
   - (c) Cardiac muscle fibres
   - (d) Autonomic muscle fibres

2. The anisotropic dark bands of muscle fibres are called
   - (a) Z bands
   - (b) I bands
   - (c) A bands
   - (d) D bands

3. The structural unit of the myofibril is
   - (a) The myofibril
   - (b) Myosin
   - (c) The A band
   - (d) The sarcomere

4. Muscle contraction is produced by shortening of all the following *except*
   - (a) Myofibrils
   - (b) Sarcomeres
   - (c) A bands
   - (d) I bands

5. Muscle contraction is initiated when
   - (a) Ca^{2+} binds to the troponin
   - (b) Actin is removed from troponin
   - (c) Actin is made available to troponin
   - (d) Ca^{2+} is removed from the troponin

6. The source of Ca^{2+} for the muscle is
   - (a) The T tubule
   - (b) The central sac
   - (c) The terminal cisternae
   - (d) The sarcoplasmic reticulum

7. In a relaxed muscle,
   - (a) Tropomyosin blocks the attachment of myosin heads to actin
   - (b) The concentration of sarcoplasmic Ca^{2+} is low
   - (c) Tropomyosin is moved out of the way so that the myosin heads can attach to actin
   - (d) Myosin ATPase is activated

8. A single motor neuron and all the skeletal muscle fibres it innervates constitute
   - (a) A motor unit
   - (b) A muscle triad
   - (c) A sarcounit
   - (d) A neuromuscular junction

9. A muscle that develops tension against some load but that does not shorten is undergoing
   - (a) Isometric contraction
   - (b) Isotonic contraction
   - (c) Neither (a) nor (b)
   - (d) Both (a) and (b)

10. Troponin is a protein that
    - (a) Is bound to myosin to form a complex that is normally inhibited in the resting muscle fibre
    - (b) Forms the binding site for the myosin heads when they attach to actin
    - (c) Has a high affinity for calcium ions
    - (d) Contains numerous molecules of ADP

Match the Following

1.	Occipitalis (unpaired)	(a)	Adducts the thumb
2.	Frontalis (unpaired)	(b)	Abducts and extends the fingers
3.	Zygomaticus	(c)	Draws scalp backwards
4.	Levator labii superioris	(d)	Raises eyebrows and wrinkles skin of forehead
5.	Levator palpebrae superioris	(e)	Involved in smiling and laughing
6.	Pterygoid	(f)	Raises the upper lip
7.	Superior rectus	(g)	Raises the eyelid
8.	Trapezius	(h)	Closes the mouth and pulls the lower jaw forward
9.	Pectoralis major	(i)	Moves eyeball upwards
10.	Brachialis	(j)	Pulls head backwards and rotates scapula
11.	Anconeus	(k)	Flexes and adducts (i.e. draws the arm forward and towards the body)
12.	Palmarus longus	(l)	Main flexor of the elbow joint
13.	Supinator	(m)	Extends the forearm
14.	Adductor pollicis	(n)	Flexes the wrist joint
15.	Dorsal interossei	(o)	Supinates the forearm

State True or False

1. Muscle tissues account for approximately 40% of a person's weight.
2. Actin is found only in the striated fibres of cardiac and skeletal muscle tissues.
3. Slow-twitch muscle fibres are more resistant to fatigue than the other muscle fibre types.
4. Fasciculi are enclosed in a covering of perimysium.
5. A sarcomere is the region of a myofibril that lies between two consecutive Z lines.
6. An action potential in a muscle fibre is initiated by stimulation across the neuromuscular junction.
7. Sustained contractions of skeletal muscle is known as tetanus.
8. Fast-twitch muscle fibres are primarily used in endurance activities.
9. A muscle triad consists of a sarcoplasmic reticulum, a T tubule and a terminal cisternum.
10. A motor unit consists of a single motor neuron and the muscle fibres it innervates.
11. Lifting a dumbbell is an example of isometric contraction.
12. Thin myofilaments are primarily composed of myosin proteins.
13. An accumulation of lactic acid is the principal cause of sore muscles.
14. To initiate muscle contraction, calcium ions bind to and change the shape of the troponin protein molecules, which then pull the tropomyosin proteins off the myosin binding sites of the actin helix.

15. Synergistic muscles work together to perform a certain motion or action. Antagonistic muscles work in opposition to another group of muscles.

16. The strength of a muscle contraction is increased by recruiting more muscle fibres within a motor unit.

17. During muscle contraction, the I bands get smaller and the Z lines get closer together, but the A bands do not change in size.

18. The energy provided by ATP molecules allows the myosin head to bind to the exposed binding site on the actin molecule.

19. The transverse tubules (T tubules) store calcium ions needed for muscle contraction.

20. A tendon is a structure that binds the fascia of a muscle to the periosteum of a bone.

Fill in the Blanks

1. The three muscles involved in respiration are_____ and _____.

2. The _____ muscle can open the mouth or elevate the hyoid bone.

3. Sustained contractions of the skeletal muscle are known as _____.

4. Thin myofilaments are composed of _____ proteins.

5. _____is the region of the myofibril that lies between two consecutive Z lines.

Careers in the Muscular System

✓ Physicians can specialize in sports-related problems and sports medicine and treat various injuries of muscles, bones and joints.

✓ Massage therapists increase the blood circulation to the muscles by manipulating them through stroking, kneading and rubbing. This manipulation brings relaxation to the patient and improves the muscle tone.

Chapter 4

5   The Nervous System

CHAPTER OUTLINE

- Overview of the Nervous System
- Histology of Nervous Tissue
- The Physiology of Nerve Impulse
- The Synaptic Transmission
- Response of Nervous Tissue to Injury

- Brain
- Spinal Cord
- The Autonomic Nervous System
- The Pain Pathway
- Disorders Associated with the Nervous System

STUDY OBJECTIVES

- ✓ To describe the structure and basic functions of the nervous system.
- ✓ To discuss the organization of the nervous system.
- ✓ To describe the structure and classification of neurons and discuss the characteristics of neuroglia and the significance of myelination.
- ✓ To discuss the transmission of impulses in the neurons and describe the events of signal transmission at synapse.
- ✓ To identify the principal parts of the brain and discuss how the brain is protected.

- ✓ To describe the flow of cerebrospinal fluid in the brain and to discuss the various functions of cerebrospinal fluid.
- ✓ To describe the blood supply to brain.
- ✓ To outline the sensory and motor areas of the cerebrum and discuss the functions of cerebrum.
- ✓ To discuss the location and functions of various areas of cerebral cortex and describe the components and functions of diencephalon and brain stem.
- ✓ To outline the functions of 12 cranial nerves.
- ✓ To describe the anatomy and physiology of spinal cord.
- ✓ To explain the events of a reflex arc and discuss various spinal nerves.

INTRODUCTION

The nervous system is the communication network and control centre of the body. It detects the changes occurring in the internal and external environment and then responds by directing the functions of the body's organs and systems.

The nervous system and the endocrine system share the responsibility for maintaining homeostasis and controlling important aspects of the body function, but their means of achieving this objective differ. The nervous system stimulation provides immediate response to the stimuli by transmitting nerve impulses, whereas the endocrine response of releasing hormones is slower and more prolonged.

The study of normal functioning and disorders of the nervous system is known as *neurology*.

OVERVIEW OF THE NERVOUS SYSTEM

The nervous system is the most complicated and highly organized of the various systems that make up the human body. It is mainly involved in the correlation and integration of various bodily processes and the adjustment with the environment.

The nervous system contains a network of specialized cells called neurons that transmit the signals between different parts of the body. The various structures that make up the nervous system include the brain, cranial nerves and their branches, the spinal cord, the spinal nerves and their branches, and sensory receptors (Fig. 5.1).

DO YOU KNOW

- The human brain alone consists of about a 100 billion neurons and if all these neurons were to be lined up, it would form a 600-mile-long line.
- In humans, the right side of the brain controls the left side of the body, whereas the left side of the brain controls the right side.
- In a child developing inside the womb, neurons grow at the rate of 250,000 neurons per minute.
- A newborn baby's brain grows almost three times during the course of its first year.
- The weight of the brain in average adult males is 1375 g, whereas in females it is 1275 g.
- The nervous system is very quick; it can transmit impulses at a tremendous speed of 100 m/s. The speed of message transmission to the brain can be as high as 180 miles/h .
- When we touch something, we send a message to our brain at 124 m/h.
- Of all the cells in the human brain, we use only about 4%, keeping the remaining 96% as reserve.

MEDICAL TERMINOLOGY

- **Adipose tissue**: It is a kind of body tissue containing stored fat.
- **Anoxia**: It is a condition characterized by the absence of oxygen.
- **Ascending tract**: It conducts impulses up towards the spinal cord.
- **Atrophy**: It is a decrease in size of an organ caused by disease or disuse.
- **Convolution**: It is a form or part that is folded or coiled.
- **Degeneration**: It is a process by which a tissue deteriorates, loses functional activity and may become converted into or replaced by other kinds of tissue.
- **Dendrites**: They are the branched projections of a neuron.
- **Descending tract**: It conducts impulses down the spinal cord.
- **Foramen magnum**: It is the large opening at the base of the cranium through which the spinal cord passes.
- **Ganglia**: They are nerve cell bodies that group together outside the CNS.
- **Homeostasis**: It is the body's ability to physiologically regulate its inner environment to ensure its stability in response to fluctuations in the outside environment and the weather.
- **Hypoglycaemia**: It is the condition of abnormally low blood sugar.
- **Hypoxia**: It is a condition characterized by oxygen deficiency.
- **Multiple sclerosis**: it is a chronic progressive nervous disorder involving loss of myelin sheath around certain nerve fibres.
- **Necrosis**: It is the localized death of living cells.

The brain is housed within the skull and contains about 100 billion neurons. Twelve pairs of cranial nerves (right and left), numbered I to XII, emerge from the base of the brain. The spinal cord is lodged in the vertebral canal and is connected to the brain through the foramen magnum of the skull. Thirty-one pairs of spinal nerves emerge from the spinal cord, and each one of them serves a specific region on the right or left side of the body. These spinal nerves and cranial nerves are collectively termed as *cerebrospinal nerves* and are associated with the functions of special and general senses and with the voluntary movements of the body.

The sensory receptors are either specialized cells or the dendrites of sensory neurons and have a role in monitoring changes in the internal and external environment of the body.

FUNCTIONS OF THE NERVOUS SYSTEM

The basic functions of the nervous system include the following:

1. **Neural signalling**: At the most basic level, the function of the nervous system is to send signals from one cell to another or from one part of the body to another. The neurons project their axons to specific target areas and make synaptic connections with specific target cells. This neural signalling is highly specific and fast.

   The fastest nerve signal travels at a speed of more than 100 m/s.

2. **Integrative function**: The major function of the nervous system is to control the body, which it does with the help of sensory receptors that detect the internal or external stimuli. The sensory neurons

---

MEDICAL TERMINOLOGY

- ❏ **Nerve impulse**: It is the electrical discharge that travels along a nerve fibre.
- ❏ **Neuron**: It is a cell that is specialized to conduct nerve impulses.
- ❏ **Phagocyte**: A cell, such as a white blood cell, that engulfs and absorbs waste material, harmful microorganisms or other foreign bodies in the bloodstream and tissues.
- ❏ **Pineal gland**: It is an endocrine gland that secretes melatonin, which affects our mood and behaviour.
- ❏ **Protrusion**: It is something that bulges out.
- ❏ **Regeneration**: It is the process of growth anew of lost tissue or destroyed parts or an organ.
- ❏ **Rough endoplasmic reticulum**: It is a subcellular structure in the cytoplasm of a cell where proteins destined for export are assembled.
- ❏ **Synapse**: It is the junction between two neurons (axon to dendrite) or between a neuron and a muscle.
- ❏ **Tract**: It is a bundle of nerve fibres inside the CNS.
- ❏ **Trauma**: It is a serious injury or shock to the body.
- ❏ **Vertebral foramina**: It is the opening formed by a neural arch through which the spinal cord passes.
- ❏ **Visceral organs**: They are the internal organs of the body, specifically those within the chest (as the heart or lungs) or abdomen (as the liver, pancreas or intestines).
- ❏ **Voluntary movement**: It is the movement directed by the person's willpower.

Chapter 5

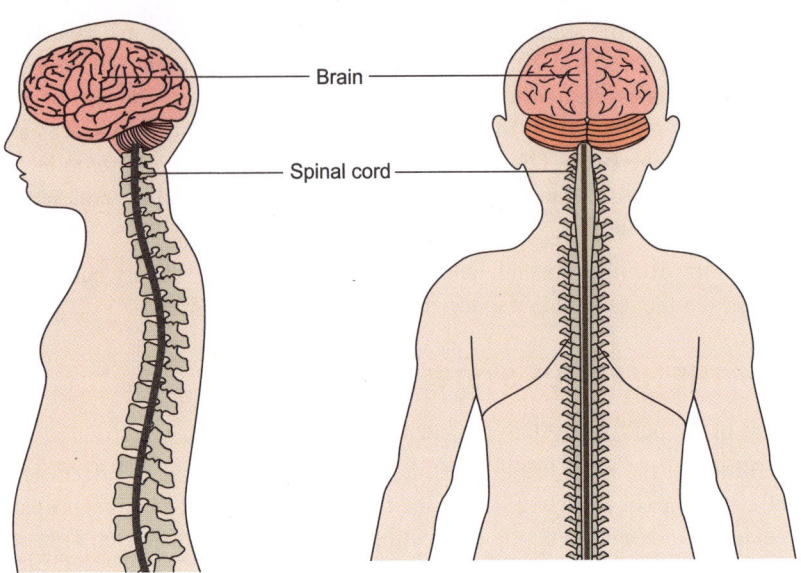

Figure 5.1 Overview of the brain and the spinal cord.

then send these signals to the central nervous system (CNS) where the information is processed and the output signals are sent to muscle/glands to activate the response.

Thus, the nervous system integrates sensory information and makes decisions regarding the appropriate response to a particular stimulus.

3. **Perception**: The nervous system is responsible for advanced perception abilities such as vision, coordination of organ systems and complex social interactions. The various features of human society that exist presently would not exist without the sophistication of the human brain.

Neurons that carry information from sensory receptors to the brain and spinal cord are called *sensory/afferent neurons*. The neurons that carry information out of the brain and spinal cord are called *motor/efferent neurons*.

ORGANIZATION OF THE NERVOUS SYSTEM

The nervous system can be grouped into the following two major categories (Fig. 5.2):

I. Central nervous system (CNS)

The central nervous system is the control centre consisting of the brain and spinal cord.

The CNS integrates and correlates the sensory information coming from receptors and sensory organs and is also the source of thoughts, emotions and memories.

II. Peripheral nervous system

The peripheral nervous system (PNS) consists of all the nerves outside the brain and spinal cord that connect with sensory receptors, muscles and glands.

The PNS can be subdivided into the following two subcategories:

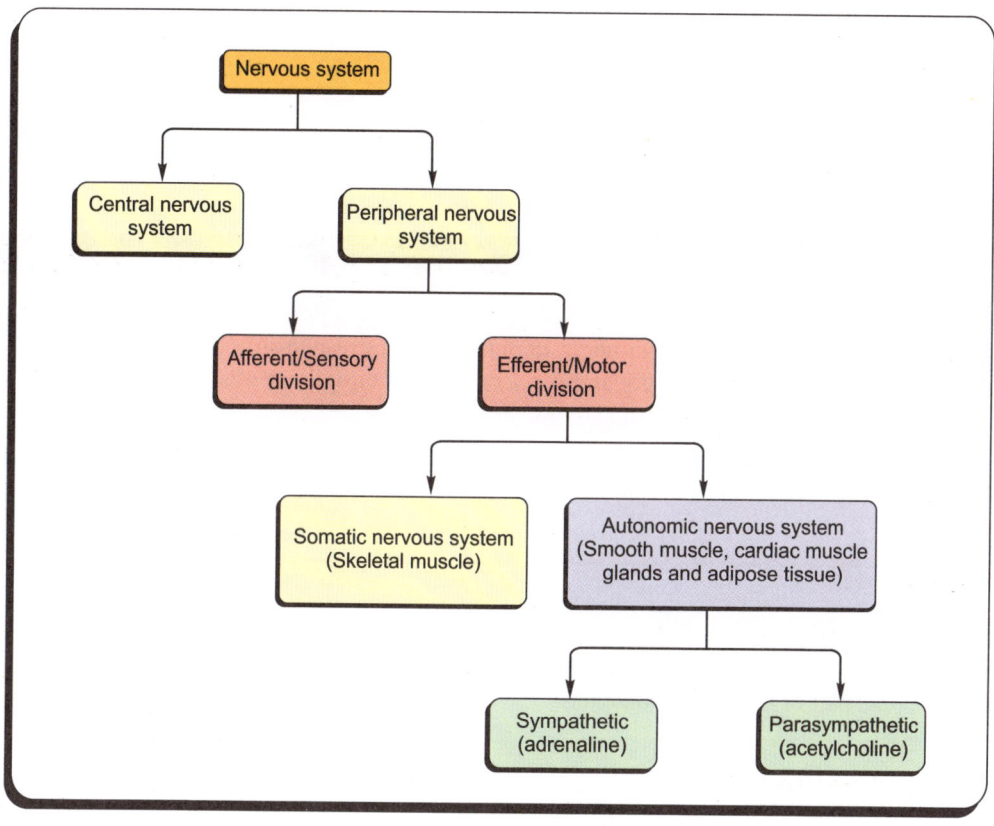

Figure 5.2 Organization of the nervous system.

(a) Somatic nervous system

The somatic nervous system (SNS) consists of the following:

1. Sensory or afferent neurons that convey information from the skin, skeletal muscles and joints to the CNS.
2. Motor/efferent neurons that conduct impulses from the brain and spinal cord to skeletal muscles only. These motor responses can be consciously controlled and play an important role in responding towards change in the external environment. The motor response of the SNS is voluntary.

(b) Autonomic nervous system

The autonomic nervous system (ANS) consists of the following:

1. Sensory or afferent neurons that convey information from the visceral organs to the CNS.
2. Motor neurons that conduct impulses from the brain and spinal cord to smooth muscle (like the intestinal smooth muscles push food through digestive tract), cardiac muscle of the heart, glands and adipose tissue. Since the motor responses of ANS are not under conscious control normally, the action of this part is considered to be involuntary.

Chapter 5

ANS has the following two divisions:

1. Sympathetic
2. Parasympathetic

The sympathetic division (neurotransmitter–adrenaline) and the parasympathetic division (acetyl-choline as neurotransmitter) have opposing actions.

HISTOLOGY OF NERVOUS TISSUE

The nervous tissue consists of two types of cells: *neurons* and *neuroglia*. Neurons are the group of nerve cells that transmit information through nerve impulses and are responsible for special functions like thinking, remembering and regulating glandular secretions. Neuroglia or glial cells constitute 60% of all brain cells, and they support, nourish and protect the neurons.

The neurons cannot divide, and for survival, they need a continuous supply of oxygen and glucose, but neuroglia continue to replicate throughout life.

NEURONS

The neurons have the property of electrical excitability and conductivity. Electrical excitability is the ability to initiate nerve impulses in response to stimuli, and conductivity is the ability to transmit the impulse from one part of the body to another.

Structure of neurons

The neurons have three parts: cell body, dendrites and an axon (Fig. 5.3).

The dendrites and axon are the nerve fibres in the nerve cell.

The cell body contains a single nucleus surrounded by the cytoplasm (soma), which includes organelles such as mitochondria, Golgi bodies, lysosomes and a network of threads called *neurofibrils* that extend into the axon part of the cell. The cell body also contains clusters of rough endoplasmic reticulum (ER), which are referred to as Nissl bodies.

The cell bodies form the *grey matter* of the nervous system and are found at the periphery of the brain.

There are two kinds of nerve fibres on the nerve cell: dendrites and axons. These nerve fibres are the extension of the cell bodies and form the *white matter* of the nervous system.

Dendrites are the short and branched extensions of the cell body (like trees) that receive and carry the incoming impulses towards cell bodies.

The second kind of nerve fibres is the *axons*, which carry the nerve impulses away from the cell body. They are usually longer than dendrites, sometimes as long as 100 cm. An axon is a single long extension that begins as a slight enlargement of the cell body called *axonal hillock*. The cytoplasm in the axon, called *axoplasm*, is surrounded by a plasma membrane known as *axolemma*. An axon contains numerous mitochondria and neurofibrils but does not contain rough ER; thus, protein synthesis does not occur in the axon.

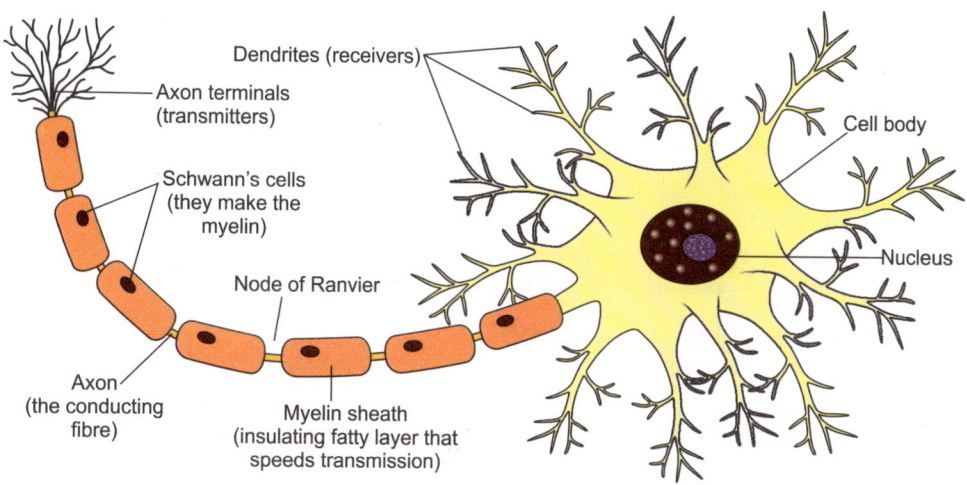

Dendrites (receivers)
Axon terminals (transmitters)
Schwann's cells (they make the myelin)
Node of Ranvier
Axon (the conducting fibre)
Myelin sheath (insulating fatty layer that speeds transmission)
Cell body
Nucleus

Figure 5.3 Structure of a neuron.

The axon begins singly but may branch, and it has many fine extensions at its end called *axon terminals* that contact with the dendrites of other neurons. The site of communication between two neurons is called a *synapse*.

The large peripheral neurons are surrounded by the myelin sheath produced by the Schwann cells (neuroglia). This myelin sheath consists of a series of Schwann cells arranged along the length of the axon that produce fatty sheets of lipoprotein called *myelin*.

The outermost layer of the Schwann cell plasma membrane is called *neurilemma*. There are some narrow gaps in the myelin sheaths, called *nodes of Ranvier*, which help in the rapid transmission of nerve impulses in myelinated neurons.

Classification of neurons

Neurons display great diversity in size, shape and functions. They can be classified on the basis of structural and functional features.

Structural classification of neurons

Structurally, neurons can be classified into the following three types (Fig. 5.4):

1. **Multipolar neurons** are neurons having several dendrites and one axon. Most neurons in the brain and spinal cord are of this type.
2. **Bipolar neurons** have one dendrite and one axon, and they function as receptor cells in special sense organs. They are found in only three areas of the body: the retina of the eye, the inner ear and the olfactory area of the nose.
3. **Unipolar neurons** have only one extension from the cell body. This single extension divides into two branches: a central branch that functions as an axon and a peripheral branch that functions as a dendrite. Most sensory neurons are unipolar neurons. The central branch (axon) enters the brain or spinal cord, and the peripheral branch (dendrite) connects to the peripheral part of the body.

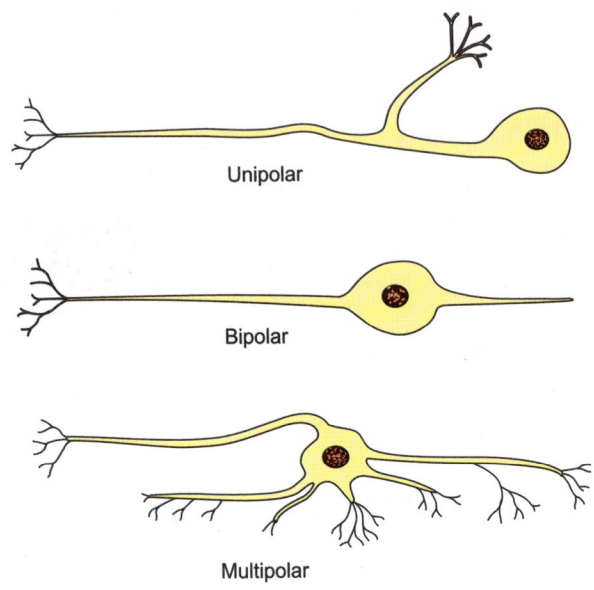

Unipolar

Bipolar

Multipolar

Figure 5.4 Types of neuron.

Functional classification of neurons

Functionally, neurons can be classified into the following three types:

1. **Sensory/afferent neurons**: As discussed previously in the organization of the nervous system, these nerves transmit the impulses from the peripheral parts of the body to the brain and spinal cord (Fig. 5.5). These neurons are unipolar in nature.

    Different stimuli (changes) inside and outside the body stimulate the sensory receptors (i.e. the specialized endings of the sensory neurons), which then transmit the impulses to the spinal cord and brain through the sensory nerve fibres.

2. **Motor/efferent neurons**: The motor nerves originate in the brain and spinal cord and they transmit the impulses to the effector organs (i.e. muscle and glands) (Fig. 5.5). The motor neuron is of the multipolar type, and it is responsible for bringing out the response to the original stimulus.

    There are two types of motor neurons:

    (a) *Somatic nerves*: They are involved in skeletal muscle contraction.

    (b) *Autonomic nerves (sympathetic and parasympathetic)*: They are involved in cardiac and smooth muscle contraction and glandular secretion.

3. **Mixed neurons**: In the spinal cord, sensory and motor nerves are arranged in separate groups or tracts. However, outside the spinal cord, when the sensory and motor nerves are enclosed within the same sheath of connective tissue, they are called *mixed nerves*.

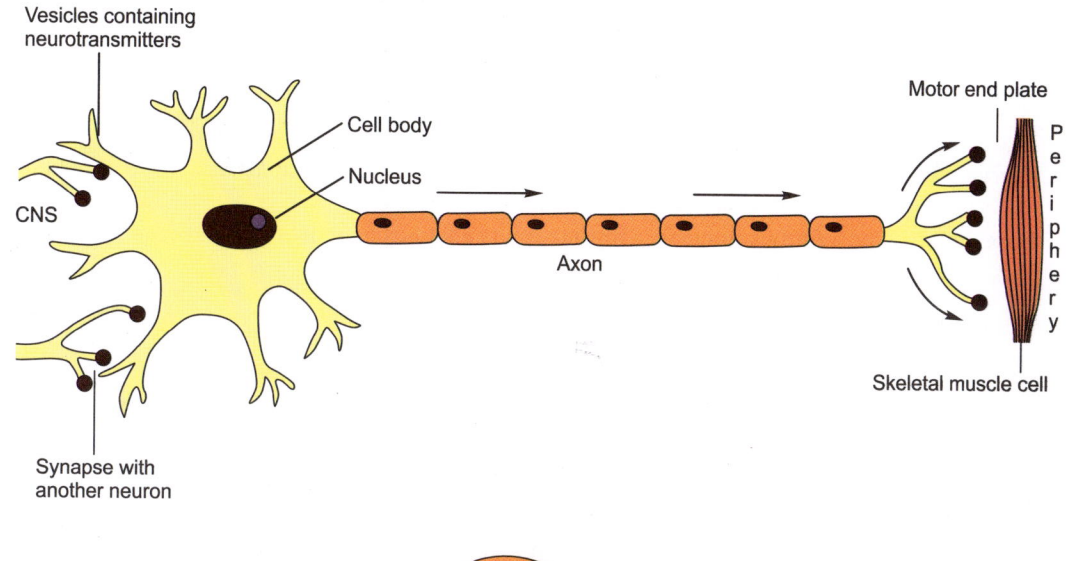

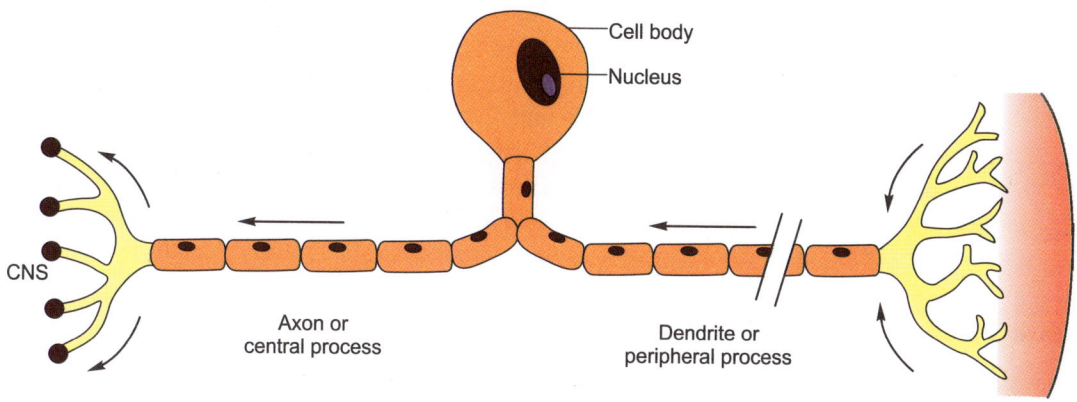

Figure 5.5 (a) Motor neuron; (b) Sensory neuron.

SENSORY RECEPTORS

Sensory receptors respond to different types of stimuli, such as:

1. Cutaneous, which originates in the skin due to pain, touch, heat and cold.
2. Proprioceptor, which originates in muscles and joints and is responsible for the maintenance of balance and posture.
3. Special senses, i.e. sight, hearing, balance, smell and taste.

Connective tissue coverings of nerves

Each nerve consists of numerous nerve fibres collected into bundles. Each nerve bundle has protective coverings of connective tissue as follows:

1. **Endoneurium (innermost layer)**: It is a delicate tissue that surrounds each nerve fibre.
2. **Perineurium (middle layer)**: The nerves are arranged in bundles called *fascicles*, and each bundle of nerve fibre (fascicle) is wrapped in perineurium.
3. **Epineurium**: It is a fibrous tissue that surrounds and encloses a number of bundles of nerve fibres. This is the outermost covering over the entire nerve.

Myelination

The axons of most mammalian neurons are surrounded by a multilayered lipid and protein covering called the *myelin sheath* that is produced by neuroglia. The sheath increases the speed of nerve impulse conduction. Axons with such covering are said to be myelinated, whereas those without the covering are unmyelinated.

Two types of neuroglia produce myelin sheaths, which are as follows:

1. **Schwann cells**: They produce myelin sheath around nerves in the PNS.
2. **Oligodendrocytes**: They produce and maintain myelin sheath around nerves in the CNS.

   ❏ The amount of myelin sheath increases from birth to maturity and its presence greatly increases the speed of nerve impulse conduction. An impulse on a myelinated nerve fibre can travel about 120 m/s, whereas on an unmyelinated fibre it would travel only 0.5 m/s.
   ❏ The conduction of nerve impulse in unmyelinated fibre is slower than that along myelinated fibre. As the myelinated fibre is insulated by the myelin sheath, the impulse jumps from node to node, and this fast conduction from one node to the next is called saltatory conduction.

NEUROGLIA

Neuroglia or glial cells constitute about half the volume of the CNS. They hold the nervous tissue together and have an active role in the operation of the nervous system. Generally, neuroglia are smaller than neurons and are 5–50 times more in number. In case of injury or disease, they multiply to fill in the spaces formerly occupied by neurons.

There are five different types of neuroglia, which are as follows (Fig. 5.6):

1. **Astrocytes**
   ❏ They are star-shaped cells that wrap around the nerve cells and serve as the major supporting tissue of the CNS. They provide nutrients to the neurons and help in maintaining the appropriate chemical environment for the generation of nerve impulse by maintaining the proper balance of Ca^+ and K^+ ions.
   ❏ They also help in the formation of the blood–brain barrier (BBB).
2. **Oligodendrocytes**: These cells are smaller than astrocytes and form a supporting network around CNS neurons. They produce and maintain myelin sheath (for insulation) on the neurons in the brain and spinal cord, and they have a similar function as Schwann cells in peripheral nerves.
3. **Microglia**: These are small cells derived from monocytes that migrate from the blood into the nervous system before birth. They protect CNS cells from disease by engulfing the invading microbes and clear away the debris of dead cells.

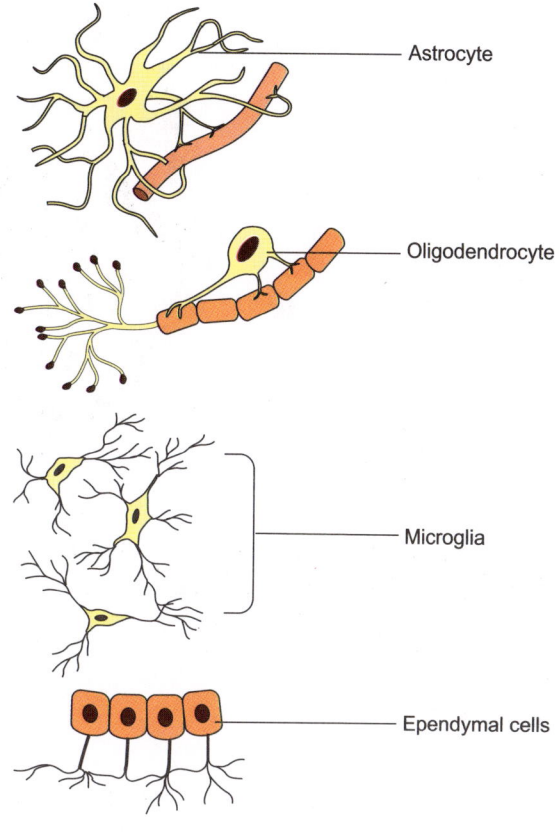

Figure 5.6 Neuroglial cells of the CNS.

4. **Ependymal cells**: These cells form the epithelial lining of the ventricles of the brain. They produce cerebrospinal fluid (CSF) and help in its circulation.
5. **Schwann cells**: They form myelin sheaths around nerve fibres in the PNS.

GREY AND WHITE MATTER

Some white and grey regions are observed in a freshly dissected section of the brain and spinal cord. The white matter/region is the collection of the myelinated neurons, and it appears whitish due to the white colour of the myelin. The grey matter of the nervous system contains cell bodies of neurons, dendrites, unmyelinated axons and neuroglia. It looks greyish due to the absence of myelin in these areas.

In the spinal cord, the white matter surrounds the inner core of the grey matter like the letter H/ butterfly, as shown in Figure 5.7. Thus, in the spinal cord, grey matter is inside and white matter is outside, whereas in the brain it is mostly the reverse.

In brain, a thin shell of grey matter covers the surface of the brain's largest portion, namely the cerebrum and the cerebellum.

Chapter 5

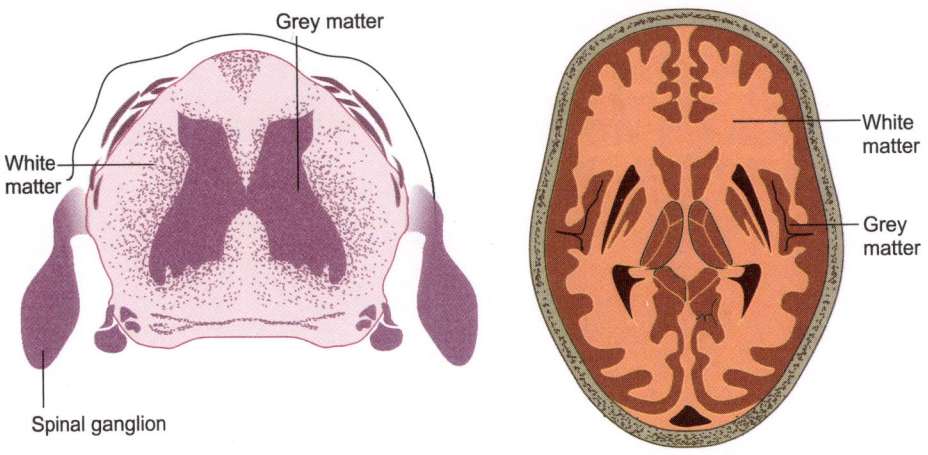

Figure 5.7 Grey and white matter in the spinal cord and brain.

THE PHYSIOLOGY OF NERVE IMPULSE (ACTION POTENTIAL)

Nerve impulse is a self-propagating wave that moves down the nerve fibre. A nerve impulse or action potential is initiated by the stimulation of sensory receptors that further stimulates sensory nerves. This impulse or action potential is then transmitted to another nerve due to the movement of ions across the nerve cell membrane.

Similar to the muscle cell, the nerve cell has ion concentration inside and outside the cell membrane. Positively charged Na^+ ions are in greater concentration outside the cell, whereas K^+ ions are more concentrated inside the cell. This situation is maintained by the cell membrane's Na^+–K^+ pump.

In addition to the K^+ ions, nerve cell consists of negatively charged (Cl^-) ions and other negatively charged organic molecules. Thus, at the resting condition, the charge is positive outside and negative inside.

There are three phases of membrane potential in the nerves, which are as follows (Fig. 5.8):

1. **Resting phase**
   - ❑ In this phase, there is a different electrical charge on each side of the membrane, which is called the *resting membrane potential*.
   - ❑ In this condition, the outside is positively charged (Na^+), whereas the inside is negatively charged (K^+ and Cl^-).

2. **Depolarization phase**
   - ❑ When the nerve is stimulated, the permeability of the nerve cell membrane to Na^+ ions changes. The Na^+ ion rushes inside, causing a change from negative to positive charge inside the nerve membrane. This reversal of electrical charge is called *depolarization*, which creates a nerve impulse or action potential (Fig. 5.9).
   - ❑ This depolarization is very rapid and the nerve impulse is conducted in one direction along the entire length of the neuron in a few milliseconds (ms).

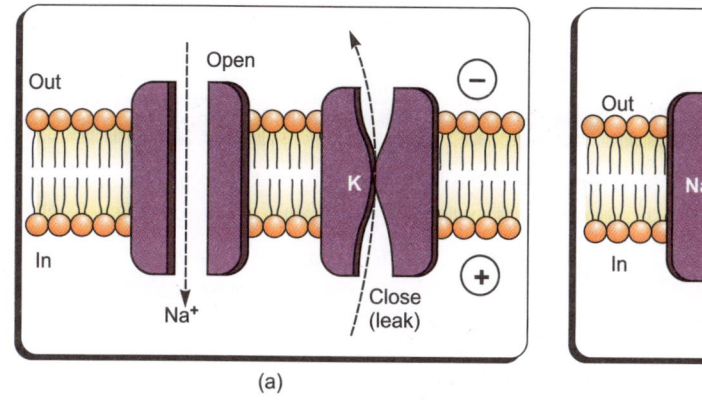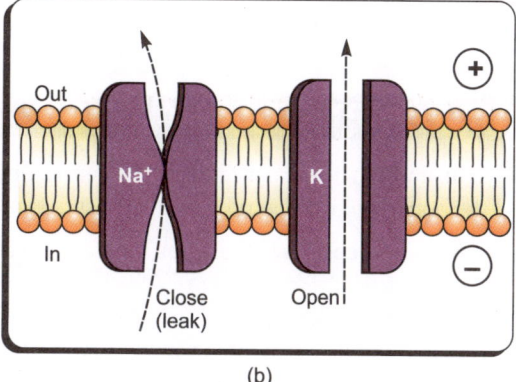

Figure 5.8 Phases of membrane potential in nerves.

3. **Repolarization phase/refractory period**

   ❏ After action potential, the K⁺ ions begin to move outside to restore the resting membrane potential. This is called the *refractory phase* and re-stimulation is not possible during this period.

   ❏ After this phase, the Na⁺–K⁺ pump begins to function, expelling Na⁺ from the cell in exchange of K⁺ ions; thus, the neuron returns to its original resting state.

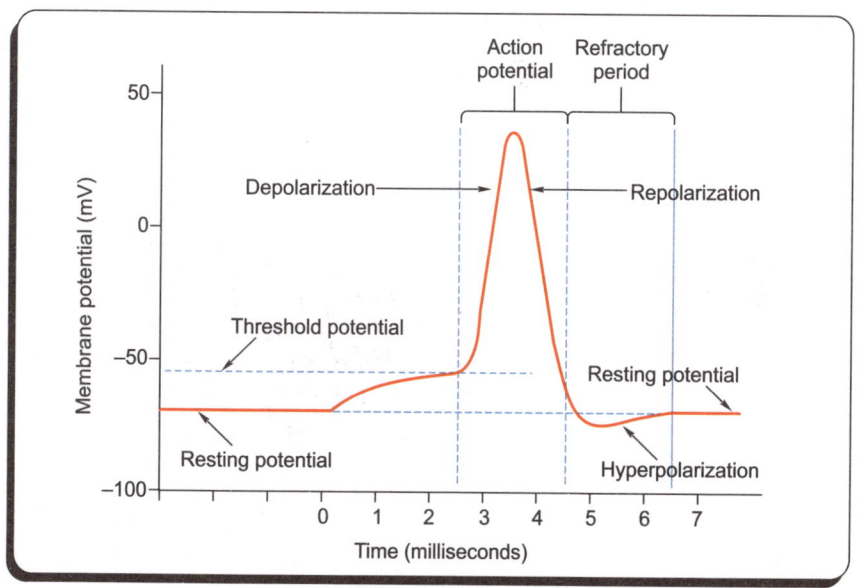

Figure 5.9 Action potential in a neuron.

This process continues along the nerve fibre and acts like the electrical current that carries the nerve impulse along the fibre.

THE SYNAPTIC TRANSMISSION

The transmission of the nerve impulse from its origin to the destination involves more than one neuron, and the point where the nerve impulse passes from one nerve to another is called *synapse* (Fig. 5.10).

Thus, the synapses are the areas where the terminal branch of an axon (the axon terminals) of one neuron passes the information or is close to the ends of the dendrites of another neuron. At the synapse between neurons, the neuron that sends the impulse is called the *presynaptic neuron* and the neuron that receives that impulse is termed as the *postsynaptic neuron*.

The other areas of synapses are between the axon endings and the muscles (somatic nerves carry impulses directly to synapses at the skeletal muscle) or between axon endings and glands (sympathetic and parasympathetic nerves).

The axon terminal (or the free end) of the presynaptic neuron breaks into minute branches that end in small swellings called the *synaptic knob*. These synaptic knobs are close to the dendrites of the

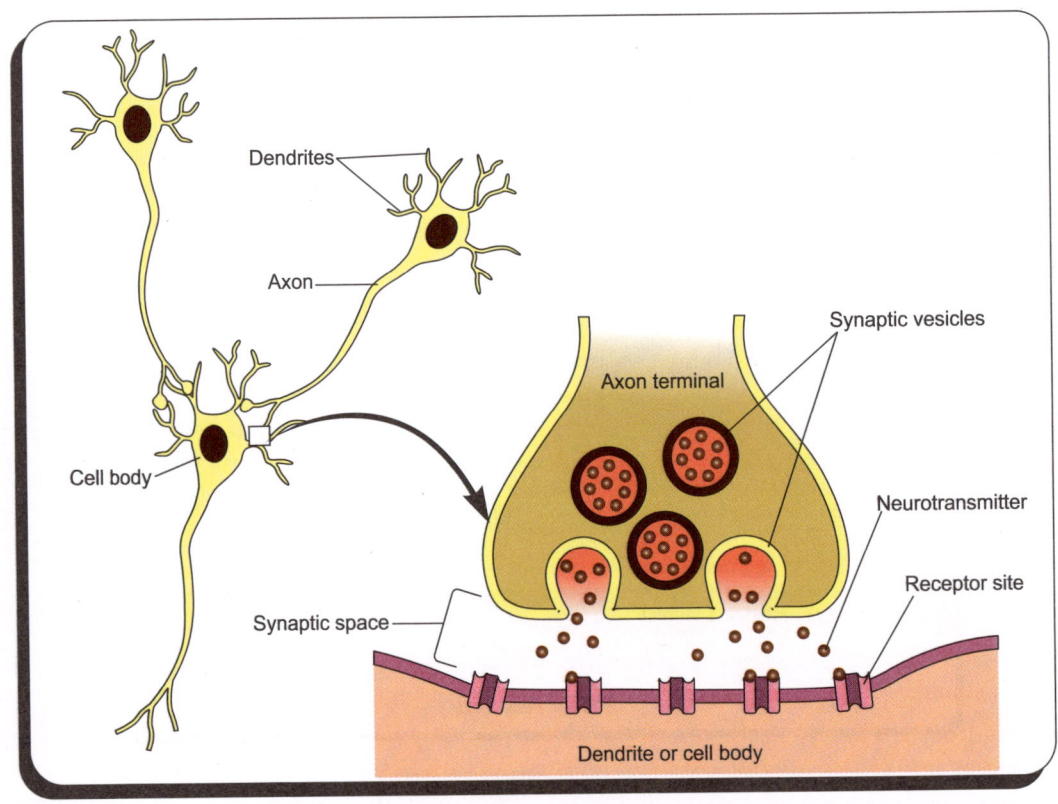

Figure 5.10 Synapse.

postsynaptic neuron and the space between these synaptic knobs and dendrites is called the *synaptic cleft*.

The synaptic knob consists of spherical synaptic vesicles that contain a chemical, the neurotransmitter which is synthesized by nerve cells and stored in the synaptic vesicles. They are released in response to the action potential into the synaptic cleft where they act on the specific receptor sites present on postsynaptic membranes. The action of the neurotransmitter is short lived because immediately after binding to receptor sites and causing stimulation, they are either inactivated by enzymes or taken back into the synaptic knob.

Neurotransmitters: The neurotransmitters in the brain and spinal cord include noradrenaline (norepinephrine), adrenaline (epinephrine), dopamine, histamine, serotonin, γ-amino butyric acid (GABA) and acetylcholine. Usually, these neurotransmitters have a stimulatory effect at the synapse, but sometimes they are inhibitory.

RESPONSE OF NERVOUS TISSUE TO INJURY

Mammalian neurons have very limited power of regeneration as they have very less capacity to replicate themselves. In the PNS, damage to dendrites and myelinated axons may be repaired if the cell body remains intact, but in CNS, even when the cell body remains intact, damaged axons cannot be repaired or regrown. The damage to nervous tissue may occur due to hypoxia, anoxia, nutritional deficiency, poisons (organic lead), trauma, infections, hypoglycaemia or ageing.

REPAIR OF NEURONS IN THE PNS

The axons and dendrites of peripheral nerves may undergo repair or regenerate if the cell body is intact, but generally it takes several months to recover.

The portion of the axon and myelin sheath that is distal to the site of injury disintegrates and is removed by macrophages, but the Schwann cells survive and proliferate within the neurilemma (the outermost layer of the Schwann cell plasma membrane). The Schwann cells then multiply by mitosis and grow towards each other and form a regeneration tube across the injured area that grows along the original track. New regenerating axons then begin to invade the tube formed by Schwann cells and grow at a rate of about 1.5 mm/day across the area of damage. The function is restored when satisfactory connections are established with the end organ.

In severe conditions, when neurilemma is destroyed, the sprouting axon and Schwann cells form a tumour-like cluster that produces severe pain, for example due to fracture and amputation of limbs.

REPAIR OF NEUROGLIA

Astrocytes: When severely damaged, the astrocytes undergo necrosis and disintegrate; however, in less severe condition, the astrocytes may proliferate.

Oligodendrocytes: These cells form and maintain myelin; thus, they increase in number around the degenerating neurons but get destroyed in demyelinating diseases such as multiple sclerosis.

Microglia: Microglia increase in size and become phagocytic during inflammation and cell destruction.

Chapter 5

BRAIN

The brain is one of the largest organs of the body. It weighs about 1.4 kg (3 lbs) and has a volume of 1200 cc (71 inch³) in an average adult. The adult human brain has almost 97% of the total body's neuronal tissues.

Brain size varies considerably among individuals. Because of the difference in average body weight of males and females, males have 10% larger brain than those of females (on average). However, it is a fact that there is no correlation between the brain size and intelligence. An individual with the smallest brain (750 cc) and the other with the larger brain (2100 cc) both function normally and may have similar intelligence.

The brain is the centre for intellect, emotions, behaviour and memory. The different regions of the brain are specialized for different functions and many parts of the brain work together to accomplish a particular function.

The human brain weighs about 1.4 kg and is the most complex of all known living structures. The physical actions and mental processes are coordinated by the joint work of about 1 trillion nerve cells. These processes set humans apart from other species.

OVERVIEW OF BRAIN ORGANIZATION

Major parts of the brain

The brain constitutes about one-fiftieth of the body weight and lies within the cranial cavity.

The brain is divided into the following three major parts (Fig. 5.11):

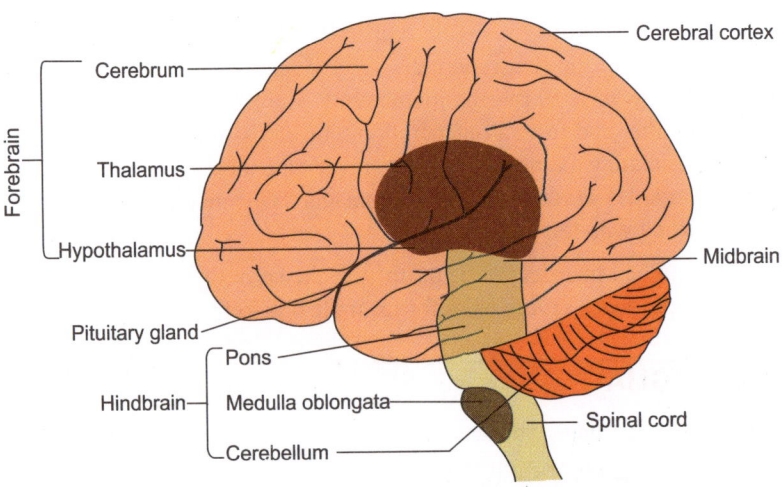

Figure 5.11 Parts of the brain: forebrain, midbrain and hindbrain.

1. **Fore brain**, which includes the cerebrum and the diencephalon
2. Midbrain
3. **Hind brain**, which includes the pons, medulla oblongata and cerebellum

Midbrain, pons and medulla oblongata are collectively termed as the *brain stem*.

The brain stem is continuous with the spinal cord and posterior to the brain stem is the cerebellum. The diencephalon, present superiorly to the brain stem, consists of the thalamus and the hypothalamus. The cerebrum spreads over the diencephalon and occupies most of the cranium (Fig. 5.12).

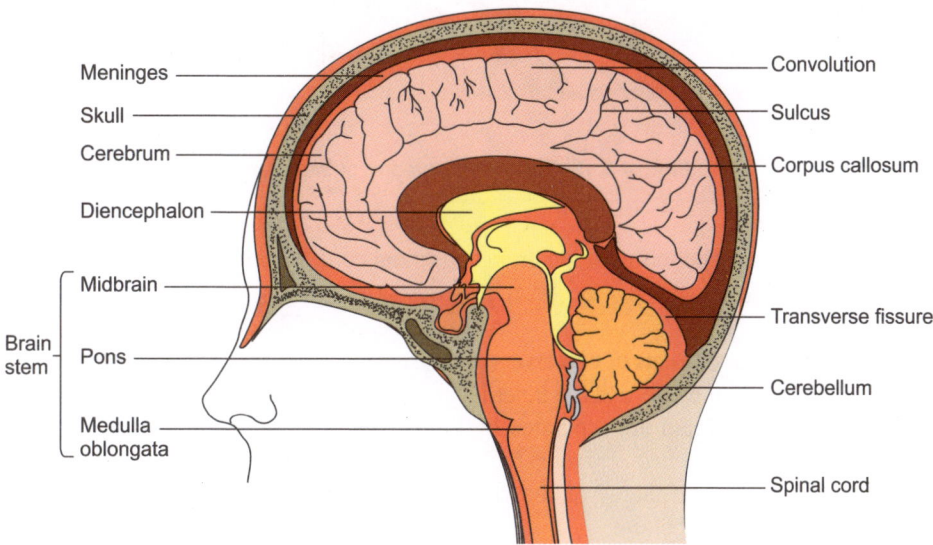

Figure 5.12 The major portions of the brain.

Protective covering of the brain

The brain is protected by the cranial bones and the cranial meninges. The meninges are the three layers of tissue that completely surround the brain and spinal cord. The meninges that protect the brain are termed as *cranial meninges* and they are present between the skull and brain. The cranial meninges are continuous with the spinal meninges that protect the spinal cord and are present between the vertebral foramina and the spinal cord.

The cranial meninges and spinal meninges have the same basic structure and bear the same names: the *outer dura mater, middle arachnoid mater* and the *inner pia mater*. The dura and arachnoid maters are separated by the subdural space, whereas the arachnoid and pia maters are separated by the subarachnoid space that contains the cerebrospinal fluid (CSF) (Fig. 5.13).

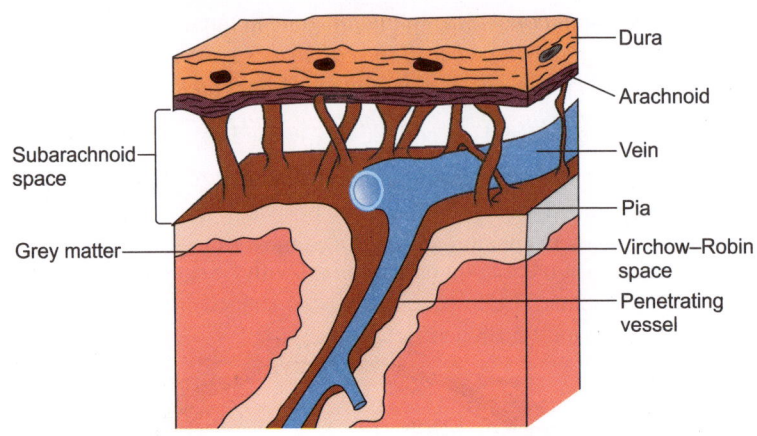

Figure 5.13 Protective covering of the brain.

1. **Dura mater**

   ❑ This is the outermost covering of the brain and spinal cord. The part enclosing the brain is called *cerebral dura mater*, whereas the other part that covers the spinal cord is called *spinal dura mater*.

   ❑ Cerebral dura mater consists of two layers of dense fibrous tissue. The outer layer firmly attaches to sutures of the skull bones and the inner layer provides a protective covering for the brain. The various parts of the brain are separated by three extensions of cerebral dura mater, which are as follows: *the falx cerebri*, separates the two hemispheres of the cerebrum; *the falx cerebelli*, separates the two hemispheres of the cerebellum; and *the tentorium cerebelli*, separates the cerebrum from the cerebellum.

   ❑ Spinal dura mater is continuous with cerebral dura mater and it forms a loose sheath around the spinal cord. There are some dural folds in the spinal dura mater, which stabilize and support the spinal cord.

2. **Arachnoid mater**

   ❑ This is a layer of fibrous tissue that lies between the dura and pia maters. It is separated from the dura mater by the subdural space and from the pia mater by the subarachnoid space containing CSF. It is a delicate membrane that passes over the convolutions (sulci and gyri) of the cerebrum and other parts of the brain and the spinal cord.

   ❑ This membrane is in contact with the inner epithelial layer of dura mater. Certain protrusions of arachnoid mater accompany the inner layer of dura mater in the formation of arachnoid villi.

3. **Pia mater**

   ❑ This is a delicate layer of connective tissue that adheres to the brain and completely covers the convolutions and various folds. Pia mater is thicker than arachnoid mater, especially over the spinal cord.

   ❑ This layer contains many minute blood vessels that penetrate into different internal portions of the brain.

Cranial meninges and cranial bones play a major role in brain protection. Let us consider a hypothetical example of the brain driving a car. If the car strikes a tree, the car protects the driver from hitting the tree. But serious injury can occur unless a seat belt protects the contact of driver with the car. Similarly, the cranial bones are like the car for the brain and the meninges act like the seat belt and protect the brain.

Ventricles of the brain

The ventricles are the cavities within the brain that are filled with CSF, which serves as a shock absorber for the CNS and circulates nutrients. There are four irregular-shaped cavities in the brain: right and left lateral ventricles, third ventricle and fourth ventricle (Fig. 5.14).

Lateral ventricles

These cavities are present in each hemisphere of the cerebrum just below the corpus callosum. The right and left ventricles are separated from each other by a thin membrane, the septum pellucidum (*pellucid*: transparent). Each lateral ventricle connects with the third ventricle by a narrow opening called the *interventricular foramen*.

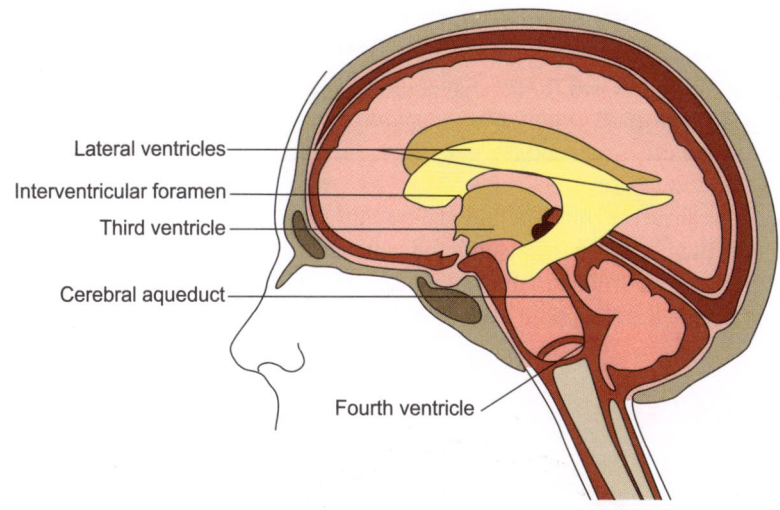

Figure 5.14 Ventricles of the brain.

The third ventricle

The third ventricle is a cavity situated below the lateral ventricles between the right and left halves of the thalamus. It connects with the fourth ventricle by a canal, known as the *cerebral aqueduct*.

The fourth ventricle

The fourth ventricle is a diamond-shaped cavity situated below and behind the third ventricle, between the cerebellum and pons. The roof of this fourth ventricle has three foramina (openings) through which it connects with the subarachnoid space of the brain and spinal meninges, thus allowing the flow of CSF through the spinal cord, the brain and the ventricles of the brain.

Cerebrospinal fluid (CSF)

CSF is a clear, colourless liquid that protects the brain and spinal cord against injuries by acting as a shock absorber; it carries oxygen, glucose and other required nutrients from the blood to neurons and neuroglia.

This fluid continuously circulates through the subarachnoid space around the brain and spinal cord as well as through cavities within the brain and spinal cord.

The sites of CSF production are the choroid plexuses, which are the networks of capillaries surrounded by ependymal cells in the linings of the ventricle walls. The CSF formed in the choroid plexuses of each lateral ventricle flows into the third ventricle through the interventricular foramen where more CSF is added by the choroid plexus present in the roof of the third ventricle. The fluid then flows into the fourth ventricle through the cerebral aqueduct where some more fluid is added by choroid plexus of the fourth ventricle. From the roof of the fourth ventricle, CSF flows through foramina (openings) into the subarachnoid space and completely surrounds the brain and spinal cord (Fig. 5.15).

The movement of CSF occurs due to the pulsation of blood vessels, respiration and positive charges.

CLINICAL ASPECT

❑ CSF samples nay be withdrawn for the diagnosis of diseases.
❑ Spinal anaesthesia is performed by injecting anaesthetic in CSF through lumbar puncture.

CSF is gradually reabsorbed into the blood through arachnoid villi (finger-like extensions of the arachnoid mater) and then further projects into the venous sinuses (a sinus is like a vein but has thinner walls). The movement of CSF from the subarachnoid space into venous sinuses depends on the difference in pressure on each side of the arachnoid villi. This difference in pressure serves the purpose of one-way valves, that is:

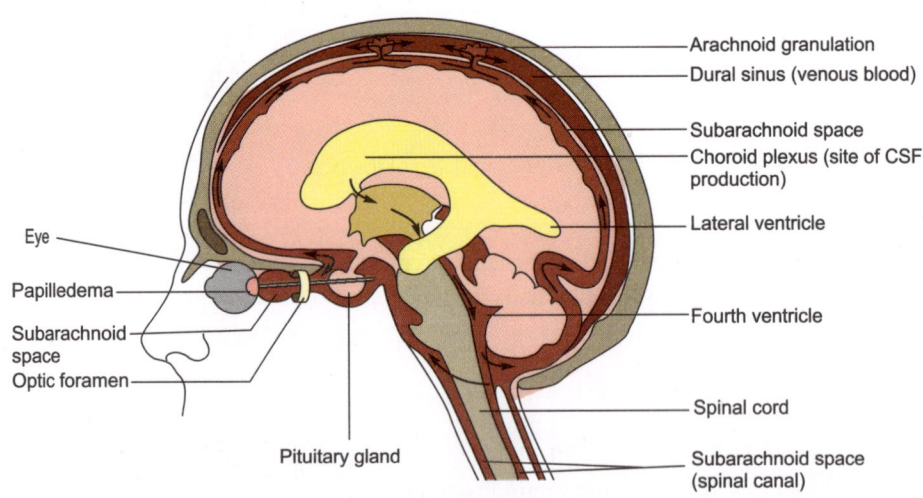

Figure 5.15 Flow of CSF.

Chapter 5

❑ When CSF pressure > Venous pressure, CSF passes into the blood.
❑ When venous pressure > CSF pressure, the arachnoid villi collapses and prevents the passage of blood constituents into the CSF.

CSF is continuously secreted at a rate of about 0.5 mL/min (i.e. 720 mL/day) but the volume remains fairly constant at about 120 mL, which means that CSF is reabsorbed as rapidly as it is formed by the choroid plexuses.

If the volume of brain tissue gets enlarged due to tumour, some compensation is made by a reduction in the amount of CSF. Conversely, when the volume of brain tissue is reduced such as in degeneration or atrophy, the volume of CSF increases.

Functions of CSF

1. It supports and protects the brain and spinal cord.
2. It acts as a fluid buffer and protects the brain from shock.
3. It is the medium for the interchange of substances such as nutrients and waste products between CSF and nerve cells.

Supply to the brain

The brain receives about 15% of the cardiac output, that is ~750 mL of blood per minute. The major part of the brain is supplied with arterial blood by an arrangement of arteries called *circulus arteriosus* or the *Circle of Willis* (Fig. 5.16).

The arrangement of various arteries in the Circle of Willis is such that the brain as a whole receives an adequate blood supply even when there is damage to a contributing artery.

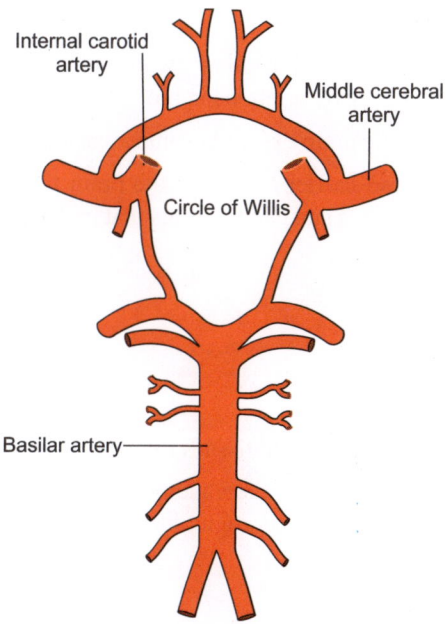

Internal carotid artery

Middle cerebral artery

Circle of Willis

Basilar artery

Figure 5.16 Circle of Willis: Blood supply to the brain.

Chapter 5

The Circle of Willis comprises four large arteries: the two internal carotid arteries and the two vertebral arteries.

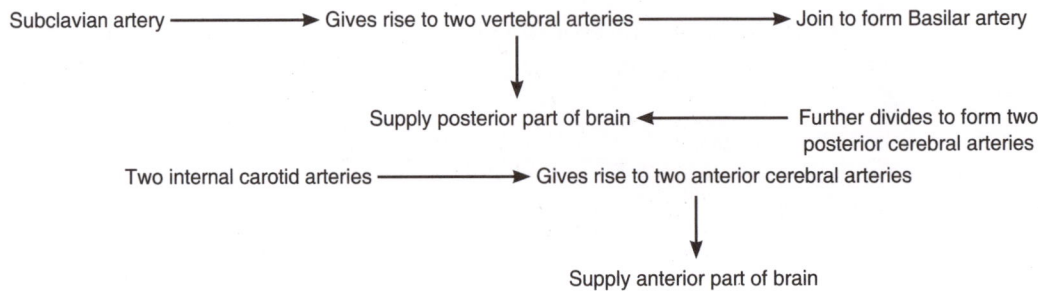

Thus, the circle of Willis is formed by the following:

1. Two anterior cerebral arteries
2. Two internal carotid arteries
3. Two posterior cerebral arteries
4. One basilar artery

Neurons produce ATP by predominantly utilizing glucose via the reactions that use oxygen, and this is achieved by the Circle of Willis and its contributing arteries, which maintain a constant supply of oxygen and glucose.

Interruption in blood flow for 1–2 min ⟶ *impairs the functions of neurons*

Deprivation of oxygen for about 4 min ⟶ *leads to permanent injury*

Blood–Brain Barrier (BBB)

The BBB is a selective barrier between the capillary wall and neurons that protects the brain from potentially toxic substances and chemical variations in blood (Fig. 5.17).

The barrier exists in all parts of the brain except in some areas of the hypothalamus.

The substances that can cross the barrier and enter the brain tissues are oxygen, carbon dioxide, water, glucose, amino acids, electrolytes and certain drugs that include sulphonamides, tetracycline and many lipid-soluble drugs.

The BBB is composed of the following:

❑ Capillary endothelium
❑ Basement membrane of the endothelium
❑ Numerous processes of astrocytes

Some harmful substances can enter the brain tissues in infants as it is not well developed in infants.

❑ **Development of BBB**: During childhood, the endothelial cells of the blood capillaries form tight junctions; simultaneously, the astrocytes (neuroglia) develop around the capillaries, which reinforce the barrier.
❑ **Significance of BBB**
   ➤ The BBB prevents the entry of injurious substances in the brain. It also prevents the entry of protein-bounded substances in the brain.

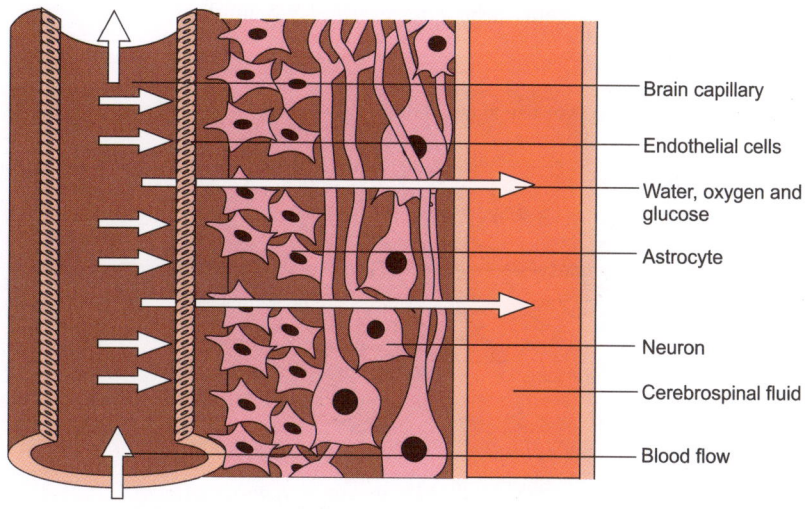

Brain capillary

Endothelial cells

Water, oxygen and glucose

Astrocyte

Neuron

Cerebrospinal fluid

Blood flow

Figure 5.17 Blood–brain barrier.

➤ It helps maintain a constant neuronal environment within the CNS by preventing the escape of neurotransmitters into the blood.

➤ Some metabolic enzymes are also present on the BBB that inactivate some toxic metabolites and prevent any damage to the brain.

➤ It prevents the adverse CNS effects of some aqueous-soluble drugs (e.g. penicillin, streptomycin and thiopentone)

➤ The entry of hormones is also restricted, thereby preventing the disturbance of normal rhythm of the body.

THE CEREBRUM

This is the largest part of the brain and is termed as 'seat of intelligence' as this part is responsible for the abilities of reading, writing, speaking, planning and imagination. The superficial part of the cerebrum is composed of nerve cell bodies or grey matter and is referred to as the *cerebral cortex*. The deeper layer of the cerebrum consists of nerve fibres/white matter.

The surface of the cerebral cortex shows many folds called *gyri* or *convolutions*, and these folds are separated by grooves called *sulci (shallow groove)* or *fissures (deep groove)*.

The most prominent fissure, the longitudinal cerebral fissure, separates the cerebrum into right and left cerebral hemispheres. The hemispheres are connected internally by a mass of white matter (nerve fibres) called the *corpus callosum*.

Each cerebral hemisphere is divided into four lobes named after the bones that cover them. These are as follows (Fig. 5.18):

1. Frontal lobe
2. Parietal lobe
3. Temporal lobe
4. Occipital lobe

Chapter 5

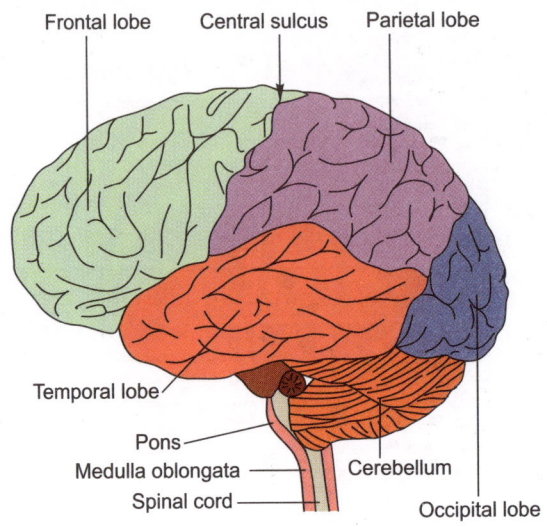

Figure 5.18 Lobes of the cerebrum.

The lobes are separated by various sulci, which are as follows (Fig. 5.19):

1. **Central sulci**: It separates the frontal lobe from the parietal lobe.
2. **Lateral sulci**: It separates the frontal lobe from the temporal lobe.
3. **Parietooccipital sulci**: It separates the parietal lobe from the occipital lobe.

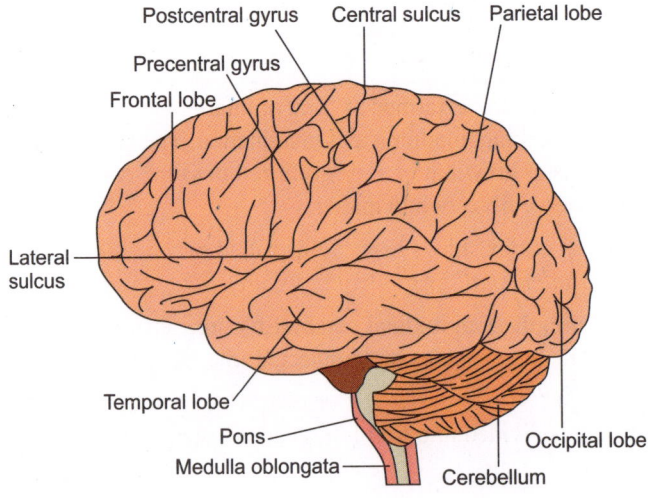

Figure 5.19 Sulci and gyri in the cerebrum.

The white matter (nerve fibres) present in the deeper layers of the cerebrum connects different parts of the brain and spinal cord. These nerve fibres are organized into tracts which are of the following three main types (Fig. 5.20):

1. **Association tracts**: They connect different parts of a cerebral hemisphere and transmit nerve impulses between gyri in the same hemisphere.
2. **Commissural tract**: It connects the corresponding areas of two cerebral hemispheres by transmitting impulses from gyri in one hemisphere to the corresponding gyri in another hemisphere (e.g. the corpus callosum).
3. **Projection tract**: It connects the cerebral cortex with the brain stem and the spinal cord. These fibres may transmit impulses either from the cerebrum to the spinal cord or from the spinal cord to the brain (e.g. internal capsule).

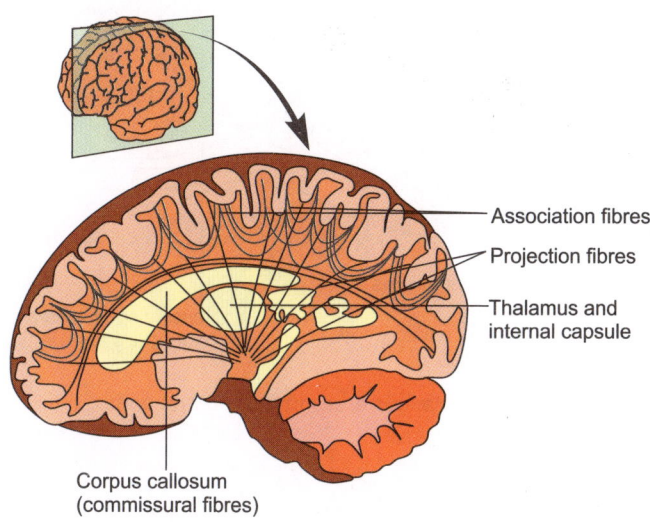

Association fibres
Projection fibres
Thalamus and internal capsule
Corpus callosum (commissural fibres)

Figure 5.20 Nerve fibre tracts (as shown in vertical section of the brain).

Cerebral cortex areas and their functions (Fig. 5.21)

The following are the functional areas of the cerebral cortex: motor area, sensory area and association area.

The cerebral cortex comprises different types of functional areas that are responsible for the various activities or functions of the cerebral cortex.

The various functions associated with cerebral cortex are as follows (Fig. 5.22):

1. **Mental activities**: The association area of the cerebral cortex deals with complex mental functions such as intelligence, memory, reasoning, judgement and emotions.
2. **Sensory perception**: The sensory area of the cerebral cortex receives and interprets sensory impulses, thus enabling sensory perception.

3. **Skeletal muscle movement**: The motor area of the cerebral cortex initiates the skeletal (voluntary) muscle movements.

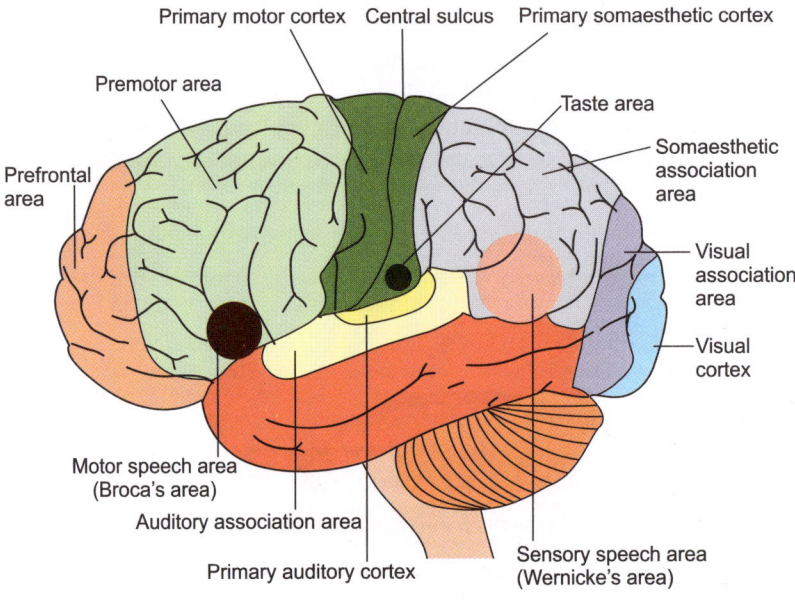

Figure 5.21 Various areas in the cerebral cortex.

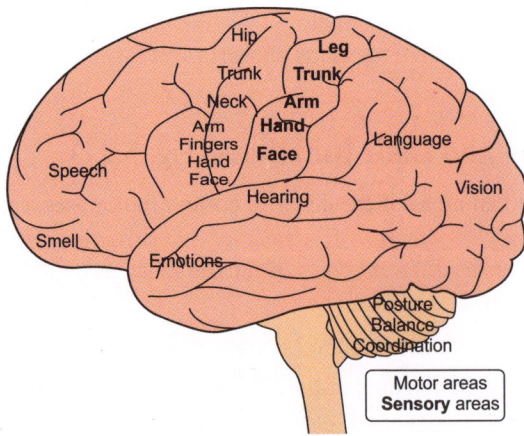

Figure 5.22 Functions of sensory and motor areas of the cerebrum.

Motor areas of the cerebral cortex

The primary motor area

It is located in the frontal lobe immediately anterior to the central sulcus and controls the voluntary contractions of specific muscles or group of muscles, especially the fine movements of fingers and hands.

The cell bodies (Betz cells) in this area initiate the contraction of skeletal muscles and a nerve fibre (upper motor neuron) from Betz cell passes it downwards to the medulla oblongata through the internal capsule. At medulla oblongata, this nerve impulse moves to the opposite side and then descends in the spinal cord where it crosses the synapse at an appropriate level to stimulate a second neuron (lower motor neuron) that finally terminates at the skeletal muscle fibre.

Thus, the nerve impulse in the primary motor area results in the contraction of specific skeletal muscle fibres on the opposite side of the body, that is the motor area of the right hemisphere of the cerebrum controls voluntary muscle movement on the left side of the body and vice versa. Damage to the neurons on either side of the cerebral hemisphere may result in paralysis.

Broca's speech area

- It is located in the frontal lobe just above the lateral sulcus and controls the muscle movements necessary for speech.
- It is dominant in the left hemisphere in right-handed people (97% of the population) and vice versa.
- The coordinated contractions of the speech and breathing muscles help us speak out our thoughts.

Note: The size of the cortical area is proportional to:

1. Complexity of the movement of body parts, that is the larger cortical area is involved for complex, skilled and delicate movements and vice versa. (e.g. movement of fingers is regulated by large cortical area).
2. Extent of sensory innervations, that is the number of receptors present on a particular body part (e.g. the larger cortical area is involved in receiving impulses from the lips and fingers, whereas the smaller area is involved in receiving impulses from the hips).

Sensory areas of the cerebral cortex

Some of the important sensory areas present in the cerebral cortex are as follows:

The somatosensory area

- It is located immediately behind the central sulcus and is also known as the *primary sensory area*.
- This area receives information about touch, pain, temperature, pressure, muscle movement and joint position.
- The primary sensory area of the right hemisphere receives impulses from the left side of the body and vice versa.

The visual area

- It is located at the posterior tip of the occipital lobe, behind the parietoccipital sulcus.
- This area receives the impulses of visual information and interprets them for visual perception (size, shape and colour of object).

Chapter 5

The auditory (hearing) area

❑ It is located within the temporal lobe, immediately below the lateral sulcus.
❑ This area receives impulses for sound and interprets them for auditory perception (pitch, intensity and properties of sound).

The olfactory (smell) area

❑ It is located in the temporal lobe.
❑ This area receives impulses for smell and interprets them for olfactory perception.

The gustatory (taste) area

❑ It is located deep within the somatosensory area, just above the lateral sulcus in the parietal lobe.
❑ This area receives impulses from taste buds receptors and interprets them for taste.

Association areas of the cerebral cortex

❑ The association areas regulate the higher cognitive abilities by coordinating the nerve impulses from the sensory and motor areas.
❑ The different association areas of the cerebral cortex are connected to each other by association tracts.
❑ The various association areas of the cerebral cortex are as follows:

Premotor area

❑ It is located in the frontal area immediately anterior to the primary motor area.
❑ This area is concerned with learned motor skills that require a sequence of movements.

For example, tying a shoe lace and writing; with repeated practice, our premotor area has learned this sequence so well that we are able to repeat it without consciously thinking about it.

Do you remember that you have learned tying a shoe lace?

It is achieved by the neurons of this area that coordinate the movements initiated by the primary motor area and generate nerve impulses that cause specific groups of muscles to contract in a sequential manner.

Prefrontal area

❑ It is located anterior to the premotor area just behind the eyes.
❑ This area is more developed in humans than in other animals and is concerned with intellectual functions that include the management of emotions, anticipation and planning for future and social behaviour.

Wernicke's (sensory speech) area

❑ It is located in the temporal area.
❑ It is concerned with the interpretation of the meaning of speech by perceiving spoken words and various sounds.

Visual association area

This area is concerned with spatial awareness (judgement of distance), interpretation of written language and the ability to name objects. We can recognize the things by touch alone because of the knowledge from past experience (memory) retained in this area.

Summary of lobes of the cerebral cortex and their functions

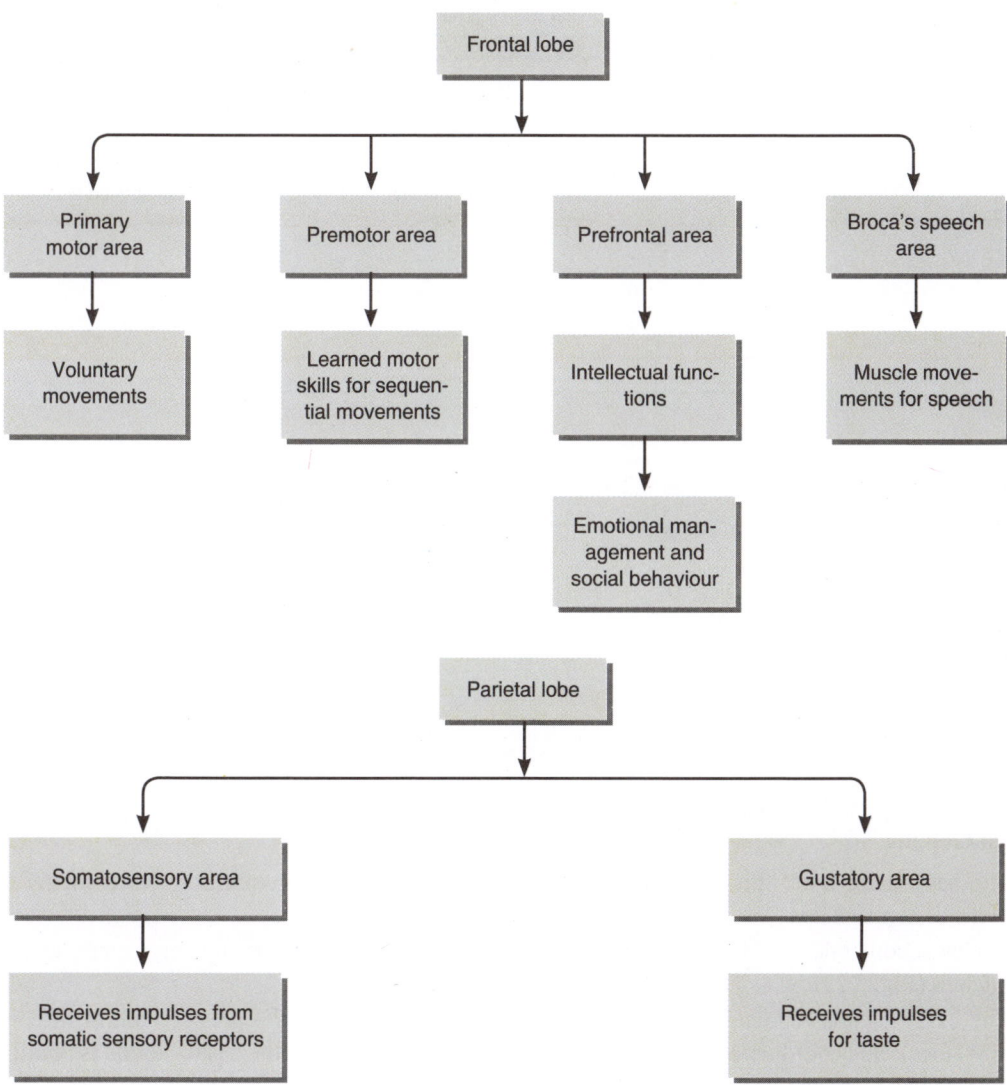

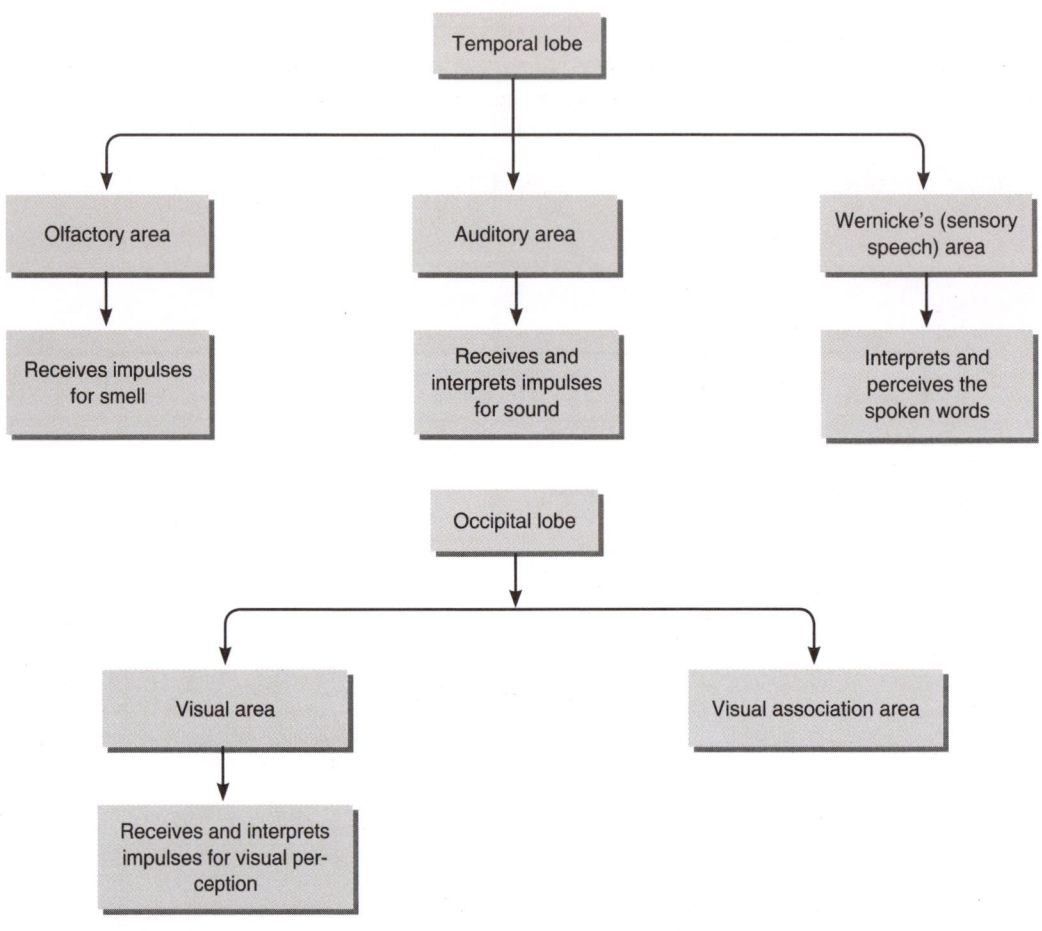

Basal Ganglia

❏ The basal ganglia are the paired masses of grey matter, lying deep within the white matter of the cerebral hemispheres.

❏ The main components of the basal ganglia are the striatum pallidum, substantia nigra and subthalamic nucleus (Fig. 5.23).

❏ The basal ganglia regulate muscle movement and are involved in the precise control of complex movements and coordinated activities. The most common disorder of the basal ganglia is Parkinson's disease in which the movements become jerky and uncoordinated.

Limbic system

❏ It is a group of cortical and subcortical structures that form a ring on the inner border of the cerebrum. It includes the hypothalamus, the hippocampus, the amygdala and several other nearby areas (Fig. 5.24). Our emotions and formation of memories are mainly influenced by this system.

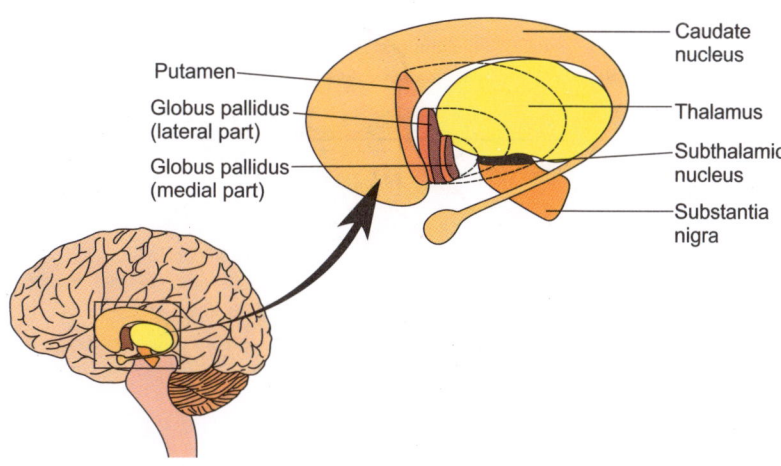

Figure 5.23 Basal ganglia.

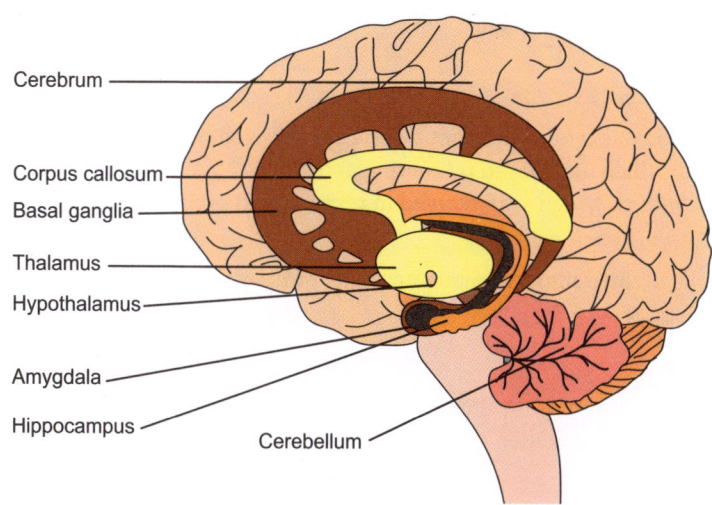

Figure 5.24 The limbic system.

❏ It plays a primary role in maintaining emotional state including pain, pleasure, affection and anger. It is also involved in olfaction (smell) and memory.

THE DIENCEPHALON

The diencephalon is present between the two cerebral hemispheres, superior to the midbrain (Fig. 5.25). It also surrounds the third ventricle.

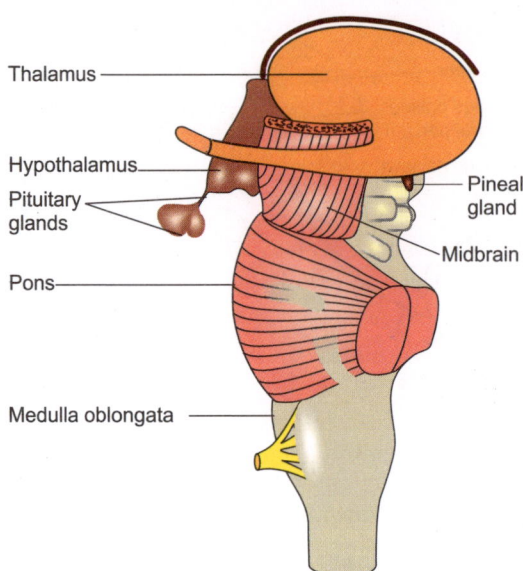

Figure 5.25 The diencephalon.

It includes the following:

1. Optic tracts and optic chiasma, where optic nerves cross each other
2. The infundibulum, which attaches to pituitary gland
3. The mammillary bodies, which are involved in responses to odour
4. Pineal gland

The diencephalon is divided into two main areas: the *thalamus* and the *hypothalamus*.

The thalamus

The thalamus is the superior part of the diencephalon and consists of paired oval masses of grey matter with interspersed tracts of white matter.

It is the principal relay station for sensory impulses that reach the cerebral cortex from the spinal cord, brain stem and parts of the cerebrum. The sensory impulses first enter the thalamus, which relays them to the cerebrum, where sensations are felt.

It also plays an important role as an interpretation centre for conscious awareness of pain, temperature, touch and pressure.

The hypothalamus

The hypothalamus is a small part of the diencephalon and is composed of a number of groups of nerve cells. It is situated below and in front of the thalamus, immediately above the pituitary gland.

The hypothalamus is linked to the posterior lobe of the pituitary gland by nerve fibres and to the anterior lobe by a complex system of blood vessels. Thus, it controls the output of hormones from both lobes of the gland.

The hypothalamus is one of the major regulators of homeostasis.

The chief functions of the hypothalamus are as follows:

1. **Control of the pituitary gland**

   Posterior pituitary hormones: The supraoptic and paraventricular nuclei of the hypothalamus secrete antidiuretic hormone (ADH) and oxytocin. These hormones are transported through axons to the posterior pituitary gland, where they are stored and released.

   Anterior pituitary hormones: The hypothalamus secretes the regulating hormones (releasing and inhibitory hormones), which are carried by the blood stream to the anterior pituitary gland, where they stimulate or inhibit the secretion of pituitary hormones.

   Examples are growth hormone–releasing hormone (GHRH), growth hormone–inhibitory hormone (GHIH), thyrotropic-releasing hormone (TRH), corticotropin-releasing hormone (CRH), gonadotropin-releasing hormone (GnRH) and prolactin-inhibitory hormone (PIH).

2. **Regulation of the autonomic nervous system (ANS)**: The hypothalamus controls and integrates the activities of ANS and regulates both the sympathetic and parasympathetic systems. Thus, it has an important role in the regulation of heart rate, blood pressure, secretion from glands, contraction of smooth and cardiac muscles and other visceral activities.

3. **Regulation of body temperature**: The hypothalamus regulates the normal body temperature in the following two ways:

   (a) If body temperature increases above normal → hypothalamus directs the ANS to stimulate activities that promote heat loss (increase sweat secretion).

   (b) If body temperature decreases below normal → hypothalamus generates impulses that promote heat production and retention (shivering).

4. **Regulation of food intake and water balance**: The hypothalamus regulates food intake through the following two centres:

   (a) *Feeding centre*
   - (i) Its stimulation leads to increased food intake (polyphagia) and leads to obesity.
   - (ii) Its destruction leads to anorexia (loss of appetite).

   (b) *Satiety centre*
   - (i) Its stimulation leads to decreased food intake.
   - (ii) Its destruction leads to hyperphagia.

   The hypothalamus regulates water balance through the following two mechanisms:

   (a) *Thirst mechanism*

   Controlled by the thirst centre present in the hypothalamus:
   - (i) Decreased extracellular fluid (ECF) volume → increases osmolality of ECF → activates thirst centre → causes thirst sensation
   - (ii) The intake of water decreases osmolality of ECF and increases ECF volume.

Chapter 5

(b) *ADH mechanism*

   (i) Decreased ECF volume → stimulates ADH release from hypothalamus

$$\downarrow$$

       ECF volume normal ← causes water reabsorption

  (ii) Increased ECF volume → ADH not secreted

$$\downarrow$$

       ECF volume normal ← increased water excretion

5. **Regulation of circadian rhythm**: The body rhythm to the 24-hr dark–light cycle is called the *circadian rhythm*. The hypothalamus regulates the circadian rhythm by regulating sleeping and wakefulness.

6. **Regulation of behavioural and emotional responses**: The hypothalamus along with the limbic system regulates the feelings of rage, aggression, pain and pleasure and the behavioural patterns related to sexual arousal.

Summary of diencephalon

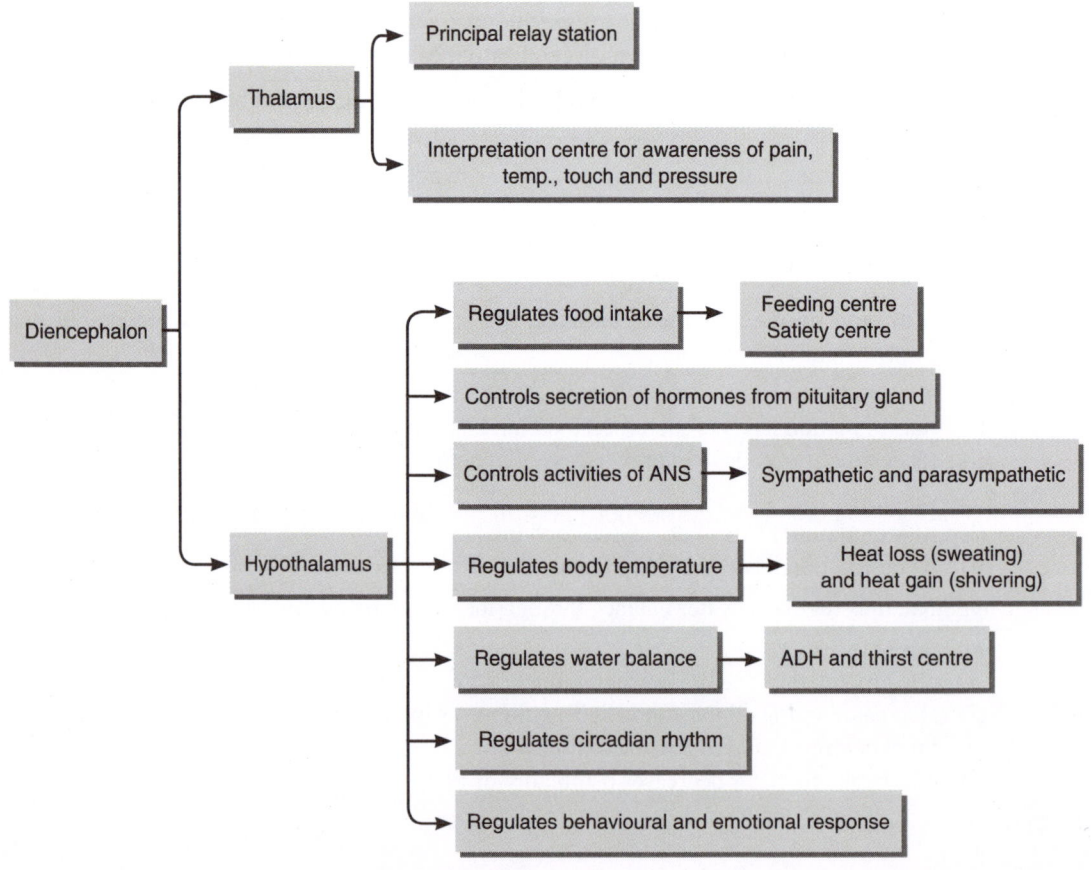

THE BRAIN STEM

The brain stem is the part of the brain between the diencephalon and the spinal cord. It is a very delicate area of the brain because damage to even small areas could result in death.

It consists of the midbrain, pons and medulla oblongata (Fig. 5.26).

The brain stem serves the following two major functions:

1. It forms the pathway for ascending and descending nerve fibres between the brain and the spinal cord.
2. It regulates the vital functions of the body as many important centres are located in this part.

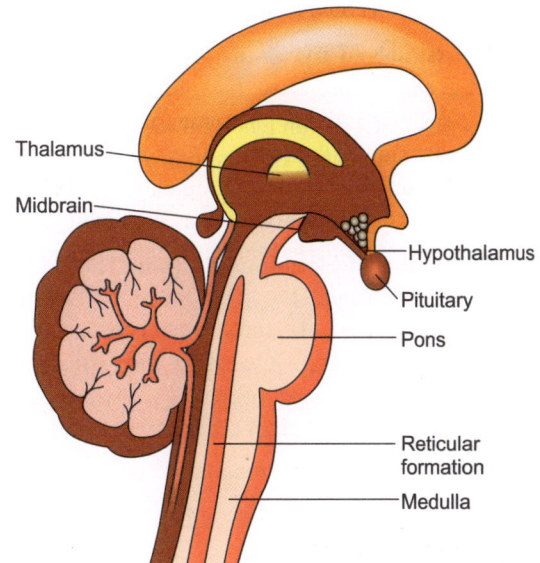

Figure 5.26 The brain stem.

The midbrain

The midbrain, also called the *mesencephalon,* is the area of brain situated below the cerebrum and above the pons. It consists of nuclei and nerve fibres (tracts) that connect the cerebrum with the lower parts of the brain and with the spinal cord.

The midbrain contains the following:

1. *Cerebral peduncles*: They conduct nerve impulses from the cerebral cortex to the pons and spinal cord.
2. *Tectum*: They serve as a reflex centre that controls the following:
   (a) Movement of eye balls and head in response to visual stimuli
   (b) Movement of head and trunk in response to auditory stimuli
3. *Substantia nigra*: They release dopamine and control subconscious muscle activities.

The pons

The pons is situated in front of the cerebellum, below the midbrain and above the medulla oblongata.

It consists mainly of nerve fibres (white matter) that form a bridge to connect the spinal cord with the brain and also to connect parts of the brain with one another. Some of the nerve fibres of the pons connect the two hemispheres of the cerebellum.

The pons also consists of *pneumotaxic* and *apneustic areas* that help regulate breathing.

The medulla oblongata

The medulla oblongata extends from the pons above and is continuous with the spinal cord below. It forms the main pathway for the ascending (sensory) and descending (motor) tracts that connect the spinal cord and various parts of the brain.

Chapter 5

The special features of medulla are as follows:

1. **Decussation of pyramids**: Some motor nerves descending from the motor area in the cerebrum to the spinal cord cross from one side to another in the medulla. This crossing of tracts is called *decussation*, and this phenomenon explains why each side of the brain controls movements on the opposite side of the body.
2. **Cardiovascular centre**: It regulates the force of cardiac contraction and heart rate.
3. **Vasomotor centre**: It regulates the diameter of blood vessels, thereby controlling blood pressure.
4. **Respiratory centre**: It controls the rate and depth of respiration (breathing).
5. **Reflex centre**: It is the centre that controls coughing, sneezing, swallowing and vomiting.

Reticular formation: The brain stem consists of a broad region where small clusters of grey matter are interspersed among the white matter and exhibits a net-like arrangement. This area is called the *reticular formation*, which consists of neural pathways that conduct ascending and descending nerve impulses between the brain and spinal cord.

The reticular formation maintains consciousness and arousal and helps regulate the muscle tone.

THE CEREBELLUM

The cerebellum (shaped like a butterfly) is the second largest portion of the brain and is situated below the posterior portion of the cerebrum and behind the pons and medulla of the brainstem.

It consists of two partially separated hemispheres connected by a narrow strip called the *vermis*. The surface of the cerebellum is composed of grey matter (nerve cell bodies), whereas the deeper layers consist of white matter (nerve fibres).

The functions of the cerebellum are mainly concerned with movements and include coordination of voluntary muscular movement and maintenance of posture, balance and equilibrium. The damage of the cerebellum can lead to tremors, loss of equilibrium and difficulty in skeletal muscle movements.

Summary of brain parts and their functions

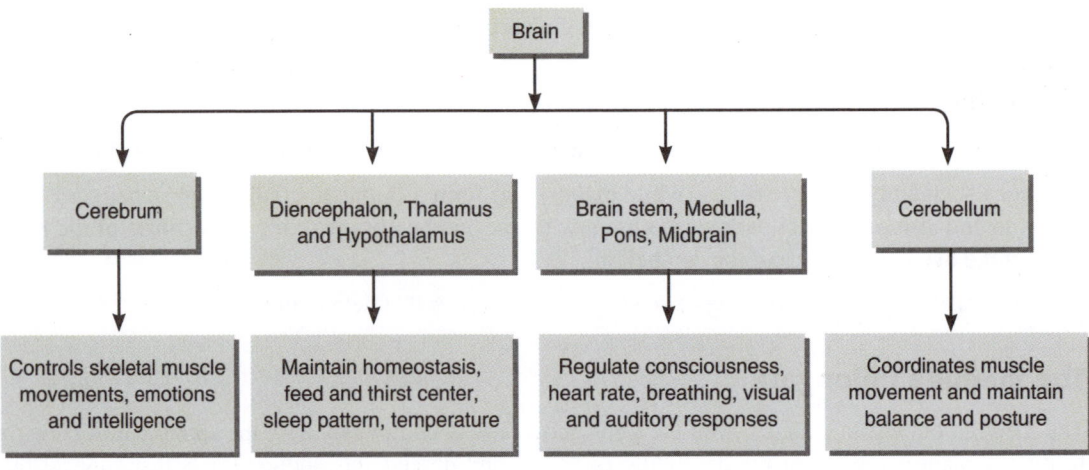

CRANIAL NERVES

There are 12 pairs of cranial nerves that leave the skull through various foramina of cranial bones.

Each cranial nerve is designated by a roman numeral (number) as well as a name. The numerals/numbers indicate the order in which the nerves arise from the brain (from anterior and posterior) and the names indicate their function and distribution. Some cranial nerves are only sensory or afferent; others are only motor or efferent. The cranial nerves with both sensory and motor functions are called *mixed nerves*.

The 12 pairs of cranial nerves are summarized in Table 1.

Table 5.1 Cranial nerves

S.no.	Nerve	Nature	Origin	Termination	Function
1.	Olfactory nerve (I)	Sensory	Olfactory lobe (roof of nose)	Temporal lobe of the cerebrum	Conducts nerve impulses for olfaction (smell)
2.	Optic nerve (II)	Sensory	Retina of eyes	Occipital lobe of the cerebrum	Conducts impulses for vision (sight)
3.	Oculomotor nerve (III)	Motor	Midbrain	Eyes	Controls movements of eyeball and eyelid Adjusts the lens for near vision and constricts the pupil in bright light Regulates proprioception
4.	Trochlear nerve (IV) (the smallest cranial nerve)	Motor	Midbrain	Eyes	Controls movements of eye ball Regulates proprioception
5.	Trigeminal nerve* (V) (the largest cranial nerve)	Mixed	**Motor:** Pons **Sensory:** Face, head and teeth	**Motor:** Chewing muscles **Sensory:** Pons	**Motor:** Contraction of chewing muscles **Sensory:** Conduct impulses of pain, temp. and touch to face, head and teeth
6.	Abducens nerve (VI)	Motor	Pons	Eyes	Controls movements of eye ball
7.	Facial nerve (VII)	Mixed	**Motor:** Pons **Sensory:** Tongue	**Motor:** Face, neck and scalp **Sensory:** Pons	**Motor:** Controls the muscles for facial expression and also controls saliva secretion **Sensory:** Conducts impulses for taste sensation

Chapter 5

S. no.	Nerve	Nature	Origin	Termination	Function
8.	Vestibulocochlear nerve (VIII) (auditory nerve)	Sensory	Inner ear	**Cochlear branch:** Temporal lobe **Vestibular branch:** Pons and Cerebellum	Cochlear branch: Conducts impulses for hearing. Vestibular branch: Conducts impulses for equilibrium.
9.	Glossopharyngeal nerve (IX)	Mixed	**Motor:** Medulla oblongata **Sensory:** Parotid gland	**Motor:** Tongue and pharynx **Sensory:** Medulla oblongata	**Motor:** Control contraction of pharynx and salivary secretion **Sensory:** Conducts impulses for taste sensation
10.	Vagus nerve (X) (major parasympathetic nerve)	Mixed	**Motor:** Medulla oblongata; **Sensory:** Pharynx, larynx, lungs, heart, GIT	**Motor:** Pharynx, larynx, lungs, heart, GIT **Sensory:** Medulla oblongata	**Motor:** Regulates GIT contraction, digestive secretions and heart rate **Sensory:** Controls skeletal muscle movements in larynx and pharynx
11.	Accessory nerve (XI)	Motor	Brain stem and spinal cord	Muscles of pharynx, larynx and neck	Regulates movement of head and controls process of swallowing
12.	Hypoglossal nerve (XII)	Motor	Medulla oblongata	Tongue muscles	Controls movement of tongue during speaking and swallowing.

* There are three branches of trigeminal nerves, which are as follows:

1. Ophthalmic, which supplies the lacrimal glands, eyes, forehead, eye lids, anterior half of scalp and nose.
2. Maxillary, which supply the cheeks, upper gums, teeth and lower eyelids.
3. Mandibular, which supplies the lower gums and teeth, ears, lower lips and tongue.

Summary of cranial nerves

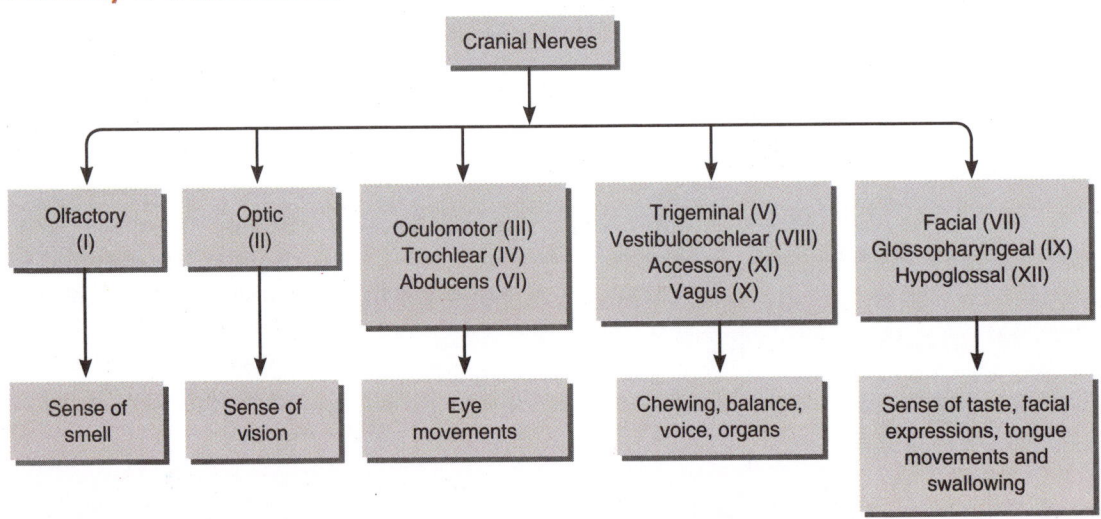

SPINAL CORD

The spinal cord is the elongated, almost cylindrical part of the CNS, which is enclosed within the vertebral canal and surrounded by the meninges and CSF.

In adults, it extends from the medulla oblongata to the superior border of the second lumbar vertebra. The length of the spinal cord ranges from 42 cm to 45 cm.

FUNCTIONS OF THE SPINAL CORD

The spinal cord is of great importance to the nervous system and to the body as a whole.

The major functions of spinal cord include the following:

1. It serves as the link between the brain and rest of the body. The ascending nerve tracts (sensory nerves) from the periphery (body parts) carry information through the spinal cord and pass it to the brain. Similarly, the descending nerve tracts (motor nerves) descend through the spinal cord and thus conduct the impulses from the brain to periphery.
2. It is responsible for spinal cord reflex (i.e. quick, automatic response to environmental changes). The spinal cord contains neuron connections between sensory and motor neurons that facilitate rapid reaction to certain stimuli (e.g. dropping a hot object when touched).

ANATOMY OF THE SPINAL CORD

External anatomy of the spinal cord

The spinal cord has two enlargements that can be viewed externally. They are as follows:

1. **Cervical enlargement**: It extends from the fourth cervical vertebra to the first thoracic vertebra. Nerves to and from the upper limbs pass through this enlargement.
2. **Lumbar enlargement**: It extends from the 9th to 12th thoracic vertebra. It serves as the passage for nerves to and from the lower limbs.

Certain external anatomical features of the spinal cord

1. **Filum terminale**: The spinal cord terminates as a tapering, conical structure called *conus medullaris* between the first and second lumbar vertebrae. From the conus medullaris, pia mater extends inferiorly and anchors the spinal cord to the coccyx. This extension of pia mater is termed *filum terminale* (Fig. 5.27).
2. **Cauda equina**: The spinal cord terminates between the first and second lumbar vertebrae but the vertebral column extends longer till the coccyx. Thus, the spinal nerves from the lumbar, sacral and coccygeal regions extend downwards from the end of the spinal cord to leave the vertebral column. These nerves are collectively named the *cauda equina* as they resemble a horse tail.

Internal anatomy of the spinal cord

Internally, the spinal cord is incompletely divided into two equal parts: anteriorly by a short median fissure and posteriorly by a deep septum, the posterior median septum.

The grey matter of the spinal cord is shaped like the letter H or a butterfly and is surrounded by the white matter.

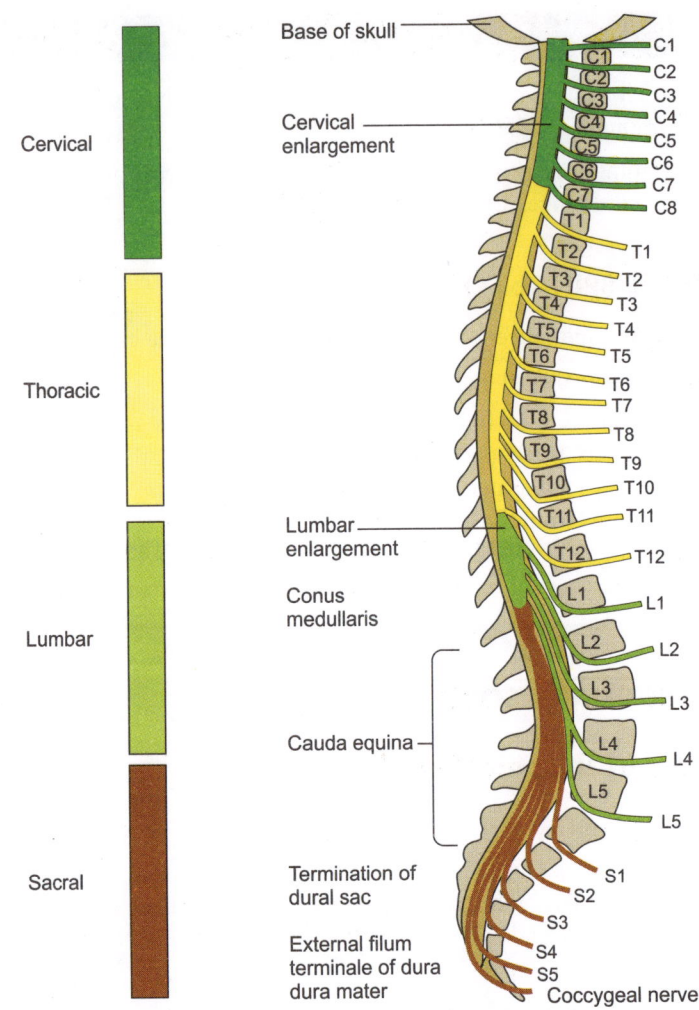

Figure 5.27 Anatomy of the spinal cord.

Arrangement of grey and white matter in the spinal cord

The nerve cell bodies in the grey matter and nerve fibres in the white matter are arranged in the following three columns (Fig. 5.28):

1. **Posterior column (dorsal root)**: It is composed of sensory nerve cell bodies and nerve fibres.
2. **Anterior column (ventral root)**: It is composed of motor nerve cell bodies and nerve fibres.
3. **Lateral column**: It is composed of connector neurons that link sensory and motor neurons to form reflex arcs.

Sensory nerve tracts in the spinal cord

Sensory/ascending/afferent tracts transmit nerve impulses through the spinal cord towards the brain.

The stimuli of sensory impulse may be as follows:

1. **Cutaneous receptors** (sensory impulses in skin): They are stimulated by pain, heat, cold, touch and pressure.
2. **Proprioceptors** (receptors in muscles, tendons and joints): They are stimulated by stretch. These receptors are associated with the maintenance of the body's balance and posture.

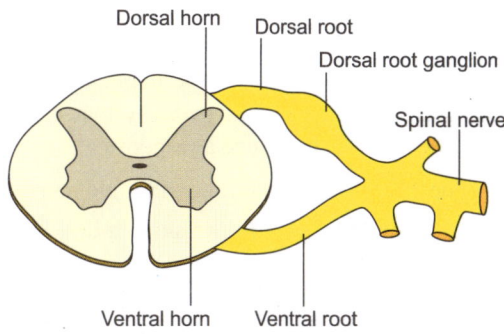

Figure 5.28 Dorsal and ventral root in the spinal cord.

Motor nerve tracts in the spinal cord

Motor/descending/efferent tracts transmit nerve impulses from the brain to the periphery. The stimulation of motor neurons is responsible for contraction of skeletal (voluntary) muscle, smooth (involuntary) muscle, cardiac muscle and secretion by glands.

The motor tracts from the brain to the periphery may follow a pyramidal or extrapyramidal pathway.

Pyramidal pathway: The pathway through which motor fibres pass through the internal capsule.

Extrapyramidal pathway: The pathway through which motor fibres do not pass through internal capsule.

Both sensory and motor nerve impulses undergo decussation (cross to the other side) either in the spinal cord or medulla and thus conduct impulse in the opposite cerebral hemisphere. Thus, the right cerebral hemisphere controls the left side of the body and vice versa.

PHYSIOLOGY OF THE SPINAL CORD

The spinal cord regulates homeostasis by the following two principal mechanisms:

1. **Propagation of nerve impulse**: As discussed previously, the sensory and motor nerve tracts travel to and from the brain through the spinal cord, which serves as a highway for nerve impulse propagation (e.g. anterior spinothalamic tract, which begins in the spinal cord and terminates in the thalamus).
2. **Integration of information**: The spinal cord serves as an integration centre for certain reflexes. A reflex is an involuntary response (i.e. fast, automatic reaction) that occurs in response to an external stimulus. Most of these reflexes are given by the spinal cord and do not depend directly on the brain. These reflexes are termed as spinal reflexes and they have a protective function.

Chapter 5

REFLEX ARC

The pathway followed by the nerve impulse that results in the reflex is called the *reflex arc*. It is the smallest and simplest pathway that can receive a stimulus, enter the spinal cord for immediate interpretation and produce a response.

The reflex arc has the following five components (Fig. 5.29):

1. **Sensory receptor in the skin**: It detects the change (stimulus) in internal or external environment and generates impulses.
2. **Sensory neuron**: It transmits the impulse from receptors to the spinal cord.
3. **Integrating centre**: Its impulse is integrated by the association neuron/connector neuron in the spinal cord.
4. **Motor neuron**: The impulse is transmitted along the motor neuron to the periphery.
5. **Effector organs**: It provides response (e.g. muscle contraction/secretion by glands).

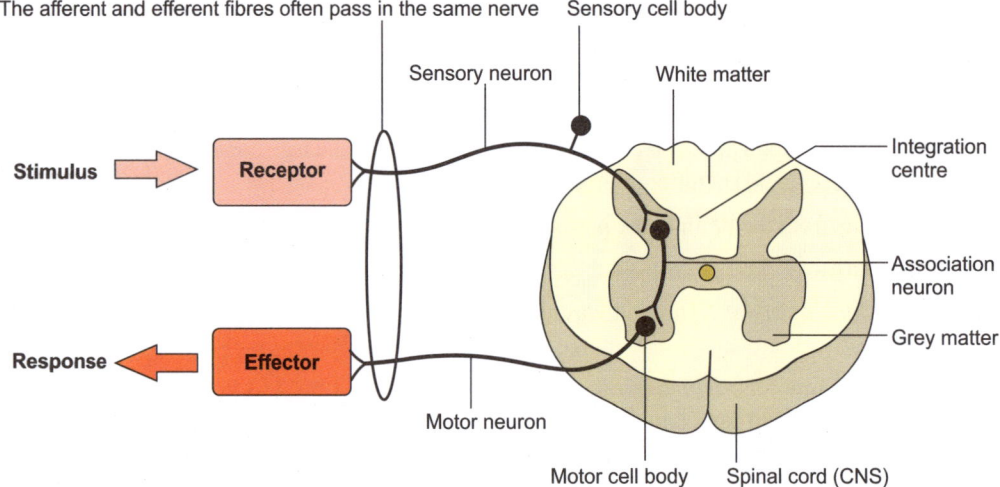

Figure 5.29 Reflex arc.

Spinal cord reflexes

Stretch reflex

A stretch reflex causes contraction of a skeletal muscle in response to the stretching of muscle (Fig. 5.30).

For example, patella (or knee jerk) reflex

Tap/slight hitting on patellar tendon (just below patella)

Causes stimulation of stretch receptors

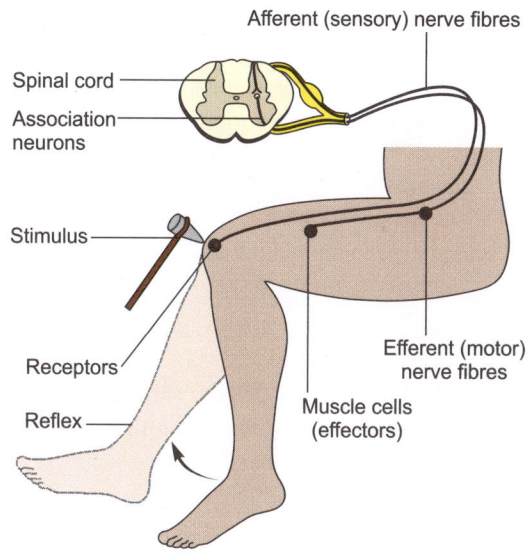

Figure 5.30 Stretch reflex.

Generates impulse that is propagated through sensory neuron to the spinal cord for interpretation

↓

In the spinal cord, the sensory neurons synapse with connector neurons, which further activate the motor neurons

↓

Motor neurons carry impulses back to the muscle and lead to muscle contraction and extension of the lower leg.

This reflex has clinical implication as it provides useful information about the health of the nervous system. The absence of stretch reflex indicates damage to sensory/motor neurons or a spinal cord injury. Thus, it may be a first step in the clinical assessment of neurological damage.

This stretch reflex also helps us maintain the body's posture.

For example,

If the body tilts to the left side

↓

The muscles in the right side of leg and trunk are stretched

↓

This initiates the stretch reflexes in the muscles and causes contraction of muscles that reestablishes the body's upright posture

Flexor reflex (or withdrawal reflex)

This reflex occurs when the stimulus is painful and can cause harm; the response of this reflex is to pull away from the danger. For example

Touching a hot plate

↓

Stimulates the sensory receptors, which send the nerve impulse through sensory neurons to the spinal cord

↓

In the spinal cord, the sensory neurons synapse with connector neurons, which in turn synapse with motor neurons

↓

Motor neurons carry impulse and produce the response due to which we pull our hand away

Autonomic reflex

Some reflexes occur inside the body to maintain homeostasis. Heart beat rate, digestion and breathing rates are maintained by these reflexes and thus help regulate the normal body functions.

These spinal reflexes automatically provide response immediately without the involvement of the brain. These immediate responses due to spinal reflexes play a major role in protecting the body from any harmful stimulus.

SPINAL NERVES

There are 31 pairs of spinal nerves that emerge from the spinal cord. These spinal nerves leave the vertebral canal by passing through the intervertebral foramina between the adjacent vertebrae.

The spinal nerves are named and numbered according to the region and level of the vertebral column from which they emerge. There are 8 pairs of cervical nerves, 12 pairs of thoracic nerves, 5 pairs of lumbar nerves, 5 pairs of sacral nerves and 1 very small coccygeal pair. The spinal nerves are numbered according to the order (starting superiorly) within the region. Thus, the 31 pairs of cranial nerves are C1–C8 (cervical), T1–T12 (thoracic), L1–L5 (lumbar), S1–S5 (sacral) and Cx (coccygeal) (Fig. 5.31).

The first cervical pair leaves the vertebral canal between the atlas (first cervical vertebrae) and occipital bone.

Nerve roots

Each spinal nerve has two connections with the spinal cord: posterior root and anterior root. The posterior nerve root consists of sensory nerve fibres and anterior nerve root consists of motor nerve fibres, which unite to form a spinal nerve that leaves the spinal cord through intervertebral foramina (Fig. 5.32).

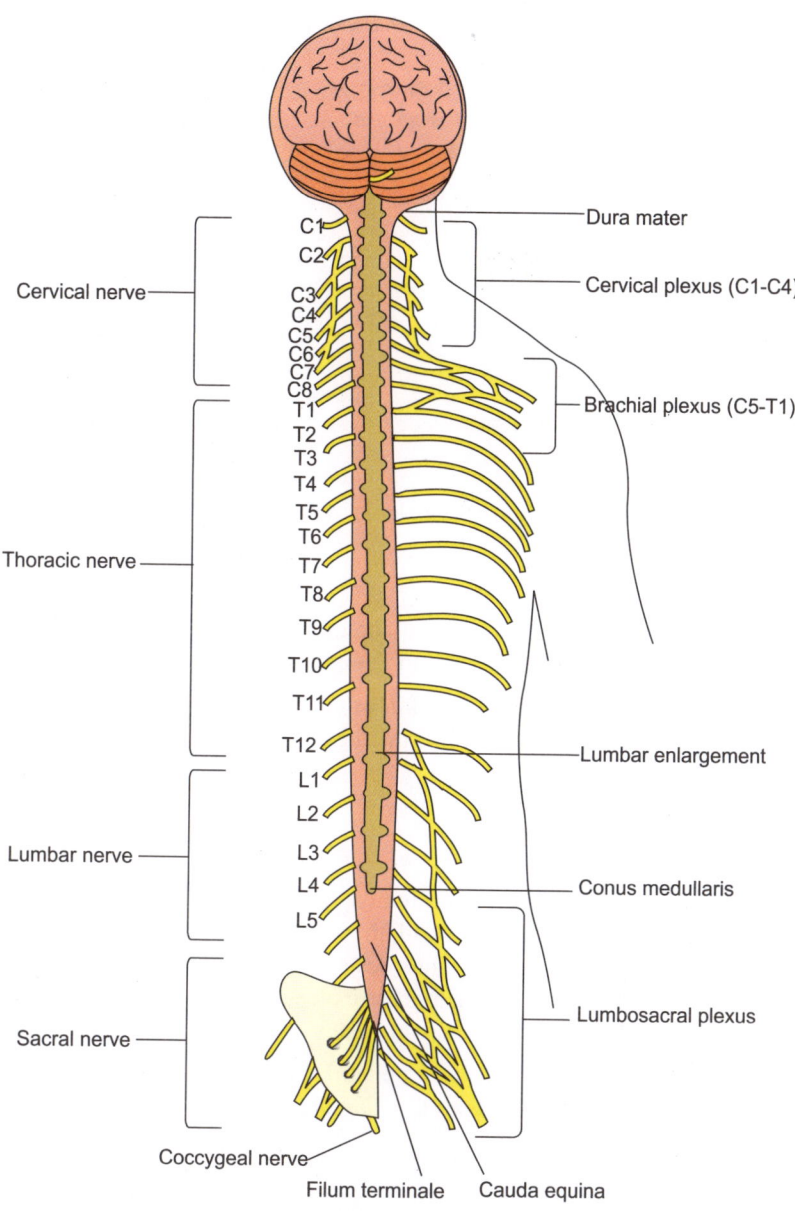

Figure 5.31 Spinal nerves.

The anterior nerve root is made up of the motor neurons that carry the impulses from the spinal cord to the muscle or glands. The posterior nerve root is made of the sensory neurons that carry impulses into the spinal cord. Just outside the spinal cord, there is an enlargement called *posterior root ganglion* that contains the cell bodies of the sensory neurons. The sensory nerve fibres pass through these ganglia before entering the spinal cord. The area of the skin that provides sensory input to CNS through nerves is called *dermatome*.

Chapter 5

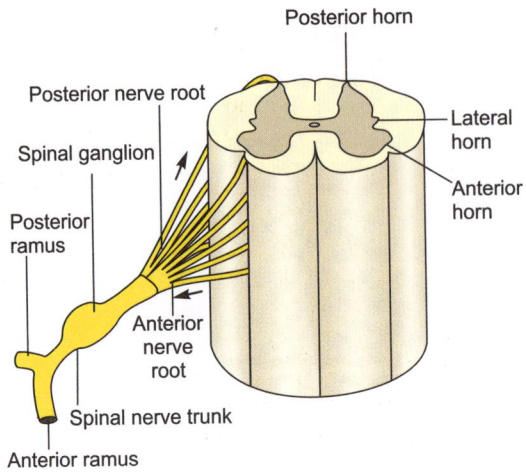

Figure 5.32 Nerve root.

Branches

Immediately after emerging from the intervertebral foramen, the spinal nerves divide into several branches or rami: posterior ramus, anterior ramus and ramus communicans.

Posterior ramus supplies the deep muscles and skin of the posterior trunk. Anterior ramus supplies the anterior and lateral (sides) portions of the trunk, and the upper and lower limbs.

Ramus communicans forms the part of the ANS.

Plexuses

The anterior rami (motor neurons) of the cervical, lumbar and sacral regions (except thoracic) do not go directly to the body structures they supply. Instead, they unite with various anterior rami of adjacent nerves and form networks on both the left and right sides of the body before proceeding to a particular area. Such a network is called a *plexus*; there are five large plexus on each side of the vertebral column: cervical plexus, brachial plexus, lumbar plexus, sacral plexus and coccygeal plexus (Fig. 5.33).

This implies that each region of the body is supplied by more than one spinal nerve; therefore, damage to one spinal nerve does not cause loss of function of a region.

Note: The anterior rami of spinal nerves (T2–T12) do not form plexus and are known as *intercostal* or *thoracic nerves*.

Spinal nerves

❑ **Cervical plexus (C1–C5)**: It supplies the head, neck, superior part of the shoulder and chest.
  ➤ *Phrenic nerve (C3–C5)*: It supplies the diaphragm.

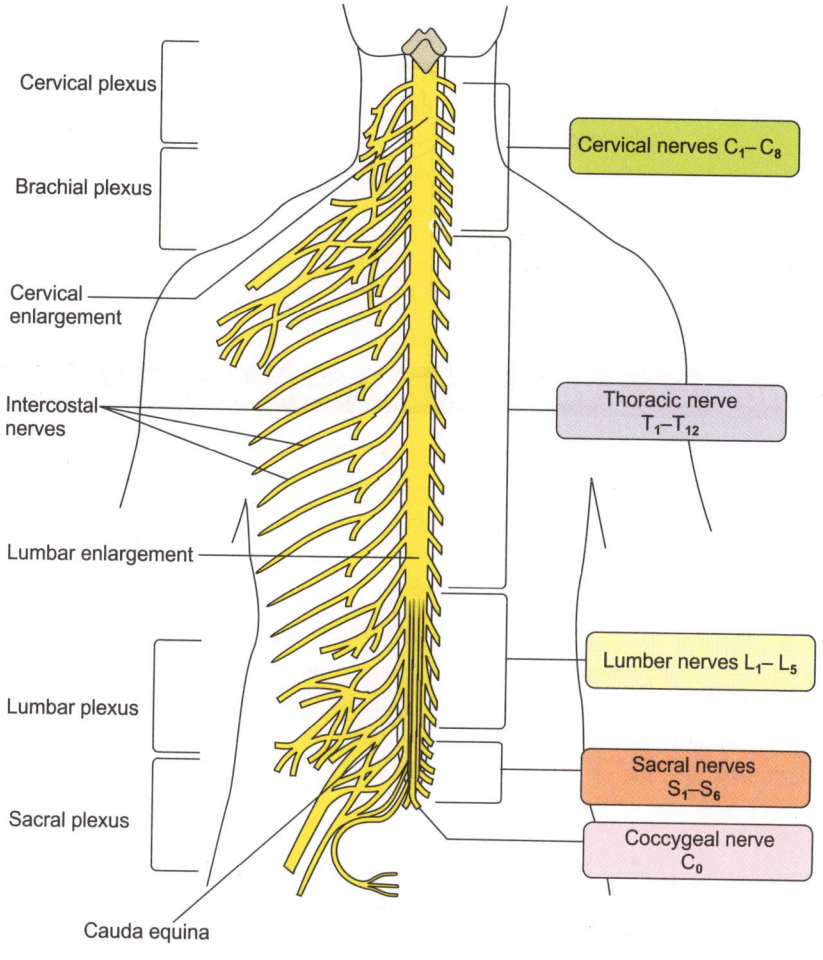

Figure 5.33 Plexuses (posterior view).

❑ **Brachial plexus (C5–C8), T1**: It supplies the upper limbs and shoulders.
  ➤ The following are the five important nerves arising from the brachial plexus:
   1. *Axillary nerve*: It supplies the deltoid muscle and shoulder joint.
   2. *Radial nerve*: It supplies the posterior arm, forearm, hand, thumb and first two fingers.
   3. *Musculocutaneous nerve*: It supplies the muscles of forearm.
   4. *Median nerve*: It supplies the anterior arm, forearm and hand.
   5. *Ulnar nerve*: It supplies the medial arm, forearm, hand, little finger and ring finger.

- ❏ **Intercostal nerves (T2–T12):** They supply the intercostals muscles, abdominal muscles and skin of the trunk.
- ❏ **Lumbar plexus (L1–L4):** It supplies the abdominal wall, external genitalis and lower limbs.
  - ➤ One of the important branches of the lumbar plexus is the femoral nerve, which supplies the anterior thigh, leg and foot.
- ❏ **Sacral plexus (L4–L5) and (S1–S4):** It supplies the pelvic organs, lower limbs and buttocks.
  - ➤ The largest nerve in the body, the sciatic nerve arises from the sacral plexus. This nerve supplies the posterior thigh, leg and foot.
- ❏ **Coccygeal plexus (S4–S5 and coccygeal nerve):** It supplies the skin around the coccyx and anal area.

THE AUTONOMIC NERVOUS SYSTEM

The autonomic or involuntary part of the nervous system functions automatically without conscious effort. The autonomic activity produces rapid effects and major effector organs include the following:

1. **Smooth muscle**: It is involved in the change in blood vessels diameter and airway.
2. **Cardiac muscle**: It is involved in the change in rate and force of heartbeat.
3. **Glands**: It is involved in the increase/decrease in secretion by glands.

   The ANS is separated into two divisions: sympathetic division and parasympathetic division.

- ❏ These two divisions have both structural and functional differences and normally work in an opposing manner. Sympathetic activity tends to predominate in stressful situations and helps deal with emergency situations, whereas the parasympathetic activity predominates during rest. Their opposing nature plays a major role in the regulation of involuntary functions. The activity of both the divisions is integrated by the hypothalamus, which ensures their appropriate response to the situation.
- ❏ An autonomic nerve pathway from the CNS to the effector organ consists of two motor neurons that synapse in a ganglion outside the CNS (Fig. 5.34). The first neuron is called the *preganglionic neuron*, from the CNS to the ganglion. The second neuron is called the *postganglionic neuron*, from the ganglion to the effector organs. The preganglionic neuron synapses with postganglionic neuron in the ganglion outside the CNS and the postganglionic neuron then conducts impulses to the effector organ.

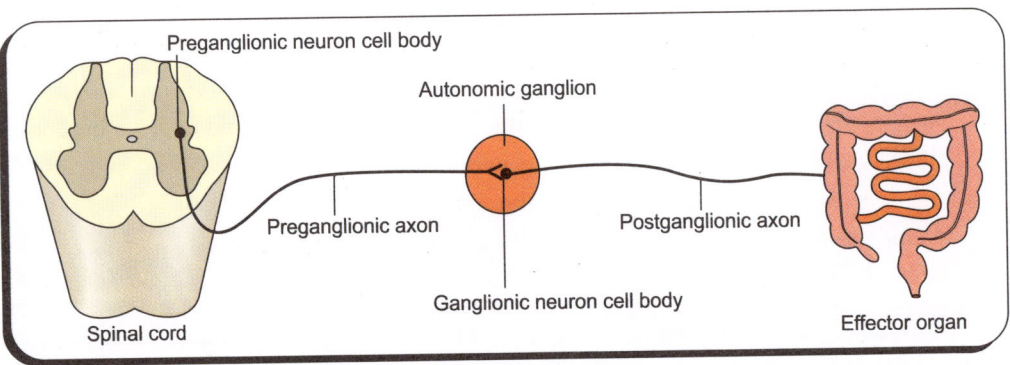

Figure 5.34 Autonomic nerve pathway.

SYMPATHETIC DIVISION

This division is also named as *thoracolumbar division*, which designates the origin of the sympathetic preganglionic neuron. The preganglionic nerve fibre leaves the spinal cord and terminates at the synapse in the sympathetic ganglia. The neurotransmitter at the sympathetic ganglia is acetylcholine. The postganglionic nerve fibre originates in ganglia and terminates in the effector organ. Noradrenaline (norepinephrine) is the neurotransmitter at the effector organ.

One preganglionic neuron often synapses with many postganglionic neurons. This anatomic arrangement has physiological importance as this brings widespread responses in many organs.

The sympathetic division is dominant in stressful situations, which include anger, fear, anxiety and exercise and prepares the body for 'fight or flight response'. The effects caused by sympathetic stimulation in stressed conditions include the following:

1. Increased heart rate
2. Vasodilation in skeletal muscle, which supplies them with more oxygen
3. Dilation in bronchioles to take more air
4. Glycogenolysis to provide energy
5. Decreased digestive secretion and decreased peristalsis
6. Vasoconstriction in skin and visceral organs such as heart, muscles and brain

All these responses enable our body to prepare for life-threatening or stressful situations.

❏ Thus in the autonomic nerve pathways, there are two synapses: one between preganglionic and postganglionic neurons and the other between postganglionic neuron and the effector organs.

❏ The neurotransmitter released by all preganglionic neurons, both sympathetic and parasympathetic neurons, is acetylcholine. The sympathetic postganglionic neurons release noradrenaline (norepinephrine) at the synapse with effector organs, whereas the parasympathetic postganglionic neuron releases acetylcholine at synapse with effector organs (Fig. 5.35).

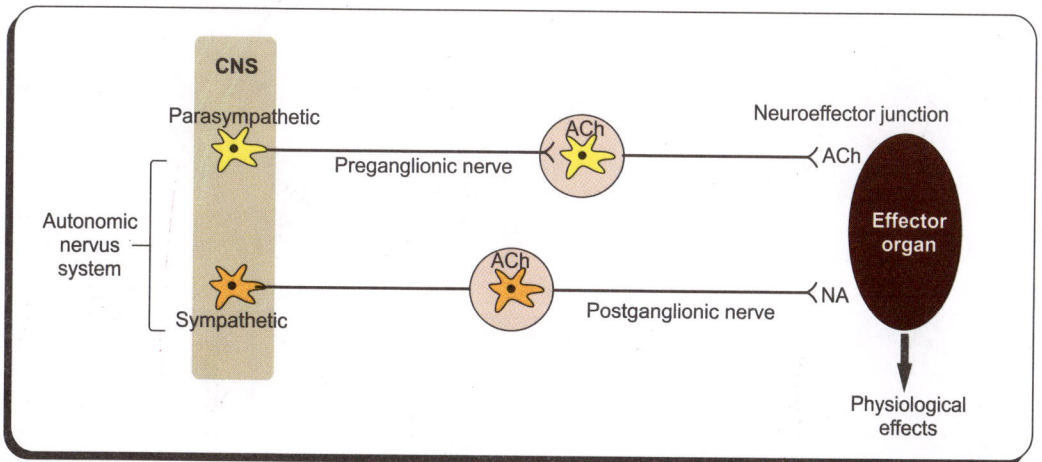

Figure 5.35 Main components of the ANS.

Chapter 5

PARASYMPATHETIC DIVISION

This division is also named as *craniosacral division*. The preganglionic neurons originate in the brain stem and sacral segments of the spinal cord and leave the spinal cord to synapse at parasympathetic ganglia, which are very close to or are in the effector organ. The postganglionic neuron is usually very short and it terminates in the effector organ.

In this division, one preganglionic neuron synapses with very few postganglionic neurons. This anatomic arrangement enables the localized response of parasympathetic division.

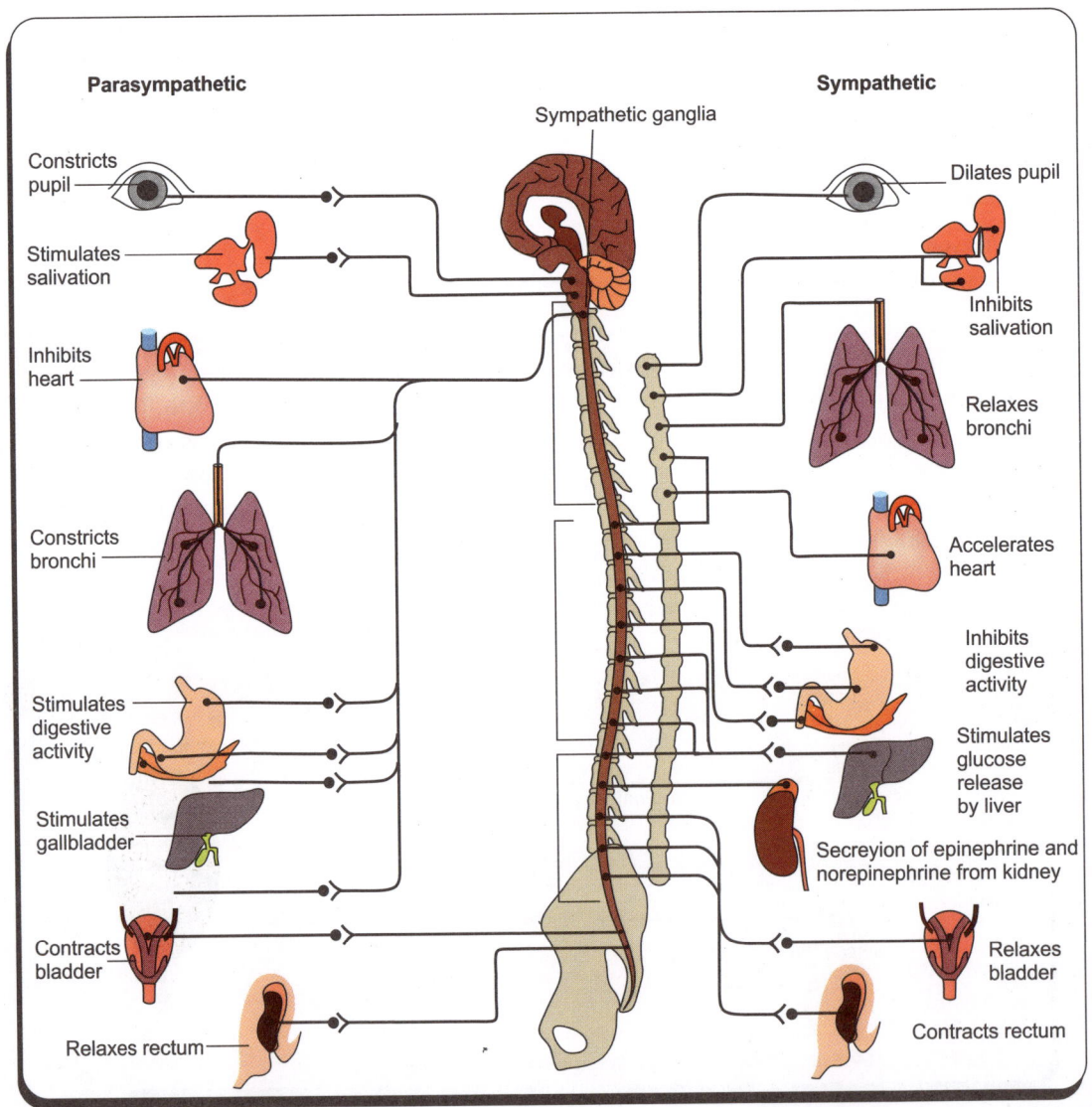

Figure 5.36 Comparison of sympathetic and parasympathetic divisions.

The parasympathetic division dominates in relaxed (nonstress) situations to promote normal functioning of the body and acts as peacemaker to restore the processes peacefully and quietly. Some of the effects caused by parasympathetic stimulation include the following:

1. Efficient digestion with increased peristalsis and increased secretions
2. Normal heart rate
3. Contraction of smooth muscles

Most of the organs of the body are supplied by both parasympathetic and sympathetic nerves, which have opposite effects. Thus, both the divisions function together to maintain balance, ensuring homeostasis (Fig. 5.36).

Exception: Some effector organs receive only sympathetic impulses, for example sweat glands. In such cases, the opposite response is brought about by a decrease in sympathetic impulse.

Neurohumoral transmission in the ANS

Neurohumoral transmission implies that nerves transmit their message across the synapses by the release of humoral, that is chemical messengers. These chemical messengers or neurotransmitters are mainly adrenaline in sympathetic nerves and acetylcholine in parasympathetic nerves. The neurotransmitters are present in the presynaptic neurons and are released in the synapse after nerve stimulation.

Steps in neurohumoral transmission

1. Impulse conduction
   Nerve stimulation causes a sudden increase in sodium (Na^+) conduction and results in depolarization.
2. Release of neurotransmitters
   The neurotransmitter is stored in the vesicle of presynaptic neuron. The depolarization causes the release of neurotransmitter from the vesicle into the synapse.
3. Neurotransmitter action
   The released neurotransmitter combines with specific receptors on the postsynaptic neuron and results in a specific response, which may be muscle contraction or secretion from a gland.

PAIN PATHWAY

Pain is defined as an unpleasant sensation and emotional experience associated with or without actual tissue damage. It mainly serves a protective function by signalling the presence of noxious, tissue-damaging conditions.

Pain may be classified as follows:

- **Cutaneous pain**: It is a sharp, bright, burning; it can have a fast or slow onset.
- **Deep somatic pain**: It stems from tendons, muscles, joints, periosteum and blood vessels.
- **Visceral pain**: It originates from internal organs; it is diffused initially and later may be localized (e.g. appendicitis).
- **Psychogenic pain**: An individual feels pain but the cause is emotional rather than physical.

Whenever a pain stimulus is applied, initially a sharp and localized pain sensation is produced. This is called the *fast pain* and is carried by A-delta (Aδ) fibres. The fast pain is followed by a dull, diffused and unpleasant pain. This is known as *slow pain* and is carried by C type of nerve fibres.

Chapter 5

Nociceptive neuron (nerve receptors that transmits pain impulses) transmits pain impulses to the spinal cord through unmyelinated C fibres and myelinated A-delta fibres. The smaller C fibres carry impulses at the rate of 0.5–2.0 m/s and the larger A-delta fibres carry impulses at the rate of 5–30 m/s.

PATHWAYS OF PAIN SENSATION

1. **Pain pathway from the skin and deeper structures**: The receptors for pain (i.e. nociceptors) are free nerve endings and they are distributed throughout the body. Intense thermal, mechanical or chemical stimuli activate the nociceptors (Fig. 5.37).

Mechanical, chemical or thermal stimuli

↓

Activate pain receptors (nociceptors)

↓

Nerve impulse from nociceptors passed to the posterior column of the spinal cord

First-order neurons
{ Fast pain – carried by Aδ fibres

Slow pain – carried by C-type fibres }

↓

Second-order neurons { The nerve fibres in the spinal cord carry the impulses from the spinal cord towards the thalamus by the lateral spinothalamic tract

↓

Third-order neurons { The third-order neurons are neurons of the thalamus and these nerve fibres pass the impulse to the sensory area of the cerebral cortex where the pain is perceived

Thus, the nerve impulse for pain is carried from nociceptors to cerebral cortex through first-, second- and third-order neurons, and Substance P is thought to be responsible for the transmission of pain-producing impulses.

2. **Pain pathway from viscera and face**
   (a) Pain sensation from thoracic and abdominal viscera is carried by sympathetic nerves.
   (b) Pain from the oesophagus, trachea and pharynx is transmitted by the vagus nerve.
   (c) Pain sensation from the face is carried by the trigeminal nerve.

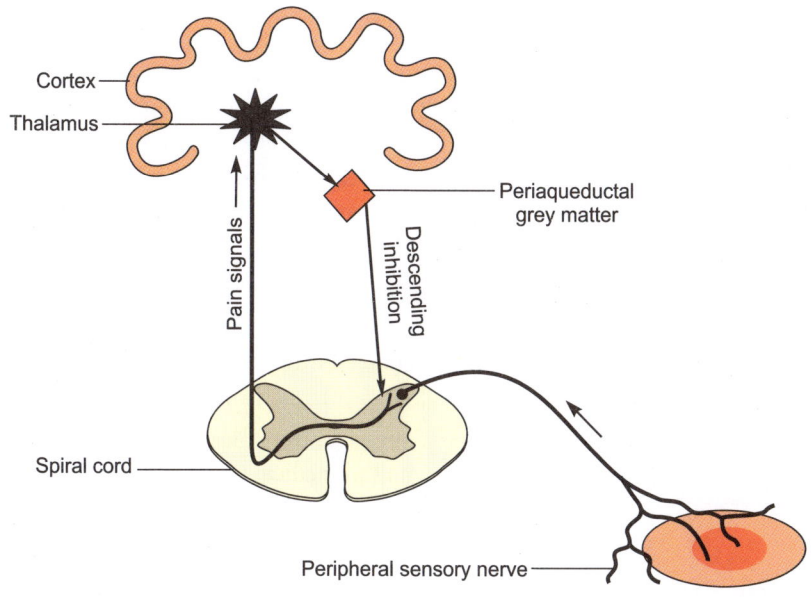

Figure 5.37 Pain pathway.

REFERRED PAIN

The pain sensation produced in some parts of the body is felt in other structures away from the site of origin. This is called *referred pain* (e.g. cardiac pain is felt in the left arm and the left shoulder and pain in diaphragm is felt in right shoulder).

DISORDERS ASSOCIATED WITH THE NERVOUS SYSTEM

STROKE (CEREBROVASCULAR ACCIDENT)

Stroke is a general term for a sudden neurological event that results in the onset of neurological symptoms such as paralysis or loss of sensation, which arise from the destruction of brain tissue. It is the common cause of death and disability, especially in the elderly.

Causes: It can be caused by hypertension, emboli (blood clots), cigarette smoking, diabetes mellitus and atherosclerosis (formation of cholesterol-containing plaques that block blood flow). In this disease, the blood flow to the brain is suddenly interrupted, causing hypoxia.

Symptoms: Symptoms include paralysis or loss of sensation, weakness, speech defect or the inability to speak. In severe conditions, it can also result in death.

Treatment: Treatment includes supportive (like oxygen supply, IV fluid) and medical (like tissue plasminogen activator [TPA] and heparin and aspirin) aid.

Chapter 5

EPILEPSY

Epilepsy is a common chronic neurological disorder characterized by recurrent unprovoked seizures. Seizures are an abnormal overactivity of the cells of the brain, which can affect variable regions of the CNS, primarily in the forebrain. These seizures are initiated by abnormal, synchronous electrical discharges from millions of neurons in the brain. However, it almost never affects intelligence. Epilepsy is more likely to occur in young children or in people over the age of 65; however, it can occur at any time.

Causes: Any injury to the brain can lead to seizures, including trauma, tumours, vascular lesions, haemorrhage and developmental anomalies.

Symptoms: Symptoms include physical convulsions, sensory hallucinations, alteration or loss of consciousness and drop attacks.

Treatment: It includes medication by antiepileptic drugs (barbiturates, benzodiazepines, ethosuximide, phenytoin, etc.) and surgery. Only those patients who fail medical treatment or who have some specific causes of epilepsy are referred for surgical treatment.

PARKINSON'S DISEASE

It is a degenerative disease process (associated with ageing) that affects the basal ganglia of the brain. In this disease, there is gradual degeneration of dopamine-releasing neurons in the extrapyramidal system.

Causes: It is associated with a deficiency of the neurotransmitter dopamine and with ageing.

Symptoms: Symptoms include tremor, rigidity of voluntary muscles and lack of control and coordination of muscle movement.

Treatment: It includes treatment with drugs such as levodopa, selegiline and anticholinergic drugs such as benzotropine and trihexyphenidyl.

NEURITIS

It is a disease of the peripheral nerves showing the pathological changes of inflammation.

Causes: Causes include infection, chemical injury, physical injury, radiation and poisons such as carbon monoxide, heavy metals and some drugs.

Symptoms: Symptoms include inflammation of the nerves, which may be painful, hypoaesthesia (numbness), paralysis and disappearance of the reflexes.

Treatment: It includes treatment with drugs such as tricyclic antidepressant (such as amitriptyline) and antiepileptic therapies such as gabapentin or sodium valproate.

ALZHEIMER'S DISEASE

It is a slowly progressive disease and is the common form of dementia of the brain that is characterized by impairment of memory and eventually by disturbances in reasoning, planning, language and perception.

It usually affects older people but may begin in middle age with symptoms of memory loss and behavioural changes.

Causes: It can be caused by head injury, hereditary factors resulting in the loss of neurons in the cerebral cortex and decrease in brain size.

Symptoms: Symptoms include memory loss, confusion, restlessness, decrease in intellectual capacity and, occasionally, speech disturbances.

Treatment: Drugs such as tacrine, memantine, rivastigmine and piracetam.

MULTIPLE SCLEROSIS

It is a progressive destruction of myelin sheaths in the CNS that results in slow conduction of nerve impulses.

Causes: It can be caused by genetic factors and immune factors.

Symptoms: Symptoms include weakness of skeletal muscles, lack of coordination and movement, visual disturbances and may cause paralysis.

Treatment: Treatment includes corticosteroids and interferons.

TETANUS

It is a prolonged painful muscle spasm that occurs due to disruption in the action of motor neurons.

Causes: It can be caused by bacteria *Clostridium tetani* that produces a neurotoxin that affects the motor neurons in the spinal cord and brain stem.

Death may occur due to spasm of respiratory muscles and diaphragm.

Symptoms: Symptoms include restlessness, headache, and irritability. The tetanus neurotoxin causes the muscles to tighten up into a continuous ('tetanic' or 'tonic') contraction or spasm. The jaw is 'locked' by muscle spasms, giving the name *lockjaw* (also called 'trismus').

Treatment: Treatment includes antibiotics (e.g. metronidazole) to kill the bacteria; tetanus booster shot; if necessary, and occasionally, antitoxin to neutralize the toxin.

POLIOMYELITIS

This neurological disorder is characterized by fever, severe headache, stiffness of neck and back, muscle pain and weakness, and loss of certain reflexes.

Causes: It can be caused by a virus called poliovirus, hormonal deficiencies and environmental toxins.

Symptoms: Symptoms include fever, severe headache, stiff neck and back, deep muscle pain and weakness and loss of certain somatic reflexes.

Treatment: Treatment includes administration of pyridostigmine to increase the action of acetylcholine in stimulating muscle contraction, nerve growth factors to stimulate nerve growth and muscle-strengthening exercises.

Chapter 5

BRAIN INJURY

It is commonly associated with head trauma and results in the displacement of neuronal tissue. The effects of brain injury include increased intracranial pressure, decreased blood pressure and respiratory complications.

Brain injury may be of varied degrees, which are as follows:

Concussion: It is an abrupt loss of consciousness after sudden blow to the head. It is the most common form of head injury. Symptoms include headache, drowsiness, lack of concentration and confusion.

Contusion: It is bruising of the brain due to trauma and includes the leakage of blood. It results in immediate loss of consciousness, loss of reflexes, decreased blood pressure and transient cessation of respiration.

Laceration: It is a tear of the brain, usually from a skull fracture, that results in rupture of large blood vessels. It causes localized pooling of blood, oedema and increased intracranial pressure.

CEREBRAL PALSY

It is a group of motor disorders that causes loss of muscle control and coordination and occurs due to the damage of the motor areas of the brain during brain development at fetal life or infancy.

Causes: It can be caused by viral infection, radiation during fetal life and temporary lack of oxygen during birth.

Symptoms: Symptoms include impaired speaking, difficulty in swallowing, muscle tremors and spasms and awkward movements.

Treatment: Medications used to relieve spasticity and abnormal movements include the following:

❑ Dopaminergic drugs such as levodopa/carbidopa and trihexyphenidyl.
❑ Muscle relaxants such as baclofen
❑ Benzodiazepines such as diazepam
❑ Botulinum toxin type A such as BOTOX

MENINGITIS

It is a life-threatening inflammation of the meninges, the tough layer of tissue that surrounds the brain and the spinal cord. If left untreated, it may lead to brain swelling, permanent disability, coma and even death.

Causes: It is caused by bacteria (the most serious) or viral infection.

Symptoms: Symptoms include headache, fever, stiff neck, confusion, seizures and in severe conditions it may result in paralysis, coma and death.

Treatment: Treatment includes the following:

❑ For viral meningitis, it includes acetaminophen and other pain medications.
❑ For bacterial meningitis, it includes intravenous antibiotics, an IV line is inserted and fluids are administered.
❑ Steroids may be given to try to decrease the severity of the disease.

ENCEPHALITIS

Encephalitis is an acute infection and inflammation of the brain tissue.

Causes: It is caused by viral infection. The viruses gain entry into the CNS and damage the neurons by multiplying within them or stimulating an immune reaction.

Symptoms: Symptoms include coma, fever and convulsions and could result in death.

Treatment: Treatment includes the following:

- ❑ For herpes encephalitis: Acyclovir.
- ❑ Other than herpes encephalitis: People infected with viral encephalitis are hydrated with IV fluids while monitoring for brain swelling. Anticonvulsants can be given for seizure control.

HYDROCEPHALUS

It is a condition characterized by elevated CSF pressure caused due to brain abnormalities such as tumour, inflammation or developmental malformation. These abnormalities interfere with the drainage of CSF from the ventricles and lead to its accumulation.

Other diseases of the nervous system include the following:

1. **Myelitis**: It is the inflammation of the spinal cord.

2. **Neuralgia**: It is pain in nerves.

3. **Neuritis**: It is the inflammation of nerves that may be due to injury, bone fracture or infections.

4. **Paraesthesia**: It is a disorder of the sensory nerve that results in abnormal sensation such as burning, tickling or tingling.

5. **Hemiplegia**: It is the paralysis of the upper limb trunk and lower limb on one side of the body.

6. **Monoplagia**: It is the paralysis of only one limb.

7. **Schizophrenia**: It is a severe psychiatric illness with severe distortion of thought, behaviour and the capacity to recognize reality, which results in hallucination and the inability to think coherently.

8. **Mania**: It is characterized by hyperactivity, uncontrollable thought and speech, irritable mood and reduced sleep.

Chapter 5

Electroencephalogram

❑ The recording of electrical activities of the brain is called the *electroencephalogram* (*EEG*). German psychiatrist Hans Berger was the first one to analyze the EEG waves systematically, and hence EEG waves are also referred to as *Berger's waves*.

❑ **Significance of EEG**: EEG is useful in the diagnosis of neurological and sleep disorders. The common neurological disorders that cause changes in the EEG pattern are epilepsy and disorders of the midbrain.

❑ **Method of recording EEG**: EEG can be recorded by using scalp electrodes, which are placed over the brain after opening the skull, or by piercing into the brain.

❑ **Waves of EEG**: In normal persons, EEG has three frequency bands: (1) Alpha rhythm (2) Beta rhythm (3) Delta rhythm

❑ **Alpha rhythm**: This is obtained in an inattentive brain or mind as in drowsiness, light sleep or narcosis with closed eyes. This is abolished by visual stimuli or any other type of stimuli or by mental effort. Hence, it is diminished when the eyes are opened.

❑ **Beta rhythm**: This is recorded during mental activity or mental tension or arousal state. It is not affected by the opening of the eyes.

❑ **Delta rhythm**: This commonly occurs in early childhood during waking hours. In adults, it appears mostly during deep sleep. The presence of delta waves in adults during conditions other than sleep indicates pathological processes in the brain such as tumour, epilepsy, increased intracranial pressure and mental deficiency or depression. These waves are not affected by the opening of the eyes.

Lumbar Puncture or Spinal Tap

❑ It is a diagnostic and therapeutic procedure that is performed to collect a sample of cerebrospinal fluid (CSF) for the biochemical, microbiological and cytological analysis.

❑ It is performed by giving local anaesthetic and inserting a needle into the subarachnoid space in the spinal cord.

Ageing and Nervous System

❑ Ageing is associated with various changes in the nervous system such as the following:
1. Decreased brain size
2. Loss of neurons in the outer part of the cerebral cortex
3. Loss of synapses and neurotransmitters

❑ These changes result in the following:
1. Decreased capacity to send impulses to and from the brain
2. Decreased processing of information
3. Slowing of voluntary muscular movements
4. Increased reflex time

❑ All these age-related factors along with the reduction in the size of arteries supplying the brain make the elderly much more susceptible to strokes.

Embryonic Development of Nervous System

- ❏ Development of the nervous system begins in the third week of gestation.
- ❏ **3rd week**: The ectoderm thickens and develops into a neural plate. The plate folds inwards and forms a neural groove. The raised edges of the plate are called neural folds, which form a tube called the neural tube.
- ❏ The covering of the neural tube differentiates into three layers of cells, which are as follows:
  - ➤ Outer layer, which develops into white matter
  - ➤ Middle layer, which develops into grey matter
  - ➤ Inner layer, which develops into lining of the spinal cord and ventricles of the brain
- ❏ **4th week**: Neural tube develops into prosencephalon, or forebrain; mesencephalon or midbrain; and rhombocephalon or hindbrain.
- ❏ **5th week**: Prosencephalon develops into the following:
  - ➤ Telencephalon, which forms the cerebral hemisphere
  - ➤ Diencephalon, which forms the thalamus and hypothalamus
- ❏ Rhombocephalon develops into the following:
  - ➤ Metencephalon, which forms pons and medulla
  - ➤ Myelencephalon, which forms medulla oblongata

HOW TO KEEP YOUR BRAIN HEALTHY

1. Get out and get some physical exercise. Aerobic exercise produces oxygen that is used by brain for energy that helps stimulate the growth of new brain cells.
2. Exercise the brain's mental abilities by doing mental exercises like reading, playing cards and solving crossword puzzles.
3. Try to avoid sugar, saturated fats, trans fats, preservatives, alcohol, caffeine
4. Eat more fish, colourful fruits and vegetables, nuts, whole grains, egg yolks, olive oil.
5. Take saunas and steam baths to promote sweating, which helps eliminate toxins through the skin.
6. Take plenty of rest as it relaxes the body, mind and spirit.

Chapter 5

Review Questions

Long Answer Questions

1. Describe the structure and functions of the central nervous system.
2. Discuss the anatomy of a neuron with the help of a well-labelled diagram.
3. Explain the external and internal anatomy of the spinal cord.
4. List the principal structures in each of the five regions of the brain and indicate their general functions.

5. Describe the location and structure of the diencephalon and explain its autonomic functions.

6. Review the organization of the autonomic nervous system and distinguish between the sympathetic and parasympathetic divisions.

7. Name the 12 pairs of *cranial nerves* and their functions.

8. What specific physiological activities are regulated by the ANS?

9. Explain the various functions of the hypothalamus.

10. Discuss the reflex arc.

Multiple Choice Questions

1. The white matter of the central nervous system (CNS) is always
   - (a) Deep to the grey matter
   - (b) Unmyelinated
   - (c) Arranged into tracts
   - (d) Composed of sensory fibres only

2. Which of the following are the three initial developmental regions of the brain?
   - (a) Telencephalon, prosencephalon, rhombencephalon
   - (b) Rhombencephalon, prosencephalon, mesencephalon
   - (c) Metencephalon, myelencephalon, prosencephalon
   - (d) Prosencephalon, diencephalon, mesencephalon

3. The third ventricle is located in
   - (a) The cerebrum
   - (b) The forebrain
   - (c) The hindbrain
   - (d) The midbrain
   - (e) The cerebellum

4. Neuropeptides are
   - (a) Neurotransmitter chemicals
   - (b) Neuroglia
   - (c) Products of the choroid plexuses
   - (d) Nutrients for brain tissue
   - (e) Both (a) and (c)

5. The thalamus is located in
   - (a) The telencephalon
   - (b) The mesencephalon
   - (c) The diencephalon
   - (d) The metencephalon
   - (e) The myelencephalon

6. Regarding the cerebrum, which of the following is a *false* statement?
   - (a) It accounts for about 80% of the brain's mass
   - (b) It consists of four paired lobes
   - (c) It contains a thin superficial layer of convoluted grey matter
   - (d) It is located within the telencephalonic region of the brain

7. Which is *not* a lobe of the cerebrum?

   (a) Parietal lobe　　　　　　　(b) Insula

   (c) Occipital lobe　　　　　　(d) Temporal lobe

   (e) Sphenoidal lobe

8. Which lobe–function pairing is *incorrect*?

   (a) Frontal lobe–sensory interpretation

   (b) Parietal lobe–speech patterns

   (c) Occipital lobe–vision

   (d) Temporal lobe–memory

   (e) Parietal lobe–somaesthetic interpretation

9. The basal nuclei form all of the following *except*

   (a) The putamen　　　　　　(b) The caudate nucleus

   (c) The globus pallidus　　　(d) The infundibulum

10. Clusters of neuron cell bodies embedded in the white matter of the brain are referred to as

    (a) Nuclei　　　　　　　　(b) Gyri

    (c) Sulci　　　　　　　　　(d) Ganglia

    (e) Fasciculi

11. Tracts of white matter that connect the right and left cerebral hemispheres are composed of

    (a) Decussation fibres　　　　(b) Association fibres

    (c) Commissural fibres　　　(d) Projection fibres

12. The primary motor cortex, Broca's area, and the premotor area are located in which lobe?

    (a) Frontal　　　　　　　　(b) Parietal

    (c) Temporal　　　　　　　(d) Occipital

13 The innermost layer of the meninges, delicate and closely apposed to the brain tissue, is the

    (a) Dura mater　　　　　　(b) Corpus callosum

    (c) Arachnoid　　　　　　(d) Pia mater

14. CSF is formed by

    (a) Arachnoid villi　　　　　(b) The dura mater

    (c) Choroid plexuses　　　　(d) All of these

15. Fibre tracts that allow neurons within the same cerebral hemisphere to communicate are

    (a) Association tracts

    (b) Commissures

    (c) Projection tracts

Chapter 5

16. The chemical transmitter between sympathetic postganglionic fibres and the effector organs is
    (a) Norepinephrine
    (b) Acetylcholine
    (c) Adrenaline
    (d) Epinephrine

17. Most body organs are innervated by
    (a) The parasympathetic division of the autonomic nervous system (ANS)
    (b) The sympathetic division of the ANS
    (c) Both divisions of the ANS
    (d) The central nervous system (CNS)

18. The connective tissue sheath that surrounds a fascicle of nerve fibres is the
    (a) Epineurium
    (b) Endoneurium
    (c) Perineurium
    (d) Neurilemma

19. Which brain structure–autonomic function pairing is *incorrect*?
    (a) Pons–respiration
    (b) Corpus callosum–blood pressure
    (c) Medulla oblongata–respiration
    (d) Thalamus–intense pain
    (e) Hypothalamus–body temperature

20. An abnormal production of antidiuretic hormone (ADH) could result from a dysfunction of
    (a) The hypothalamus
    (b) The choroid plexus
    (c) The medulla oblongata
    (d) The reticular activation system
    (e) The pineal gland

Fill in the Blanks

1. A _____ is the area of the skin innervated by all the cutaneous neurons of a given spinal or cranial nerve.

2. The _____ cranial nerve innervates the lateral rectus (ocular) muscle.

3. _____ is a disorder of the trigeminal (fifth cranial) nerve characterized by severe recurring pain on one side of the face.

4. The _____ nerve is the branch of the trigeminal (fifth cranial) nerve that innervates the lower jaw and teeth, skin over the lower jaw and the tongue.

5. There are _____ cervical nerves, _____ thoracic nerves, _____ lumbar nerves, _____ sacral nerves and _____ coccygeal nerve

6. The autonomic nervous system is divided into the _____ or adrenergic, division and the _____ or cholinergic, division.

7. _____ receptors are located at the ganglia in both sympathetic and parasympathetic divisions of the ANS.

8. _____ fibres do not synapse after they leave the CNS.

9. The portion of the ANS that is thoracolumbar in its origin is the_____ division.

10. The _____ cranial nerve conveys sensations from the retina of the eye to the thalamus.

11. The _____ is a diamond-shaped "soft spot" on the top of a newborn's skull that facilitates childbirth and permits brain growth.

12. Separating the diaphysis and epiphysis of a child's long bone is a_____, which permits linear bone growth.

13. The _____ foramen is an opening in the mandible on the lateral side below the second premolar tooth.

14. The _____ and the perpendicular plate of the _____ bone compose the bony framework of the nasal septum.

15. In an adult, the ilium, ischium and pubis are fused to form the _____ or hipbone.

16. The foot contains _____tarsal bones, _____metatarsal bones and_____ phalanges.

Careers in Neurology

✓ Anaesthesiologists are physicians who administer anaesthesia directly to patients during surgery or supervise nurse anaesthetists in giving anaesthesia.

✓ Neurosurgeons are physicians specialized in surgery of the brain, spinal cord and the peripheral nerves.

✓ Psychiatrists are physicians specialized in the diagnosis, prevention and the treatment of mental disorders.

✓ Psychologists are health specialists who provide counselling for patients with emotional and mental disorders.

The Endocrine System

STUDY OBJECTIVES

- ✓ To discuss the different types of glands in the body.
- ✓ To define hormones and describe the mechanism of hormone action.
- ✓ To describe the structure of the hypothalamus and pituitary glands and discuss the various hormones secreted by the hypothalamus and the anterior pituitary and posterior pituitary glands.
- ✓ To describe the anatomical structure and function of various hormones secreted by the pineal, thyroid and parathyroid glands.
- ✓ To describe the anatomical structure of adrenal gland and discuss the various hormones secreted from the adrenal cortex and the adrenal medulla.
- ✓ To describe the anatomical structure and function of various hormones secreted by pancreas, gonads and the gastrointestinal system.

INTRODUCTION

Endocrine system (Greek word: *endon*: within, *krinien*: to separate) works in coordination with the nervous system to maintain homeostasis and to perform the basic functions of internal communication and regulation of all body systems. However, there are some basic differences between the two controlling systems. The nervous system stimulation provides immediate response to the stimuli by transmitting nerve impulses, whereas the endocrine system releases mediator molecules called *hormones* (Greek word: *hormaein*: to excite), and their response is usually slow but more prolonged.

To summarize, the nervous and endocrine systems share a unique partnership to coordinate the body functions. Therefore, the two systems are often collectively called the *neuroendocrine* system. This chapter mainly emphasizes the endocrine system, the various major endocrine glands and their role in coordinating body activities. The study of endocrine glands and the role of their secretions is called *endocrinology*.

The body contains the following two types of glands (Fig. 6.1):

1. **Exocrine glands**
   - ❏ These glands secrete their products into ducts that carry these secretions into body cavities, into lumen of an organ or to the outer surface of the body.
   - ❏ Exocrine glands include sebaceous (oil), sweat, salivary and gastric glands.

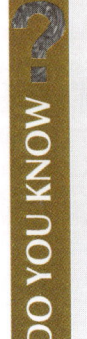

DO YOU KNOW?

- ❏ The endocrine system produces almost 30 hormones in our body.
- ❏ The hormone melatonin controls the sleep cycle of our body and is produced by the pineal gland.
- ❏ The hypothalamus gland in our body triggers the sense of thirst and hunger.
- ❏ The thyroid gland is responsible for activities such as overactivity or sluggishness of an individual.
- ❏ The endocrine system significantly influences the behaviour and the characteristics of a person.

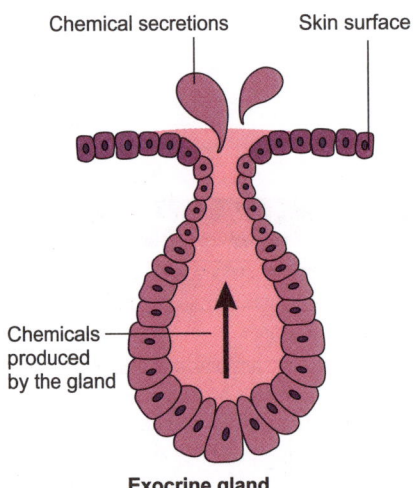

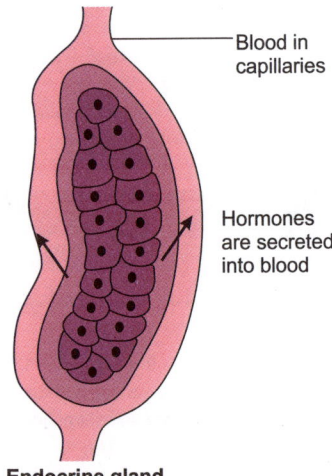

Figure 6.1 Exocrine and endocrine glands.

MEDICAL TERMINOLOGY

- ❏ **Antidiuretic**: It is a drug that limits the formation of urine.
- ❏ **Circadian rhythm**: It is the 'internal body clock' that regulates the (roughly) 24-hour cycle of biological processes.
- ❏ **Corpus luteum**: It is a yellow body that forms in the ovary on the site where an egg has been released and that produces progesterone to facilitate a pregnancy.
- ❏ **Glands**: It is a cell, a tissue or an organ that secretes certain chemical compounds useful for our body.
- ❏ **Homeostasis**: It is the body's ability to physiologically regulate its inner environment to ensure its stability in response to fluctuations in the outside environment and the weather.

2. **Endocrine glands or ductless glands**
   - ❏ These glands lack ducts and therefore secrete their products directly into the bloodstream. The blood circulatory system then carries these products to the target organs.
   - ❏ The secretions of these glands are known as *hormones*, and these are secreted in response to changes in the external or internal environment.
   - ❏ Endocrine glands include the pituitary, thyroid, parathyroid, adrenal and pineal glands.

Although there are many endocrine glands located throughout the body, only major endocrine glands are discussed in this chapter.

Figure 6.2 shows the location of major endocrine glands.

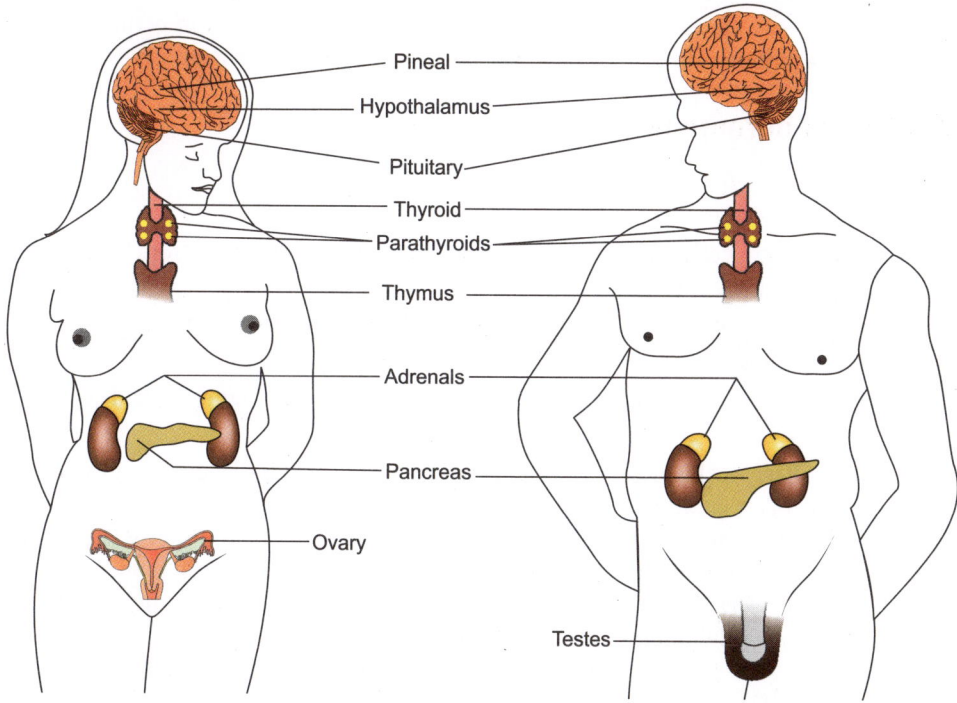

Figure 6.2 The major endocrine glands.

MEDICAL TERMINOLOGY

- ❏ **Nerve impulse**: It is the electrical discharge that travels along a nerve fibre.
- ❏ **Osmoreceptors**: It is a specialized nerve cell responsible for monitoring the osmotic pressure of the blood and extracellular fluid.
- ❏ **Ovulation**: It is the process in a female's menstrual cycle by which a mature ovarian follicle ruptures and discharges an ovum.
- ❏ **Receptors**: It is a structure on the surface of a cell (or inside a cell) that selectively receives and binds a specific substance.

HORMONES

Hormones are the chemical messengers secreted by endocrine glands that regulate the physiological processes in the body.

The first hormone was discovered in 1903 by two physiologists: William M. Bayliss and Ernest H. Starling. The term *hormone* was coined by Starling in 1905.

The hormones secreted by the endocrine gland travel throughout the body, but they affect only the *target cells* because only the target cells for a given hormone have receptors that bind and recognize that hormone. The nontarget cells lack these receptors and therefore they do not respond to the circulating hormones.

The hormone binds to the receptor on the target cell and changes the shape of the receptor. The receptor's new shape sets up certain changes in the cell—such as alteration in permeability, enzyme activity or gene transcription—which results in physiological responses in the target cells.

Classification of hormones

The hormones can be classified into the following two categories:

1. **Steroid hormones**
   - ❏ These hormones are derived from cholesterol and include the hormones from the adrenal cortex, testes, ovaries and placenta.
   - ❏ Examples include oestrogen, aldosterone, hydrocortisone, testosterone and progesterone.

2. **Nonsteroid hormones**
   - ❏ These hormones may be proteins (polypeptides), peptides, amino acid derivatives or glycoproteins.
     - (a) *Proteins*: They include adrenocorticotropic hormone (ACTH), calcitonin, insulin, glucagon, prolactin, parathyroid hormone (PTH) and growth hormone (GH).
     - (b) *Peptides*: They include gonadotropin-releasing hormone, thyrotropin-releasing hormone, somatostatin, oxytocin, melanocyte-stimulating hormone and antidiuretic hormone.
     - (c) *Amino acid derivatives*: They include epinephrine, norepinephrine, melatonin, thyroxine (T_4) and triiodothyronine (T_3).
     - (d) *Glycoproteins*: They include thyroid-stimulating hormone (TSH), follicle-stimulating hormone (FSH), luteinizing hormone (LH) and chorionic gonadotropin.

In addition to the above classification, the hormones can also be classified into two groups according to the distance between the site of production and target site:

Circulating hormones: Hormones that are secreted into the blood and act on distant target cells are called *circulating hormones*.

Local hormones: These hormones act locally without first entering the bloodstream. Among local hormones are those that act on neighbouring cells, called *paracrines* (*para*: near), and those that act on the same cell that secreted them, are termed *autocrines* (*auto*: self).

Mechanism of hormone action

The mechanism of hormonal action differs in different categories of hormones. For example, catecholamines (adrenaline and noradrenaline) and pancreatic (protein) hormones are lipid insoluble and thus cannot diffuse through the lipid bilayer of the plasma membrane. On the other hand, steroid hormones and thyroid hormones are lipid soluble and thus readily pass through the plasma membrane of target cells to enter the cytoplasm.

Thus, the molecular mechanism of hormone action can be described by the following two ways.

1. Mode of hormone action through extracellular receptors

The lipid-insoluble hormones such as catecholamines and pancreatic hormones cannot enter the target cell, and therefore they bind to the specific receptor molecules present on the surface of the cell membrane. In this case, the hormone acts as the first messenger and causes the production of a second messenger inside the cell, where specific responses takes place. The examples of second messenger are cyclic adenosine monophosphate (cAMP), inositol triphosphate (IP_3), diacyl glycerol (DAG), calcium ions (Ca^+) and cyclic guanosine monophosphate (cGMP) (Fig. 6.3a).

The various steps of the mechanism of hormonal action are as follows:

1. **Formation of the hormone–receptor complex**: The lipid-insoluble hormone binds to the receptor present at the surface of the target cell's membrane. The hormone–receptor complex activates a membrane protein called a *G protein* that causes the releases of an enzyme *adenylate cyclase* from the receptor site.

2. **Formation of second messenger**: Adenylate cyclase converts ATP into cAMP, which activates the protein kinases present in the cell. [Protein kinases are the enzymes that phosphorylates (adds a phosphate group) the other cellular proteins.] The activated protein kinases phosphorylate the cellular proteins and trigger the reactions that produce physiological responses.

3. **Inactivation of second messenger**: After some time, an enzyme called *phosphodiesterase* inactivates cAMP, resulting in the inhibition of response.

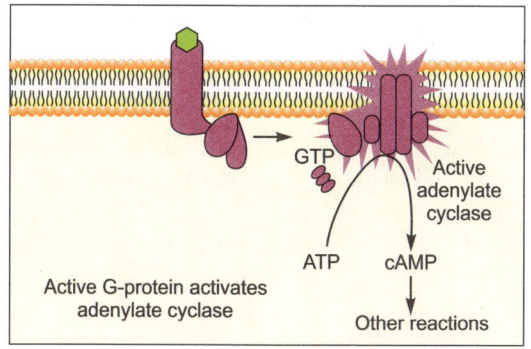
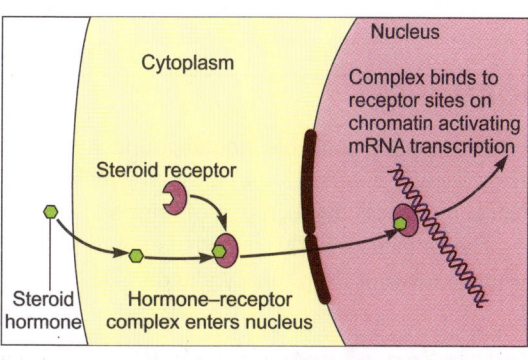

Figure 6.3 Hormone action by (a) extracellular and (b) intracellular receptors.

Hormones that bind to the plasma membrane receptors can induce their effects at very low concentration as they initiate a cascade of chain reaction.

For example: Binding of a single epinephrine molecule to the receptor activates hundreds of G proteins, each of which activates an adenylate cyclase molecule. Each adenylate cyclase produces around 1000 cAMP, and each cAMP may act on thousands of substrate molecules. Thus, the response is the result of the amplification of signal.

❑ **Synergistic effect**: When the effect of two hormones acting together is greater or extensive than the effect of each hormone acting alone, the two hormones are said to have the synergistic effect.

❑ **Antagonistic effect**: When one hormone opposes the actions of the other hormone, the two hormones are said to have the antagonistic effect.

2. Mode of hormone action through extracellular receptors

The lipid-soluble hormones, such as steroid hormone and thyroid hormone, bind to receptors within target cells (Fig. 6.3b).

Their mechanism of action is as follows:

1. The lipid-soluble hormone diffuses through the cell membrane and binds to the receptor located in the cytoplasm or nucleus.
2. The receptor–hormone complex then alters gene expression by activating certain genes.
3. The activated genes transcribe the mRNA, which directs the synthesis of a new protein (often an enzyme) on the ribosomes.
4. The new protein promotes the metabolic reactions in the cell and alters the cell activity.

HYPOTHALAMUS

ANATOMICAL STRUCTURE

The hypothalamus is a small part of the diencephalon and is composed of a number of groups of nerve cells. It is situated below and in front of the thalamus and immediately above the pituitary gland and serves as the major link between the nervous system and the endocrine system. For more details, see Chapter 5.

HORMONES

Hypothalamus is connected to the pituitary gland through a funnel-shaped stalk called the *infundibulum* (also called as *pituitary stalk*) through which it sends neural and chemical signals to the pituitary gland. Hence, it controls the secretion of hormones from the pituitary gland.

The influence of the hypothalamus on the release of hormones is different in the anterior and posterior lobes of the pituitary gland.

Regulation of anterior pituitary hormones

The hypothalamus contains some specialized nerve cells called *neurosecretory cells* that synthesize and secrete certain releasing and inhibitory hormones. These hormones are immediately taken into a complex network of blood vessels that form the hypophyseal portal system, which transports these hormones from the hypothalamus into the infundibulum and then directly to the anterior pituitary.

These releasing and inhibitory hormones either stimulate or inhibit the release of a particular hormone from the anterior pituitary gland.

The releasing and inhibitory hormones secreted by the hypothalamus are summarized in Table 6.1.

Table 6.1 Hypothalamic hormones

Hypothalamic hormones	Functions
Thyrotropin-releasing hormone (TRH)	Triggers the release of thyroid-stimulating hormone (TSH) or thyrotropin from anterior pituitary
Prolactin-releasing hormone (PRH)	Triggers the release of prolactin from the anterior pituitary
Prolactin-inhibiting hormone (PIH)	Inhibits the release of prolactin from the anterior pituitary
Growth hormone–releasing hormone (GHRH)	Triggers the release of growth hormone (GH) from the anterior pituitary
Somatostatin /Growth hormone–inhibiting hormone (SS/GHIH)	Inhibits the release of GH from anterior pituitary
Gonadotropin-releasing hormone (GnRH)	Triggers the release of follicle-stimulating hormone (FSH) and luteinizing hormone (LH) from the anterior pituitary
Corticotropin-releasing hormone (CRH)	Triggers the release of adrenocorticotropic hormone (ACTH) or adrenocorticotropin from the anterior pituitary

Regulation of posterior pituitary hormones

The hormones secreted by the posterior lobe of the pituitary gland are actually synthesized by specialized neurons of the hypothalamus. These hormones are transported to the posterior pituitary through the nerve fibres of the hypothalamohypophyseal tract by means of axonic flow and then stored in the vesicles within the axon terminals in the posterior pituitary.

Nerve impulses from the hypothalamus trigger their release from the posterior pituitary by exocytosis.

To summarize, the hypothalamus is linked to the posterior lobe of the pituitary gland by nerve fibres and to the anterior lobe by a complex system of blood vessels. This hypothalamic–pituitary system plays an important role in homeostasis as it regulates the activities of most of the other endocrine glands (Fig. 6.4).

PITUITARY GLAND

The pituitary gland, or hypophysis, was initially called the *master* endocrine gland because it secretes several hormones that control other endocrine glands. However, now, it is clear that the pituitary gland itself is regulated by the hypothalamus.

ANATOMICAL STRUCTURE

The pituitary is a small, pea-shaped gland, about 1.2–1.6 cm in length, located in the depression of the sphenoid bone below the hypothalamus. It is attached to the hypothalamus of the brain through a stalk or infundibulum.

The pituitary gland is divided into the following two lobes:

1. **Anterior lobe or pars anterior**: It is also called *adenohypophysis* (adeno gland).
2. **Posterior lobe or pars nervosa**: It is also referred to as *neurohypophysis*.

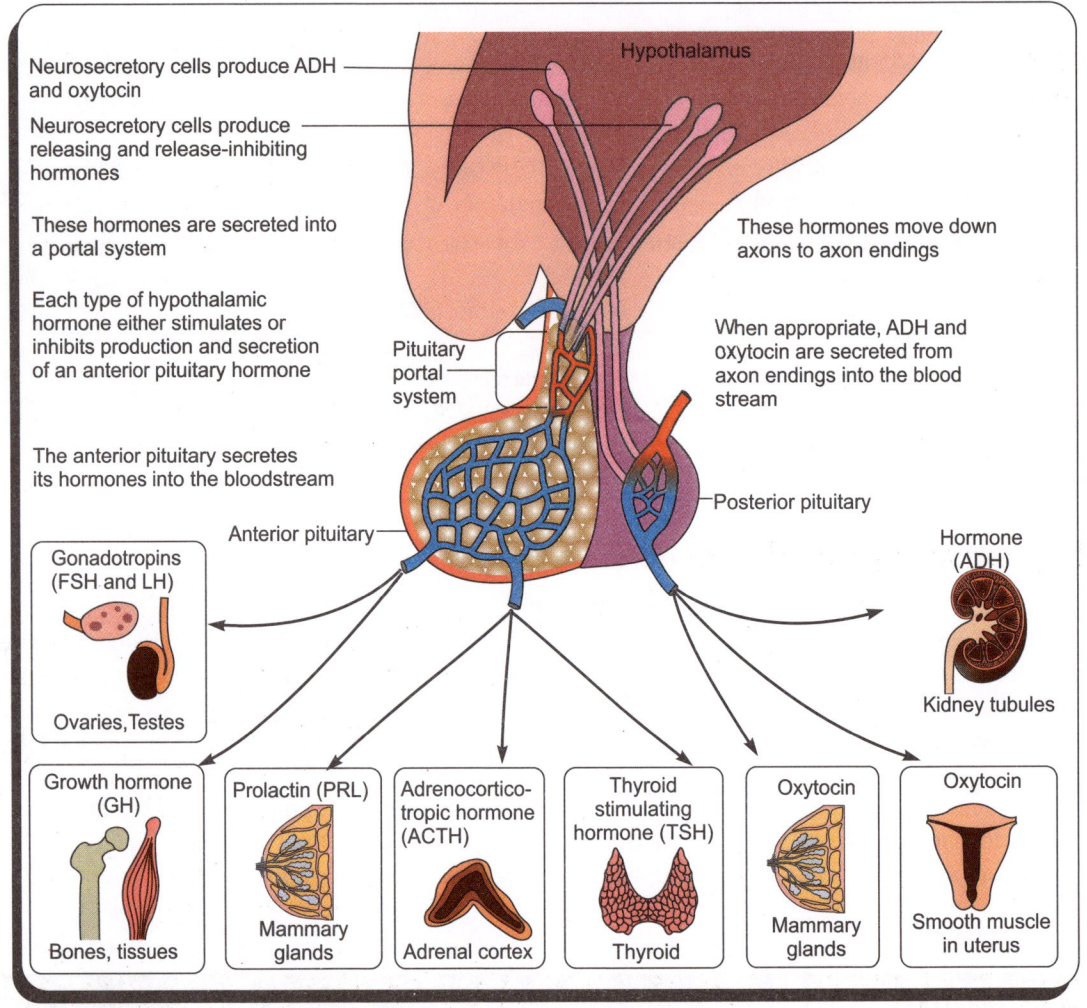

Neurosecretory cells produce ADH and oxytocin

Neurosecretory cells produce releasing and release-inhibiting hormones

These hormones are secreted into a portal system

Each type of hypothalamic hormone either stimulates or inhibits production and secretion of an anterior pituitary hormone

The anterior pituitary secretes its hormones into the bloodstream

Hypothalamus

These hormones move down axons to axon endings

When appropriate, ADH and oxytocin are secreted from axon endings into the blood stream

Pituitary portal system

Anterior pituitary

Posterior pituitary

Hormone (ADH)

Gonadotropins (FSH and LH)

Ovaries, Testes

Kidney tubules

Growth hormone (GH)

Bones, tissues

Prolactin (PRL)

Mammary glands

Adrenocortico-tropic hormone (ACTH)

Adrenal cortex

Thyroid stimulating hormone (TSH)

Thyroid

Oxytocin

Mammary glands

Oxytocin

Smooth muscle in uterus

Figure 6.4 Hypothalamic–pituitary system.

(a) Between these two lobes, there is an intermediate lobe that atrophies during human fetal development and does not exist as a separate lobe. Its role in humans is not known.

(b) The anterior pituitary develops as an upwards growth from the pharyngeal epithelium, and the posterior pituitary is the downgrowth of nervous tissue from the brain.

ANTERIOR PITUITARY

Anterior pituitary consists of the following five types of secretory cells that secrete various hormones:

1. **Somatotrophs**: These secretory cells secrete GH or somatotropin (*somato*: body; *tropin*: change).
2. **Thyrotrophs**: These secretory cells secrete TSH or thyrotropin.
3. **Corticotrophs**: These secretory cells secrete ACTH or corticotrophin.

4. **Gonadotrophs**: These secretory cells secrete two hormones: FSH and LH.
5. **Lactotrophs**: These secretory cells secrete prolactin.

Most of the hormones of the anterior pituitary are *tropic hormones* or *tropin* (i.e. the hormones that stimulate other endocrine glands). The FSH and LH are collectively called *gonadotropins* as they specifically regulate the functions of the gonads. Thyrotropin stimulates the thyroid gland and the corticotrophin acts on the cortex of the adrenal gland.

As discussed previously, the release of anterior pituitary hormones is regulated by the secretion of releasing and inhibitory hormones from the hypothalamus. This whole system is controlled by a *negative feedback system*, that is when the concentration of a particular hormone reaches a certain level in the body, it inhibits the gland to release further hormones, and later when the concentration falls below normal, the inhibition on the gland ceases and it begins to release the hormones again. This system helps regulate the concentration of hormones in our body. Figure 6.5 shows an example of the negative feedback system.

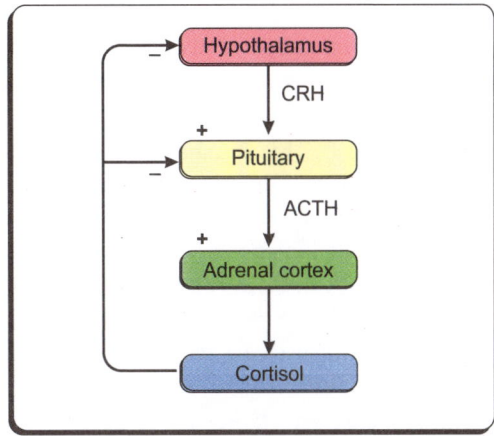

Figure 6.5 Negative feedback system.

Note: Increased cortisol secretion inhibits the hypo-thalamus and pituitary to secrete CRH and ACTH, respectively.

Hormones of anterior pituitary

The anterior pituitary lobe secretes the following hormones:

❑ Growth hormone (GH)
❑ Prolactin
❑ Thyroid-stimulating hormone (TSH)
❑ Adrenocorticotropic hormone (ACTH)
❑ Follicle-stimulating hormone (FSH)
❑ Luteinizing hormone (LH)

Growth hormone (GH)

❑ It is the most abundant hormone synthesized by anterior pituitary and is responsible for the general growth of the body.
❑ Body growth in response to GH secretion is evident during childhood and adolescence, and thereafter, secretion of GH maintains the mass of bones and skeletal muscles.
❑ GH stimulates the liver to secrete small protein hormones called *insulin-like growth factors (IGFs)*, or *somatomedins*, that stimulate the growth of the body by:
  ➤ Stimulating growth and division of most of the body cells, especially of bones and skeletal muscles
  ➤ Increasing protein synthesis by enhancing the uptake of amino acids into cells and increasing transcription and translation

Chapter 6

➤ Promoting mobilization of fats from adipose tissue and accelerating their catabolism, which results in the release of free fatty acids that can be used for ATP production by body cells

❑ GH also increases blood glucose levels by decreasing glucose uptake, which decreases the use of glucose for ATP production in the cells

❑ The release of GH is stimulated by growth hormone–releasing hormone (GHRH) and suppressed by growth hormone–inhibiting hormone (GHIH), both of which are secreted by the hypothalamus. The secretion of GH is greater during periods of sleep, exercise and fasting (hypoglycaemia). The secretion is also inhibited by increased levels of GH itself through the negative feedback mechanism.

❑ The deficiency of GH in children causes stunted growth leading to *dwarfism*, whereas the excessive secretion of GH causes enormous growth of the body leading to *gigantism*. The excessive secretion of GH may also cause *diabetogenic effect* (i.e. condition of diabetes mellitus due to persistent hyperglycaemia).

❑ **Diabetogenic effect**: Persistent hyperglycaemia due to excessive GH stimulates the pancreas to secrete insulin continually. Such excessive stimulation for prolonged periods may cause *beta cells burnout* (i.e. decreased capacity of beta cells of pancreas to secrete insulin, resulting in the condition of *diabetes mellitus*).

Prolactin

❑ It is also known as *luteotrophic/lactogenic hormone*.

❑ It promotes the development of mammary glands during pregnancy and stimulates *lactation* (milk production) after parturition (childbirth).

❑ The release of prolactin is stimulated by the prolactin-releasing hormone (PRH) from the hypothalamus and the suckling action of a nursing infant. The secretion is lowered by prolactin-inhibiting hormone (PIH, or dopamine) and by an increased blood level of prolactin (negative feedback). In non-nursing mothers and males, PIH secreted by hypothalamus inhibits the production of prolactin hormone.

Thyroid-stimulating hormone (TSH)

❑ It stimulates and maintains the growth and development of the thyroid gland. It also stimulates the thyroid gland to secrete thyroid hormones—T_4 and T_3.

❑ The release of TSH is stimulated by thyrotropin-releasing hormone (TRH) from the hypothalamus and is suppressed by increased levels of T_3 and T_4 through the negative feedback mechanism.

Adrenocorticotropic hormone (ACTH)

❑ ACTH promotes and maintains the growth of the adrenal cortex and stimulates the adrenal cortex to secrete glucocorticoids (mainly cortisol) and mineralocorticoids.

❑ ACTH secretion is stimulated by corticotrophin-releasing hormone (CRH) produced by the hypothalamus and is suppressed by the negative feedback mechanism when the blood level of ACTH rises.

Follicle-stimulating hormone (FSH)

❑ In females, FSH stimulates the development of the follicles in the ovaries of females. It also stimulates follicular cells to secrete *oestrogens* (female sex hormones).

❑ In males, it promotes the development of testes and stimulates spermatogenesis (production of sperms).

- The release of FSH is stimulated by gonadotropin-releasing hormone (GnRH) from the hypothalamus and is suppressed by the negative feedback mechanism by oestrogen (in females) and testosterone (in males).

Luteinizing hormone (LH)

- In females, LH functions as follows:
  - Stimulates ovulation and forms corpus luteum in the ovary. It also stimulates the secretion of progesterone from corpus luteum.
  - FSH and LH together stimulate the secretion of oestrogen by ovarian cells.
- In males, LH is also known as interstitial cell–stimulating hormone (ICSH) because it stimulates the interstitial cells of Leydig in testes to synthesize and secrete the male sex hormone *testosterone*.
- Secretion of LH, similar to that of FSH, is regulated by GnRH from the hypothalamus.

POSTERIOR PITUITARY

Posterior pituitary is formed from nervous tissue and consists primarily of nerve cells surrounded by specialized neuroglial cells called *pituicytes*. These neurons in the posterior pituitary have their cell bodies in the supraoptic and paraventricular nuclei of the hypothalamus, and their axons form the hypothalamo-hypophyseal tract, which begins in the hypothalamus and ends in the posterior pituitary.

Posterior pituitary hormones are synthesized in the nerve cell bodies of the hypothalamus and are transported along the axons to be stored within the axon terminals in the posterior pituitary. Thus, posterior pituitary only stores the hormones and releases them when stimulated by nerve impulses from the hypothalamus.

Hormones of posterior pituitary

The posterior pituitary lobe stores and releases the following two hormones:

- Vasopressin/antidiuretic hormone (VP/ADH)
- Oxytocin (OT)

Vasopressin/antidiuretic hormone (VP/ADH)

- It maintains the body's water balance by promoting increased water reabsorption in the distal convoluted and collecting tubules of the nephrons of the kidneys, resulting in decreased urine output. If secreted in large amounts, VP/ADH leads to constriction of blood vessels and thus increased blood pressure; hence, it is also referred to as *vasopressin*.
- The hypothalamus regulates ADH secretion through osmoreceptors that detect changes in the osmotic pressure of body fluids. Conditions such as decreased extracellular fluid (ECF) volume or high osmotic pressure due to dehydration like in diarrhoea, excessive sweating or haemorrhage stimulate osmoreceptors in the hypothalamus, which further stimulate the posterior pituitary to release ADH to prevent fluid loss from the body.
- Conversely, low osmotic pressure of blood (or increased blood volume) due to excessive fluid intake inhibits ADH release by the negative feedback mechanism.

Oxytocin (OT)

- It causes the contraction of the uterine smooth muscles to facilitate labour at the time of childbirth (parturition). Hence, it is popularly known as *birth hormone*.

Chapter 6

❑ It also causes the initiation of the 'milk ejection reflex' upon suckling by baby and stimulates the contraction of cells in the mammary glands, leading to milk ejection. Hence, it is also called *milk-ejecting hormone*.

❑ Oxytocin is released in response to the stimulation of uterine stretch receptors because of uterine distension during childbirth and suckling by baby after childbirth.

PINEAL GLAND

ANATOMICAL STRUCTURE

Pineal gland is also called as *pineal body*.

It is a small, pine-shaped gland attached to the roof of the third ventricle and is present between the two cerebral hemispheres of the brain.

HORMONES

The hormone secreted by the pineal gland is *melatonin*.

Melatonin regulates the biological clock of the body and affects our circadian (sleep–wake pattern) rhythm. The secretion of melatonin is controlled by daylight, and its levels fluctuate during each 24-h period, being lesser in bright light (day) and higher in darkness (night). This is because the nerve impulses in the retina of eyes send light information to the pineal gland. In dark or dim light, nerve impulses from the eyes decrease, which causes increased melatonin secretion that results in sleepiness.

It also inhibits growth and development of the sex organs before puberty, possibly by inhibiting the secretion of gonadotropin hormones (FSH and LH) from the anterior pituitary gland.

THYROID GLAND

ANATOMICAL STRUCTURE

The thyroid gland is a highly vascular, large endocrine gland weighing about 20–40 gm in an adult. It is situated in the neck just inferior to the larynx and consists of two lobes, one on either side of the trachea, that are connected in the middle by an isthmus (Fig. 6.6).

The thyroid gland is composed of a large number of thyroid follicles. The wall of each follicle consists primarily of cuboidal epithelial cells called *follicular cells*. The follicular cells produce two hormones: T_4 or *tetraiodothyronine* that contains four atoms of iodine and T_3 or *tri-iodothyronine* that contains three atoms of iodine; *the iodine atoms in these hormones indicate that iodine is essential for the formation of thyroid hormones.*

Between the follicles, there are other cells called *parafollicular cells* or *C cells*, which secrete the hormone *calcitonin*.

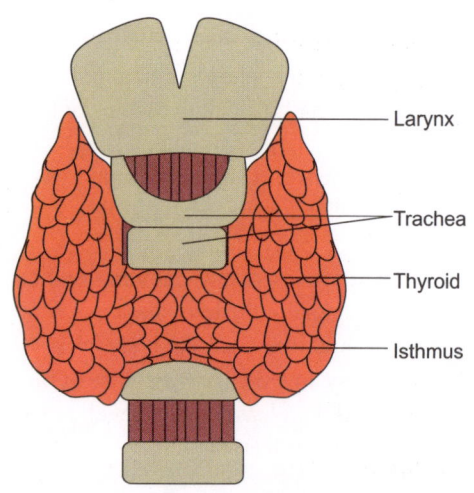

Larynx

Trachea

Thyroid

Isthmus

Figure 6.6 Anatomical location of the thyroid gland.

HORMONES

The thyroid gland secretes three hormones: T_3, T_4 and *calcitonin*.

T_4 and T_3

T_4 and T_3 exert their effects throughout the body as most of the body cells have receptors for thyroid hormones. The various actions of thyroid gland include the following:

1. Thyroid hormones increase the basal metabolic rate (BMR) by stimulating the production and oxidation of ATP. When the basal metabolic rate increases, the metabolism of carbohydrates, fats and proteins is also stimulated.
2. Increased BMR and cellular metabolic processes increases the heat production in the body and leads to rise in body temperature. This phenomenon is called as the *calorigenic effect*. In this way, thyroid hormones play an important role in the maintenance of normal body temperature.
3. Thyroid hormones are necessary for normal body growth and development, especially the growth of the nervous system and the skeletal system. They accelerate growth by increasing the use of carbohydrates and lipids for ATP production and by stimulating protein synthesis. Deficiency of thyroid hormones during fetal development, infancy or childhood causes severe mental retardation and stunted bone growth.

The secretion of thyroid hormones is controlled by the anterior pituitary through the feedback mechanism. Anterior pituitary secretes thyroid-stimulating hormone (TSH) under the influence of thyrotropin-releasing hormone (TRH) from the hypothalamus. TSH stimulates thyroid to release the thyroid hormones in conditions of stress, malnutrition, cold, pregnancy, high altitude and low thyroid hormone levels. Conversely, TSH and TRH secretions are inhibited in response to high thyroid hormone levels by the negative feedback mechanism.

Calcitonin

Calcitonin controls the calcium and phosphorus balance and lowers the concentration of calcium and phosphorus in the blood by:

1. Inhibiting bone resorption (breakdown of the bone extracellular matrix) by osteoclasts and facilitating the deposition of calcium and phosphorus in bones
2. Increasing the excretion of calcium and phosphorus by the kidneys

It acts antagonistically to parathormone (PTH), the hormone released by the parathyroid gland.

Release of calcitonin is stimulated by an increase in the blood calcium level and vice versa.

PARATHYROID GLANDS

ANATOMICAL STRUCTURE

Parathyroids are small, round and flattened glands present on the posterior surface of the thyroid gland. These are usually four in number, two in each lobe of the thyroid (Fig. 6.7).

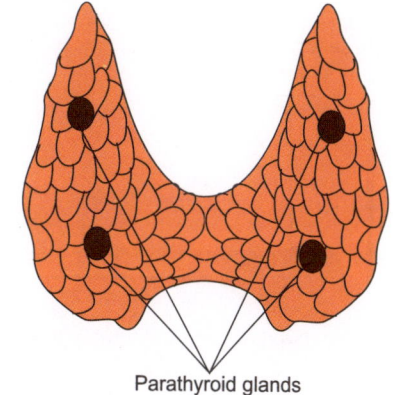

Parathyroid glands

Figure 6.7 Anatomical location of parathyroid glands.

Chapter 6

At the cellular level, parathyroid glands contain two kinds of epithelial cells: chief cells and oxyphil cells. The chief cells secrete parathormone (PTH), whereas the function of oxyphil cells is not known.

HORMONES

The parathyroid glands secrete *PTH*.

The primary action of PTH is to increase the calcium levels in the blood (Fig. 6.8). This is achieved as follows:

1. It increases the number and activity of osteoclasts and thus elevates bone resorption that releases calcium and phosphate ions into the blood.
2. It enhances active reabsorption of calcium and magnesium from kidneys.
3. It also increases the excretion of phosphate ions in the urine and thus lowers the blood phosphate levels.
4. It promotes formation of calcitriol (active form of vitamin D) in the kidneys, which increases the rate of absorption of calcium and phosphate ions from the gastrointestinal tract into the blood.

The secretion of PTH is regulated directly by the calcium levels in the blood. Decrease in the blood calcium level stimulates the secretion of PTH and vice versa.

PTH and calcitonin act in a complementary manner to maintain blood calcium levels within a narrow range. This maintenance of blood calcium levels is very essential for muscle contraction, blood clotting and transmission of nerve impulse.

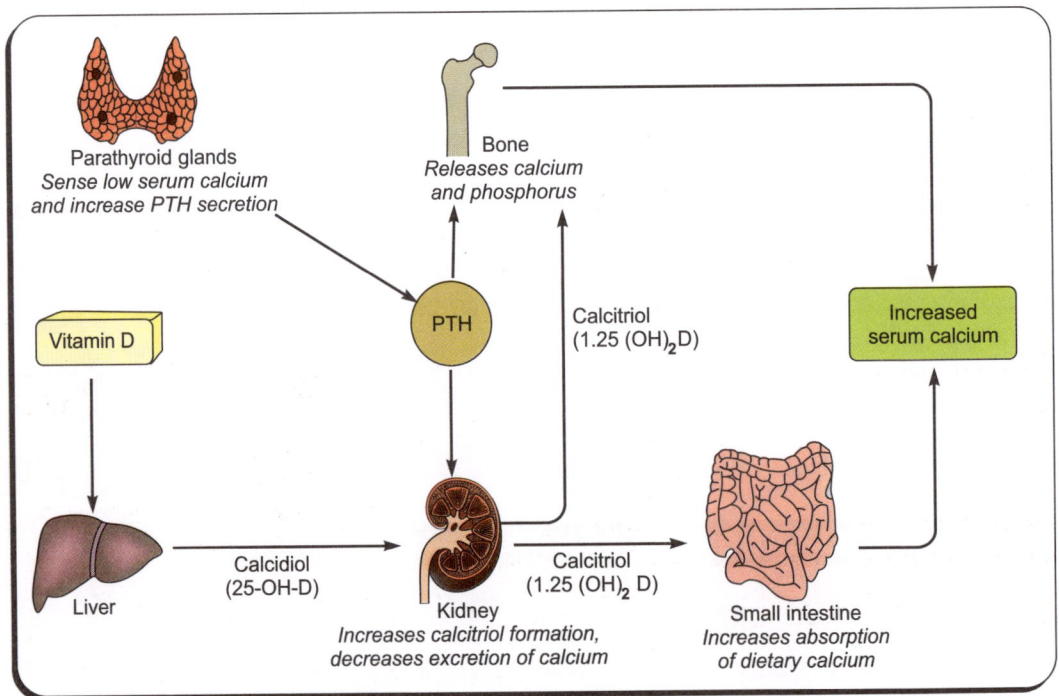

Parathyroid glands
*Sense low serum calcium
and increase PTH secretion*

Vitamin D

PTH

Bone
*Releases calcium
and phosphorus*

Calcitriol
(1.25 (OH)$_2$D)

Increased
serum calcium

Liver

Calcidiol
(25-OH-D)

Kidney
*Increases calcitriol formation,
decreases excretion of calcium*

Calcitriol
(1.25 (OH)$_2$ D)

Small intestine
*Increases absorption
of dietary calcium*

Figure 6.8 Role of parathormone in calcium regulation.

ADRENAL GLANDS

ANATOMICAL STRUCTURE

Adrenal glands are also known as the suprarenal glands. There are two adrenal glands situated on the upper pole (top) of each kidney.

Each gland is made of two parts: *adrenal cortex*—the outer part—and *adrenal medulla*—the inner part. These two parts are structurally and functionally different from each other (Fig. 6.9).

ADRENAL CORTEX

The adrenal cortex is subdivided into three zones: *zona glomerulosa*—the outer zone, *zona fasciculata*—the middle zone and *zona reticulata*—the inner zone.

Each of these zones secretes different hormones: the outer zone, the zona glomerulosa, secretes hormones called mineralocorticoids; the middle zone, the zona fasciculata, secretes mainly glucocorticoids; and the inner zone, the zona reticulata, secretes mainly gonadocorticoids (sex hormones).

The adrenal cortex is essential for life. The damage or destruction of the adrenal cortex may lead to death due to electrolyte imbalances and dehydration.

Hormones of the adrenal cortex

The hormones of the adrenal cortex are collectively known as *adrenocortical hormones* or *corticosteroids*. All adrenocortical hormones are steroid in nature and are synthesized mainly from the cholesterol.

The adrenocortical hormones include *mineralocorticoids*, *glucocorticoids* and *gonadocorticoids* (sex hormones).

Mineralocorticoids

The major mineralocorticoid is *aldosterone*, and it is very essential for life. Thus, it is usually called *life-saving hormone*.

The major function of aldosterone involves regulation of the water and electrolyte balance and blood volume in the body. It regulates this balance by increasing the reabsorption of sodium and water from renal tubules to reduce their loss from the body. It also stimulates the kidneys to increase the secretion of K^+ and H^+ into the urine.

The increased water reabsorption by kidneys causes persistent increase in blood volume, which finally leads to increase in blood pressure.

The secretion of aldosterone from the adrenal cortex is regulated by the following factors:

1. **The blood potassium level**: The increase in the blood potassium level increases the aldosterone secretion and vice versa.
2. **The renin–angiotensin–aldosterone system (RAAS)**
   - ❑ The decrease in the sodium ion concentration or blood volume stimulates the *juxtaglomerular cells* in the kidneys to secrete *renin*.
   - ❑ Renin converts *angiotensinogen*, produced by the liver, to *angiotensin I*, which is further converted to *angiotensin II* by *angiotensin-converting enzyme (ACE)*.
   - ❑ Angiotensin II stimulates the adrenal cortex to secrete aldosterone. It also causes vasoconstriction and increases the blood pressure. (For more details, see chapter The Urinary System.)

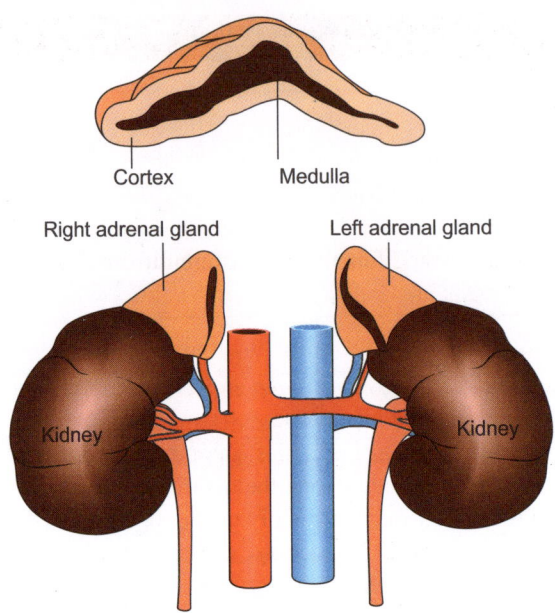

Figure 6.9 Anatomical location of adrenal glands.

Glucocorticoids

Glucocorticoids include cortisol (or hydrocortisone), corticosterone and cortisone. The major and most abundant of them is *cortisol*, which is usually referred to as *life-protecting hormone*. They are very essential for life as they regulate the metabolism of carbohydrates, proteins and fats and also help withstand stress and trauma.

The various effects of glucocorticoids include the following:

1. **Glucose formation**: The glucocorticoids increase the blood glucose level by promoting gluconeogenesis in the liver from amino acids and by inhibiting glucose uptake and utilization by peripheral cells.

2. **Metabolism of proteins and lipids**: The glucocorticoids stimulate the breakdown of proteins and lipids to release amino acids and fatty acids, respectively, into the bloodstream. The amino acids can be used by body cells to synthesize new proteins (e.g. enzymes). Both amino acids and fatty acids may also be taken up by tissues for ATP production as a quick source of energy.

3. **Resistance to stress**: The glucocorticoids provide resistance to stress in many ways: the fatty acids released from cells and glucose in liver cells serve as a quick source of energy during stressful conditions such as exercise, fasting, infection, trauma and disease. In case of excessive bleeding, glucocorticoids constrict blood vessels to counterbalance the drop in blood pressure due to blood loss.

4. **Anti-inflammatory effects**: Glucocorticoids prevent the inflammatory changes in the cells caused by injury or infection. They inhibit the migration of leukocytes (white blood cells) to the affected area and prevent the rush of blood to the injured area by causing vasoconstriction. By these effects, glucocorticoids also retard tissue repair and slow down wound healing.

5. **Immunosuppressive effects**: Glucocorticoids suppress the immune system of the body by decreasing the number of T-lymphocytes. Thus, they are used to prevent tissue rejection during organ transplantation.

The secretion of glucocorticoids is regulated through the negative feedback mechanism involving the hypothalamus and anterior pituitary. The stressful conditions and the low level of cortisol stimulate the hypothalamus to secrete *CRH*. CRH, in turn, stimulates the secretion of *ACTH* from the anterior pituitary. ACTH flows towards adrenal cortex through blood, where it stimulates glucocorticoid (cortisol) secretion. Conversely, high levels of cortisol inhibit the release of corticotropin-releasing hormone (CRH) from the hypothalamus and ACTH from the anterior pituitary.

Gonadocorticoids (sex hormones)

Most of the gonadocorticoids secreted by the adrenal cortex are male sex hormones (androgens). They are secreted in very small amounts in both males and females, and the major androgen secreted is *dehydroepiandrosterone (DHEA)*. The androgens, in general, are responsible for the development of male sexual characteristics, but the amount of androgens secreted by the adrenal cortex is usually so low that their effects are insignificant.

They stimulate the growth of pubic and axillary hair in both males and females. They also promote libido (sex drive) and are converted to oestrogens by other body tissues.

ADRENAL MEDULLA

Medulla is the inner part of the adrenal gland. It mainly consists of the hormone-producing cells called *chromaffin cells* that release the hormones after stimulation by the sympathetic division of the autonomic nervous system (ANS).

Hormones of adrenal medulla

Unlike the hormones of the adrenal cortex, the medullary hormones are not essential for life as they only intensify the responses of the sympathetic nervous system.

The two major hormones synthesized by adrenal medulla include *epinephrine* (or *adrenaline*) and *norepinephrine* (or *noradrenaline*). Both these hormones are structurally very similar and thus also have similar effects.

Effects of epinephrine and norepinephrine

Epinephrine and norepinephrine prepare our body for stressful situations such as injury, exercise, trauma, anger, fear, pain and danger; hence, they are commonly referred to as *fight or flight hormones*.

The various actions of these hormones include the following:
1. Increase in heart rate and force of contraction that leads to increased cardiac output and blood pressure
2. Increased blood flow to essential organs including the heart, liver, brain and skeletal muscles by dilating their blood vessels and constricting those of less-essential organs, such as skin
3. Increased metabolic rate and increased breakdown of glycogen (glycogenolysis) and lipids (lipolysis) to release glucose and fatty acids in the bloodstream for ATP synthesis
4. Increased rate and force of respiration

Chapter 6

All these changes prepare our body to either fight or flee the stressful situation and thus these responses are collectively termed as *flight* or *fight responses*.

The release of these hormones is regulated by the hypothalamus and stressful situations that cause the stimulation of the sympathetic nervous system to further stimulate the adrenal medulla to release epinephrine and norepinephrine.

Response to stress

Stressful conditions such as infection, emotional disturbance, fasting and exercise stimulate an immediate response called short-term response' by the release of flight or fight hormones. However, in the longer term, ACTH from the anterior pituitary stimulates the release of glucocorticoids and mineralocorticoids from the adrenal cortex, resulting in longer term response to stress.

PANCREAS

ANATOMICAL STRUCTURE

The pancreas is a flattened, elongated organ located in the epigastric and hypochondriac (left) regions of the abdomen. (For more details, see the chapter The Digestive System).

Pancreas mainly consists of lobules or acini that secrete the pancreatic juice, which flows into the gastrointestinal tract through a network of ducts (exocrine function of pancreas). Interspersed at random among the acini are tiny clusters of endocrine tissues called *pancreatic islets* or *islets of Langerhans* that secrete the pancreatic hormones directly into the bloodstream (endocrine function of pancreas) (Fig. 6.10).

HORMONES

The islets of Langerhans consist of the following four main types of cells:

- ❏ Alpha cells, which secrete the hormone *glucagon*
- ❏ Beta cells, which secrete the hormone *insulin*
- ❏ Delta cells, which secrete the hormone *somatostatin*
- ❏ PP cells, which secrete the hormone *pancreatic polypeptide (PP)*
- ❏ Insulin and glucagon are the important pancreatic hormones and have antagonistic effects on *blood glucose levels*; glucagon increases blood glucose levels and insulin lowers them.

Insulin

The various functions of insulin are as follows:

1. **Increased glucose uptake**: Insulin accelerates the transport of glucose into cells by increasing the permeability of cell membrane to glucose. It enhances the uptake and use of glucose by all the tissues, especially by the liver, skeletal muscle and adipose tissue.
2. **Increased glycogenesis**: Insulin promotes the rapid conversion of glucose into glycogen (glycogenesis), especially in the muscles and liver.
3. **Increased lipogenesis**: Insulin promotes the synthesis of fatty acids and storage of fats in adipose tissue.

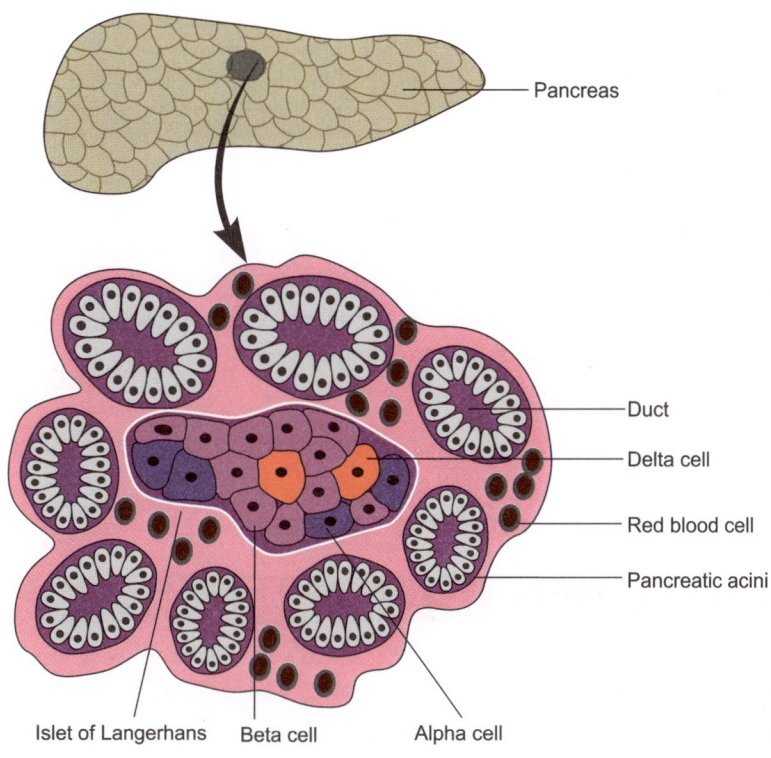

Figure 6.10 Anatomical structure of pancreas (close-up view of an islet of Langerhans).

4. **Increased protein synthesis**: Insulin accelerates the uptake of amino acids by cells and stimulates protein synthesis.

5. **Decreased proteolysis, lipolysis and gluconeogenesis**
   ❑ Insulin prevents the breakdown of proteins and fats and inhibits gluconeogenesis (i.e. formation of glucose from nonsugar substrates such as proteins).
   ❑ Insulin also inhibits glycogenolysis (i.e. breakdown of glycogen into glucose in the muscles and liver).

Secretion of insulin is stimulated by increased blood glucose level, increased blood amino acid and fatty acids levels, parasympathetic stimulation (acetylcholine) and gastrointestinal hormones (e.g. gastrin, secretin and cholecystokinin). Secretion is inhibited by glucagon, sympathetic stimulation (adrenaline) and somatostatin.

Glucagon

Glucagon increases the blood glucose levels and is released when the blood glucose level falls drastically.

The effects of glucagon in increasing the blood sugar level are as follows:

1. It accelerates the breakdown of glycogen into glucose in the liver (*glycogenolysis*), which is released into the bloodstream.
2. It promotes gluconeogenesis (i.e. the formation of glucose from nonsugar substrates such as proteins and fats).

Chapter 6

3. It promotes lipolysis (i.e. breakdown of fats to provide an alternative energy source).

Thus, glucagon and insulin are part of a feedback system that maintains the correct blood glucose level (Fig. 6.11). Secretion of glucagon is stimulated by low blood glucose level and exercise, and it is decreased by somatostatin and insulin.

Somatostatin

Somatostatin performs the following functions:

1. It inhibits the secretion of both insulin and glucagon.
2. It inhibits the release of GH and TSH from the anterior pituitary.
3. It also decreases the smooth muscle contractions and flow of blood in the intestine. Thus, it decreases the rate of nutrient absorption from the gastrointestinal tract.

Pancreatic polypeptide (PP)

The principal actions of PP include the following:

1. It inhibits somatostatin secretion and gall bladder contraction.
2. It also inhibits the release of pancreatic juice.

GONADS

ANATOMICAL STRUCTURE

Gonads are the structures that produce gametes—sperm in males and oocyte in females. The anatomical structures of male (testes) and female gonads (ovaries) are discussed in the chapter The Reproductive System.

HORMONES

The hormones secreted by the gonads include the following:

- ❑ Testosterone (secreted by testes)
- ❑ Oestrogen (secreted by ovaries)
- ❑ Progesterone (secreted by ovaries)
- ❑ Relaxin (secreted by ovaries)

Testosterone

- ❑ Testosterone is the male sex hormone.
- ❑ It is responsible for the development of male reproductive structures, and at puberty, for the enlargement of testes and penis.
- ❑ It stimulates the formation of sperms (spermatogenesis) in the seminiferous tubules.
- ❑ It also promotes the development of accessory male sexual characters such as growth of facial and chest hair, deepening of the voice, muscular development and bone growth.

Oestrogen

- ❑ Oestrogen is the female sex hormone.
- ❑ It is responsible for the development and growth of female reproductive structures: the uterus, vagina and fallopian tubes.

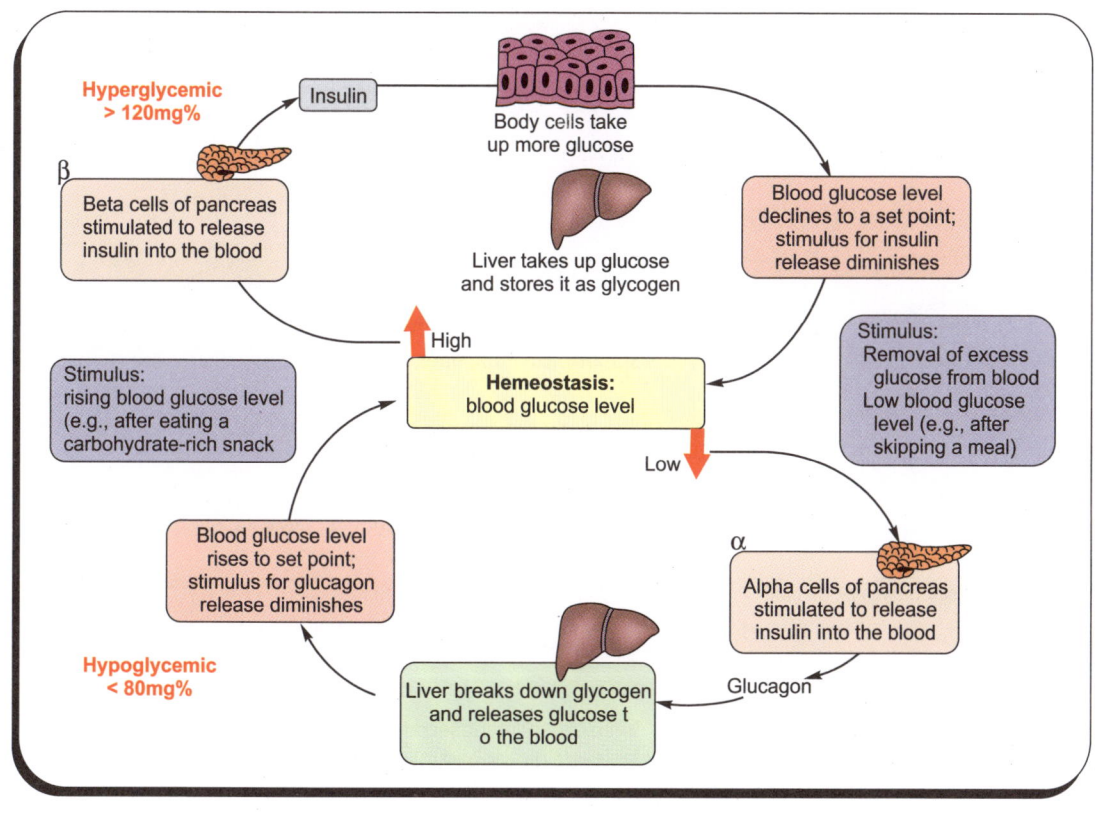

Figure 6.11 Regulation of pancreatic hormones insulin and glucagon.

❑ It stimulates the differentiation of ova (oogenesis) in the ovary.
❑ It promotes the development of accessory female sexual characters such as enlargement of breasts, growth of pubic and axillary hair, deposition of fat in the thighs and onset of menstrual cycle.

Progesterone

❑ Progesterone is also called *hormone of pregnancy*.
❑ It plays a major role in implanting the fetus to the uterine wall, forming the placenta and regulating the development of fetus in the uterus.

Relaxin

Relaxin is believed to increase the flexibility of pubic symphysis during pregnancy and widen the pubic symphysis at the time of birth.

All the hormones produced by gonads are discussed in details in the chapter The Reproductive System.

Chapter 6

GASTROINTESTINAL HORMONES

The anatomy and physiology of the gastrointestinal (GI) system have been discussed in the chapter The Digestive System.

The GI hormones are summarized in Table 6.2.

Table 6.2 Gastrointestinal hormones

Agent	Effect
Gastrin	Stimulates HCl gastric secretion Stimulates mucosal cell growth Stimulates contractions of oesophageal sphincter and stomach
Cholecystokinin (CCK)	Stimulates contraction of gall bladder; inhibits gastric emptying Stimulates pancreatic secretion of enzymes Inhibits gastric secretion of HCl
Secretin	Stimulates pancreatic secretion of fluid Stimulates bile-salt-independent biliary secretion Inhibits gastric emptying
Gastric-inhibitory polypeptide (GIP)	Inhibits gastric secretion of HCL Stimulates intestinal secretion of Cl^- Inhibits intestinal absorption of Na^+
Enteroglucagons	Inhibit gastric secretion of HCl
Pancreatic polypeptide	Inhibits pancreatic secretion of HCO_3^- and enzymes Increases gastric and intestinal motility

OTHER ENDOCRINE GLANDS

Some other organs, which also perform glandular function, are listed in Table 6.3.

Table 6.3 Other endocrine glands

S. no.	Hormone	Principal actions
1.	**Heart** Atrial natriuretic peptide (ANP)	Decreases blood pressure
2.	**Placenta** Human chorionic gonado-tropin (HCG)	Stimulates the corpus luteum in the mother's ovary to continue the secretion of oestrogen and progesterone to maintain pregnancy
3.	**Thymus gland** Thymosin	Promotes the maturation of T-lymphocytes
4.	**Kidney** (a) Renin (b) Erythropoietin	(a) Converts angiotensinogen to angiotensin that raises blood pressure by vasoconstriction and aldosterone secretion (b) Increases the rate of RBC production

DISORDERS ASSOCIATED WITH THE ENDOCRINE SYSTEM

ADDISON'S DISEASE

Addison's disease is a chronic endocrine disorder in which the adrenal glands produce insufficient steroid hormones—glucocorticoids and mineralocorticoids.

The most common cause is autoimmune disorder in which antibodies destroy the adrenal cortex or block the binding of ACTH to its receptors.

The most common symptoms include fatigue, mental lethargy, anorexia, muscle weakness, fever, weight loss and gastrointestinal disturbances including nausea, vomiting and diarrhoea.

Treatment consists of replacing glucocorticoids and mineralocorticoids and increasing sodium in the diet.

DIABETES MELLITUS

Diabetes mellitus is a very common disorder manifested by high blood sugar (glucose). The classical symptoms of diabetes mellitus include polyuria (frequent urination), polydipsia (increased thirst) and polyphagia (increased hunger).

There are two main types of diabetes as follows:

❏ **Type 1 diabetes** or **IDDM (insulin-dependent diabetes mellitus)**: It occurs due to the deficiency or absence of insulin.
❏ **Type 2 diabetes** or **NIDDM (non-insulin-dependent diabetes mellitus)**: It is the most common form of diabetes that occurs due to insulin resistance, a condition in which cells fail to use insulin properly. It usually develops after 40 years due to genetic factors, obesity or sedentary lifestyle.

DIABETES INSIPIDUS

Diabetes insipidus is the most common abnormality associated with the dysfunction of the posterior pituitary and mainly occurs due to deficiency of antidiuretic hormone (ADH).

The symptoms include excretion of large amounts of severely diluted urine, resulting in excessive thirst and dehydration.

Treatment involves mainly hormone replacement therapy.

GOITRE

This is enlargement of thyroid gland that leads to the swelling of the neck or larynx. It is caused by reduced levels of T_3 and T_4 that stimulate the secretion of TSH, resulting in hyperplasia of the thyroid gland.

The main reason of goitre is low dietary intake of iodine, which results in inadequate synthesis of thyroid hormones.

HYPERTHYROIDISM

Hyperthyroidism is also known as thyrotoxicosis and refers to the increased thyroid hormones (T_4 and/ or T_3) in the blood.

Chapter 6

The symptoms of hyperthyroidism include nervousness, irritability, anxiety, thinning of the skin, fine brittle hair and muscular weakness.

The causes of hyperthyroidism include Grave's disease (autoimmune disorder in which an antibody functions similar to TSH and results in increased release of T_4 and T_3) or toxic nodular goitre (the nodules of gland secrete excess T_4 and T_3).

HYPOTHYROIDISM

Hypothyroidism refers to the deficiency of thyroid hormone and occurs due to an abnormality in the thyroid gland or, less commonly, the pituitary gland or hypothalamus.

Cretinism is a form of hypothyroidism occurring in infants. Its symptoms include poor muscle tone (muscle hypotonia), fatigue, dry, itchy and puffy skin, especially on the face and abnormal menstrual cycles.

Myxoedema is the condition of hypothyroidism in adults and results in an abnormally low metabolic rate.

ACROMEGALY

Acromegaly is a syndrome in which the pituitary gland produces excess GH after the epiphyseal plate closure at puberty.

It mostly affects adults in middle age and results in severe disfigurement of the body parts, especially the face, enlarged tongue and excessive large hands and feet.

The treatment for acromegaly includes irradiation, radioisotope implantation or surgical removal of the tumour or pituitary gland.

GIGANTISM

Gigantism is a condition manifested by abnormal excessive growth and height that is significantly above average.

It is caused by an overproduction of human GH, usually by a hormone-secreting pituitary tumour.

The treatment for gigantism includes surgical removal of the tumour or the pituitary gland (hypophysectomy).

PITUITARY DWARFISM

Pituitary dwarfism is the condition characterized by hyposecretion of GH during the growth years.

It leads to the slowing of bone growth and closure of the epiphyseal plates before normal height is reached.

The symptoms include small body, but normally proportioned; mild obesity with lack of appetite; tender, thin skin.

The treatment includes GH injections.

CUSHING'S DISEASE

Cushing's disease is characterized by the increased secretion of ACTH from the anterior pituitary.

Its symptoms include rapid weight gain, moon-like face, shape of back and neck resembles a buffalo hump, hyperhidrosis (excess sweating), telangiectasia (dilation of capillaries) and thinning of the skin.

Its treatment includes surgical removal of portions of the pituitary gland or adrenal glands, irradiation and hormone replacement therapy.

GRAVE'S DISEASE (THYROTOXICOSIS)

Grave's disease is characterized by hyperthyroid secretion (excessive secretion by the thyroid gland).

Its symptoms include loss of weight, rapid pulse, warm and moist skin, increased appetite, increased BMR, tremor, goitre, exophthalmos (bulging eyes) and muscular weakness.

Its treatment includes removal of a portion of the thyroid gland, radioiodine and antithyroid drugs.

MYXOEDEMA

Myxoedema is characterized by hypothyroid secretion (insufficient secretion of the thyroid gland) in adults.

Its symptoms include weight gain, slow pulse, dry and brittle hair, decreased BMR, lack of energy, sensation of coldness, diminished perspiration and weakness.

Its treatment includes thyroid hormone (T3 and T4) administration.

CRETINISM

Cretinism is characterized by hypothyroid secretion (severe insufficiency of thyroid gland secretion) in infants and children.

Its symptoms include stunted growth, thickened facial features, large and protruding tongue, abnormal bone growth, mental retardation, decreased BMR and general lethargy.

Its treatment includes thyroid hormone administration.

Summary of major hormones

Major hormones, alongwith their position and functions, are listed in Table 6.4.

Table 6.4 Summary of major hormones

S. no.	Gland	Position	Hormones and their nature	Functions
1.	Thyroid	In the neck inferior to larynx	i) Thyroxine (T$_4$) ii) Triiodothyronine (T$_3$) iii) Calcitonin (CT) (peptide)	i) Increase basal metabolic rate; excess of the hormone causes Grave's disease; deficiency produces cretinism in children and myxoedema in adults. iii) Calcitonin controls the calcium and phosphorus balance.
2.	Parathyroids	In the back of thyroid	i) Parathormone (PTH) (peptide)	i) Regulates the calcium–phosphorus balance in blood; deficiency causes cramps and convulsions; excess of the hormone weakens bones.
3.	Adrenals a) Cortex	On top of kidneys	i) Glucocorticoids, e.g. cortisol (steroid) ii) Mineralocorticoid, e.g. Aldosterone (steroid) iii) Sex corticoids (steroids)	i) Regulates carbohydrate, fat and protein metabolism; controls the electrolyte and water balance; deficiency causes Addison's disease. ii) Produces accessory sex characters; excess in early life causes early abnormal sexual maturity. iii) Prepare the body for emergency by increasing heart beat, blood pressure, respiratory rate, blood sugar level, etc.
	b) Medulla		i) Adrenaline (amine) ii) Noradrenaline (amine)	
4.	Hypothalamus	Base of diencephalon	i) Releaser hormones (peptides) ii) Inhibiting hormones (peptides)	i) Stimulate anterior pituitary to secrete hormones. ii) Inhibit anterior pituitary to secrete hormones.
5.	Pituitary a) Anterior lobe	Beneath brain	i) Follicle-stimulating hormone (FSH) (protein) ii) Luteinizing hormone LH (protein) iii) Growth Hormone (GH) (protein) iv) Prolactin (protein) v) Adrenocorticotrophin (ACTH) (peptide) vi) Thyrotrophin (TSH) (protein)	i) Stimulates spermatogenesis in males and growth of ovarian follicle in female; promotes ovulation and secretion of oestrogen and progesterone in females; induces testosterone secretion in males iii) Regulates protein metabolism and growth of bones; deficiency causes dwarfism; excess hormones leads to gigantism in young and acromegaly in adults. iv) Controls the development of milk glands. v) Stimulates secretion of hormones of the adrenal cortex. vi) Stimulates secretion of thyroid hormones.

S. no.	Gland	Position	Hormones and their nature	Functions
	b) Posterior lobe		i) Oxytocin (peptide) ii) Vasopressin/ADH (peptide)	i) Regulates uterine contractions and release of milk ii) Reduces loss of water in urine
6.	Pineal	Roof of brain	i) Melatonin (amine)	i) Regulates sleep-awake pattern.
7.	Pancreas	Below stomach	i) Insulin (protein) ii) Glucagon (protein) iii) Somatostatin (SS) iv) Pancreatic polypeptide	i) Controls carbohydrate metabolism, increases glucose uptake, lipogenesis, glycogenesis and protein synthesis; its deficiency causes diabetes mellitus. ii) Increases the blood sugar level. iii) Inhibits secretion of both insulin and glucagon. iv) Inhibits the release of pancreatic juice.
10.	Gonads a) Testes	In scrotal sacs	i) Testosterone (steroid)	i) Develops male reproductive organs and accessory sexual characters.
	b) Ovaries	Lower abdomen	i) Oestrogen or oestradiol (steroid) ii) Progesterone (steroid) iii) Relaxin (protein)	i) Develops female genital organs and accessory sexual characters. ii) Attaches fetus to uterine wall. iii) Widening of pelvis at birth.

Chapter 6

Ageing and the Endocrine System

❑ With age, the endocrine glands shrink and may release lesser amount of hormones.
  ➤ Growth hormone (GH) production decreases ⟶ leads to muscle atrophy and decreased bone mass
  ➤ Thyroid hormone decreases ⟶ leads to decreased BMR, increased body fat and hypothyroidism
  ➤ Pancreatic hormones decrease ⟶ insulin release gets slower
  ➤ Ovaries reduce in size ⟶ leads to decreased release of oestrogen
  ➤ Testes function decreases ⟶ decreased release of testosterone
  ➤ Melatonin secretion decreases ⟶ cause change in the sleep–wake pattern
❑ All these age-related changes in the endocrine system make the elderly more susceptible to diabetes, osteoporosis, high blood cholesterol and atherosclerosis.

Embryonic Development of the Endocrine System

❑ About the third week: Pituitary gland begins to develop from two different regions of ectoderm.
  1. **Outgrowth of ectoderm**: Neurohypophyseal bud ⟶ forms posterior pituitary on the floor of hypothalamus.
  2. **Outgrowth of ectoderm**: from roof ⟶ forms anterior pituitary.
❑ Fourth week: Thyroid gland develops as an outgrowth of the endoderm called *thyroid diverticulum* from the floor of the pharynx.
❑ Fourth week: Parathyroid gland ⟶ develops from endoderm as an outgrowth from pharyngeal pouches.
❑ Fifth week: Adrenal cortex develops from mesoderm; adrenal medulla develops from ectoderm.
❑ Fifth to seventh week: Pancreas develops as an outgrowth of endoderm from the foregut.

TIPS TO BALANCE HORMONES NATURALLY

1. **Healthy diet**: Diet should contain low-fat protein, vegetables, fruits, whole grains and nuts.
2. **Stress Management**: Prolonged stress and tension leads to adrenal exhaustion. Practicing relaxation techniques such as meditation and yoga, plus getting enough rest and exercise, makes a huge positive difference.
3. **Daily Exercise**: Moderate regular exercise like daily half-hour walk helps balance hormones.
4. **Drinking more water**: Increase the intake of water as no other liquid provides the benefits of water.
5. **Intake of supplements**: Diet may not be enough to balance hormones naturally. Good-quality health supplements, high in B-complex, can fill in the gaps.
6. **Healthy lifestyle**: Avoid bad habits such as unhealthy foods, smoking, drinking alcohol, excessive coffee and sodas to balance your hormones naturally.
7. **Think positively**: Learning to steer your mind in a positive direction, irrespective of what is going on in your body or your life, can have a major positive effect on your health, your endocrine system and how you feel.

Review Questions

Long Answer Questions

1. Define hormone and describe the various classes of hormones.
2. Explain the principal endocrine glands and list their secretions.
3. Describe the structure of the pituitary gland and explain the secretory cells of the anterior pituitary.
4. What are the mechanisms by which growth hormone (GH) stimulates the growth of body cells?
5. What are the mechanisms that stimulate oxytocin and ADH release?
6. Describe the anatomy and physiology of the thyroid gland.
7. Describe the actions of thyroid hormones T_3 and T_4.
8. Describe the anatomy and physiology of the parathyroid glands.
9. Describe the anatomy and physiology of the adrenal gland.
10. Explain the pancreatic hormones and discuss their physiological effects.
11. What are the endocrine functions of the pineal gland?

Multiple Choice Questions

1. A hormone is best described as
   (a) An internal secretion that is transported through ducts
   (b) An internal secretion with many effects
   (c) A chemical secreted by a gland
   (d) A chemical produced in one part of the body that is transported in the blood to another place, where it acts in a regulatory capacity

2. Which of the following is *not* a steroid hormone?
   (a) Oestrogen
   (b) Cortisone
   (c) Adrenaline
   (d) Testosterone
   (e) None of the above

3. The alpha cells of the pancreas secrete
   (a) Insulin
   (b) Enzymes
   (c) Glucagon
   (d) None of the above

4. The group of adrenocortical hormones concerned with electrolyte balance is
   (a) The glucocorticoids
   (b) The mineralocorticoids
   (c) The androgens
   (d) Epinephrine and norepinephrine

Chapter 6

5. The adrenal medulla secretes
   - (a) Cortisone
   - (b) Cortisol
   - (c) Epinephrine
   - (d) Acetylcholine

6. The secretion of ACTH from the pituitary stimulates the release of
   - (a) Aldosterone from the adrenal medulla
   - (b) Cortisol from the adrenal cortex
   - (c) Epinephrine from the adrenal medulla
   - (d) Renin from the kidney

7. Oxytocin and antidiuretic hormone (ADH) are stored in
   - (a) The adenohypophysis
   - (b) The anterior pituitary
   - (c) The posterior pituitary
   - (d) The kidneys

8. Hypersecretion of growth hormone after closure of the epiphyseal plates causes
   - (a) Acromegaly
   - (b) Myxedema
   - (c) Addison's disease
   - (d) Gigantism
   - (c) None of the above

9. A marked deficiency of hormone secretion by the thyroid gland in a young child causes
   - (a) Acromegaly
   - (b) Repressed mental and physical growth
   - (c) Bulging eyes
   - (d) High basal metabolic rate
   - (e) All of the above

10. Which of the following is *not* a pituitary hormone?
    - (a) Growth hormone (GH)
    - (b) LH
    - (c) prolactin (PRL)
    - (d) Testosterone
    - (e) Oxytocin

11. Calcium levels in the blood are increased by
    - (a) Calcitonin
    - (b) Heparin
    - (c) Dicumarol
    - (d) Parathyroid hormone
    - (e) Vitamin E

12. Milk ejection from the mammary gland is assisted by

   (a) Oxygen

   (b) Prolactin-releasing hormone

   (c) Oxytocin

   (d) Prostate hormone

   (e) ADH

13. Releasing hormones are synthesized in

   (a) The hypothalamus

   (b) The hypophysis

   (c) The pancreas

   (d) The posterior pituitary

   (e) The ovary

14. The hormone whose action resembles stimulation through the sympathetic division of the autonomic nervous system is

   (a) Epinephrine

   (b) Cortisol

   (c) Androgens

   (d) Aldosterone

   (e) Melatonin

15. Which of the following statements about glucocorticoids is *true*?

   (a) The major glucocorticoid in humans is cortisol

   (b) They are secreted by the zona fasciculata of the adrenal cortex

   (c) Secretion of these hormones is decreased in Addison's disease

   (d) All of the above are true

16. The basal metabolic rate can reflect the dysfunction of

   (a) The pituitary gland

   (b) The parathyroid glands

   (c) The adrenal gland

   (d) The thyroid gland

   (e) The pancreas

17. A symptom of diabetes mellitus is

   (a) Glycaemia

   (b) Polydipsia

   (c) Weight gain

   (d) Hypoglycaemia

Chapter 6

18. Through the negative feedback, a hormone may shut off the secretion of an anterior pituitary hormone by
    (a) Stimulating the release of a (hypothalamic) releasing hormone
    (b) Inhibiting the release of a (hypothalamic) inhibiting hormone
    (c) Inhibiting the release of a (hypothalamic) releasing hormone
    (d) All of the above

19. Stimulation of the mother's nipples by a nursing baby initiates sensory impulses that pass into the central nervous system and eventually reach the hypothalamus. These impulses result in
    (a) Synthesis and release of prolactin from the posterior pituitary
    (b) Release of lactogenic hormone from the anterior pituitary
    (c) Release of oxytocin from the posterior pituitary
    (d) Release of prolactin-inhibiting factor

State True or False

1. Inhibition or stimulation of transport across the cell membrane is one of the major hormonal actions.
2. The major mode of action of steroid hormones is to increase protein synthesis in specific target organ cells.
3. The adrenal medulla secretes adrenaline and noradrenaline.
4. An enlarged thyroid gland is referred to as a goitre.
5. The cells of a parathyroid gland respond directly to the glucose concentration in the blood.

Fill in the Blanks

1. Antidiuretic hormone, or ADH, is also known as _____.
2. Hormones that cross the cell membrane are said to be _____, whereas those that cannot are _____.
3. The _____ gland and the _____ function together as an integrated unit.
4. The technical name of the posterior pituitary is _____, and the technical name of the anterior pituitary is _____.
5. _____ enhances breast development and milk production in females and _____ allows for the let-down of milk and causes uterine contractions.
6. Hyperthyroid secretion in infants and children is known as _____.

7. Sex hormones, in addition to being produced in the ovaries and testes, are also produced in minimal amounts in the _____ .

3. The _____ is a diamond-shaped 'soft spot' on the top of a newborn's skull that facilitates childbirth and permits brain growth.

4. Separating the diaphysis and epiphysis of a child's long bone is a_____, which permits linear bone growth.

5. The _____ foramen is an opening in the mandible on the lateral side below the second premolar tooth.

6. The _____ and the perpendicular plate of the _____ bone compose the bony framework of the nasal septum.

9. In an adult, the ilium, ischium and pubis are fused to form the _____ or hipbone.

10. The foot contains _____tarsal bones, _____ metatarsal bones and _____ phalanges.

Careers in the Endocrine System

✓ Endocrinologists are physicians who specialize in the endocrine system and the treatment of endocrine problems.

✓ Diabetes dieticians are trained dieticians who specialize in counselling and planning of balanced meal for patients with diabetes mellitus.

7 | The Blood

STUDY OBJECTIVES

✓ To describe the functions and components of blood.
✓ To discuss the structure, functions and formation of red blood cells, white blood cells and platelets.

✓ To explain the different blood groups.
✓ To discuss the process of blood coagulation.

INTRODUCTION

Blood is a uniquely specialized connective tissue. It provides means of communication between the cells of different parts of the body and the external environment. It is considered as the fluid of life (carries oxygen from lungs to all body parts), fluid of growth (carries nutrients and hormones) and fluid of health (protects the body against diseases). The branch of science concerned with the study of blood, blood-forming tissues and the disorders associated with blood is termed as *haematology* (*haem*: blood; *logy*: study).

Blood accounts for about 7% of the total body weight. An average male has approximately 6 L of blood in the body, whereas an average female has about 5 L of blood.

Blood in the blood vessels is always mobile due to the pumping action of the heart. This continuous mobility of blood maintains a constant environment for the body cells.

PROPERTIES OF BLOOD

Blood is an opaque and somewhat sticky fluid connective tissue.

The various properties of blood include the following:

1. **Colour**: It is bright red when oxygenated and purple red when deoxygenated.
2. **pH**: It has a slightly alkaline pH ranging from 7.35 to 7.45 and has a saltish taste.
3. **Specific gravity**: It has a specific gravity of 1.06 and is slightly heavier than water.
4. **Viscosity**: Blood is five times more viscous than water because of the presence of red blood cells and plasma proteins.

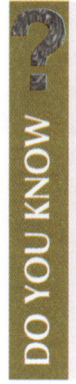

DO YOU KNOW ?

- ❑ Two million red blood cells die every second.
- ❑ Each day almost 400 gallons of recycled blood is pumped through the kidneys.
- ❑ Seven percent of a human's body weight is made up of blood.

FUNCTIONS OF BLOOD

Blood plays a vital role in the body. Its various functions include the following:

1. Transportation

- ❑ Blood transports oxygen from the lungs to different tissues and carbon dioxide from tissues to the lungs.
- ❑ Blood carries nutrients like glucose, amino acids, lipids and vitamins from the gastrointestinal tract to the body cells and transports waste products and heat formed during various metabolic activities away from the cells.
- ❑ Blood also carries various hormones from the endocrine glands to target organs in the body.

2. Regulation

- ❑ Blood helps regulate the water balance of the body as it supplies water to the tissues when needed and receives the excess water formed in metabolic processes.

MEDICAL TERMINOLOGY

- ❑ **Antibodies**: They are a specialized immune protein, produced because of the introduction of an antigen into the body and which possesses the remarkable ability to combine with the very antigen that triggered its production.
- ❑ **Blasts**: Cells that secrete extracellular matrix.
- ❑ **Cytes**: cells in any tissue that maintain the tissue.
- ❑ **Ligaments**: Tough connective tissue structures that attaches bones to bones.
- ❑ **Osmotic Pressure**: It is the pressure necessary to prevent osmosis into a given solution when the solution is separated from the pure solvent by a semipermeable membrane.
- ❑ **Phagocytosis**: The process of engulfing and ingestion of particles by the cell or a phagocyte (e.g. macrophage).
- ❑ **Red Bone Marrow**: It is connective tissue present in trabeculae of spongy bone tissue. It is present mainly in the bones of axial skeleton, pectoral and pelvic girdles, and the proximal epiphyses of the humerus and femur.
- ❑ **Tendons**: Structures that attach muscle to bone.

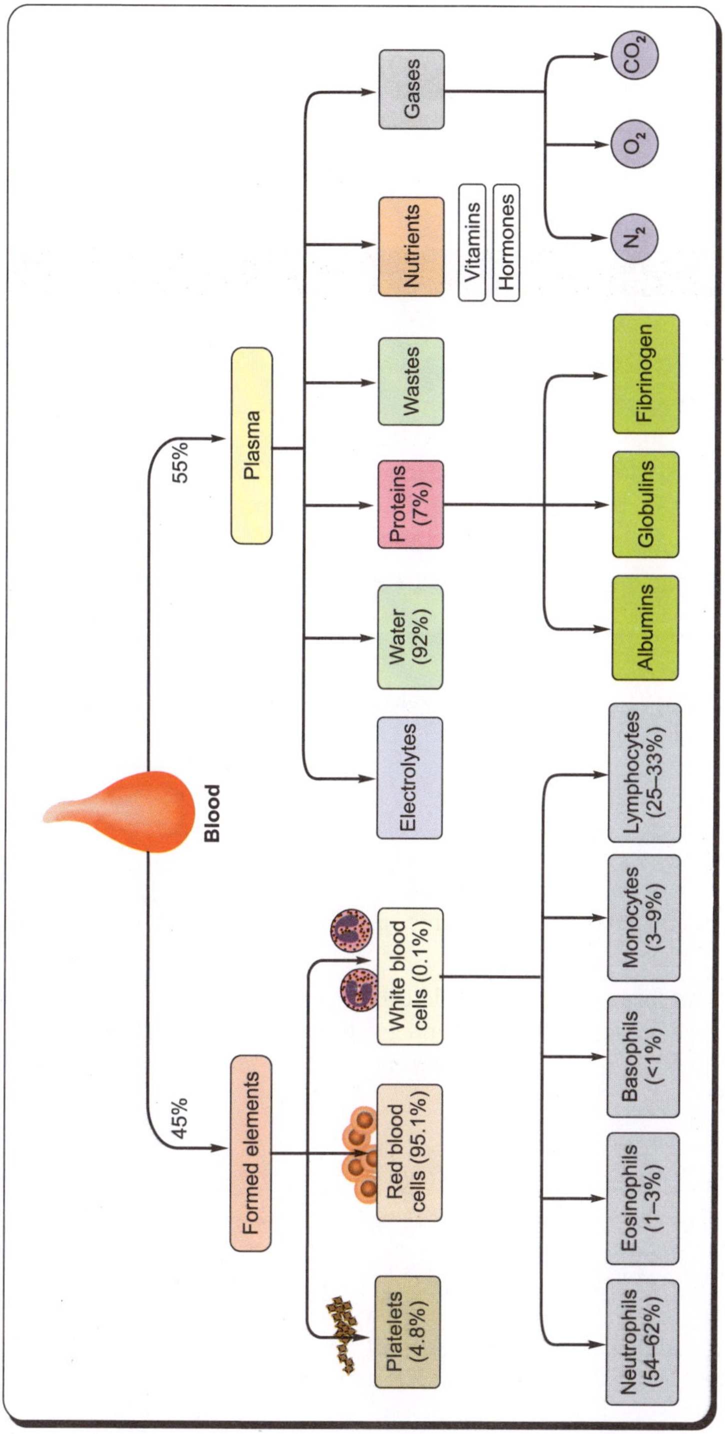

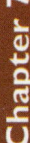

Figure 7.1 Components of blood.

❑ Blood helps regulate body pH through plasma proteins and buffers present in the blood.

❑ Blood also plays a role in the regulation of normal body temperature because of the heat-absorbing and coolant properties of the water in plasma.

3. Defence: The white blood cells (WBCs) protect the body against the disease-causing microorganisms and toxins by carrying on phagocytosis and production of proteins called *antibodies*.

4. Blood clotting: The platelets play a role in blood clotting and thus prevent excessive loss of blood from the body after an injury.

COMPONENTS OF BLOOD

Blood consists of two components: the fluid part of blood or plasma that accounts for about 55% of blood and the formed elements of blood or the blood cells that constitute about 45% of the total volume of blood (Fig. 7.1).

If a blood sample is centrifuged in a small glass tube, the red blood cells (RBCs) settle down at the bottom of the tube, while the clear plasma forms a layer at the top (Fig. 7.2). The WBCs and platelets form a very thin layer, called the *buffy coat*, between the RBCs and plasma in centrifuged blood.

The percentage of total blood volume occupied by RBCs is called the *haematocrit value*. The normal range of haematocrit for adult females and males is 38–46% and 40–54%, respectively.

PLASMA

Plasma is a straw-coloured, slightly alkaline clear liquid. It consists of about 92% water and 8–9% of solutes, most of which (7% of weight) are proteins (Fig. 7.3).

Plasma proteins

Plasma proteins, which constitute about 7% of plasma, are mainly produced by the liver. The plasma proteins play a vital role in maintaining normal osmotic pressure of the blood (25 mm Hg) as they are unable to pass through the capillary membrane due to their large size and remain within the blood and exert colloidal osmotic pressure.

Osmotic pressure is a very important factor involved in fluid exchange across capillary walls. If the plasma protein level falls due to reduced production or loss from blood vessels, osmotic pressure is also reduced. This condition results in excessive filtration of water from the blood into the tissues, causing oedema (swelling) of the extremities.

The major proteins in the plasma are as follows:

1. **Albumin**: The molecular weight of plasma albumin is 69,000.
2. **Globulin**: The molecular weight of globulins varies in the range 90,000–1,300,000. The globulins are a mixture of several proteins, which can be separated by electrophoresis.
   (a) α_1–α_2 *globulin* (Mol. wt.: 41,000–200,000)
   (b) β *globulin* (Mol. wt.: 90,000–1,300,000): β-Lipoprotein helps in carrying lipid, steroid and carotene, while the globulin portion helps in the transport of iron.
   (c) γ *globulin* (Mol. wt.: 150,000–190,000)

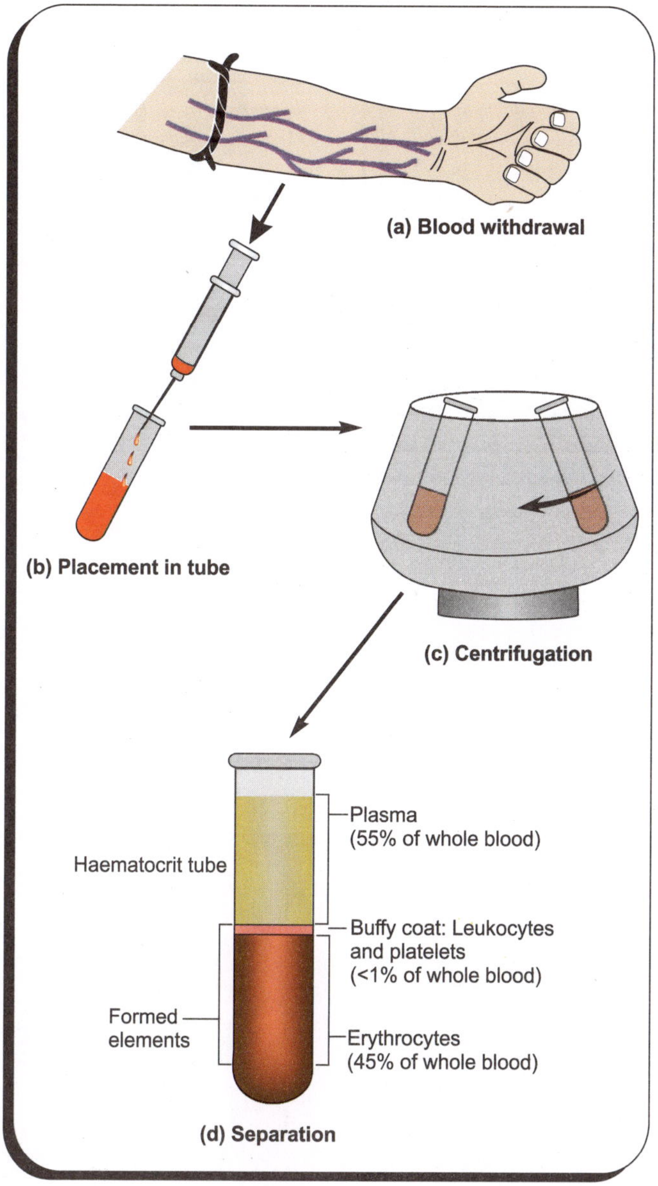

Figure 7.2 Separation of blood after centrifugation.

3. **Fibrinogen**: The molecular weight of fibrinogen is 3,45,000. It is involved in blood clotting.

The average normal concentration of the plasma proteins are serum albumin (4.8 g%), serum globulin (2.3 g%) and fibrinogen (0.3 g%).

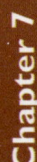

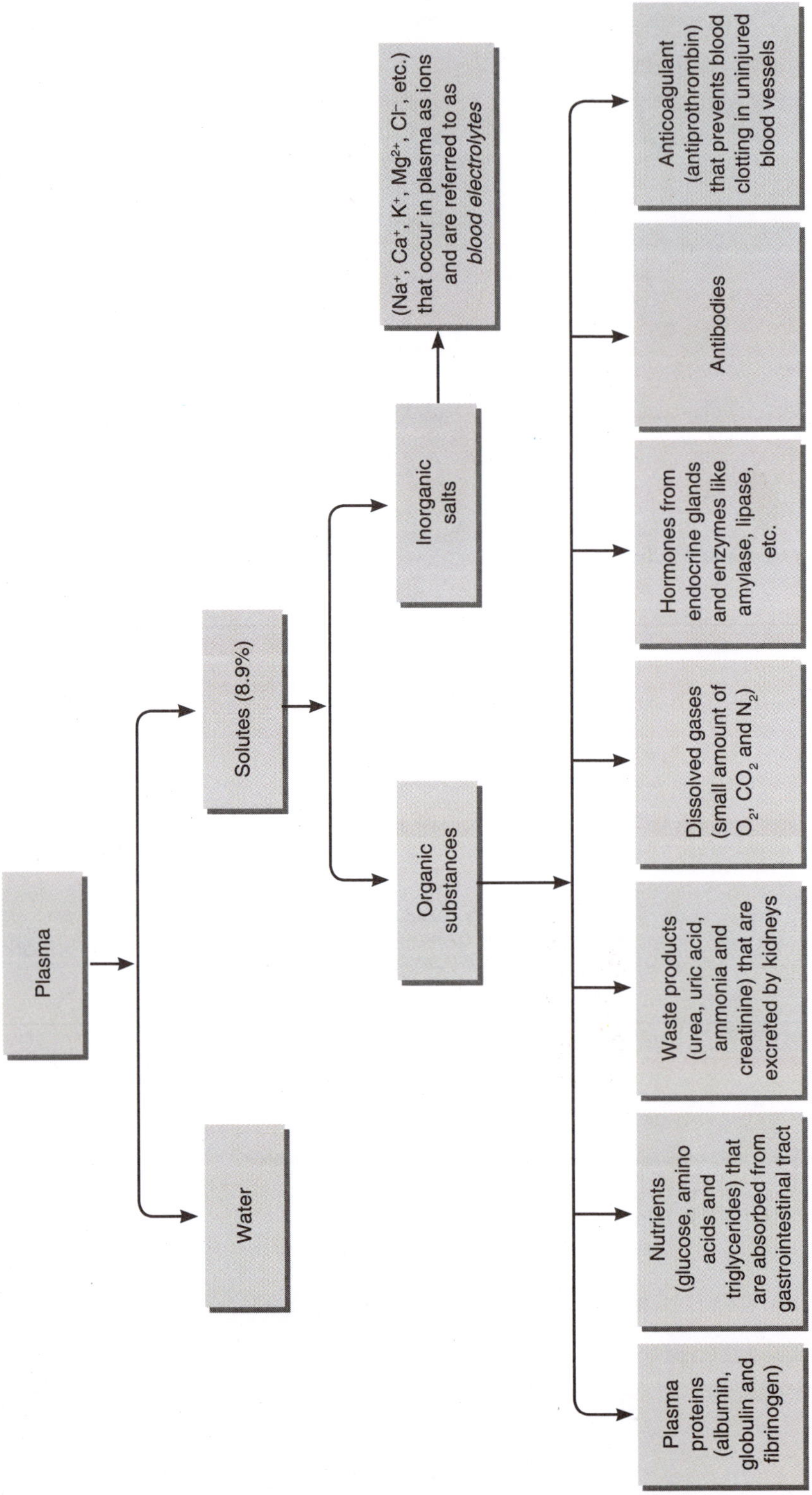

Plasma

Water

Solutes (8.9%)

Inorganic salts

(Na⁺, Ca²⁺, K⁺, Mg²⁺, Cl⁻, etc.) that occur in plasma as ions and are referred to as *blood electrolytes*

Organic substances

Plasma proteins (albumin, globulin and fibrinogen)

Nutrients (glucose, amino acids and triglycerides) that are absorbed from gastrointestinal tract

Waste products (urea, uric acid, ammonia and creatinine) that are excreted by kidneys

Dissolved gases (small amount of O_2, CO_2 and N_2)

Hormones from endocrine glands and enzymes like amylase, lipase, etc.

Antibodies

Anticoagulant (antiprothrombin) that prevents blood clotting in uninjured blood vessels

Figure 7.3 Components of plasma.

DIFFERENCE BETWEEN SERUM AND PLASMA

❑ Serum is a straw-coloured fluid that contains all the other constituents of plasma except fibrinogen.

Thus, serum = plasma – fibrinogen.

❑ Owing to this, albumin and globulin are usually referred to as *serum albumin* and *serum globulin*, respectively.

Functions of plasma proteins

1. **Regulation**

   (a) *Acid–base balance*: Plasma proteins (particularly albumin) act as buffers and maintain pH of the blood.

   (b) *Osmotic pressure*: Albumin and globulin maintain the osmotic pressure of the blood and thus keep the plasma fluid within circulation.

2. **Transportation**: Plasma proteins are essential for the transport of various substances in the blood. For example, albumins act as the carrier molecules for lipids and steroid hormones, and globulins carry the hormone thyroxine and insulin to the target organs.

3. **Defence**: Some globulins, called *immunoglobulins* (IG), also called *antibodies*, play an important role in the defence mechanism of the body. These proteins are produced in response to the entry of foreign microorganisms such as bacteria and viruses (antigens) and result in the production of antigen–antibody complexes, which disable the invading antigen.

4. **Blood coagulation**: Fibrinogen plays a vital role in blood coagulation as it converts into fibrin and forms the blood clot.

5. **Reserve proteins**: During conditions like fasting or inadequate food intake, the plasma proteins are utilized by the body tissues for their routine activities and thus the plasma proteins are also referred to as *reserve proteins*.

BLOOD CELLS

There are three types of blood cells, which are as follows (Fig. 7.4):

1. **Erythrocytes or RBCs**: They make up about 95% of the volume of blood cells.
2. **Leukocytes or WBCs**: They are divided into the following two categories:
   (a) *Granular leukocytes or granulocytes*: They have granules in their cytoplasm. They are of the following three types:
      (i) Neutrophils: They make up 60–70% of WBCs.
      (ii) Eosinophils: They make up 2–4% of WBCs.
      (iii) Basophils: They make up 0.5–1% of WBCs.
   (b) *Agranular leukocytes or agranulocytes*: They do not have granules in their cytoplasm. They are of the following two types:
      (i) Monocytes: They make up 3–8% of WBCs.
      (ii) Lymphocytes: They make up 20–25% of WBCs.

Chapter 7

3. **Thrombocytes or platelets**

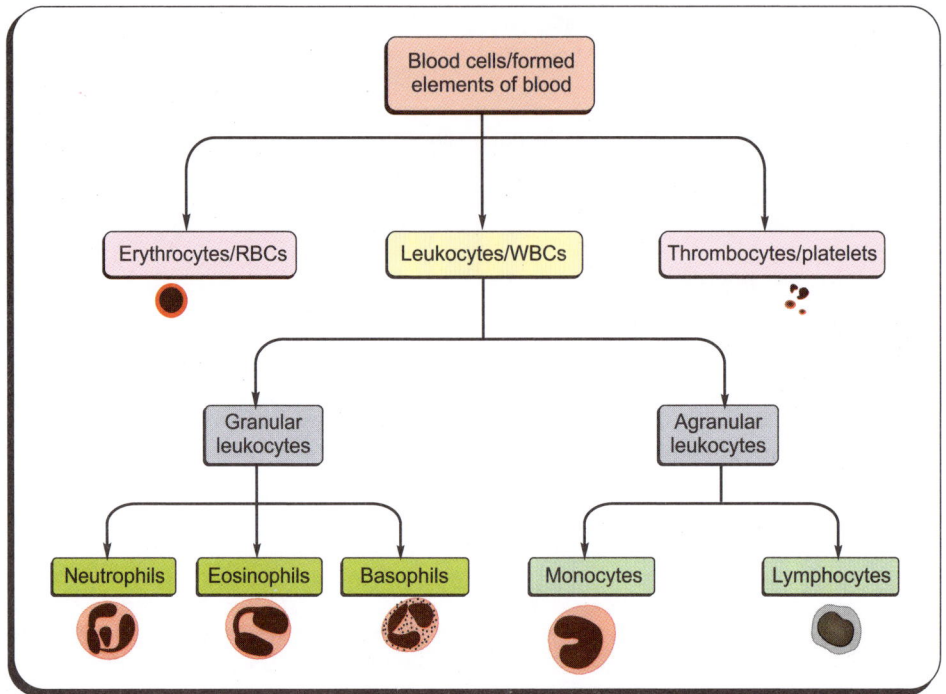

Figure 7.4 Types of blood cells.

Formation of blood cells

The process of development of blood cells is termed as *haemopoiesis* or *haematopoiesis*. Before birth, haemopoiesis first takes place in the yolk sac of an embryo and later in the liver, spleen, thymus and lymph nodes of the fetus. In the last 3 months before birth, red bone marrow becomes the primary site of haemopoiesis and this continues as the main source of blood cells after birth and throughout life.

The blood cells develop from the primitive cells in the bone marrow. These primitive cells are called the *stem cells* and they have the capacity to develop into different types of blood cells; hence, they are also called *pluripotent haemopoietic stem cells*.

The pluripotent haemopoietic stem cells develop into the following two further types of stem cells (Fig. 7.5):

1. **Lymphoid stem cells (LSCs)**: These cells give rise to lymphocytes.
2. **Myeloid stem cells (MSCs)**: These cells give rise to the blood cells other than lymphocytes by forming different colony-forming units (CFUs).

The different CFUs are as follows:

1. **CFU-erythrocytes (CFU-E)**: They develop into erythrocytes.
2. **CFU-granulocytes/monocytes (CFU-GM)**: They develop into granulocytes (neutrophils, basophils and eosinophils) and monocytes.
3. **CFU-megakaryocytes (CFU-M)**: They develop into platelets.

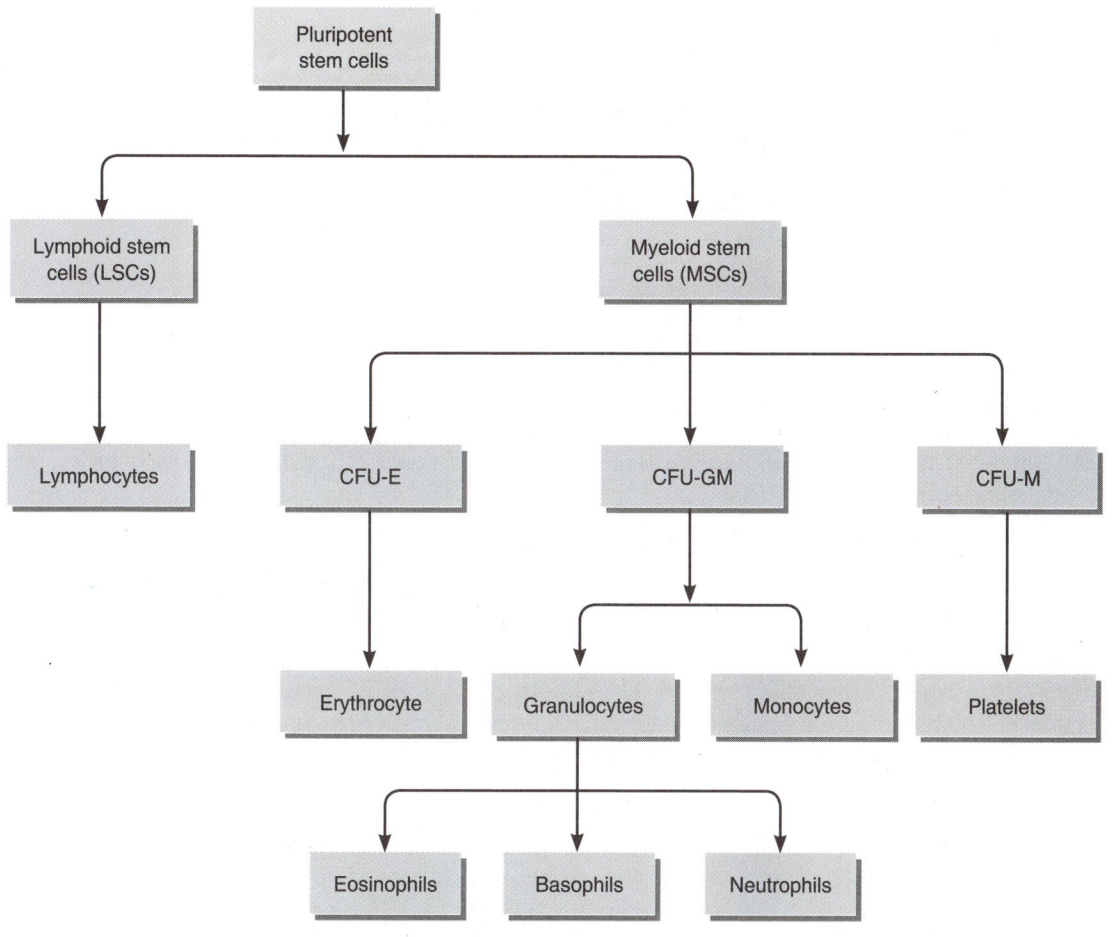

Figure 7.5 Formation of blood cells.

Erythrocytes or RBCs

RBCs are the most numerous formed elements of the blood. A unique feature of RBCs is the presence of a red, oxygen-carrying pigment, the *haemoglobin*, in their cytoplasm.

Morphology of RBCs

1. **Normal size**: RBCs are smaller than WBCs and their diameter is about 7 μm.
2. **Normal shape**: They are biconcave, denucleated discs with a thinner central part compared to the margins. This characteristic shape provides flexibility and increases the surface area, which facilitates quick diffusion of gases (Fig. 7.6).

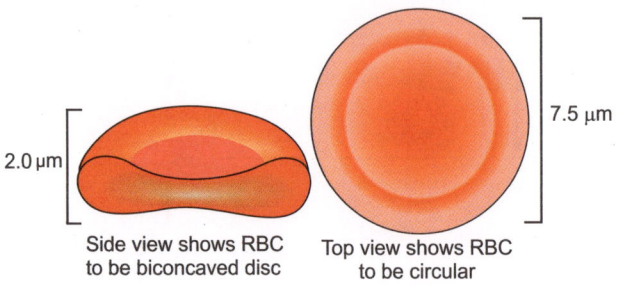

Figure 7.6 Shape of RBC.

3. **Number**: A healthy adult male and female have about 5 and 4.5 million RBCs per cubic meter of blood, respectively.
4. **Colour**: The blood appears red in colour due to the presence of a red, oxygen-carrying protein haemoglobin (Hb) in the RBCs.
5. **Structure**: RBCs are bounded by an elastic and semipermeable plasma membrane, which is both strong and flexible and allows them to squeeze through narrow capillaries without rupturing. Moreover, RBCs lack nucleus and other intracellular organelles, thus leaving more space for Hb.

Haemoglobin (Hb)

The average range of Hb in males and females is 14–18 g/dL and 12–15.5 g/dL, respectively. Hb level is high in newborns (23 g/dL) because they remain in the state of relative hypoxia, which serves as a potent stimulus for erythropoietin secretion. With age, the Hb level decreases to the normal level.

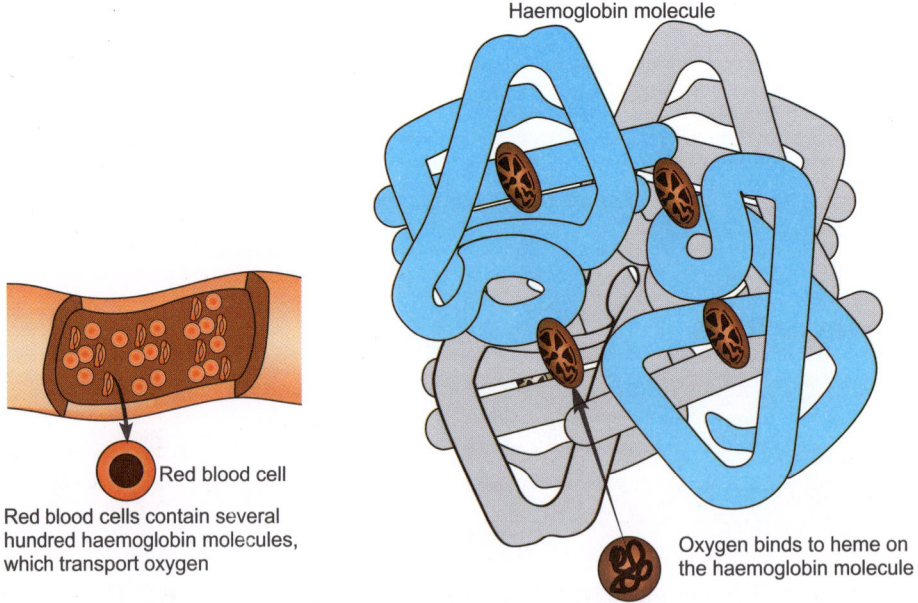

Figure 7.7 Haemoglobin molecule.

Hb is a large, complex protein consisting of four molecules of globin protein joined to four pigmented iron-containing complexes called *haem*. Each haem molecule contains four iron ions (Fe^{2+}), each of which can combine reversibly with one oxygen molecule (Fig. 7.7).

Haemoglobin (Hb) = 4 Haem + 4 Globin (protein)

↓

Consists of 4 Fe^{2+} atoms that can combine with 4 O_2 molecules.

An average RBC carries about 280 million Hb molecules; thus, one RBC can carry over a billion oxygen molecules.

In the lungs, due to the high partial pressure of oxygen, Hb takes up oxygen and changes to bright red oxyhaemoglobin (HbO), which is transported to other body tissues.

Haemoglobin (Hb) + oxygen (O_2) → Oxyhaemoglobin (HbO)

In the body tissues, due to the low partial pressure of oxygen, HbO releases its oxygen readily. After oxygen is released, the protein globin now combines with the carbon dioxide from the interstitial fluid and carries it to the lungs where it is released.

Properties of RBCs

1. **Rouleaux formation**: The property of adhering together and piling up of RBCs above one another when taken out of the blood vessel is termed as *rouleaux formation* (Fig. 7.8).

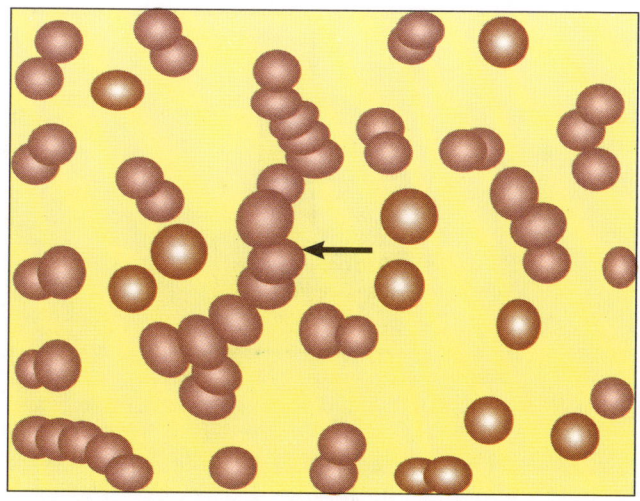

Figure 7.8 Rouleaux formation in RBCs.

2. **Haematocrit or packed cell volume**: The percentage of total blood volume occupied by RBCs settled at the bottom when the blood is centrifuged is called *packed cell volume (PCV)* or *haematocrit*. In normal conditions, the RBCs form 45% of the total blood.

3. **Suspension stability**: The property of RBCs owing to which it remains uniformly suspended in blood during circulation is termed as *suspension stability*.

Functions of RBCs

1. RBCs are highly specialized for their oxygen transport function. The primary function of RBCs is to combine with oxygen in the lungs and to transport it to the various tissues of the body.
2. RBCs combine with carbon dioxide in the tissues and transport it to the lungs for expulsion from the body.
3. RBCs carry the blood group antigens A, B and Rh factor, which help determine the blood group and play a vital role in the transfusion of blood.

Lifespan and fate of RBCs

The average lifespan of RBCs is about 120 days. As the cells become older (120 days), their plasma membranes become more and more fragile and eventually gets destroyed while trying to squeeze

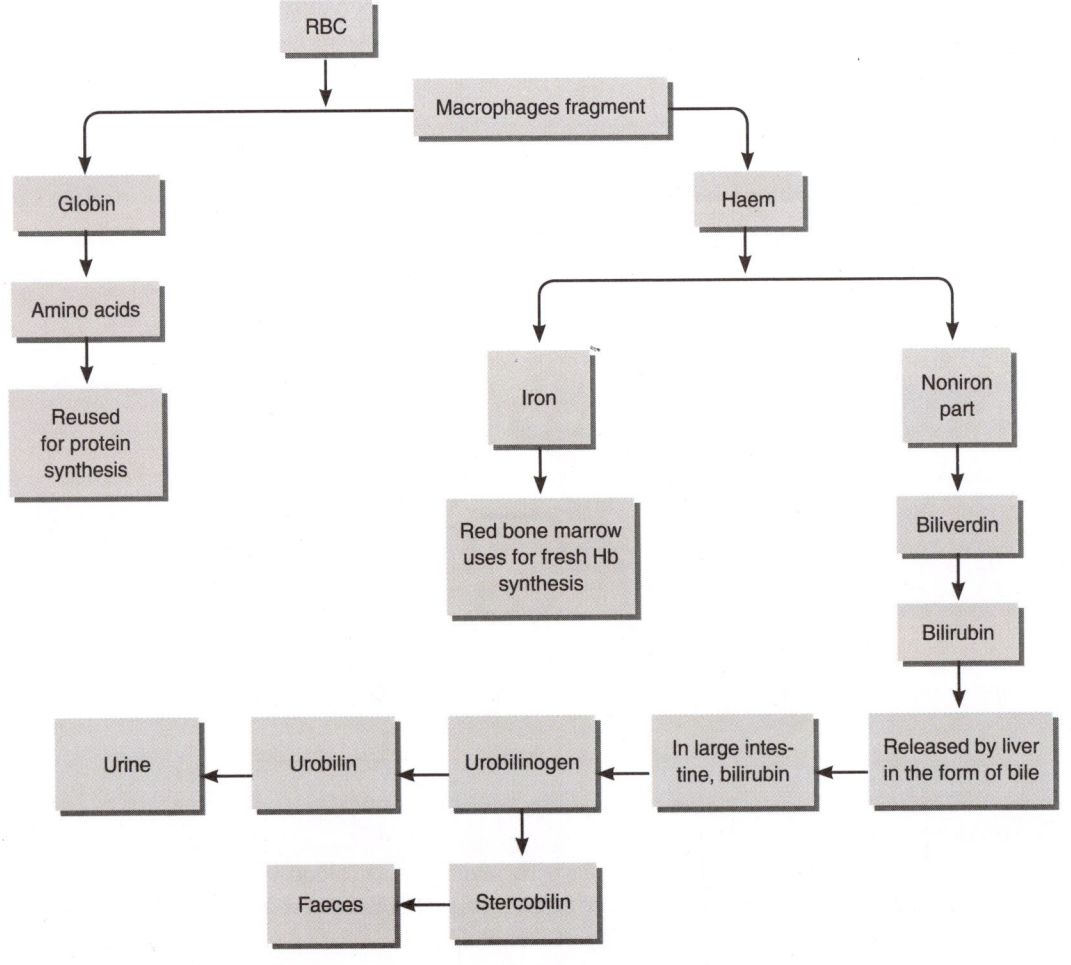

Figure 7.9 Destruction of RBC.

through the narrow capillaries. The destruction occurs mostly in the capillaries of the spleen as they have thin lumen. Hence, the spleen is usually called the *graveyard of RBCs*. Haemolysis is carried out by phagocytic reticuloendothelial cells mainly in the spleen, bone marrow and liver.

The breakdown products of worn-out RBCs are recycled as follows (Fig. 7.9):

1. Macrophages in the spleen, liver and bone marrow carry out haemolysis and thereby split the globin and haem portions of Hb.
2. Globin is broken down into amino acids that can be reused to synthesize other proteins.
3. Iron is removed from the haem portion and is returned to the red bone marrow for reuse in the synthesis of fresh Hb.
4. When iron is removed from haem, the noniron portion of haem is converted to biliverdin, a green pigment, which is almost completely reduced to the yellow pigment, bilirubin.
5. Bilirubin enters the blood and is transported to the liver where it is excreted into bile. The bile secreted from the liver passes into the small intestine and then into the large intestine.
6. In the large intestine, bacteria converts bilirubin into urobilinogen, most of which is eliminated in faeces in the form of a brown pigment called *stercobilin*; this gives faeces its characteristic colour. Some urobilinogen is absorbed back into the blood and converted to a yellow pigment called *urobilin*, which is excreted in urine.

Variations in RBCs

1. **Variations in number of RBCs**

   The variation in RBC count may occur both physiologically and pathologically.

   Increased RBC count

   The RBC count may increase physiologically due to the following factors:

   (a) **High altitude**: Hypoxia at high altitude stimulates the kidneys to release erythropoietin, which in turn stimulates the bone marrow to produce more RBCs.

   (b) **Muscular exercise**: RBC count may increase due to hypoxia.

   (c) **Emotional conditions such as anxiety**: This is due to sympathetic stimulation.

   The abnormal increase in RBC count in pathological condition is termed as *polycythaemia*.

   Decreased RBC count

   The RBC count may decrease physiologically due to the following factors:

   (a) High barometric pressure, like in deep sea.

   (b) During pregnancy, due to increased ECF volume.

   Abnormal decrease in RBC count is called *anaemia*.

2. **Variations in size of RBC**

   (a) *Microcytes:* These are small-sized RBCs that occur mostly due to iron deficiency (anaemia).

   (b) *Macrocytes:* These are large-sized RBCs that occur mainly due to megaloblastic anaemia.

   (c) *Anisocytes:* These are unequal-sized RBCs that occur due to pernicious anaemia.

3. **Variations in shape of RBC**

   RBCs may adopt some abnormal shapes due to various pathological conditions. These shapes may be crenation (shrink), spherocytosis (globular), elliptocytosis (elliptical) and sickle cell shape (crescent shaped).

Chapter 7

4. **Variations in structure of RBC**
   (a) **Goblet ring**: It is the appearance of ring-shaped strands of some basophilic material at the periphery of RBC.
   (b) **Howell Jolly bodies**: It is the appearance of some nuclear fragments in the ectoplasm of RBC.

Erythropoiesis

The process of development of RBCs is called *erythropoiesis*. It occurs in the liver and spleen in fetus and in the red bone marrow after birth.

The stem cells of the colony-forming unit (CFU-E) pass through different stages and finally become matured RBCs. (The process of CFU-E formation has already been discussed in the section Formation of Blood Cells).

The detailed steps in erythropoiesis are as follows (Fig. 7.10):

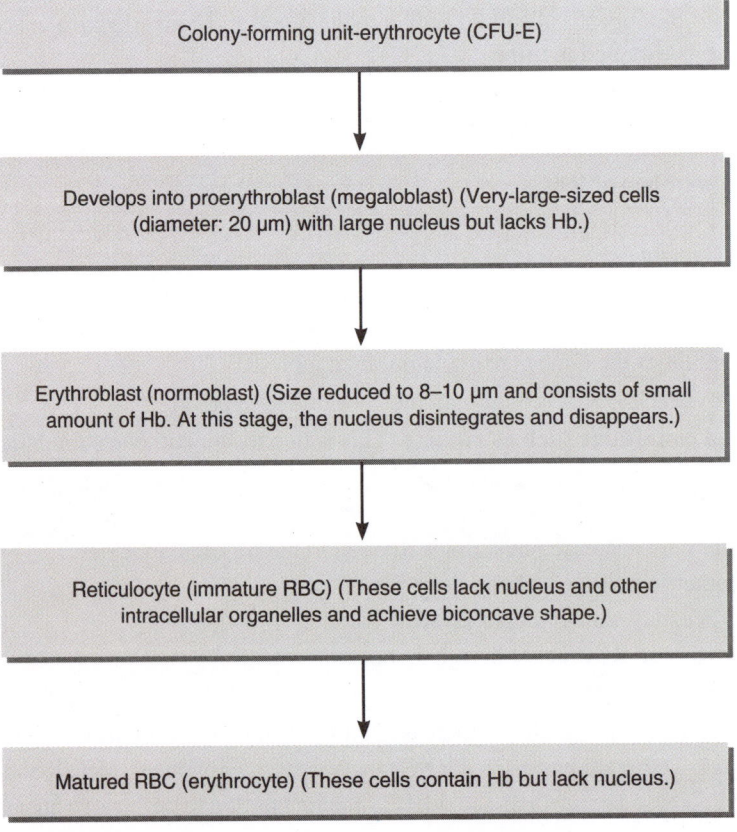

Figure 7.10 Steps in erythropoiesis.

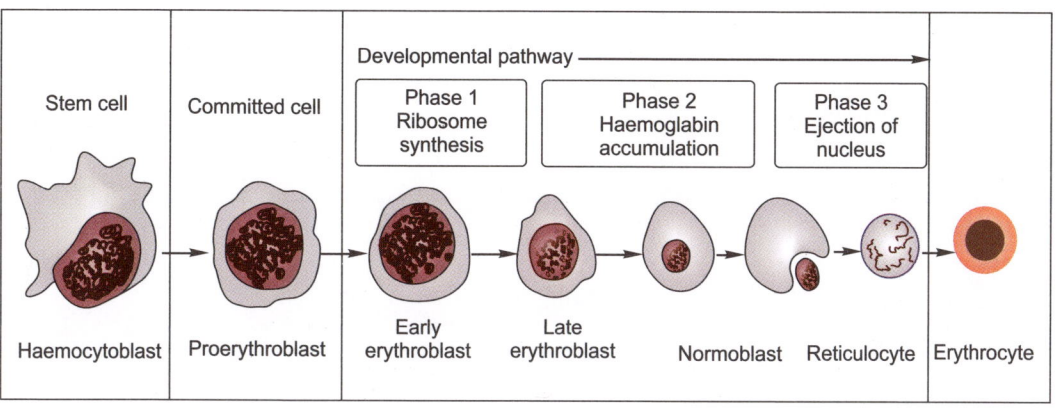

Figure 7.11 Various steps in erythropoiesis.

It requires seven days for the development of matured RBC from proerythroblast. The development of immature RBC or reticulocyte takes place in five days; the reticulocyte then takes two more days to become the matured RBC (Fig. 7.11).

Factors necessary for erythropoiesis

Erythropoiesis is regulated by a number of factors, including the following:

1. **Erythropoietin/erythrocyte stimulating factor (ESF)**: It is the hormone released from kidneys in response to hypoxia. Erythropoietin increases the production of proerythroblasts and stimulates the development of proerythroblasts into matured RBCs. These changes increase the oxygen-carrying capacity of blood and reverses hypoxia.

2. **Thyroxine**: It accelerates erythropoiesis.

3. **Cytokines**: Cytokines are small glycoproteins that are produced by red bone marrow cells, leukocytes, macrophages and endothelial cells. They stimulate the proliferation of pluripotent stem cells and CFUs. The major cytokines that regulate erythropoiesis include interleukins (IL), especially IL-3, IL-6, IL-11 and colony-stimulating factors (CSFs).

4. **Vitamin B_{12} and folic acid**: Vitamin B_{12} and folic acid are very essential for the maturation of RBCs. Both of these are absorbed from the intestine, although vitamin B_{12} requires the presence of intrinsic factor of castle for its absorption.

5. **Iron and copper**: Iron is necessary for the formation of the haem part of Hb, and copper is essential for the iron absorption from the gastrointestinal tract.

Regulation of erythropoiesis

Normally, erythropoiesis and RBC destruction proceeds at roughly the same pace, and thus the number of RBC remains fairly constant. This is regulated due to a homeostatic negative feedback mechanism, which is described in figure 7.12.

Chapter 7

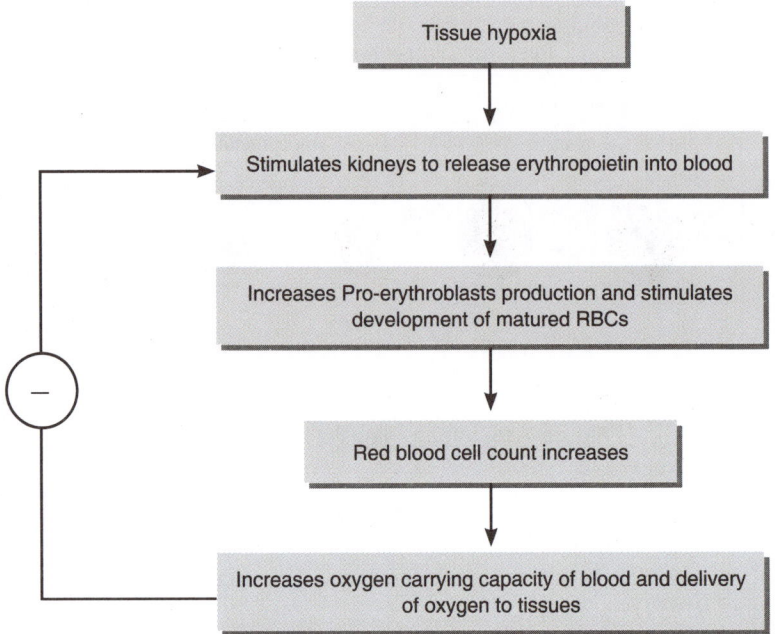

Figure 7.12 Negative feedback regulation in erythropoiesis.

Thus, the negative feedback regulation maintains the RBC count in the body. Hypoxia-like condition stimulates erythropoietin release and increases RBC count but when the tissue hypoxia is overcome, erythropoietin production declines.

Leukocytes or WBCs

WBC or leukocyte is the colourless (lacks Hb) and nucleated formed element of the blood. They are the largest blood cells and account for about 1% of the total blood volume.

WBCs play a very important role in defending the body against microbes and other foreign materials.

Morphology of WBCs

1. **Normal size**: WBCs are larger than RBCs with their diameter ranging from 12 to 20 μm.
2. **Normal shape**: They are rounded or irregular shaped and have the ability to change their shape, which enables them to squeeze out of the capillaries into the tissues.
3. **Number**: WBCs are far less numerous than RBCs in the range 4000–11,000/m³ of blood. Abnormal increase in WBC count is called *leukocytosis*, whereas abnormal decrease in WBC count is termed *leukopenia*. Abnormal uncontrolled increase in leukocyte count up to 10,00,000/m³ is termed *leukaemia*.
4. **Structure**: These are nucleated cells containing other intracellular organelles such as the golgi apparatus, mitochondria and centrioles.

5. **Lifespan and disposal**: The leukocytes survive only for a few (2–6) days in the blood. Dead WBCs are phagocytized in the blood, liver and lymph nodes.

Properties of WBCs

1. **Diapedesis**: The ability of WBCs to squeeze out of the capillaries to reach the area of infection is termed as *diapedesis* or *emigration* (Fig. 7.13). In this process, WBCs roll along the endothelium, stick to it and then squeeze between endothelial cells to reach the area of infection.

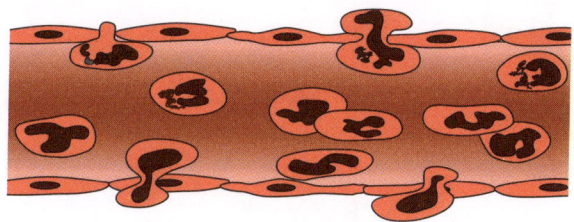

Figure 7.13 Diapedesis.

2. **Chemotaxis**: The property of WBCs owing to which they get attracted towards any infected area due to the chemical substances released by microbes and damaged cells is termed as *chemotaxis*. The substances that provide stimuli for chemotaxis are called *chemotaxens*; they include toxins produced by microbes and inflamed tissues.

3. **Phagocytosis** (*phago*: **eating;** *cytosis*: **cell**): Neutrophils and monocytes are active in phagocytosis; they ingest the microbes and thereby kill them.

Types of WBCs

The WBCs are classified into the following two types:

1. **Granulocytes (contain granules)**: They include neutrophils, eosinophils and basophils.
2. **Agranulocytes (without granules)**: They include monocytes and lymphocytes.

Differential leukocyte count (DLC): It can be defined as the count on a stained blood smear of the proportion of different types of leukocytes, expressed in percentages (as shown in Fig. 7.14).

Granulocytes or granular leukocytes

All granulocytes have multilobed nuclei and contain granules that can be made visible by staining. As these cells age, the number of nuclear lobes increases, which attain different shapes; hence, these cells are also called *polymorphonuclear leukocytes*.

These cells are produced in the red bone marrow and the process of their formation is called *granulopoiesis*.

They have three subtypes: neutrophils, eosinophils and basophils.

1. **Neutrophils**
   (a) Neutrophils have fine granules in their cytoplasm that stain equally well with both acidic and basic dyes.

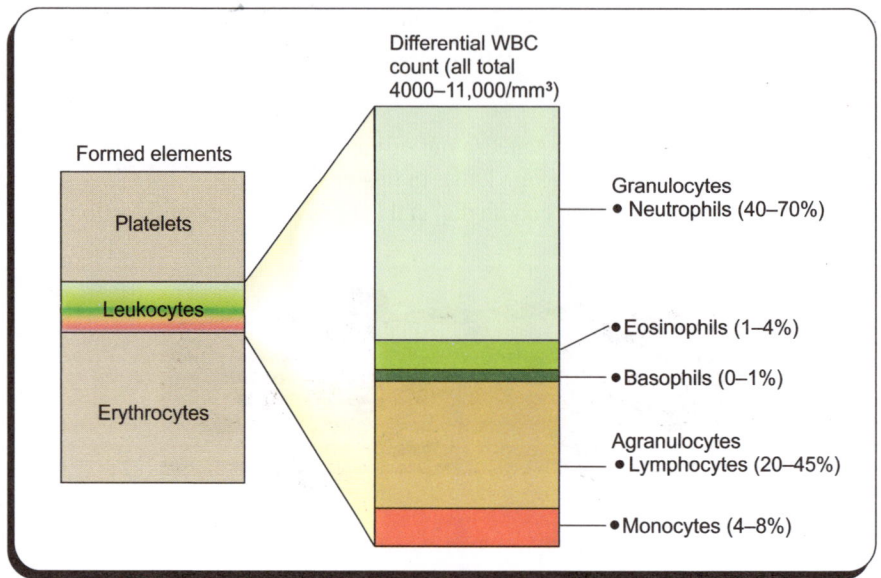

Figure 7.14 Differential leukocyte count.

(b) Their main function is to protect against foreign bodies and microorganisms and to remove waste materials, for example cell debris. These are the first cells among WBCs to respond against any tissue destruction by bacteria.

  (i) The neutrophils are attracted to the site of infection by chemotaxis, and they reach the site readily through diapedesis. Thereafter, they engulf the microbes by phagocytosis and kill them by releasing several chemicals stored in their granules. These chemicals include the hydrolytic enzyme *lysozyme*, which destroys the bacteria; antibody-like substances *defensins*; and strong oxidants such as hydrogen peroxide (H_2O_2).

  (ii) Pus that is formed in the infected area consists of dead tissue cells (cell debris), plasma leaked from blood vessels and dead WBCs.

(c) The neutrophils may increase physiologically after exercise, in emotional conditions and in later stages of pregnancy. The abnormal increase in neutrophil count in pathological condition is called *neutrophilic leukocytosis*, and this may occur in acute infections, extensive tissue damage or after acute haemorrhage.

2. **Eosinophils**

  (a) The granules in the eosinophils are eosinophilic (eosin loving), that is they stain red-orange with the acidic dye eosin.

  (b) The following are the major functions of eosinophils:

   (i) *Elimination of parasites:* Their granules contain certain cytotoxic substances such as eosinophil peroxidase (EP) and eosinophilic cationic protein, which are released over the invading organisms to destroy them.

   (ii) *Role in allergic conditions:* The eosinophils contain the enzyme histaminase, which breaks down histamine (an inflammatory agent) produced in inflammation during allergic conditions, and thus combats the allergic inflammatory conditions such as asthma and skin allergy.

(c) The abnormal increase in eosinophil count is called ***eosinophilia***, and it mainly occurs in allergic conditions, asthma and blood parasitism (malaria, filariasis, etc.).

3. **Basophils**
   (a) The granules of the basophils are basophilic (base loving), that is they stain purple blue with basic dyes such as methylene blue.
   (b) Basophils play an important role in inflammation and allergic reactions. At the site of inflammation, basophils bind with the allergen (an antigen that causes allergy and inflammation) and release granules that contain histamine (an inflammatory agent), heparin (an anticoagulant) and other substances that promote inflammation. Thus, these substances intensify the inflammatory reactions and are involved in acute hypersensitivity reactions (allergy).
      (i) Similar to basophils, mast cell is a large cell found in the tissues but is absent in blood circulation. Mast cells release their contents within seconds of binding an allergen, thus resulting in the rapid onset of allergic symptoms on exposure to an allergen (e.g. pollen).
   (c) The abnormal increase in basophil count is termed as *basophilia*, and it occurs in conditions such as small pox or chicken pox.

Agranulocytes or agranular leukocytes

These leukocytes lack granules in the cytoplasm and have nonlobed nucleus. There are two subtypes of agranular leukocytes: monocytes and lymphocytes. The monocytes are produced in the bone marrow, whereas the lymphocyte subtypes, that is B and T lymphocytes, are produced in the bone marrow and thymus, respectively. The process of formation of agranulocytes is termed as *agranulopoiesis*.

1. **Monocytes**
   (a) These are the largest leukocytes, with kidney-shaped or horseshoe-shaped nucleus and are produced in the bone marrow. Some monocytes circulate in blood and are phagocytic, whereas others migrate from the blood into the tissues, where they enlarge and develop into macrophages (For more details, see the chapter Immunity).
   (b) The monocyte–macrophage system is called the *reticuloendothelial system* that plays a vital role in protecting the body against invading microorganisms by phagocytosis. Both monocytes and macrophages secrete cytokines (IL-1) and CSF that stimulate the production of lymphocytes.
   (c) The abnormal increase in monocytes count is known as *monocytosis*, and it occurs in microbial infections such as tuberculosis, syphilis and malaria.

2. **Lymphocytes**
   (a) They are the smallest leukocytes and have kidney-shaped nucleus. They circulate in the blood and are present mainly in lymphatic tissues such as lymph nodes and the spleen. Functionally, the lymphocytes are classified into two types: B lymphocytes and T lymphocytes.
   (b) They play a crucial role in the immune response of the body and are involved in the production of antibodies. The antibodies destroy microbes and their toxins, reject grafts and kill tumour cells (For more details, see the chapter Immunity).

Leukopoiesis

The process of development of WBCs is called *leukopoiesis* (Fig. 7.15). It occurs in lymph nodes, spleen, thymus and red bone marrow.

The detailed steps in leukopoiesis are as follows (Fig. 7.16):

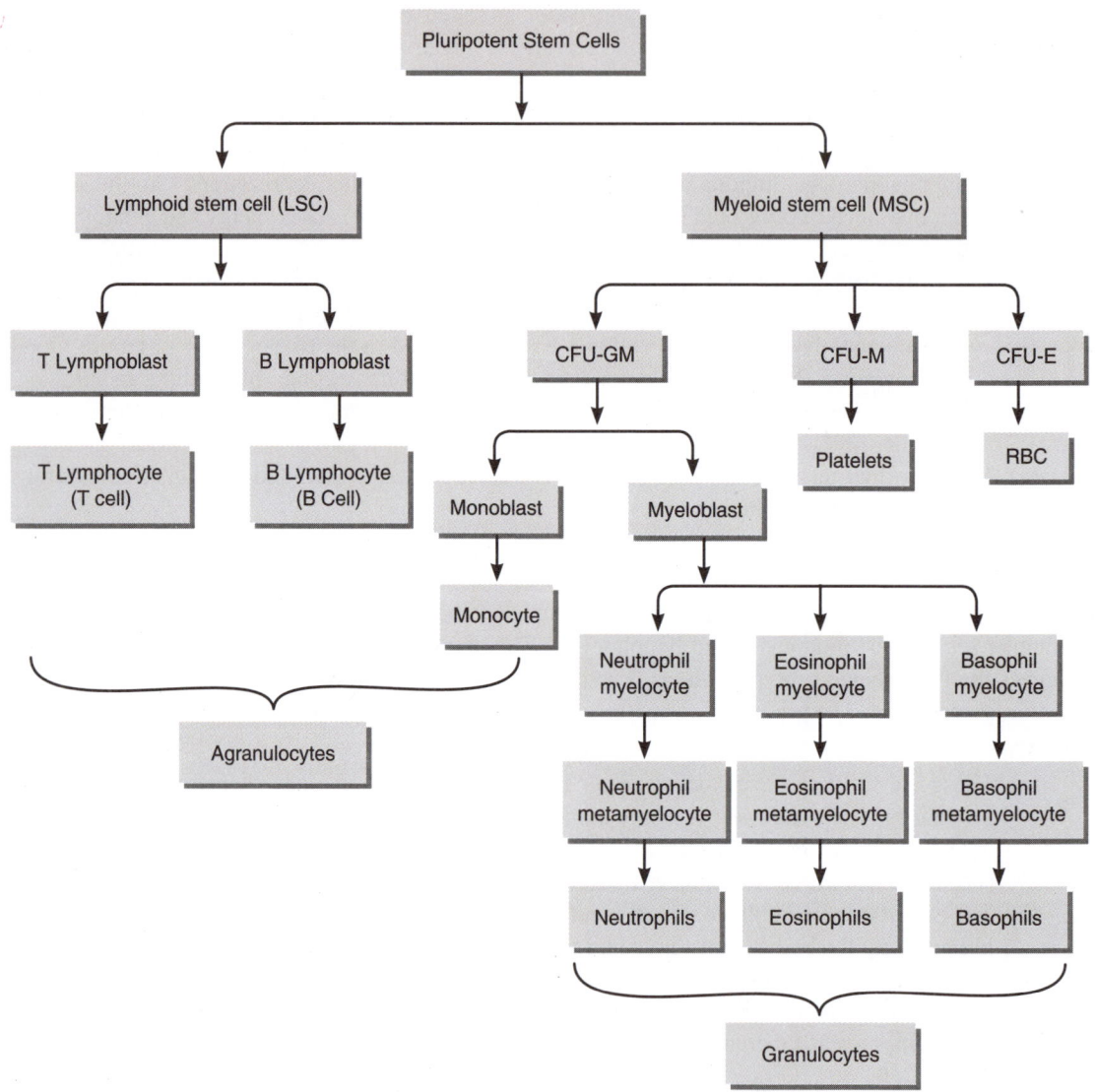

Figure 7.15 Various steps in leukopoiesis.

Platelets or thrombocytes

The platelets are small, nonnucleated formed elements of blood involved in clotting of blood.

Morphology of platelets

1. **Normal size**: They are the smallest blood cells with diameter in the range 2–5 μm.
2. **Normal shape**: The platelets are rounded or oval, disc-shaped formed elements.
3. **Number**: The platelets are fewer than RBCs and more than WBCs in number. The platelet count ranges between 2,00,000/m³ and 4,00,000/m³ of blood. Increase and decrease in the number of platelets is known as *thrombocytosis* and *thrombocytopenia*, respectively.

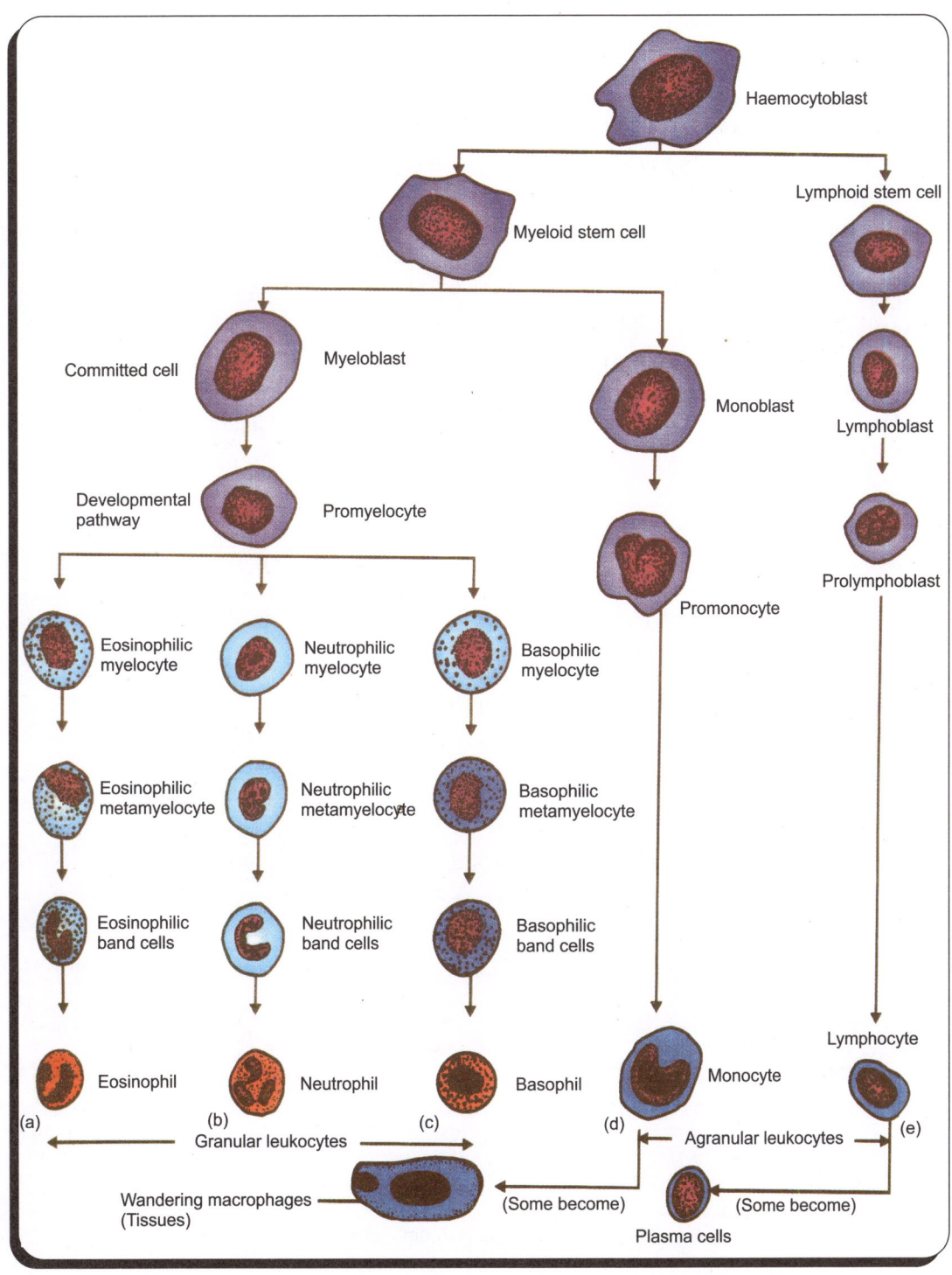

Haemocytoblast

Lymphoid stem cell

Myeloid stem cell

Committed cell   Myeloblast

Monoblast

Lymphoblast

Developmental
pathway   Promyelocyte

Promonocyte

Prolymphoblast

Eosinophilic
myelocyte

Neutrophilic
myelocyte

Basophilic
myelocyte

Eosinophilic
metamyelocyte

Neutrophilic
metamyelocyte

Basophilic
metamyelocyte

Eosinophilic
band cells

Neutrophilic
band cells

Basophilic
band cells

Lymphocyte

Eosinophil

Neutrophil

Basophil

Monocyte

Lymphocyte

(a)   (b)   (c)   (d)   (e)

Granular leukocytes   Agranular leukocytes

Wandering macrophages
(Tissues)

(Some become)   (Some become)

Plasma cells

Figure 7.16 Steps in leukopoiesis.

4. **Structure**: They are bounded by a plasma membrane and contain a few organelles in the cytoplasm. The cytoplasm contains the following chemical substances:
   (a) *Proteins* such as platelet-derived growth factor (PDGF), which repairs damaged blood vessel; platelet-activating factor (PAF), which results in platelet aggregation during injury; and Von Willebrand factor, which is responsible for platelets adherence
   (b) *Enzymes* such as adenosine triphosphatase
   (c) *Hormones* such as serotonin, which causes vasoconstriction
5. **Lifespan and disposal**: Platelets have a short lifespan, normally between 5 and 9 days. They are destroyed by macrophages, mainly in the spleen. About a third of platelets are normally stored within the spleen as an emergency store that can be released to control excessive bleeding.

Properties of platelets

1. **Adhesiveness**: The property of platelets to get activated and adhere to the rough surface (damaged endothelium) of the ruptured blood vessel is termed as *adhesiveness*.
2. **Platelet agglutination**: The clumping together of platelets at the site of injury is called *agglutination* of platelets.

Functions of platelets

1. **Blood clotting**: Platelets prevent blood loss from damaged blood vessels by initiating a chain of reactions that result in the formation of platelet plug and blood clotting.
2. **Prevention of blood loss**: Platelets secrete serotonin, which causes vasoconstriction and prevents blood loss. In addition, platelets adhere to the damaged endothelium and form a temporary plug to prevent blood loss.
3. **Repair of ruptured blood vessel**: Platelet-derived growth factor (PDGF) present in the cytoplasm of platelets is very essential for repair of endothelium.

Thrombopoiesis

The process of formation of platelets is called *thrombopoiesis*. It occurs in red bone marrow.

Steps of thrombopoiesis are as follows (Fig. 7.17):

CFU-M $\longrightarrow$ Megakaryoblasts $\longrightarrow$ Megakaryocyte $\longrightarrow$ Platelets

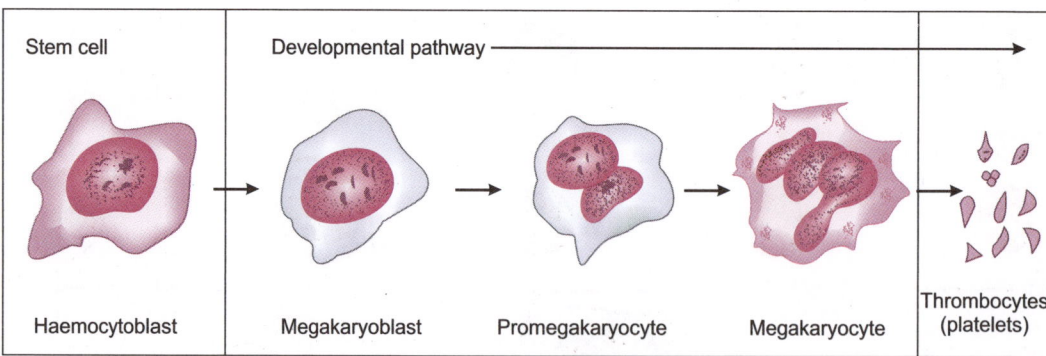

Figure 7.17 Steps in thrombopoiesis.

Thrombopoiesis is regulated mainly by a hormone released by kidneys called *thrombopoietin*, which stimulates platelet synthesis.

Table 7.1 Summary of blood cells

Cell type	Illustration	Description	Function
Red blood cells		Biconcave disk; no nucleus; contains haemoglobin, which colours the cell red; 7–5 µm in diameter	Transports oxygen and carbon dioxide
White blood cells		Spherical cell with a nucleus; white in colour because it lacks haemoglobin	Five types of white blood cells, each with specific functions
Granulocytes Neutrophil		Nucleus with two to four lobes connected by thin filaments; cytoplasmic granules stain light pink or reddish purple; 10–12 µm in diameter	Phagocytizes microorganisms and other substances
Basophil		Nucleus with two indistinct lobes; cytoplasmic granules stain blue-purple; 10–12 µm in diameter	Releases histamine, which promotes inflammation, and heparin, which prevents clot formation
Eosinophil		Nucleus often bilobed; cytoplasmic granules stain orange-red or bright red; 11–14 µm in diameter	Releases chemicals that reduce inflammation; attacks certain worm parasites
Agranulocytes Lymphocyte		Round nucleus; cytoplasm forms a thin ring around the nucleus; 6–14 µm in diameter	Produces antibodies and other chemicals responsible for destroying microorganisms; contributes to allergic reactions; graft rejection, tumour control, and regulation of the immune system
Monocyte		Nucleus round, kidney-shaped, or horseshoe-shaped; contains more cytoplasm than does lymphocyte; 12–20 µm in diameter	Phagocytic cell in the blood; leaves the blood and becomes a macrophage, which phagocytizes bacteria, dead cells, cell fragments, and other debris within tissues
Platelet		Cell fragment surrounded by a plasma membrane and containing granules; 2–4 µm in diameter	Forms platelet plugs; releases chemicals necessary for blood clotting

BLOOD GROUPS

The surface of RBCs contains a genetically determined protein molecule – the ***antigen*** – that determines an individual's blood group. There are around 20 different blood groups but the major ones are ABO blood group and Rh blood group.

ABO BLOOD GROUP

This blood group was discovered by Karl Landsteiner in 1990. He found two antigens or agglutinogens on the surface of RBCs and named them as *A antigen* and *B antigen*. In addition, he noticed the corresponding antibodies and agglutinins in the serum called as *anti-A* and *anti-B*, respectively (Fig. 7.18).

Based on this, he proposed the Landsteiner law, which states the following:

1. If the particular antigen is present on the RBCs, the corresponding antibody must be absent in the serum.
2. If the particular antigen is absent on the RBCs, the corresponding antibody must be present in the serum.

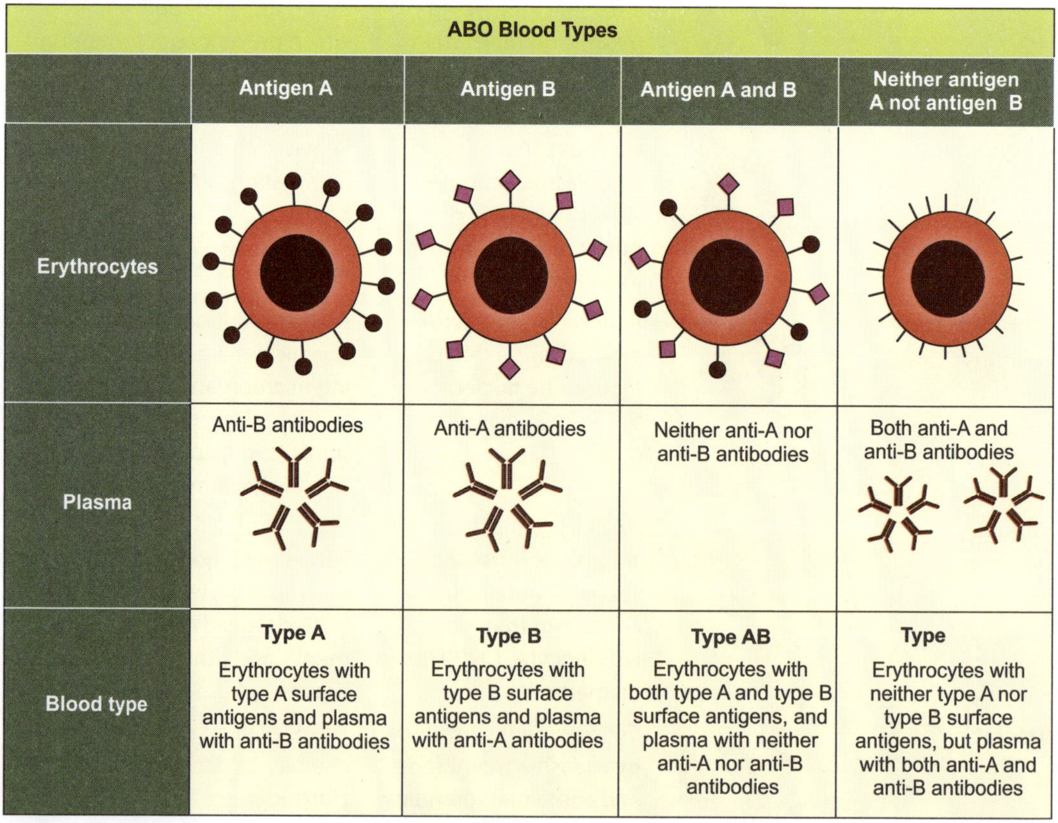

ABO Blood Types			
	Antigen A	Antigen B	Antigen A and B	Neither antigen A not antigen B
Erythrocytes				
Plasma	Anti-B antibodies	Anti-A antibodies	Neither anti-A nor anti-B antibodies	Both anti-A and anti-B antibodies
Blood type	**Type A** Erythrocytes with type A surface antigens and plasma with anti-B antibodies	**Type B** Erythrocytes with type B surface antigens and plasma with anti-A antibodies	**Type AB** Erythrocytes with both type A and type B surface antigens, and plasma with neither anti-A nor anti-B antibodies	**Type** Erythrocytes with neither type A nor type B surface antigens, but plasma with both anti-A and anti-B antibodies

Figure 7.18 Blood groups.

Thus, on the basis of the Landsteiner law, there are four types of blood groups, which are as follows:

1. **Blood group A** (having antigen A on RBC and antibody B in serum)
2. **Blood group B** (having antigen B on RBC and antibody A in serum)
3. **Blood group AB** (having both antigens A and B on RBC but no antibodies in serum)
4. **Blood group O** (having no antigen on RBC but both the antibodies A and B in serum)

Determination of ABO blood group

The process of determination of the ABO blood group is also called *blood matching* or *blood typing*. This process is based on the principle that if the blood groups are mismatched, *agglutination* or clumping of

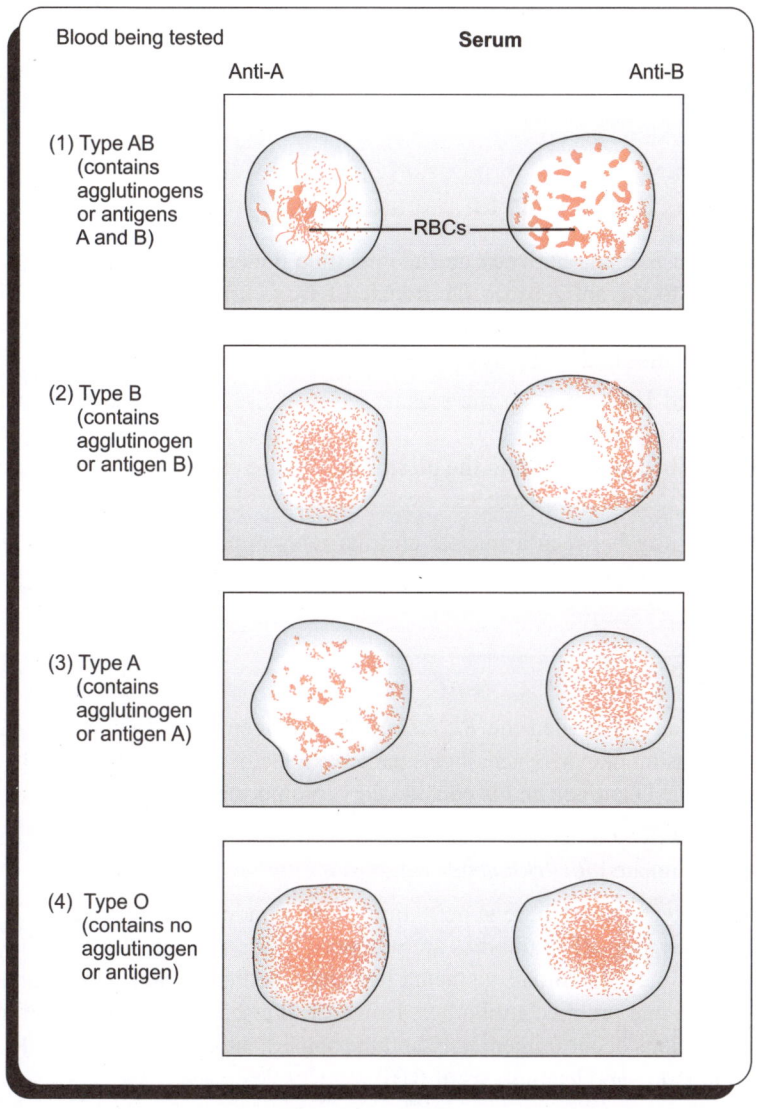

Figure 7.19 Determination of different blood groups.

RBCs will occur. Agglutination is also called *transfusion reaction* and is caused by the reaction between antibodies in the serum and antigens on the RBC surface (Fig. 7.19).

To explain:

1. If the blood sample gets agglutinated by anti-A and not by anti-B: blood group is A.
2. If blood sample gets agglutinated by anti-B and not by anti-A: blood group is B.
3. If blood sample gets agglutinated by both anti-A and anti-B: blood group is AB.
4. If blood sample does not show any reaction with both anti-A and anti-B: blood group is O.

Thus, during blood transfusion, only the compatible blood can be used, and while transfusing the blood, the antigen of the donor and the antibody of the recipient are considered important.

People with AB blood group are called *universal recipients* as they have neither anti-A nor anti-B antibodies in their serum, and thus can receive blood from donors of all four blood types.

Conversely, people with O blood group are called *universal donors* because they have neither A nor B antigens on RBC surface and thus can donate blood to all ABO blood types. However, type O people can receive only O type blood group.

Transfusion reactions due to ABO incompatibility

If the blood transfusion is made between an incompatible donor and recipient, the antibodies in the recipient's serum bind to the antigens on the donated RBCs, which results in agglutination (Ag–Ab reaction) or clumping of RBC. This reaction leads to haemolysis (rupture) of the RBCs and the release of Hb into the plasma. This condition may lead to the following complications:

1. **Jaundice**: Increased Hb content in the plasma leads to rise in bilirubin level, which may cause jaundice.
2. **Kidney damage**: The liberated Hb in the plasma may cause clogging of the filtration membrane of the kidney, leading to kidney damage.

Note: ABO incompatibility between a mother and the fetus rarely cause problems as the antibodies (anti-A and anti-B) are large sized and hence do not cross the placenta.

RH BLOOD GROUP

RBCs possess another antigen called the *Rh factor*. This antigen was discovered by Landsteiner and Weiner in 1940 in rhesus monkeys; hence, it was named Rh factor. There are many Rh antigens, but the most immunogenic is the D antigen and is considered very important.

Individuals having D (Rh) antigen on their RBC are designated *Rh⁺ (Rh positive)* and those lacking D (Rh) antigens are designated *Rh⁻ (Rh negative)*.

Unlike the ABO blood system, there is no natural corresponding antibody (anti-D) present for this D (Rh) antigen. However, anti-Rh antibodies are produced in Rh⁻ individuals when they are exposed to Rh⁺ blood for the first time. The initial mismatch has no immediate serious consequences because the body takes time to react and produce antibodies. However, if a second mismatched transfusion occurs, severe transfusion reactions occur immediately and the anti-Rh antibodies attack the Rh⁺ blood donor's RBC, causing agglutination and haemolysis of RBC.

On the other hand, Rh⁺ individuals can receive Rh⁻ blood without the risk of any complications.

Haemolytic disease of newborns

1. Erythroblastosis fetalis

❑ This is the most common problem with Rh incompatibility that may arise during pregnancy when an Rh⁻ mother carries an Rh⁺ baby. The first pregnancy is usually normal as Rh antigens cannot pass from fetal blood into the mother's blood through the placental barrier. However, at the time of delivery, the Rh antigens from fetal blood leaks into the mother's blood due to severance of the umbilical cord and leads to the formation of Rh antibody in her blood.

❑ When the mother conceives for a second time and the fetus happens to be Rh⁺ again, the Rh antibody from the mother's blood crosses the placental barrier and enters the fetal blood, leading to a condition known as *erythroblastosis fetalis*, which is characterized by agglutination and haemolysis in the fetal blood (Fig. 7.20).

❑ However, nowadays, in such conditions, the Rh⁻ woman can be given drugs called RhoGAM that contain anti-Rh antibodies. These antibodies bind to Rh⁺ fetal cells and shield them, thus preventing agglutination.

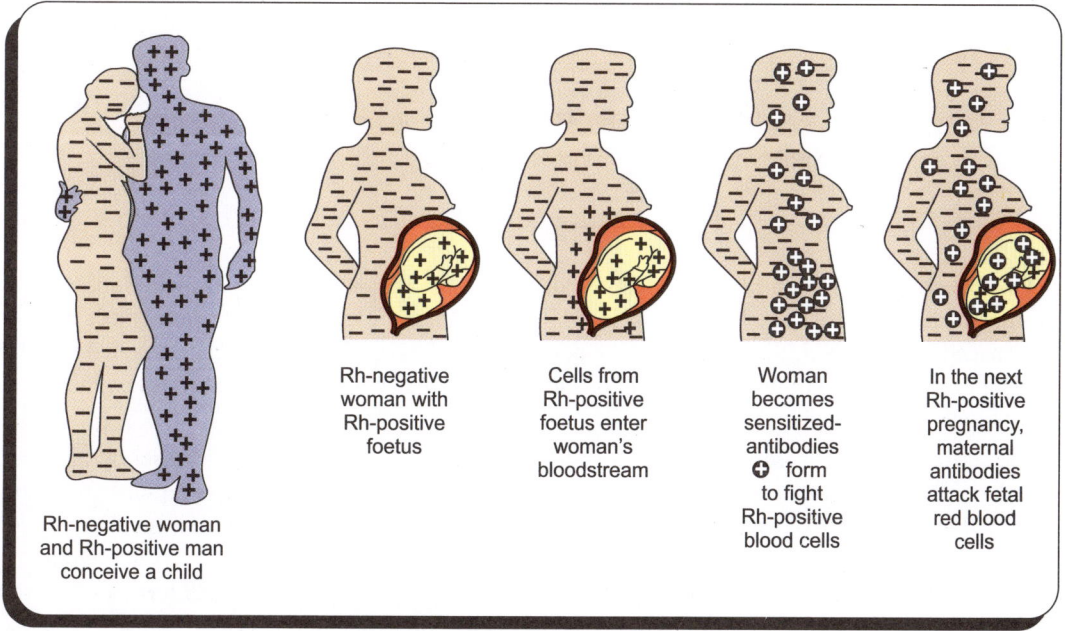

Rh-negative woman and Rh-positive man conceive a child

Rh-negative woman with Rh-positive foetus

Cells from Rh-positive foetus enter woman's bloodstream

Woman becomes sensitized-antibodies ⊕ form to fight Rh-positive blood cells

In the next Rh-positive pregnancy, maternal antibodies attack fetal red blood cells

Figure 7.20 Erythroblastosis fetalis.

2. Kernicterus:
The infant may develop some neurological problems due to agglutination reaction as haemolysis leads to high bilirubin level in the plasma. The bilirubin can enter the brain and may cause permanent brain damage.

Importance of knowing blood groups

1. Medically, it is important for blood transfusion.
2. Legally, it is helpful to sort out parental disputes.
3. Socially, it is important to prevent complications due to ABO and Rh incompatibilities.

BLOOD COAGULATION

When a blood vessel is damaged, a series of reactions are initiated near the injury to prevent the blood loss. These sequence of reactions to prevent blood loss is referred to as *haemostasis* and it includes the following three stages:

1. Vasoconstriction
2. Formation of platelet plug
3. Blood coagulation (Fig. 7.21)

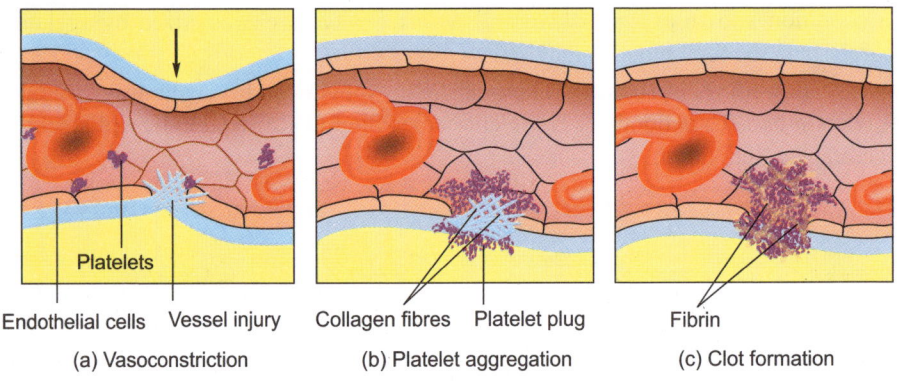

Endothelial cells   Vessel injury   Collagen fibres   Platelet plug   Fibrin

(a) Vasoconstriction   (b) Platelet aggregation   (c) Clot formation

Figure 7.21 Stages of haemostasis.

1. **Vasoconstriction**: When blood vessels are damaged, the smooth muscles in their walls contract immediately to reduce the blood loss. In addition, when the platelets come into contact with the damaged blood vessel, they adhere to the damaged wall and get activated. The activated platelets secrete serotonin and other vasoconstrictor substances, which constrict the blood vessels and reduce the blood flow through it.

2. **Formation of platelet plug**: The platelets first adhere to the damaged blood vessel by a process called *platelet adhesion* and get activated. The activated platelets then secrete some substances such as ADP and thromboxane A$_2$, which attract more platelets to the site. This phase is called *platelet release reaction*. The adherent platelets clump to each other by a process called *platelet aggregation* and, eventually, the accumulation and attachment of large numbers of platelets form a temporary seal called the *platelet plug*, which closes the vessel and prevents blood loss.

3. **Blood coagulation**
   ❏ Coagulation of blood is a complex process that occurs through a series of reactions and results in the formation of an insoluble thread-like mesh of fibrin that traps blood cells and is much stronger than the platelet plug.
   ❏ Coagulation of blood involves several substances called *clotting factors* that are necessary for clot formation. Vitamin K plays a very important role in blood clotting as it is required for the synthesis of some clotting factors.
   ❏ Thirteen clotting factors have been identified, which are listed in Table 7.2.

Table 7.2 Blood clotting factors

I	Fibrinogen
II	Prothrombin
III	Tissue factor (thromboplastin)
IV	Calcium (Ca^{2+})
V	Labile factor, proaccelerin
VII	Stable factor
VIII	Antihaemophilic globulin (AHG)
IX	Plasma thromboplastin component (PTC)
X	Thrombokinase
XI	Plasma thromboplastin antecedent (PTA)
XII	Hageman factor
XIII	Fibrin stabilizing factor

Blood clotting is a complex cascade of enzymatic reactions in which each clotting factor activates many successive reactions one after the other, resulting in the formation of large quantity of fibrin (blood clot).

Blood clotting occurs in the following three stages (Fig. 7.22):

1. Formation of prothrombin activator
2. Conversion of prothrombin into thrombin
3. Conversion of fibrinogen into fibrin

Stage 1: Formation of prothrombin activator

Prothrombin activator can be formed by two pathways that often occur together: the extrinsic and intrinsic pathways. The *extrinsic pathway* occurs rapidly (within seconds) when there is tissue damage outside the circulation. The *intrinsic pathway* is slower (takes 3–6 min) and is triggered by damage to the endothelium.

1. **The extrinsic pathway**: It is named as the extrinsic pathway because a tissue protein called *thromboplastin* released by the damaged tissue cells enters the blood and initiates the cascade of sequences that ultimately activates the clotting factor X. Once factor X is activated, it combines with factor V in the presence of calcium to form the prothrombin activator.

2. **The intrinsic pathway**
   ❑ It is named as intrinsic pathway because its activators are either in direct contact with blood or are present within the blood.
   ❑ The injury in the blood vessel exposes the collagen fibres present around the endothelium of blood vessel, resulting in the activation of clotting factor XII. This initiates a sequence of reactions that eventually activate clotting factor X in the presence of factor IV (calcium) and platelet phospholipids. Once factor X is activated, it combines with factor V and calcium to form prothrombin activator.

Stage 2: Conversion of prothrombin into thrombin

Prothrombin activator acts on the plasma protein prothrombin and converts it into thrombin in the presence of calcium (Ca^{2+}). Thrombin itself accelerates this reaction by the positive feedback mechanism, that is it accelerates the formation of prothrombin activator by activating factor V. This, in turn, accelerates the production of more thrombin and so on.

Stage 3: Conversion of fibrinogen into fibrin

Thrombin acts on another plasma protein, fibrinogen, in the presence of calcium (Ca^{2+}) and converts it into fibrin (insoluble loose threads). This is modified later into dense tight and strengthened fibrin threads by fibrin stabilizing factor (factor XIII) in the presence of calcium (Ca^{2+}) (Fig. 7.23).

Clot retraction

After some time of clot formation, the blood clot starts shrinking. Clot retraction is the tightening of the fibrin clot in such a way that the ruptured area of the blood vessel that is attached to the fibrin threads gradually contracts and pulls the edges of the damaged vessel closer, thus decreasing the risk of further damage.

In this process, the serum (yellowish fluid) oozes out of the clot, which is blood plasma without the clotting factors.

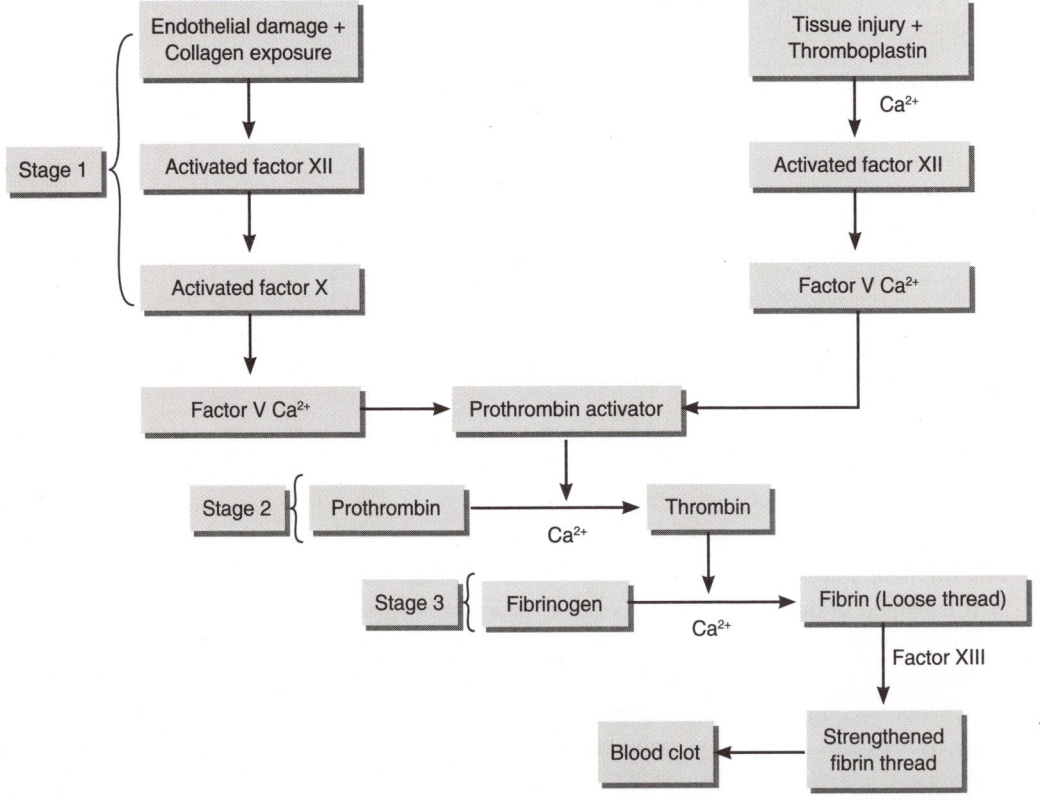

Figure 7.22 Stages of blood clotting.

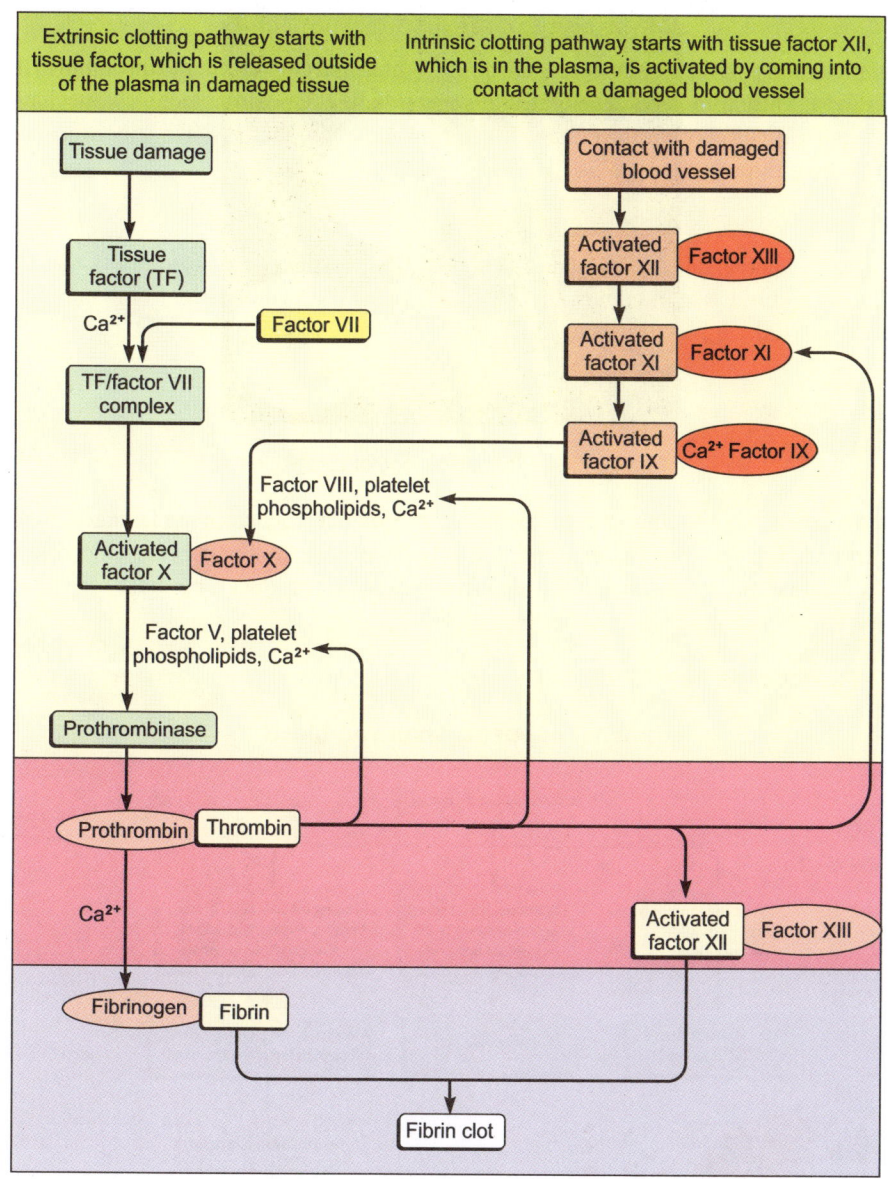

Figure 7.23 The blood-clotting cascade.

Fibrinolysis

After the clot has formed, blood vessels repair themselves by mitotic cellular division. Once the endothelial tissue is repaired, fibrinolysis or dissolution of blood clot occurs. This process is caused by an inactive substance called *plasminogen* present in the clot, which gets converted to the enzyme plasmin by tissue plasminogen activator (TPA) released from the damaged blood vessel (Fig. 7.24).

Plasmin initiates the fibrin breakdown to soluble products that are considered as waste materials and removed by phagocytosis. As the clot is removed, the integrity of blood vessel is restored.

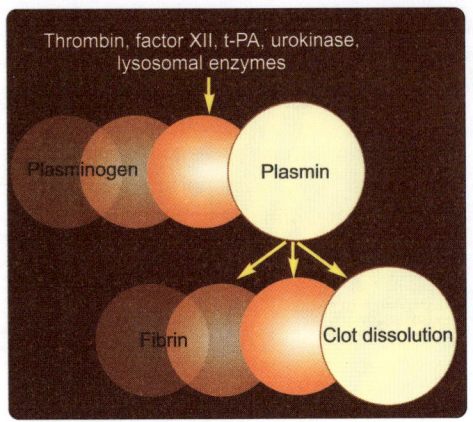

Figure 7.24 Fibrinolysis or clot dissolution.

Sometimes, unwanted clotting due to high cholesterol may occur in undamaged blood vessels. There are certain substances present in blood that may delay, suppress or prevent blood clotting. These substances are called *anticoagulants* and they include heparin (produced by mast cells) and activated protein C (APC).

Summarizing blood coagulation (Fig. 7.25)

What happens when you bleed

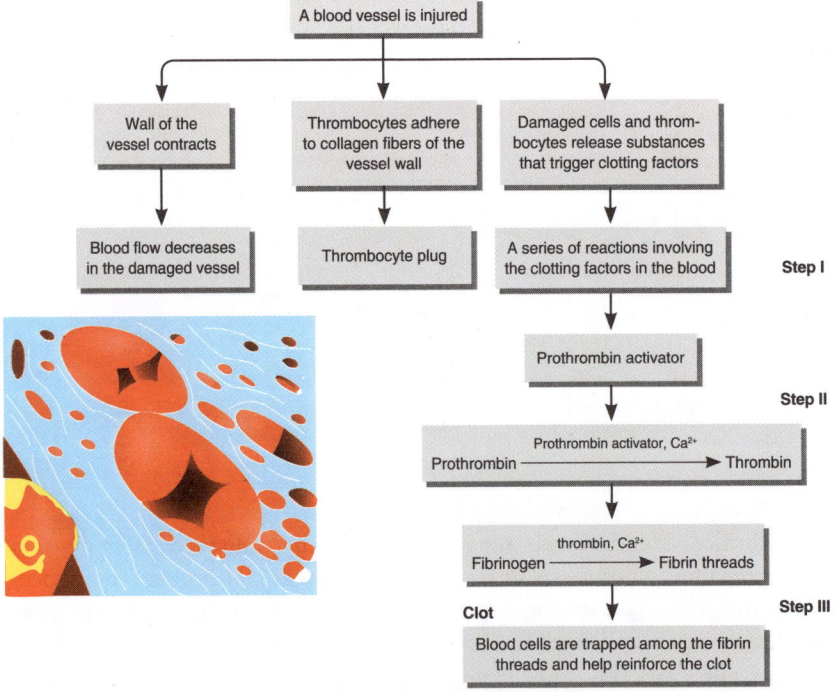

Figure 7.25 Mechanism of blood coagulation.

DISORDERS ASSOCIATED WITH BLOOD

ANAEMIA

It is the most common disorder of the blood characterized by decreased oxygen-carrying capacity of blood. In anaemia, the RBC count or Hb is less than normal. For men, anaemia is typically defined as Hb level of less than 13.5 g/100 mL, and in women as Hb level of less than 12.0 g/100 mL.

Causes: A decrease in production of RBC or Hb, or a loss or destruction of blood.

Symptoms: Patients with anaemia may feel tired, fatigue easily, appear pale, develop palpitations (feeling of heart racing) and breathlessness on exertion.

The following are the types of anaemia:

1. **Iron deficiency anaemia**: This is the most common form of anaemia caused by the inadequate absorption of iron, excessive loss of iron (menstrual blood loss), increased iron requirement (pregnancy) or insufficient intake of iron.
2. **Megaloblastic anaemia**: It is characterized by the production of abnormally large erythrocytes (megaloblasts) in red bone marrow due to the deficiency of vitamin B_{12} or folic acid.
3. **Pernicious anaemia**: This is the most common form of vitamin B_{12} deficiency anaemia that occurs due to lack of intrinsic factor (IF), which is required for the absorption of vitamin B_{12} in the gastric mucosa.
4. **Aplastic anaemia**: The destruction of red bone marrow results in aplastic anaemia due to which the enzymes required for haemopoiesis are inhibited.
5. **Thalassaemia**: It is a condition characterized by the reduced production of Hb and increased friability of the cell membrane, leading to early haemolysis and deficiency of Hb.
6. **Haemolytic anaemia**: It is an inherited condition in which RBCs are destroyed at a faster rate than normal.

SICKLE CELL ANAEMIA

It is an autosomal recessive genetic blood disorder in which RBCs become long, stiff, rod-like structures or sickle shaped. (RBCs are normally shaped like a disc).

Causes: It is caused by an abnormal type of Hb called Hb S. Hb S distorts the shape of RBCs, especially when exposed to low oxygen levels. The distorted RBCs are fragile and shaped like crescents or sickles.

Symptoms: Joint or bone pain, breathlessness, delayed growth and puberty, fatigue, fever, paleness, rapid heart rate, ulcers on the lower legs (in adolescents and adults) and yellowing of the eyes and skin (jaundice).

Treatment: It can be treated by supplements of folic acid (essential for producing RBCs). Blood transfusions are used to treat a sickle cell crisis.

HAEMOPHILIA

It is an inherited clotting disorder characterized by repeated episodes of severe and prolonged bleeding. It is associated with the expression of a recessive gene on the X chromosome inherited from the mother and passed down to male children.

Chapter 7

Symptoms: Haemorrhage after minor injury, frequent nosebleeds, haematomas in muscles and bloody urine.

LEUKAEMIA

It is a type of cancer in which there is abnormal production of WBCs. Owing to the very high rate of WBC production, these cells lack immunologic capabilities, thus making the individual highly prone to opportunistic infections.

THROMBOSIS

Thrombosis can be defined as the clotting in an unbroken blood vessel. It may be due to the roughened endothelial surface of a blood vessel due to atherosclerosis, trauma or infection. The clot formed is known as thrombus, which may dissolve spontaneously. But if it remains intact, it can be swept away by blood.

OVERVIEW OF THE BLOOD COMPONENTS AND THEIR ROLES

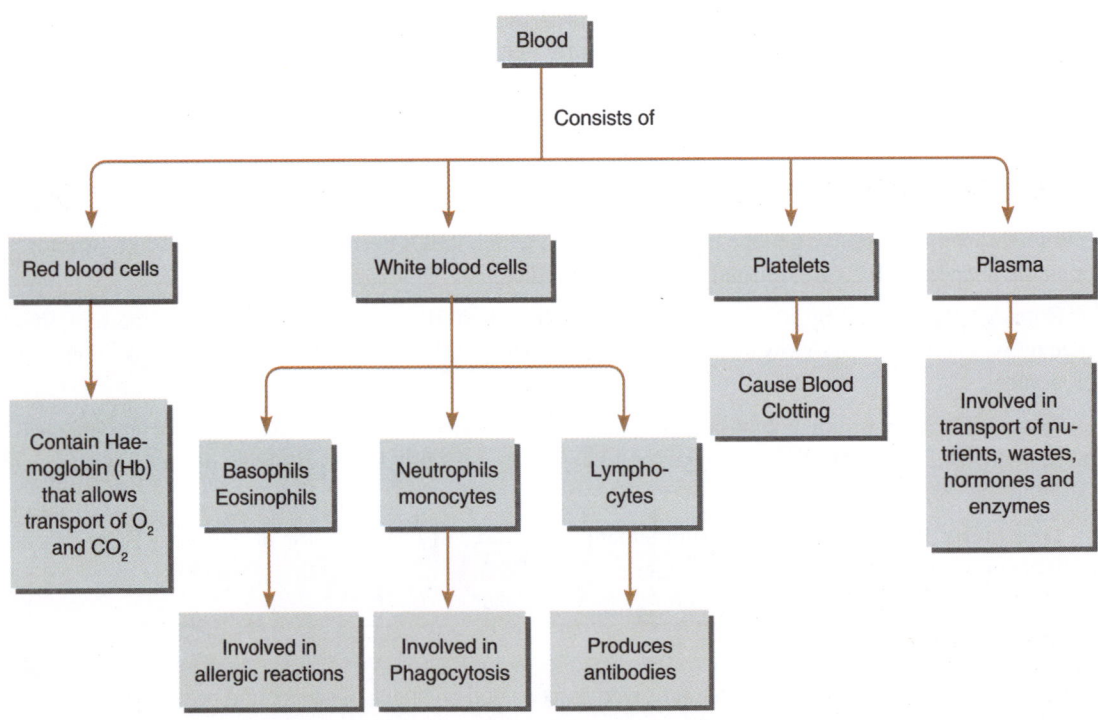

Effect of Smoking on Blood

❑ Cigarette smoke contains large amount of carbon monoxide that enters body and stays for about 6–7 h in the blood. Research suggests that these abnormally high carbon monoxide levels may play a major role in triggering heart attacks.

❑ Carbon monoxide combines with haemoglobin in blood and forms carboxyhaemoglobin, which is no longer able to transport oxygen. This means that less oxygen reaches the smoker's brain and other vital organs and results in memory loss.

❑ In addition, smoking makes the blood clot more easily and increases the chances of heart attacks and stroke.

TIPS TO MAINTAIN BLOOD CIRCULATION

1. Eat a diet high in iron to maintain healthy red blood cells.
2. Try not to eat foods with high cholesterol level as the cholesterol can lead to the formation of clots in the blood vessels. These clots lead to arterial plaque formation and block the blood flow.
3. Decrease caffeine consumption.
4. Exercise daily if possible. Regular exercise increases plasma blood volume and reduces the risk of blood clotting. Individuals who exercise regularly are at low risk of heart attacks.
5. Quit smoking as it increases fibrinogen levels in blood, increasing the possibility of unwanted clotting.

Review Questions

Long Answer Questions

1. What are the principal functions of blood?
2. Describe the composition of blood.
3. Outline the process of erythropoiesis and enlist the various factors that regulate erythropoiesis.
4. List the chemicals, or factors, involved in the clotting process.
5. Describe the two pathways that initiate clotting.
6. List the major components of blood plasma.
7. Why must blood groups be matched during blood transfusion?
8. Describe *erythrocytes* (red blood cells) in terms of origin, structure and function.
9. Discuss the fate of erythrocytes.
10. Discuss the various types of blood cells and their functions.

Multiple Choice Questions

1. Granules are not visible in
   - (a) Neutrophils
   - (b) Lymphocytes
   - (c) Eosinophils
   - (d) Basophils

2. Which of the following four components of the blood are necessary for clotting?
   - (a) Calcium, vitamin K, albumin, globulin
   - (b) Calcium, heparin, prothrombin, fibrinogen
   - (c) Calcium, prothrombin, fibrinogen, platelets
   - (d) Calcium, prothrombin, platelets, vitamin A

3. The chief function of the serum albumin in the blood is to
   - (a) Produce antibodies
   - (b) Form fibrinogen
   - (c) Maintain colloidal osmotic pressure
   - (d) Remove waste products

4. Which concentration would be an indication of anaemia?
   - (a) Thrombocytes – 300,000/mm^3
   - (b) Haematocrit – 43%
   - (c) Haemoglobin – 17 g/dL
   - (d) Erythrocytes – 3.8 million/mm^3

5. For blood clotting to occur normally,
   - (a) Heparin must be inactive
   - (b) There must be a sufficient dietary intake of vitamin C
   - (c) Tissue damage outside the vessel must occur
   - (d) The liver must have an adequate supply of vitamin K

6. Which of the following does *not* stimulate erythropoietin production?
   - (a) Haemorrhage
   - (b) Chronic emphysema
   - (c) Stress-induced release of epinephrine into the system
   - (d) Decreased oxygen delivery to the tissues

7. Insufficient vitamin B$_{12}$ in the body may result in
   - (a) Haemolytic anaemia
   - (b) Pernicious anaemia
   - (c) Aplastic anaemia
   - (d) An embolus

8. The percent volume of whole blood occupied by packed RBCs is referred to as
   - (a) The haematocrit
   - (b) The formed elements
   - (c) The Erythrocytic fraction
   - (d) the sedimentation index

9. Production of RBCs in a mature adult occurs in all of the following areas *except*

   (a) The sternum   (b) The ribs

   (c) The skull bones   (d) The vertebrae

   (e) The os coxae

10. Plasma proteins constitute what percentage of the blood plasma volume?

    (a) 17–19%   (b) 7–9%

    (c) 25–27%   (d) 52–55%

11. The general term for reactions that prevent or minimize loss of blood from the vessels if they are injured or ruptured is

    (a) Stabilization energy

    (b) Homeostasis

    (c) Syneresis

    (d) Haemostasis

12. Haemostasis does *not* involve

    (a) Contraction of smooth muscles in blood vessel walls

    (b) Adherence of platelets to damaged tissue

    (c) Clot retraction

    (d) Increased renin–angiotensin activity

13. What is the correct order of these events?

    1. Conversion of fibrinogen to fibrin

    2. Clot retraction and leakage of serum

    3. Thromboplastin production

    4. Conversion of prothrombin to thrombin

    (a) 3, 2, 1, 4   (b) 3, 4, 1, 2

    (c) 3, 4, 2, 1   (d) 4, 1, 3, 2

14. Blood minus the formed elements and clotting proteins is called

    (a) Plasma   (b) Serum

    (c) Albumin   (d) Globulin

State True or False

1. Blood functions in transport, pH balance, thermoregulation and immunity mechanisms.
2. Polycythaemia is an unusually high haematocrit.
3. The major mechanisms of haemostasis are plugging, clotting and constriction.
4. Thromboplastin is released when vascular walls or other tissue is damaged.
5. Calcium and phospholipids are required for the conversion of prothrombin to thrombin.

Fill in the Blanks

1. An excessive number of RBCs is referred to as _____.

2. _____ is the manufacture of RBCs.

3. Hb, when saturated with oxygen, is cherry red in colour and is called _____.

4. Thrombocytes are formed from giant cells called _____.

5. The _____ is activated when blood is exposed to a foreign surface.

6. In _____, the concentration of thrombocytes is too low.

7. _____ refers to the ability of leukocytes to squeeze through capillary walls.

Careers Associated with Blood

✓ Haematologists specialize in the field of blood and blood-forming tissues, and normally work in laboratory of the medical centre.

✓ Blood bank technologists are allied health professionals responsible for the blood typing of blood donors and expectant mothers to detect the presence of ABO and Rh antigens. These individuals are involved in blood transfusions and investigation of the blood abnormalities.

The Lymphatic System

STUDY OBJECTIVES

✓ To explain the components and major functions of the lymphatic system.

✓ To describe the organization of lymph vessels.

✓ To discuss the formation and flow of lymph.

✓ To describe the lymph nodes and various organs of the lymphatic system.

INTRODUCTION

The lymphatic system is closely related to the cardiovascular system as both the cardiovascular system and the lymphatic system comprise a network of vessels that transport body fluids throughout the body.

The lymphatic system is a closed system of lymph vessels that transports the lymph and helps defend the body against disease-causing agents.

The study of the lymphatic system is called *lymphatology*.

The lymphatic system consists of a fluid called *lymph*, vessels that transport the lymph called *lymphatic vessels* and lymphatic tissue that includes lymph nodes and nodules and lymph organs (e.g. the spleen and thymus gland) (Fig. 8.1).

FUNCTIONS OF THE LYMPHATIC SYSTEM

1. **Drainage of excess interstitial fluid**: Lymphatic vessels maintain the fluid balance in the body by draining the excess interstitial fluid from tissue spaces and returning the fluid to the blood. The lymphatic vessels serve an important role of returning the lost plasma to the blood without which the body would die within about 24 h.

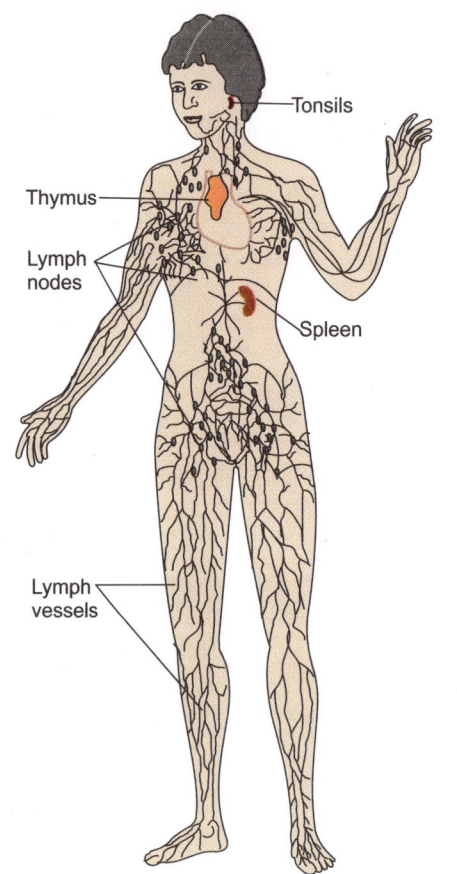

- Tonsils
- Thymus
- Lymph nodes
- Spleen
- Lymph vessels

Figure 8.1 Overview of the lymphatic system.

2. **Transport of dietary fats**: The lymphatic vessels transport fats and fat-soluble vitamins (vitamin A, D, E and K) from the gastrointestinal tract to the blood.

3. **Immunity**: The organs of the lymphatic system are involved in the production and maturation of lymphocytes (white blood cells), which help defend the body against microorganisms, foreign substances and abnormal (tumour) cells.

LYMPH

- ❏ Lymph is a fluid connective tissue consisting of plasma and blood corpuscles.
- ❏ Lymph is a clear or slightly opalescent, colourless alkaline fluid as it lacks haemoglobin containing erythrocytes. It contains proteins and fats and white blood corpuscles, especially lymphocytes, fibrinogen, nutrients, hormones, excretory materials and some blood proteins. Red blood corpuscles are absent in lymph.
- ❏ Lymphatic fluid in the intestine (called *chyle*) is milky white in colour as it contains fat.

MEDICAL TERMINOLOGY

- ❏ **Interstitial fluid**: Fluid bathing the intercellular spaces between cells and through which material is exchanged between the blood and the cells.
- ❏ **Lymphatic tissue**: Connective tissue containing lymphocytes.
- ❏ **Osmotic Pressure**: The pressure exerted by the flow of water through a semipermeable membrane separating two solutions with different concentrations.

COMPOSITION OF LYMPH

Lymph consists of 91% water and 9% solid substances. The solid substances present in the lymph have been summarized in the Table 8.1.

Table 8.1 Composition of lymph

Proteins	2–6%	Albumin, globulin, prothrombin, clotting factors, fibrinogen, antibodies and enzymes
Lipids	5–15%	In the form of chylomicrons and lipoproteins
Carbohydrates	120 mg%	Glucose
Amino acids		All amino acids of plasma
Non-protein nitrogenous	34 mg%	Urea, creatinine
Electrolytes		K, Na, Ca, Cl and bicarbonates
Cellular contents		Macrophages, monocytes, lymphocytes

FORMATION OF LYMPH

The blood pressure in the capillaries network forces some of the plasma to move out of the capillaries into the spaces between the tissue cells. When this plasma enters the space between tissue cells, it gets another name and is called *interstitial fluid*. Most of this fluid gets reabsorbed into the capillary due

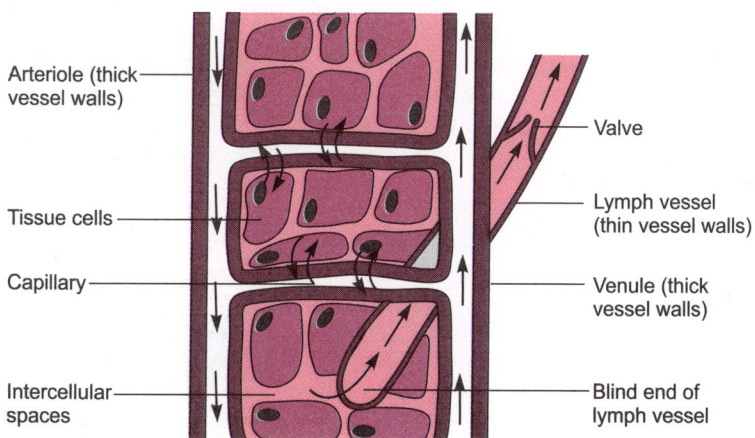

Arteriole (thick vessel walls)

Valve

Tissue cells

Lymph vessel (thin vessel walls)

Capillary

Venule (thick vessel walls)

Intercellular spaces

Blind end of lymph vessel

Figure 8.2 Schematic diagram showing lymph formation.

to the difference in osmotic pressure. However, some of the interstitial fluid left in the tissue spaces must be drained to prevent the tissues from swelling or oedema. The lymphatic capillaries drain this interstitial fluid into the lymph capillaries and after which this fluid is called *lymph* (Fig. 8.2).

Some of the proteins that leave blood plasma cannot return to blood by diffusion because of the concentration gradient (there are more proteins inside blood capillaries compared to the lesser level outside). The proteins can, however, move readily through the more permeable lymphatic capillaries into lymph.

In the small intestine, there are special lymphatic vessels called *lacteals* that absorb fats and then transport fats from the gastrointestinal tract to the blood. The presence of these fats gives the lymph a creamy-white appearance and such lymph is referred to as *chyle.*

LYMPHATIC VESSELS AND LYMPH CIRCULATION

LYMPH CAPILLARIES

Lymphatic vessels begin as lymph capillaries in the spaces between cells in most of the body parts except in the central nervous system, bones and most superficial layers of the skin.

These lymph capillaries are tiny, closed-ended tubes and occur singly or in the extensive plexuses. They have the same structure as the capillaries, that is, a single layer of endothelial cells but have thinner walls, which make them more permeable than blood capillaries. The lymph capillaries are interwoven with the blood capillaries and are much larger and also have a large number of valves, which ensure the unidirectional flow of lymph (Fig. 8.3a).

The endothelial cells of lymph capillaries are attached to the surrounding tissues by an *anchoring filament* made of elastic fibres. The ends of these endothelial cells overlap, resulting in a unique one-way structure that permits the interstitial fluid to flow into endothelial cells but not out (Fig. 8.3b).

LYMPHATIC VESSELS

Similar to blood capillaries converging to form venules and then veins, the lymphatic capillaries join to form larger lymphatic vessels called *lymphatics*.

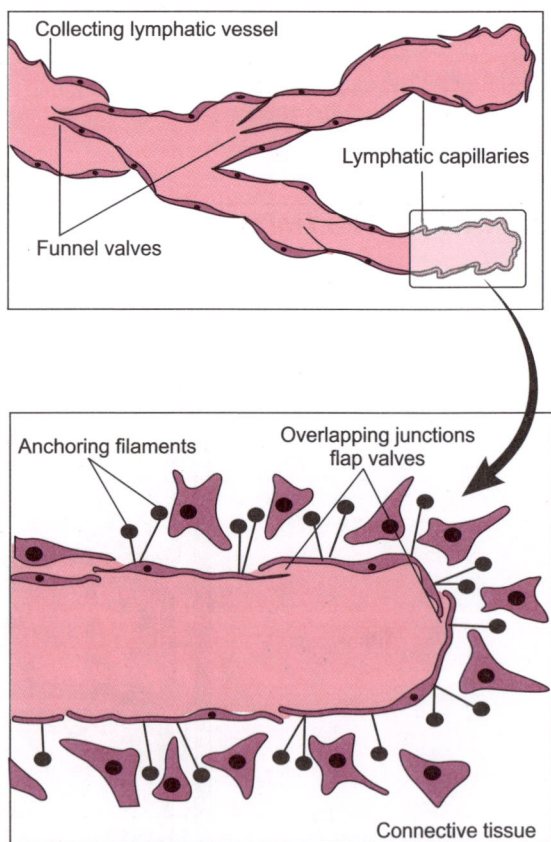

Figure 8.3 (a) Lymph capillaries; (b) Lymph valves.

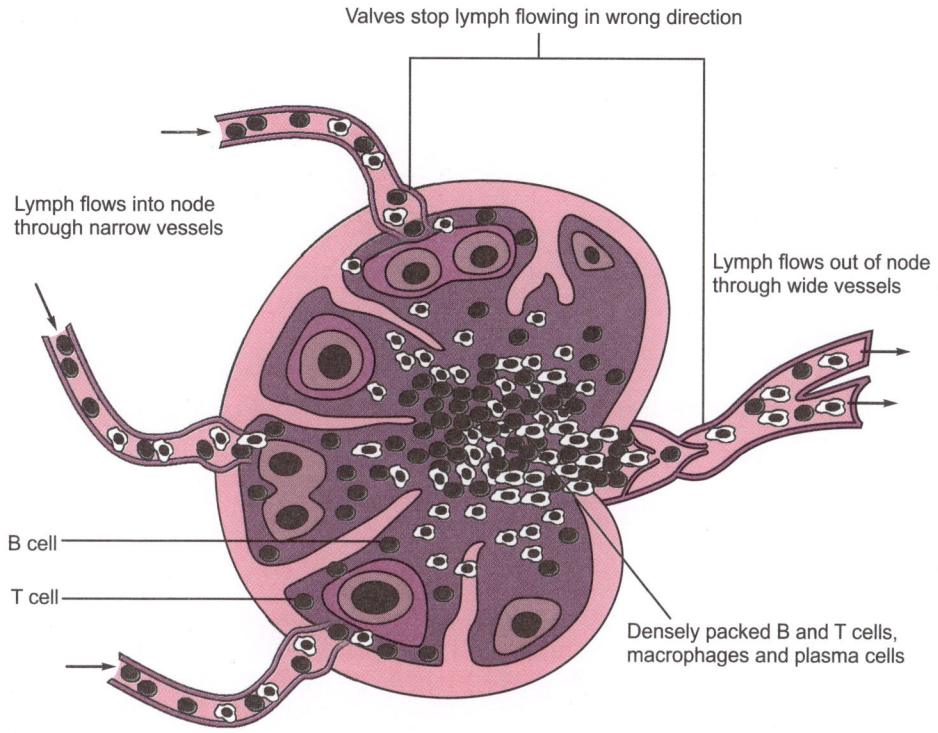

Figure 8.4 Lymph flow through lymph nodes.

The lymphatic vessels resemble veins in structure but have thinner walls and more numerous valves to prevent backflow. At intervals along the length of lymphatic vessels, lymph flows through *lymph nodes*, which are specialized lymphatic tissues consisting of masses of B cells and T cells (Fig. 8.4).

LYMPHATIC TRUNK

As lymphatic vessels leave the lymph node, they unite to form *lymphatic trunks* (Fig. 8.5).

The principal lymphatic trunks of the body are as follows:

1. **Lumbar trunk**: It drains lymph from the lower limbs, viscera of pelvis, kidney, adrenal glands and the abdominal wall.
2. **Intestinal trunk**: It drains lymph from the stomach, intestine, pancreas, spleen and parts of the liver.
3. **Bronchomediastinal trunk**: It drains lymph from the thorax, lungs and heart.
4. **Subclavian trunk**: It drains lymph from the upper limbs.
5. **Jugular trunk**: It drains lymph from the head and neck.
6. **Intercostal trunk**: It drains lymph from portions of the thorax.

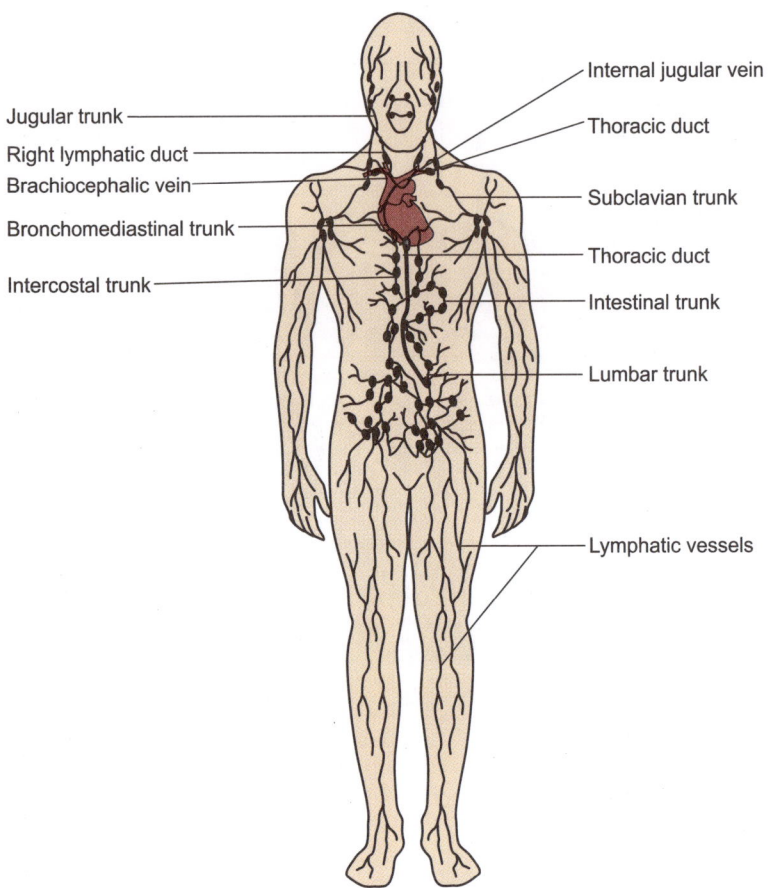

Jugular trunk

Right lymphatic duct

Brachiocephalic vein

Bronchomediastinal trunk

Intercostal trunk

Internal jugular vein

Thoracic duct

Subclavian trunk

Thoracic duct

Intestinal trunk

Lumbar trunk

Lymphatic vessels

Figure 8.5 Lymphatic trunks.

LYMPHATIC DUCTS

The principal lymphatic trunks then pass their lymph into two main ducts: the *thoracic duct* (also known as the *left lymphatic duct*) and the *right lymphatic duct*.

The thoracic duct is about 40 cm long and begins as a dilation called *cistern chyli* anterior to the second lumbar vertebra. The thoracic duct receives lymph from all parts of the body inferior to the ribs and on the left side of the body (left upper limbs and left side of the head, neck and chest) and empties into the left subclavian vein.

The lymphatic vessels of the intestine (lacteals) appear milky white and empty chyle (absorbed fats) into the thoracic duct.

The right lymphatic duct is about 1 cm long and receives lymph from the upper right side of the body (right head and neck, right area of the thorax) and empties the lymph into the right subclavian veins (Fig. 8.6).

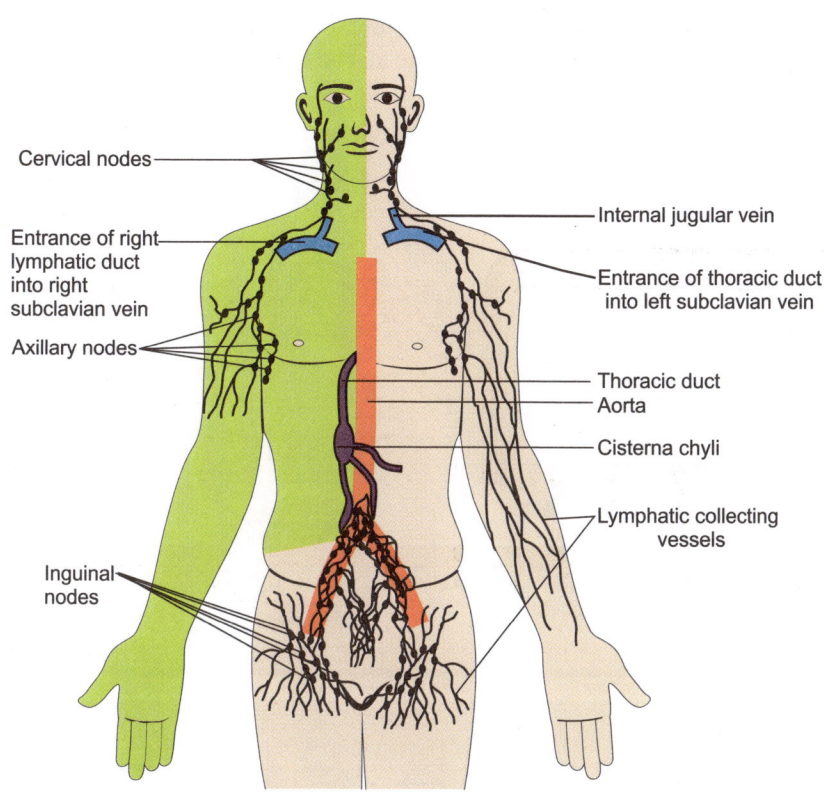

Figure 8.6 Lymphatic ducts.

The lymph circulation can be summarized by the following flowchart:

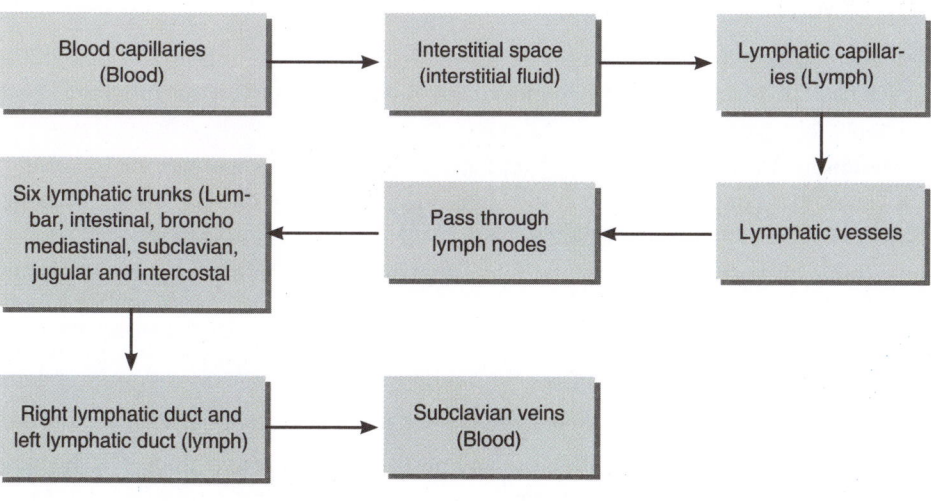

The lymph is formed from the blood plasma that diffuses out of the blood capillaries; after circulation, the lymph is eventually drained back to the blood stream and the cycle repeats itself. This circulation is continuously repeated and serves an important role to maintain the proper levels of lymph, plasma and the interstitial fluid in the body (Fig. 8.7).

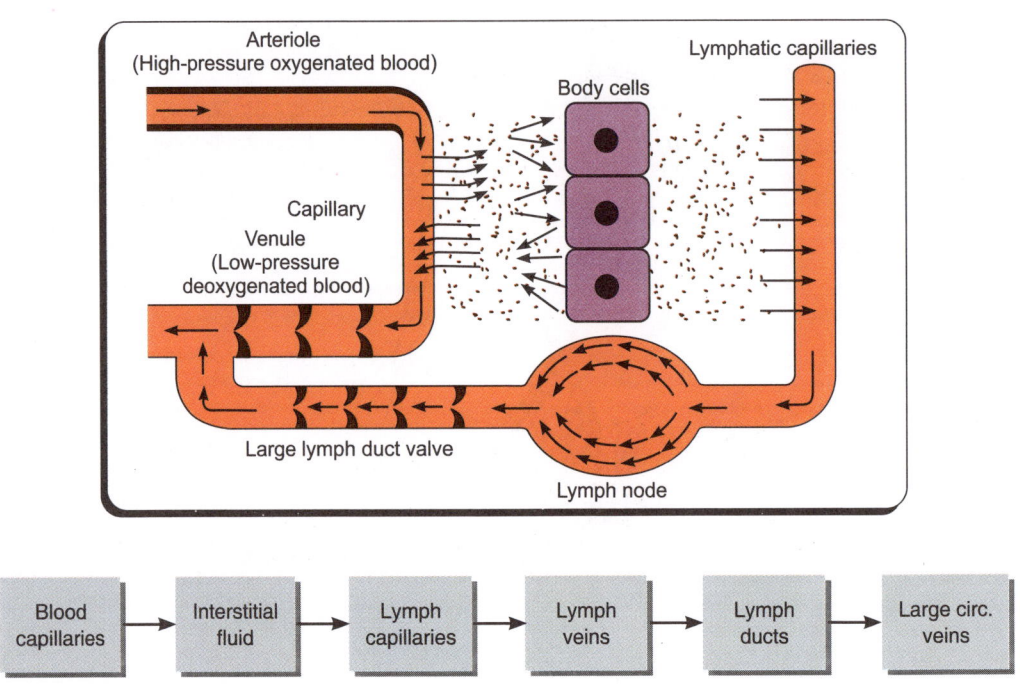

Figure 8.7 Schematic diagram depicting lymph circulation.

FLOW OF LYMPH

The lymph flows in lymphatic vessels very slowly, at the rate of 1–1.5 mL/min. Although there is no pump like the heart involved in the onward movement of lymph, the circulation of lymph is maintained by the following factors:

1. **Contraction of skeletal muscles**: Skeletal muscle contraction compresses the lymphatic vessels, which pushes the lymph in only one direction, that is, towards the subclavian veins due to the presence of valves that prevent backflow.

2. **Respiration or breathing movements**: Inhalation and exhalation causes pressure changes in the thorax, facilitating lymph movement.

3. **Contraction of smooth muscles in lymphatic vessels**: The contraction of smooth muscles pushes the lymph forward.

4. **Gravity**: It helps in moving the lymph down the lymphatic vessels of the head and the neck.

If the lymphatic vessels get blocked due to any obstruction, excessive amount of interstitial fluid develops in the tissue spaces, which might cause oedema or swelling.

LYMPH NODES

Lymph nodes are 1–25 mm long, oval- to bean-shaped structures found along the length of lymphatic vessels. They are also known as *lymph glands* or *lymphatic nodes*. They are scattered throughout the body, whereas large groups of lymph nodes are aggregated in the groin, armpits and neck (Fig. 8.8).

STRUCTURE OF THE LYMPH NODE

Each lymph node comprises of masses of lymphatic tissue covered by a capsule of fibrous connective tissue. The capsular extensions, called *trabeculae*, divide the lymph node internally into various compartments.

Lymph enters the lymph node through four or five afferent lymphatic vessels, whereas only one efferent vessel carries lymph away from the node. Each node has a slight depression on one side, called the *hilum*, where an artery enters and a vein and the efferent lymphatic vessel leaves.

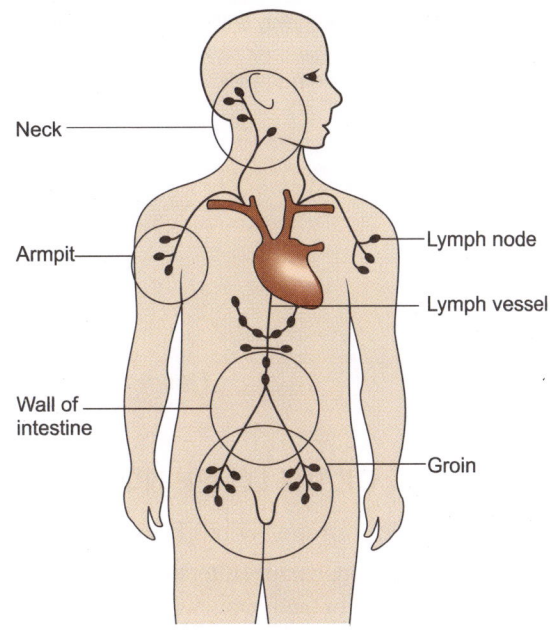

Figure 8.8 Location of aggregated lymph nodes.

The parenchyma (functional part) of the lymph node is divided into three regions: the cortex, paracortex and medulla (Fig. 8.9).

1. **Cortex**
   (a) The cortex of the lymph node consists of primary and secondary lymphatic nodules (follicles) that contain aggregates of B lymphocytes and macrophages.
   (b) The primary lymphatic nodule develops first and when some antigens enter the body and reach the lymph node, the B cells recognize them and begins to proliferate. The active proliferation of the cells occurs in a particular area of the nodule called the *germinal centre*. After the proliferation of cells, the primary nodule develops into the secondary lymphatic nodule.

2. **Paracortex (or inner cortex)**
   (a) The paracortex is present between the cortex and the medulla and does not contain lymphatic nodule.
   (b) It mainly consists of T lymphocytes.

3. **Medulla**: The medulla contains B lymphocytes, T lymphocytes and macrophages.

The lymph enters the lymph node through four or five afferent lymphatic vessels and flows in only one direction as it circulates through the cortex, paracortex and medulla. From the medulla, lymph leaves the node through one efferent lymphatic vessel. Thus, the lymph node serves as a tank where lymph stagnates for some time due to fewer outgoing and more incoming lymphatic vessels. This stagnancy gives enough time for the proliferation of lymphocytes and macrophages. The macrophages destroy some foreign substances by phagocytosis, whereas lymphocytes destroy by immune responses.

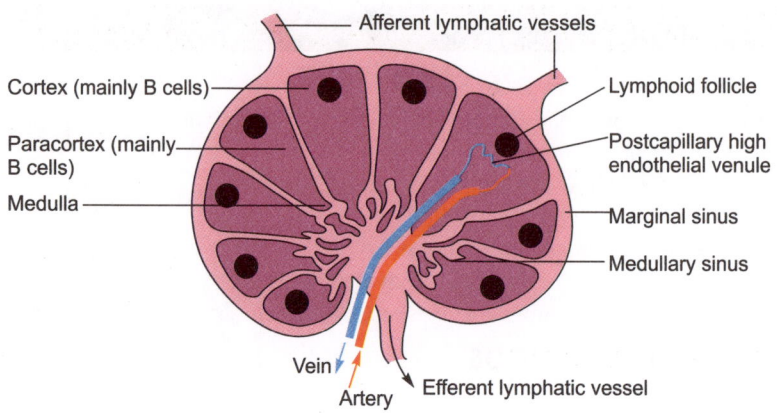

Figure 8.9 Structure of the lymph node.

FUNCTIONS OF THE LYMPH NODES

The lymph nodes perform various functions, which include the following:

1. **Filtration:** Lymph nodes filter the lymph before it is returned to the circulatory system. Macrophages and antibodies in the lymph node destroy the microbes, worn out or damaged tissue cells and cells from malignant tumours (Fig. 8.10). Thus, when the lymph enters blood after passing through successive lymph nodes, it is usually cleared of the foreign matter and cell debris.

2. **Phagocytosis**: The macrophages of the lymph nodes destroy and engulf the microorganisms, cellular debris and other toxic substances present in the lymph.

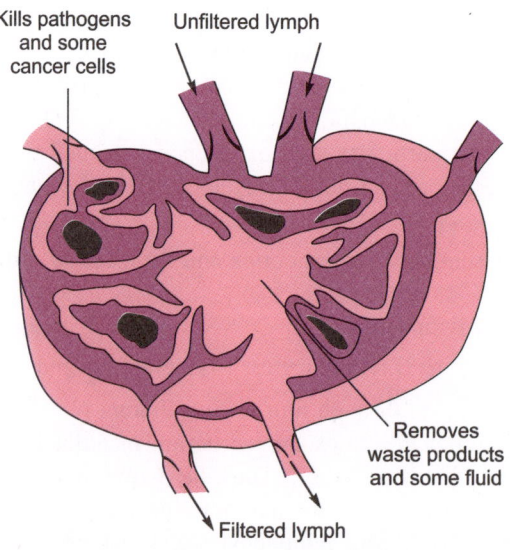

Figure 8.10 Filtration by lymph node.

3. **Destruction of cancer cells**: Lymph nodes can detect and destroy cancer cells. They can also trap cancer cells and slow the spread of cancer until they are overwhelmed of it.

ORGANS OF THE LYMPHATIC SYSTEM

SPLEEN

The spleen is the largest lymphatic organ in the body weighing about 200 g in adults. It is located in the left hypochondrial region of the abdominal cavity between the stomach and the diaphragm. It is purplish in colour and varies in size in different individuals, but is usually about 10 cm long in adults.

Structure of the Spleen

The spleen is slightly oval in shape with the hilum on one side similar to the lymph nodes, through which the splenic artery, splenic vein and efferent lymphatic vessels pass. It is enclosed by a capsule of fibrous connective tissue and the capsular extensions called *trabeculae* extend inward and form a network.

The parenchyma (functional part) of the spleen is composed of two different kinds of tissue called *white pulp* and *red pulp*. The red pulp has small patches of white pulp scattered in it (Fig. 8.11).

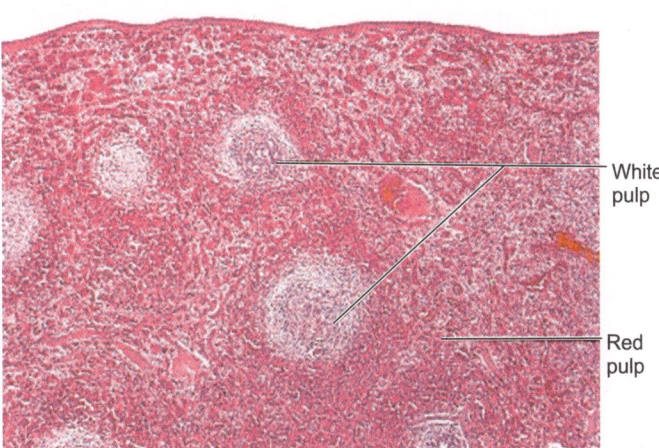

White pulp

Red pulp

Figure 8.11 White pulp and red pulp in spleen.

The white pulp is lymphatic tissue and consists of splenic corpuscles (or Malpighian corpuscles) present around the branches of the splenic artery called *central arteries*. The splenic corpuscles contain lymphocytes and macrophages. The red pulp is closely associated with the veins and consists of blood-filled venous sinuses and cords of splenic tissue called *splenic cords*. The splenic cords consist of a large quantity of concentrated red blood cells (RBCs), macrophages and lymphocytes (Fig. 8.12).

Note: Unlike the lymph nodes, the spleen does not have afferent lymphatics entering it; hence, it is not exposed to diseases spread by the lymph.

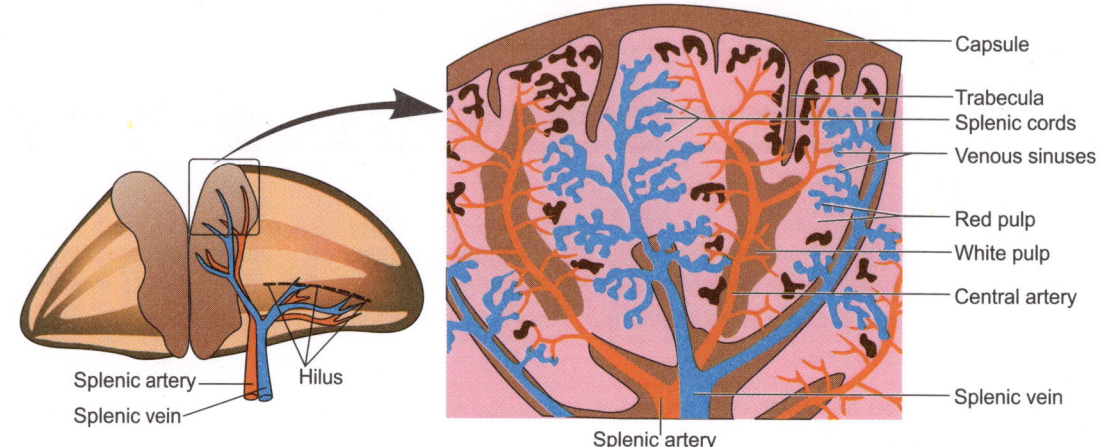

Figure 8.12 Structure of spleen.

Functions of spleen

The various functions of spleen are as follows:

1. **Destruction of worn-out blood cells**: The old and abnormal red blood corpuscles, lymphocytes and thrombocytes are phagocytized by the macrophages present in spleen. When the RBCs become old (120 days), their cell wall becomes fragile and gets damaged while squeezing through capillaries. It mostly occurs in spleen as splenic capillaries have a thin lumen. On this account, spleen is often referred to as the *graveyard of red blood cells*.

2. **Reservoir for RBCs**: In animals, the spleen stores RBCs when the animal is at rest and needs less oxygen. The RBCs are released into the blood stream during times of emergency like hypoxia and haemorrhage. However, this function is not significant in humans.

3. **Storage of iron**: Spleen stores the iron released from the haemoglobin of worn-out RBCs and sends it to the liver for reutilization.

4. **Immune response and defence of body**: The spleen contains T and B lymphocytes, which are activated by the presence of antigens, for example, in infection. The macrophages present in the spleen phagocytize the microorganisms and other foreign bodies.

5. **Eryhthropoiesis**: The spleen and liver are important sites of fetal blood cells production, and the spleen can perform this function when required.

THYMUS GLAND

The thymus gland is a bilobed organ located in the mediastinum between the sternum and the aorta (Fig. 8.13a). It weighs about 10–15 g at birth and grows until puberty. After puberty, adipose and areolar connective tissues begins to replace the thymic tissue and it begins to atrophy. In older individuals, it becomes very small and may weigh only 3 g.

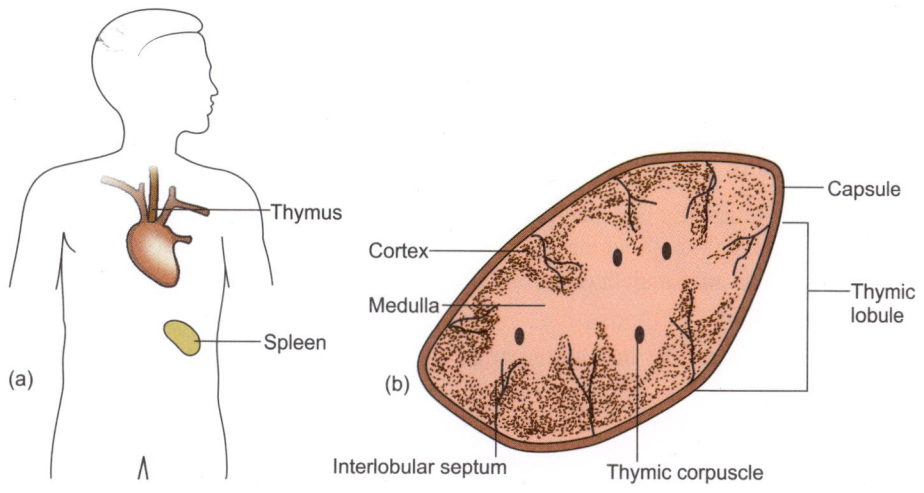

Figure 8.13 (a) Location of thymus; (b) Structure of thymus.

Structure of the thymus gland

The thymus consists of two lobes joined by areolar connective tissue. The lobes are enclosed by a capsule of fibrous connective tissue, and the capsular extensions called *trabeculae* extend inward and divide each lobe into lobules.

Each lobule of the thymus consists of the outer cortex and the inner medulla (Fig. 8.13b). The cortex consists of a large number of T lymphocytes, dendritic cells, epithelial cells and macrophages.

Immature T lymphocytes from the bone marrow migrate to the cortex of thymus where they proliferate and begin to mature. Dendritic cells assist in the maturation of T lymphocytes, and epithelial cells produce the hormones thymopoietin and thymosin, which stimulate their maturation. The macrophages clear out the debris of dead and dying cells. Most of the maturing T cells die in the cortex, whereas the surviving T cells leave the cortex and enter the medulla.

The medulla consists of mature T cells, epithelial cells, dendritic cells and macrophages. The mature T lymphocytes leave the thymus to enter the lymph nodes, spleen or other lymphatic tissues where they colonize parts of these organs and tissues.

Functions of the thymus gland

The various functions of spleen are as follows:

1. **Production of T lymphocytes**: The thymus is the site of production of T lymphocytes in the fetus and in infants for a few months after birth.
2. **Maturation of T lymphocytes**: The thymus gland is responsible for the maturation of T lymphocytes, which protect the body against foreign substances and harmful microorganisms.

3. **Specification of T lymphocytes**: Thymus educates the T lymphocytes in the fetus to distinguish body cells from foreign cells and also provides each T lymphocyte the ability to react to only one specific antigen.

LYMPHATIC NODULE

Lymphatic nodules (follicles) are egg-shaped small masses of lymphoid tissue that are not enclosed by a capsule. They are present throughout the mucous membrane that lines the gastrointestinal, respiratory, urinary and reproductive tract and thus are also referred to as *mucosa-associated lymphatic tissue (MALT)*.

The lymphatic nodules present in large aggregation in specific body parts include the tonsils and Peyer's patches.

Tonsils

Tonsils are the masses of lymphoid tissue present in the pharyngeal region. There are three groups of tonsils (Fig. 8.14):

1. **Pharyngeal or adenoid tonsils**: They are located in the posterior wall of the nasopharynx.
2. **Palatine tonsils**: They are located at the posterior region of the oral cavity, one on either side. These are the ones commonly removed in tonsillectomy (removal of tonsils).
3. **Lingual tonsils**: They are located on the back surface of the base of the tongue.

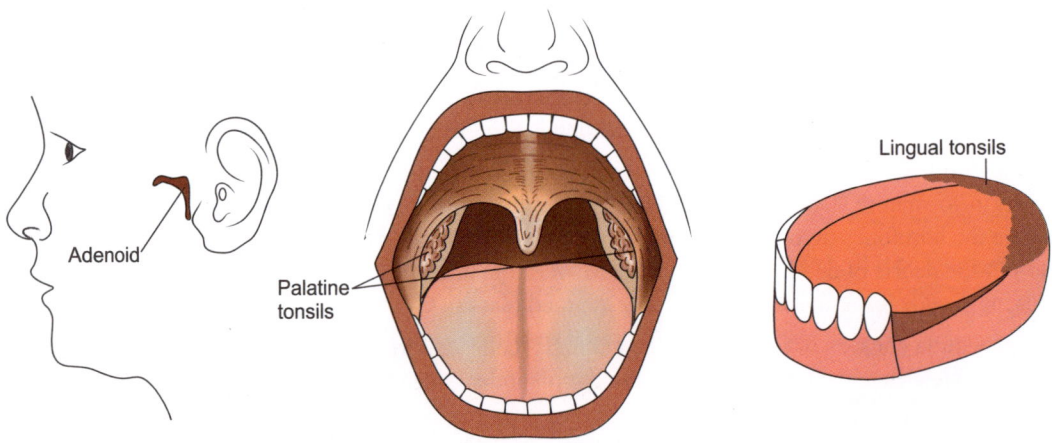

Figure 8.14 Three groups of tonsils: (a) Adenoid; (b) Palatine; (c) Lingual.

Note: These tonsils protect the body against harmful microorganisms that might enter the nose or the oral cavity.

Peyer's patches

Peyer's patches are the aggregated lymphoid tissues located in the wall of the small intestine. They mostly contain macrophages that protect the intestine from bacterial infection.

The lymph nodes and various organs of the lymphatic system can be summarized in Figure 8.15:

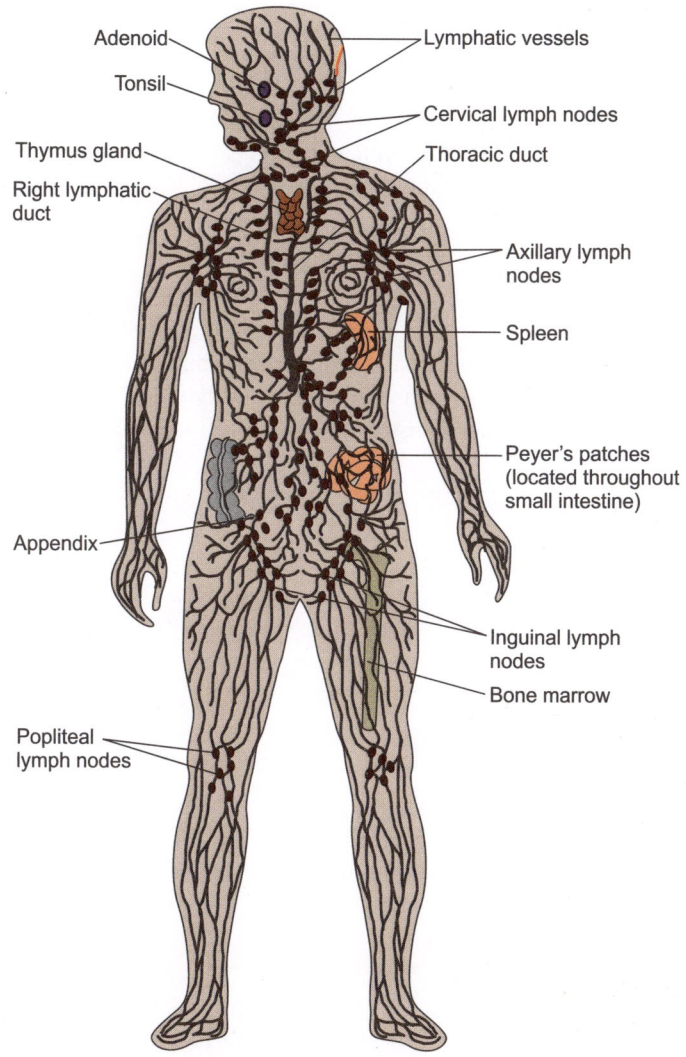

Figure 8.15 Summary of the lymphatic system.

DISORDERS ASSOCIATED WITH THE LYMPHATIC SYSTEM

LYMPHOID LEUKAEMIA

It is a form of cancer characterized by the uncontrolled production of lymphocytes that remain immature. These leukaemic cells eventually appear in such great numbers that they crowd out the normal, functioning cells.

Chemotherapeutic drugs are fairly effective in treating lymphoid leukaemia.

HODGKIN'S LYMPHOMA

It is a malignant disorder of the lymph nodes; there is progressive enlargement of the lymph nodes but the actual cause is unknown. The enlarged lymph nodes may compress the adjacent tissues and organs.

The first symptom is usually a swollen but painless lymph node, often in the neck region. The disease leads to reduced immunity due to depressed lymphocyte function.

This disease is often curable if diagnosed early and treated properly.

LYMPHOEDEMA

It is a kind of oedema developed due to lymphatic obstruction in diseases such as filariasis. The parasitic worm lives in lymphatic vessels and obstructs the drainage of lymph, causing prominent swellings of the legs and scrotum. Severe form of such obstruction may lead to elephantiasis.

ACUTE LYMPHADENITIS

It is the acute infection of lymph nodes caused by microbes reaching via lymph, draining the infected areas of the body. The infection within the lymph nodes attracts a large number of phagocytes, making them inflamed and enlarged.

NON-HODGKIN'S LYMPHOMA

It is more common than Hodgkin's lymphoma. It includes all cancers of lymphoid tissues except Hodgkin's disease.

It is characterized by the presence of uncontrolled multiplication and metastasis of undifferentiated lymphocytes, with swelling of the lymph nodes and spleen. A low-grade type, which affects the elderly, is resistant to chemotherapy and so is often fatal.

SPLENOMEGALY (*MEGA*: LARGE)

It is characterized by the enlargement of the spleen due to certain pathological conditions. Conditions like inflammatory disorders, liver and blood diseases lead to the accumulation of infectious microorganisms, often causing increased activity of the spleen, which in turn causes spleen enlargement.

TONSILLITIS

It is characterized by the inflammation of the tonsils, typically due to bacterial infection; they become red, swollen and sore.

BUBONIC PLAGUE

It is also called *black plague* and is a serious disease caused by a bacterium and spreads by fleas from rats or rodents to people. It got its 'black' name from 'buboes,' which are dark swellings found in the groin or armpit of people with plague.

OVERVIEW OF THE LYMPHATIC SYSTEM

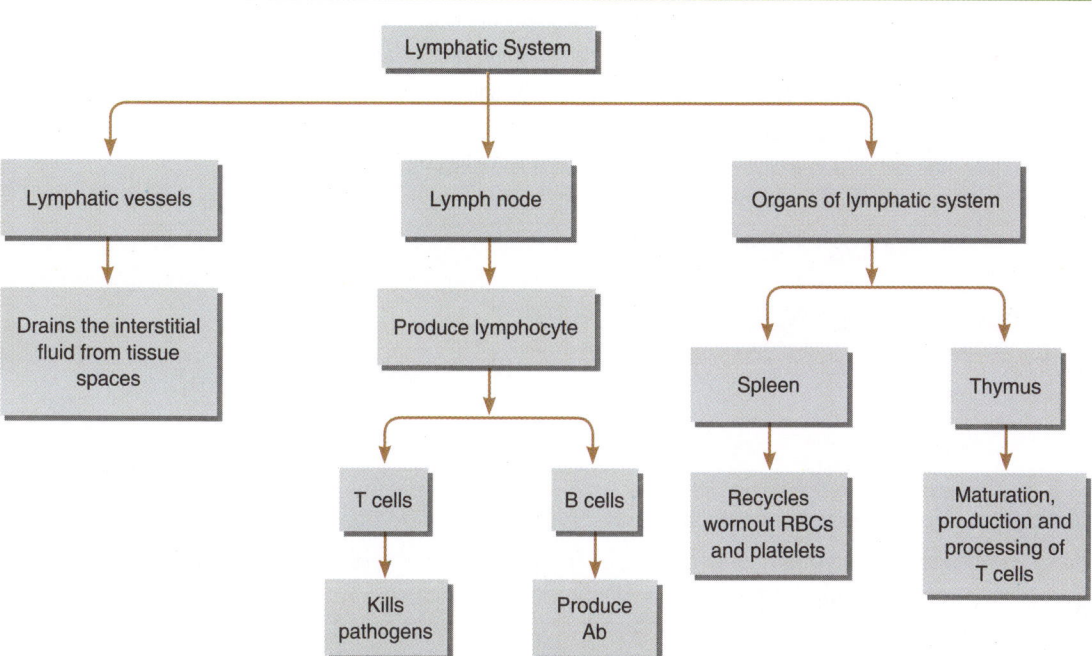

Embryonic Development of the Lymphatic System

- ❏ End of 5th week: Marks the beginning of the development of the lymphatic system.
  - ➤ Mesoderm forms developing veins → gives rise to lymph sacs → forms lymphatic vessels
  - ➤ I Lymph sac: *Jugular lymph sac* → gives rise to lymph capillaries in the thorax, upper limbs, neck and head.
  - ➤ II Lymph sac: *Retroperitoneal lymph sac* → forms lymph capillaries in abdominal viscera.
  - ➤ III Lymph sac: *Cisterna chyli* → forms thoracic duct and cysterna chyli of thoracic duct.
  - ➤ IV Lymph sac: *Posterior lymph sac* → forms lymph vessels in abdominal wall, pelvic region and lower limbs.
- ❏ The mesenchymal cells invade all the lymph sacs except the cistern chyli and convert into groups of lymph nodes.
- ❏ Mesenchymal cells between layers of stomach form spleen.
- ❏ Outgrowth of the 3rd pharyngeal pouch forms the thymus gland.

Ageing and Lymphatic System

- ❏ With age, the thymus gland decreases in size and gets replaced by adipose tissue. The secretion of thymic hormones also decreases, resulting in fewer T cells for responding to infections.
- ❏ As the T cells decrease with age, the B cells also become less responsive. Thus, the elderly are more susceptible to various infections.

Review Questions

Long Answer Questions

1. Explain the relationships among plasma, tissue fluid and lymph. Compare and contrast blood, interstitial fluid and lymph in terms of the movement of water throughout the body.

2. Describe the system of lymph vessels. Explain how lymph is kept moving in these vessels. Into which vein is lymph emptied?

3. State the locations of the major groups of lymph nodes and explain their functions.

4. Describe the location of the spleen and explain its functions.

5. Explain the function of the thymus.

6. Compare the structure and functions of a lymph node with those of the spleen.

Multiple Choice Questions

1. Lymphatic vessels
   (a) Serve as sites for immune surveillance
   (b) Filter lymph
   (c) Transport leaked plasma proteins and fluids to the cardiovascular system
   (d) Are represented by vessels that resemble arteries, capillaries and veins

2. The saclike initial portion of the thoracic duct is the
   (a) Lacteal
   (b) Right lymphatic duct
   (c) Cisterna chyli
   (d) Lymph sac

3. Entry of lymph into the lymphatic capillaries is promoted by which of the following?
   (a) One-way mini valves formed by overlapping endothelial cells
   (b) The respiratory pump, (c) the skeletal muscle pump
   (d) Greater fluid pressure in the interstitial space

4. The structural framework of lymphoid organs is
   (a) Areolar connective tissue
   (b) Hematopoietic tissue
   (c) Reticular tissue
   (d) Adipose tissue

5. Lymph nodes are densely clustered in all of the following body areas except
   (a) The brain
   (b) The axillae
   (c) The groin
   (d) The cervical region

6. The germinal centres in lymph nodes are largely sites of
   (a) Macrophages
   (b) Proliferating B lymphocytes
   (c) T lymphocytes
   (d) All of these

7. The red pulp areas of the spleen are sites of
   (a) Venous sinuses, macrophages and red blood cells
   (b) Clustered lymphocytes
   (c) Connective tissue septa

8. The lymphoid organ that functions primarily during youth and then begins to atrophy is the
   (a) Spleen
   (b) Thymus
   (c) Palatine tonsils
   (d) Bone marrow

9. Which of the following is *not* a major organ of the lymphatic system?
   (a) Lymph nodes
   (b) Thymus
   (c) Kidney
   (d) Spleen

10. A dilation of the lymphatic duct in the lumbar region that marks the beginning of the thoracic duct is

   (a) The cisterna chyli
   (b) The right lymphatic duct
   (c) The hilum
   (d) The mesenteric lymph node

11. The spleen does *not*

   (a) House lymphocytes
   (b) Filter foreign particles, damaged red blood cells and cellular debris from the blood
   (c) Contain phagocytes
   (d) Change undifferentiated lymphocytes into T lymphocytes

Fill in the Blanks

1. Specialized bands of connective tissue, called _____, divide the lymph nodes.

2. Clusters of _____ (Peyer's patches) are associated with the small intestine.

3. The _____ is located in the anterior thorax, near the manubrium of the sternum.

4. _____ is an enzyme in tears, saliva and blood plasma that breaks down bacterial cell walls.

Careers in Lymphatic System

✓ Lymphoedema therapists are trained professionals who relieve the swellings caused by blockage of lymph vessels. They use massage therapy, exercises and bandaging to relieve such swellings.

✓ Immunologists are physicians who specialize in the body's immune system to counteract any pathological condition.

The Immune System

STUDY OBJECTIVES

✓ To describe the various components of nonspecific resistance to disease.

✓ To discuss the role of different T lymphocytes in providing cell-mediated immunity.

✓ To describe the process of antibody-mediated immunity.

✓ To explain passive immunity and active immunity.

INTRODUCTION

Immunity is the ability of the body to resist infection from disease-causing microorganisms or pathogens and damage from foreign substances and harmful chemicals.

The branch of science that deals with the response of the body against microorganisms or foreign substances is called *immunology*.

Every individual is under constant threat from an enormous range of potentially harmful invaders that include attack from bacteria, viruses, cancer cells, parasites and foreign cells (tissue transplant). This threat starts in the womb and continues till the end of life. In response to this, the body has developed many protective measures, which can be termed as *immunity or resistance for infections*.

The resistance or immunity of the body is of the following two types:

1. **Nonspecific resistance or innate (natural) immunity**: This resistance is present at birth and provides immediate protection against a wide variety of pathogens and foreign substances. The mechanisms of nonspecific resistance involve epithelial barriers, antimicrobial proteins, natural killer cells, phagocytes, etc.

2. **Specific resistance or acquired immunity**
   - ❑ It is the ability of the body to resist itself against specific invading agents such as pathogens, toxins and foreign tissues. This resistance is a powerful mechanism to protect the body against microorganisms and toxic substances.
   - ❑ Acquired immunity includes the cells and tissues that carry out immune response (i.e. B lymphocytes and T lymphocytes) (Fig. 9.1).

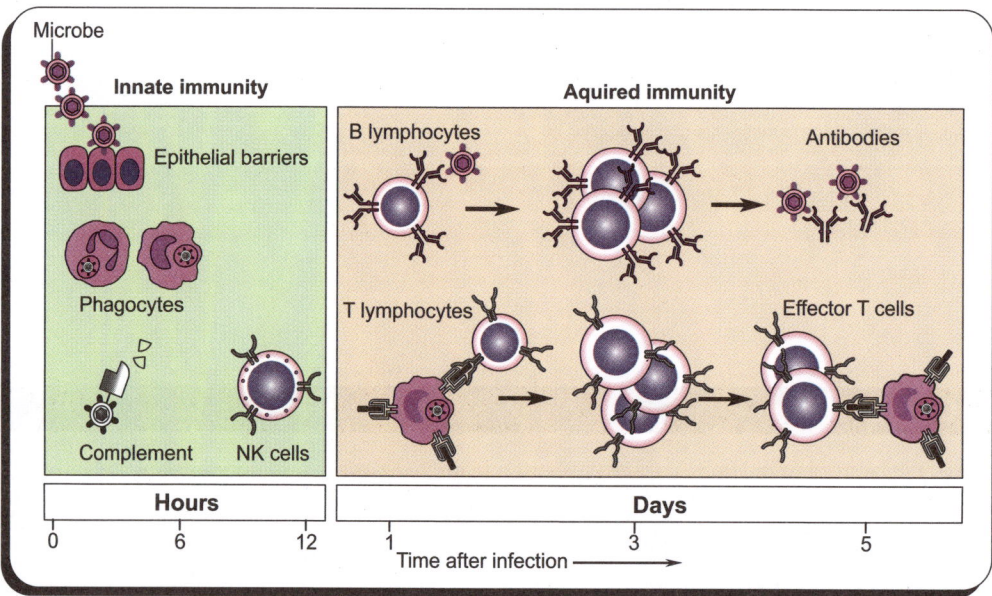

Figure 9.1 Overview of (a) innate Immunity and (b) acquired Immunity.

MEDICAL TERMINOLOGY

- ❑ **Antigen**: Any substance that causes the immune system to produce antibodies against it.
- ❑ **Parasite**: An organism that lives on or in an organism of another species known as the *host*, from the body of which it obtains nutriment, while causing harm to the host.
- ❑ **Pathogen**: A microorganism such as a virus, bacterium, prior or fungus, that causes disease in its animal or plant host.

NONSPECIFIC RESISTANCE/INNATE IMMUNITY

The various components of innate immunity are discussed in Figure 9.2.

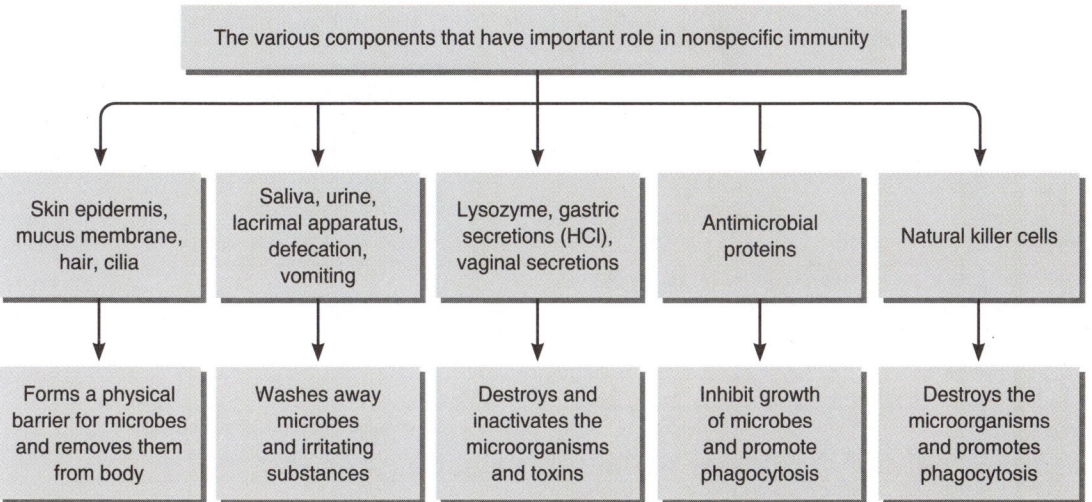

Figure 9.2 Components of innate immunity.

SPECIFIC RESISTANCE/ACQUIRED IMMUNITY

There are two types of acquired immunity, which are as follows:

1. Cell-mediated/cellular immunity
2. Antibody (Ab)-mediated immunity/humoral immunity

CELL-MEDIATED/CELLULAR IMMUNITY

This is a major defence mechanism against infection by virus, fungi, bacteria and some cancer cells.

It is developed by the activation of *T lymphocytes* in response to a specific antigen. Once the T cell gets activated, it undergoes proliferation and differentiation to form a population of identical T cells (clonal expansion) that can recognize the same antigen (Ag) and carry out immune response (Fig. 9.3).

Development of T lymphocytes

In the fetus, *T lymphocytes* develop in bone marrow and then migrate to the thymus gland for processing. T lymphocytes are called so because of their processing in thymus, which occurs just before birth and a few months after birth.

The thymus gland secretes a hormone, *thymosin*, that is responsible for the proliferation and development of T cells into fully specialized, mature and functional T lymphocytes. A mature T lymphocyte acquires *immunologic competence*, that is each T cell is designed to be activated and to develop immune response against one type of antigen (Ag) only.

Chapter 9

Chapter 9

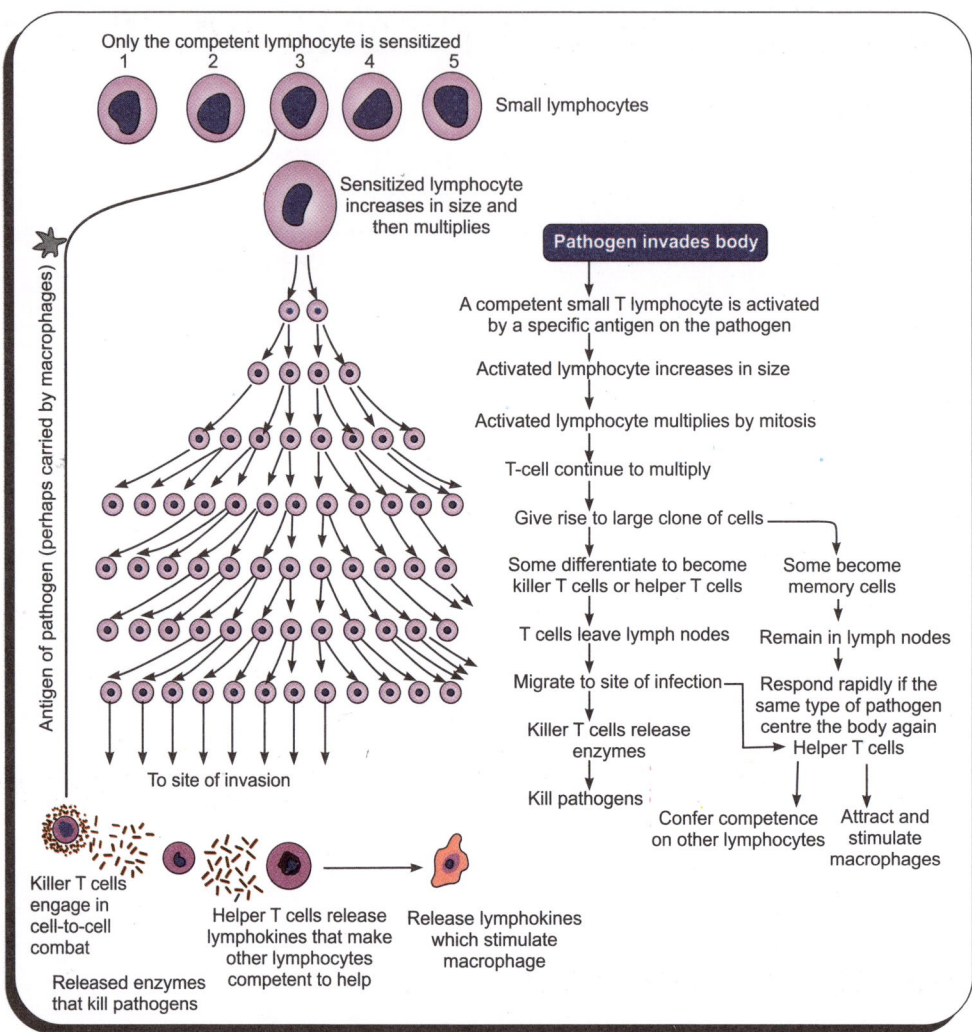

Figure 9.3 Cell-mediated immunity.

Types of T lymphocytes

During processing of T lymphocytes in the thymus gland, the T lymphocytes are transformed into the following four types:

1. Helper T cells/inducer T cells
2. Cytotoxic T cells/killer T cells
3. Suppressor T cells/regulatory T cells
4. Memory T cells

After the transformation of T lymphocytes into four types, the T lymphocytes are released into the circulation where they migrate and stay in the lymphoid tissues present in the lymph nodes, spleen and bone marrow.

1. **Helper T cells**: Helper T cells are essential for various activities of cell-mediated as well as antibody (Ab)-mediated immunity.

   The main functions of helper T cells include the following:

   (a) They are specialized in the production of special chemicals called *cytokines* (e.g. interleukins (IL-2) and interferons) that enhance the activation and proliferation of other T cells, B cells and natural killer cells. They also release certain chemicals called *lymphokines* that attract macrophages and make other lymphocytes competent to help.

   (b) B cells and T cells are required to be stimulated first by a helper T lymphocyte before initiating an immune response (i.e. production of antibodies (Abs) or cytotoxic cells).

2. **Cytotoxic T cells**: After stimulation by helper T cells, the activated cytotoxic T cells circulate through blood, lymph and lymphatic tissue and destroy the invading organisms by attacking them directly.

   The main role of cytotoxic T cells is the destruction of body cells infected by microbes, some tumour cells and cells of a tissue transplant (Fig. 9.4).

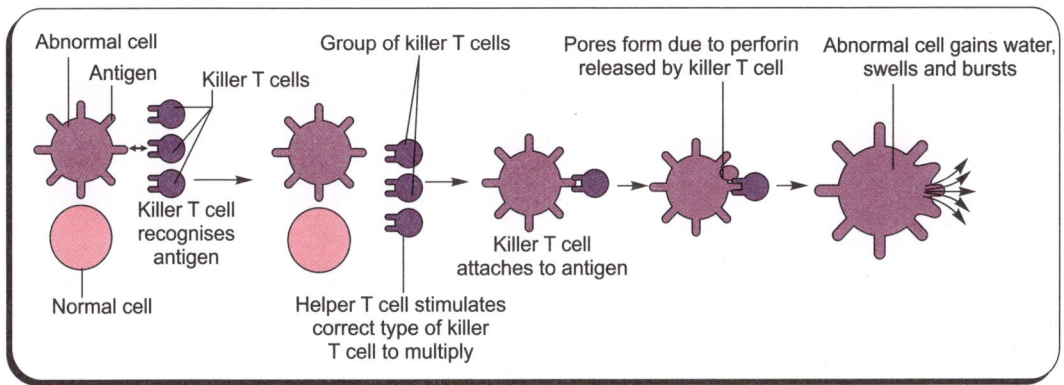

Figure 9.4 Role of cytotoxic T cells.

3. **Suppressor T cells**: The suppressor T cells suppress the activities of activated T cells and B cells and prevent them from destroying the body's own tissues, once the infection is controlled. This limits the powerful and potentially damaging effects of the immune response.

4. **Memory T cells**: Some of the activated T cells remain in the lymphoid tissue instead of entering circulation. They exist in the body for years, enabling it to respond quickly and vigorously to any future infection by the same pathogen (Fig. 9.5).

   For an immune response to occur, the T lymphocytes must recognize that a foreign Ag is present. There is a special class of cells called *Ag-presenting cells (APCs)* that process and present the foreign Ag in a certain way so that they are easily recognized by T lymphocytes. APCs include dendritic cells and macrophages. The foreign Ag is trapped by dendritic cells and is then engulfed by macrophages, where it is processed internally and then displayed on their surface. This APC then migrates to lymphatic tissue to present the Ag to T cells, which recognize it, triggering an immune response. Thus, *Ag presentation* is very important for the activation and immune response of T lymphocytes.

Chapter 9

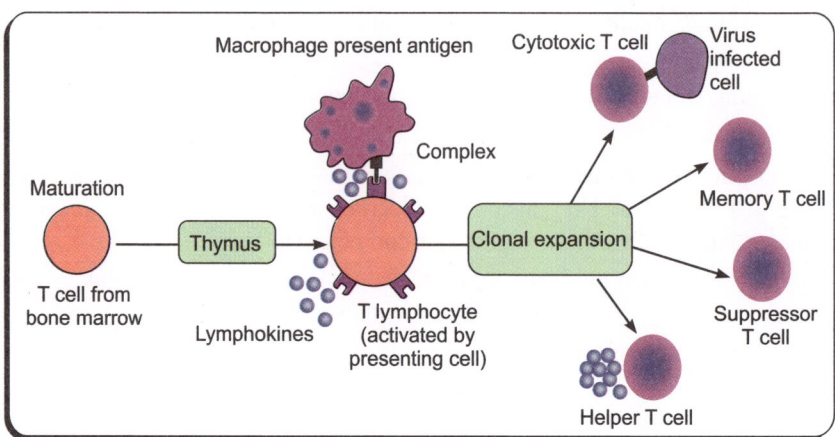

Figure 9.5 Activation and types of T lymphocytes.

ANTIBODY (AB)-MEDIATED IMMUNITY OR HUMORAL IMMUNITY

Humoral immunity plays an important role in the defence mechanism against bacterial and viral infections.

It is developed by the activation of *B lymphocytes* in response to a specific Ag. Once activated, the B lymphocytes enlarge and undergo proliferation and differentiation to produce two functionally distinct types of cells: plasma cells and memory B cells.

Development of B lymphocytes

In the fetus, B lymphocytes develop in bone marrow and then migrate and are processed in the liver during fetal life. After birth, they are produced as well as developed in bone marrow. B lymphocytes are named so because of their processing in bone narrow.

Types of B lymphocytes

During processing of B lymphocytes in bone narrow, the B lymphocytes are transformed into the following two types: plasma cells and memory B cells.

After the transformation, B lymphocytes migrate and stay in the lymphoid tissues present in the lymph nodes, spleen and bone narrow.

1. **Plasma cells**: After exposure to an Ag, the plasma cells produce antibodies (Abs) or immunoglobulins (Igs). The rate of Ab production is very high (i.e. each plasma cell produces 2000 molecules of Abs per second). The Abs are released into lymph and then transported into circulation. The Abs are produced until the end of the lifespan of each plasma cell, that is from several days to several weeks.

2. **Memory B cells**: Some of the B lymphocytes activated by Ag are transformed into memory B cells and occupy the lymphoid tissues throughout the body. The memory cells remain in an inactive state until the body is exposed to the same Ag for the second time. During second exposure, the memory cells get stimulated by Ag and they produce more quantity of Abs at a faster rate, thereby protecting the body from any future infection.

Ag presentation is also important for the activation and immune response of B lymphocytes, as discussed earlier (Fig. 9.6).

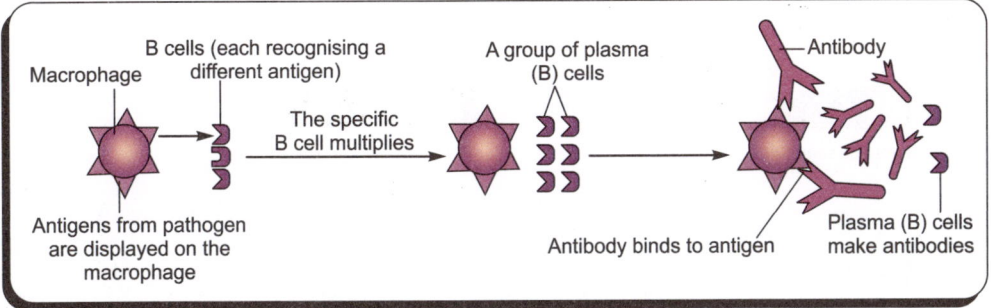

Figure 9.6 Activation of B lymphocytes.

The accelerated, more intense response by memory cells after subsequent exposure to the same Ag is called *secondary response* (Fig. 9.7).

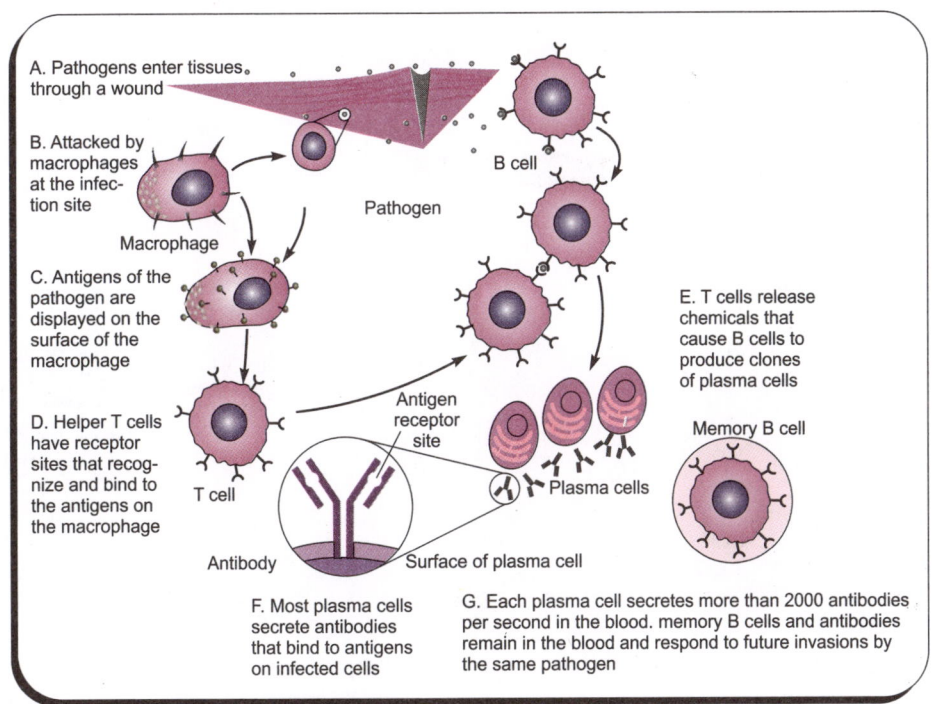

Figure 9.7 Pictorial representation of Ab-mediated immunity.

The different roles of B-lymphocytes and T-lymphocytes in cell mediated and humoral immunity have been summarised in Figures 9.8 and 9.9

Chapter 9

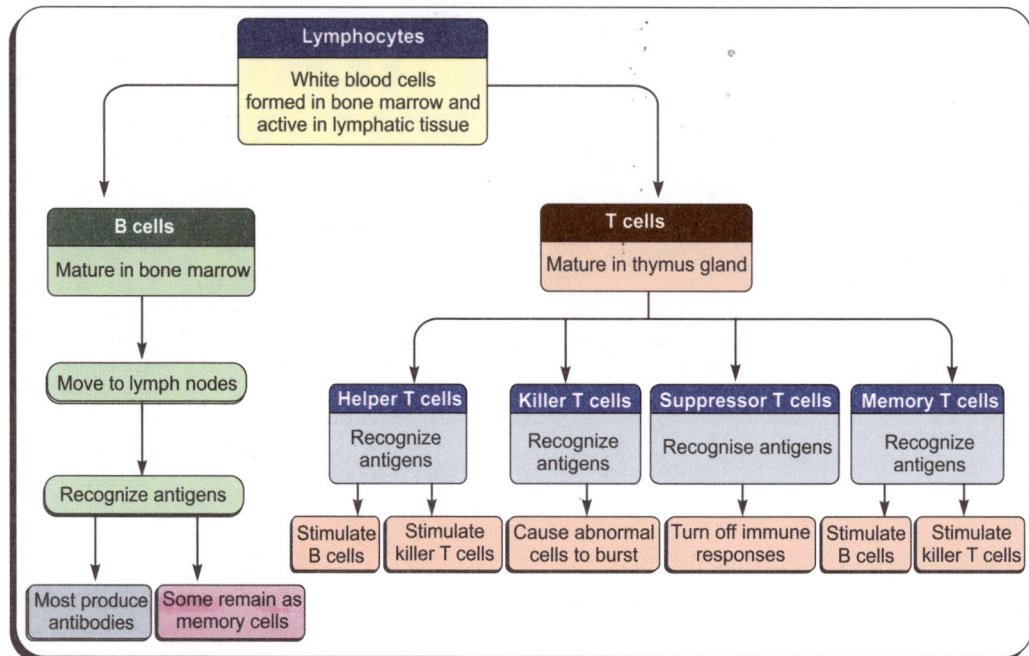

Figure 9.8 Summary of B lymphocytes and T lymphocytes.

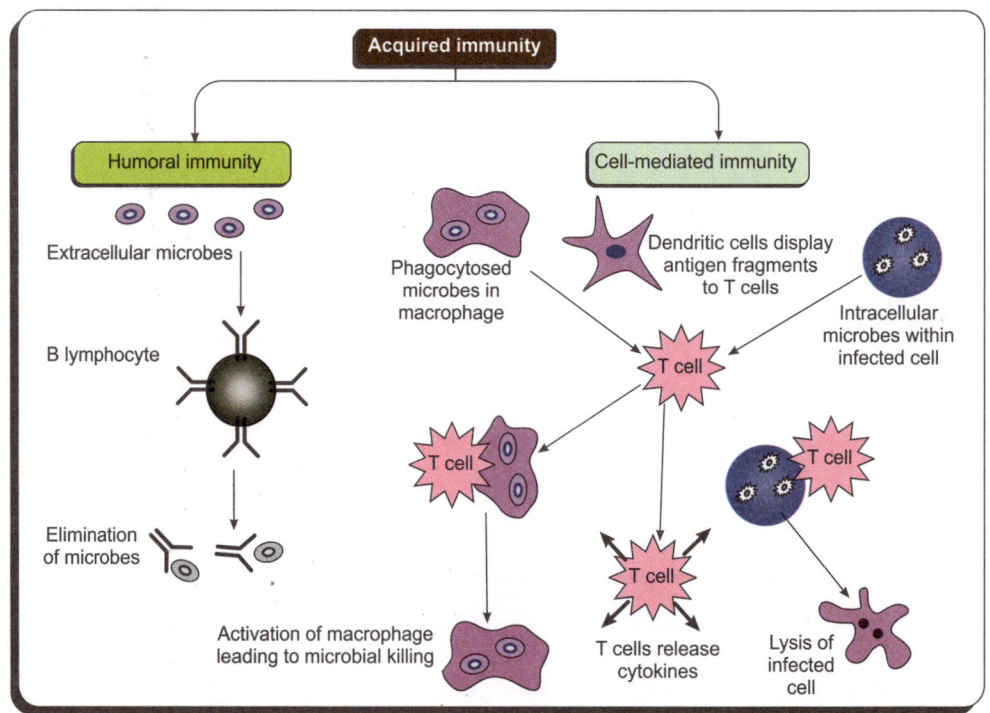

Figure 9.9 Summary of cell-mediated and humoral immunity.

IMMUNIZATION

Immunization is defined as the technique of preparing the body against a specific disease. It is done by subjecting the individual to an Ag in order to produce antibodies (Abs) in the body against that Ag (Fig. 9.10).

Immunization or immunity can be of two types: passive immunity and active immunity.

PASSIVE IMMUNITY

Passive immunization/immunity is produced without challenging the immune system of the body. This is done by administration of immunoglobulins (Igs) or Abs from a person who is already immunized to a nonimmune person.

Passive immunity can be acquired naturally or artificially (Fig. 9.11).

Naturally acquired passive immunity

This type of immunity is acquired from the mother before and after birth. Before birth the fetus receives its mother's Abs (mostly IgG) through the placenta, and after birth through breast milk (IgA).

The baby's lymphocytes are not stimulated and the Abs received from the mother are metabolized soon. Thus, passive immunity is shortlived.

Artificially acquired passive immunity

This type of immunity is developed by injecting readymade Abs produced in human or animal serum. The Abs are obtained from an individual who has recovered from an infection or animals, commonly horses, that have been artificially actively immunized.

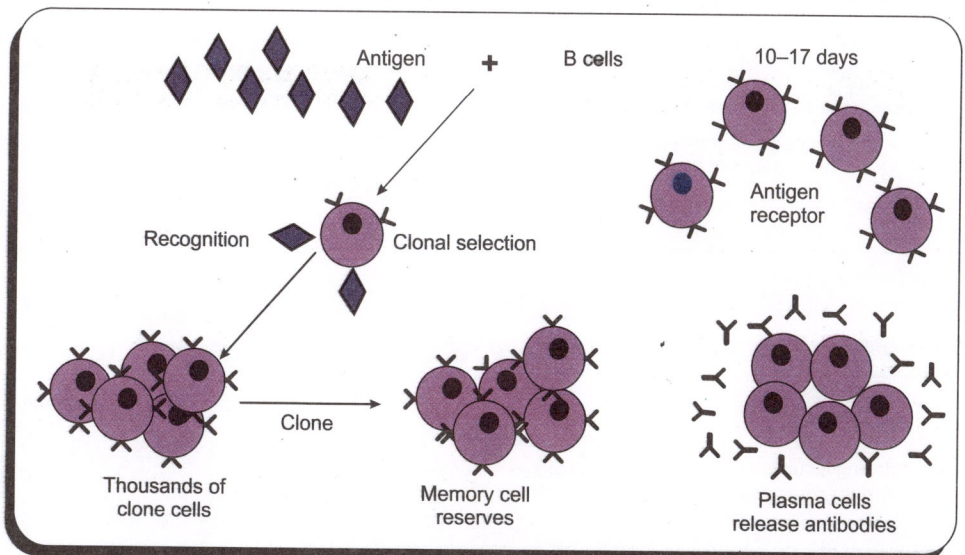

Figure 9.10 Immune response.

Specific Abs (antiserum) may be administered prophylactically to prevent the development of disease in people who may be exposed to the infection in a later period, or therapeutically after the disease has developed.

This type of immunity provides immediate protection but it only lasts for 2–3 weeks.

ACTIVE IMMUNITY

Active immunity/immunization is acquired by activating the immune system of the body. It is developed when the body is exposed to Ag, and the body responds by producing Abs, activating lymphocytes and forming memory cells.

Active immunity can be acquired either naturally or artificially.

Naturally acquired active immunity

This type of immunity involves activation of the immune system to produce Abs by the following ways:

1. **Clinical infection**: During a disease, B lymphocytes develop into plasma cells that produce sufficient quantities of Abs to overcome the infection. After recovery, memory cells retain the ability to produce Abs against the specific Ags invaded previously.

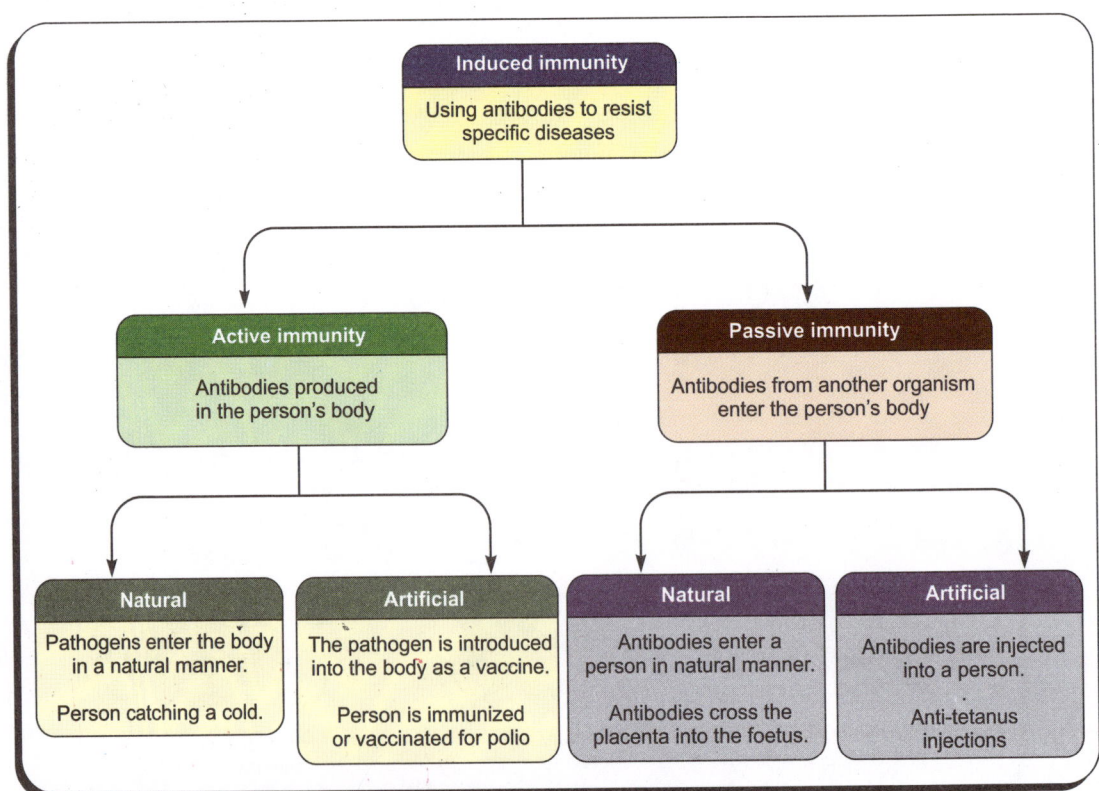

Figure 9.11 Summary of immunization or immunity.

2. **Subclinical infection**: Sometimes, the disease may not be sufficiently severe to cause a clinical disease, but it stimulates sufficient B cells to establish immunity.

Artificially acquired active immunity

This type of immunity involves the administration of dead or live artificially weakened microbes (vaccines) or deactivated toxins (toxoids). The vaccines and toxoids retain the antigenic properties that stimulate the development of immunity, but they cannot cause the disease. Artificial immunization is currently available to prevent many infectious diseases such as measles, chickenpox, small pox, polio, tetanus, diphtheria and various strains of flu.

TERMINOLOGY RELATED TO IMMUNITY

ANTIGENS (Ags)

Ags are the substances that the body recognizes as foreign and thus provokes immune response in the body. They are mostly the conjugated proteins such as lipoproteins, glycoproteins and nucleoproteins.

Ags are of two types: self-Ag and nonself-Ag

Self-Ag or MHC Ag

❑ Self-Ag is also called as the *major histocompatibility complex* (MHC) Ag (Fig. 9.12a). These are located in the plasma membrane of each body cell except RBC. These are also called human leukocyte Ags (HLA) as they were first identified on white blood cells. MHC Ags are unique for each individual.

❑ These MHCs are responsible for the rejection of a transplanted organ.

Nonself-Ag

❑ Nonself-Ags are the foreign proteins that gain access to our bodies via cuts and scrapes, through the digestive or circulatory systems or through the urinary and reproductive systems. These foreign proteins can be microbes, toxins, chemical components of pollen, egg white, incompatible blood cells and transplanted tissues and organs (Fig. 9.12b).

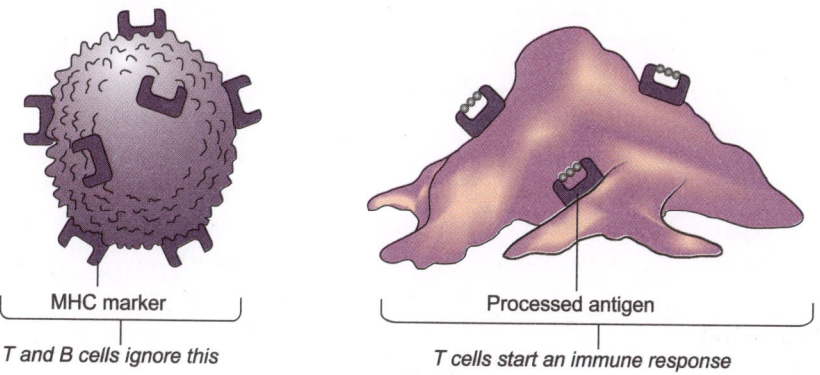

MHC marker

T and B cells ignore this

Processed antigen

T cells start an immune response

Figure 9.12 (a) Self-Ag; (b) Nonself-Ag.

❑ Certain small parts of the Ag molecule called *epitopes* or *antigenic determinants* act as the triggers for immune responses, leading to the production of Abs or Igs (Fig. 9.13).

Note: Each invading Ag is recognized and defended by a specific T and B lymphocyte. Therefore, there are millions of T and B lymphocytes in the body, each capable of responding to only one Ag.

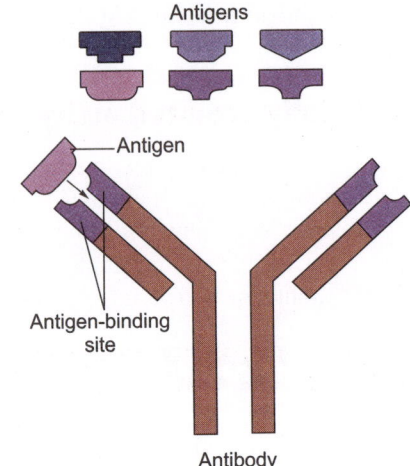

Figure 9.13 Capability of Ab to join a specific Ag.

ANTIMICROBIAL PROTEINS

Blood and interstitial fluids contain three types of antimicrobial proteins: interferons, the complement system and transferrin.

1. **Interferons**: Lymphocytes and macrophages infected with virus produce proteins called *interferons*. These interferons induce the synthesis of antiviral proteins that interfere with the viral replication within infected cells and inhibit the spread of viruses to healthy cells.

2. **Complement system**: These are a group of about 20 inactive proteins found in blood plasma and plasma membrane. When they are activated, they stimulate immune response by causing cytolysis of microbes and promoting phagocytosis.

3. **Transferrin**: These are the iron-binding proteins that inhibit the growth of bacteria by reducing the amount of available iron.

NATURAL KILLER CELLS

These are the cells present in the spleen and bone marrow that have the ability to kill a wide variety of infected body cells and certain tumour cells. They kill the infected cells by causing cytolysis or by inducing the target cell to undergo apoptosis.

PHAGOCYTES

These are the specialized cells that perform phagocytosis (cell eating), that is, the ingestion of microbes or other particles such as cellular debris (Fig. 9.14).

There are two major types of phagocytes: neutrophils and macrophages.

The neutrophils and monocytes migrate to the infected area when an infection occurs. During migration, the monocytes enlarge and develop into wandering macrophages, while other macrophages remain fixed in the specific tissues such as the liver (Kupffer cells), lungs, nervous system (microglia), spleen (reticular cells) and lymph nodes (reticular cells). This monocyte–macrophage system is also called the *reticuloendothelial system*, and it plays a vital role in immunity.

ANTIBODIES (Abs)

Abs or Igs are produced by plasma cells in response to a specific Ag. They are known as *Igs* as they belong to a group of glycoproteins called *globulins*.

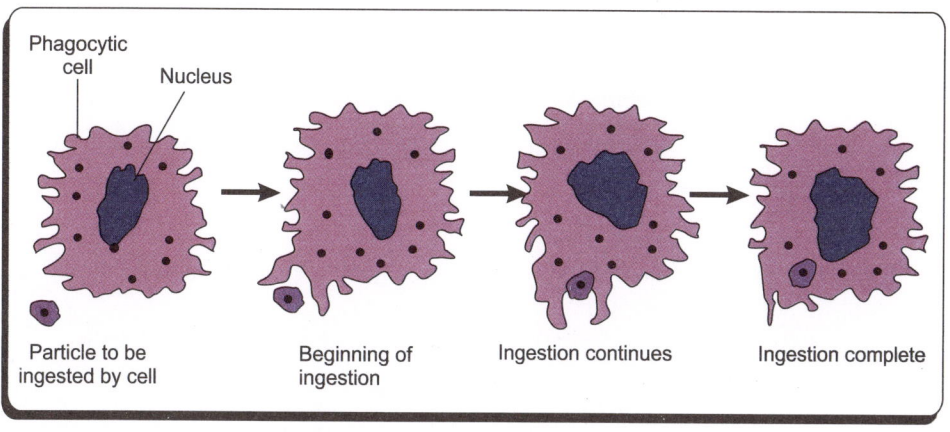

Figure 9.14 Stages of phagocytosis.

Structure of Abs

Abs are gamma globulins with a molecular weight in the range of 150,000–900,000.

Abs have a basic structure consisting of four amino acid chains linked together by disulphide bonds. The four amino acid chains include one pair of heavy (H) or long chains and one pair of light (L) or short chains. Each heavy chain consists of about 450 amino acids, and each light chain consists of about 220 amino acids. A disulphide bond (S–S) holds each light chain to a heavy chain. Two disulphide bonds also link the mid-region of the two heavy chains, and this midregion is called the *hinge region* as it allows the movement of the amino acid chains (Fig. 9.15).

Each chain of the Ab includes two regions: (1) variable region and (2) constant region.

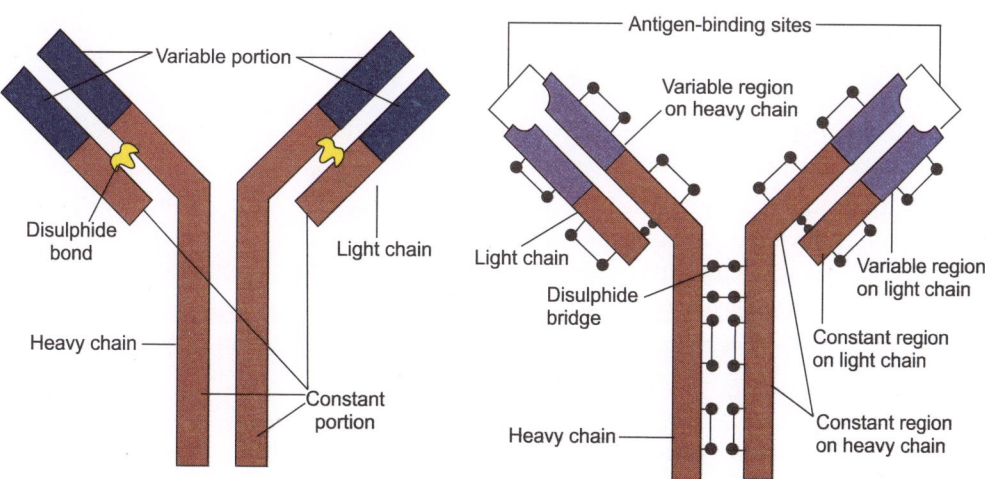

Figure 9.15 Structure of an antibody.

Variable region

The tips of the H and L chains are the variable region and it consists of the *Ag-binding site* (i.e. the site that recognizes and attaches to a specific Ag).

The number and sequence of amino acids present in this region are different in each Ab; therefore, this region is different for each kind of Ab.

Constant region

The remainder of each H and L chain is the constant region and it is responsible for the occurrence of specific types of Ag–Ab reaction.

The number and sequence of amino acids present in this region are similar in all Abs; therefore, this region is similar in all the Abs of the same class.

Types of Abs

The following are five main types of Abs:

1. **IgA**: It is found in exocrine gland secretions, nasal fluid, tears, bile, breast milk and urine. It provides localized protection by preventing the Ags from crossing the epithelial membranes.
2. **IgD**: It is found on the surface of B lymphocytes and is important in B-cell activation.
3. **IgE**: It is found on basophils and mast cells and is involved in allergic and hypersensitivity reactions.
4. **IgG**: This is the largest and most abundant Ab and is found in tissues fluids and plasma. It protects against bacteria and viruses by enhancing phagocytosis, neutralizing toxins and stimulating the complement system.
   It is the only class of Ab that crosses the placenta from the mother to the fetus.
5. **IgM**: It is found in blood and lymph. It is the first Ab class to be secreted by plasma cells in the primary response and is a potent activator of the complement system.

Actions of Abs

The following are the various actions of Abs:

1. **Neutralization**: The Ab neutralizes some bacterial toxins and also prevents the attachment of some viruses to body cells.
2. **Immobilization**: The Ab causes the bacteria with cilia or flagella to lose their mobility and thus limits their spread to nearby tissues.
3. **Agglutination and precipitation**: The Ag–Ab reaction causes the cross-linking of pathogens, resulting in agglutination (clumping). These agglutinated microbes are more easily ingested by phagocytes. Similarly, the soluble Ags are converted into insoluble form and then precipitated, which are readily phagocytized.
4. **Activation of the complement system**: The Ag–Ab reaction initiates and activates the complement pathway, which results in cytolysis, agglutination, precipitation, chemotaxis and neutralization of the microbes.
5. **Enhancement of phagocytosis**: The Ag–Ab reaction stimulates agglutination and precipitation and activates a complement, which enhances the activity of phagocytes. This process makes the pathogens more susceptible to phagocytosis, and this process is called *opsonization* (Fig. 9.16)

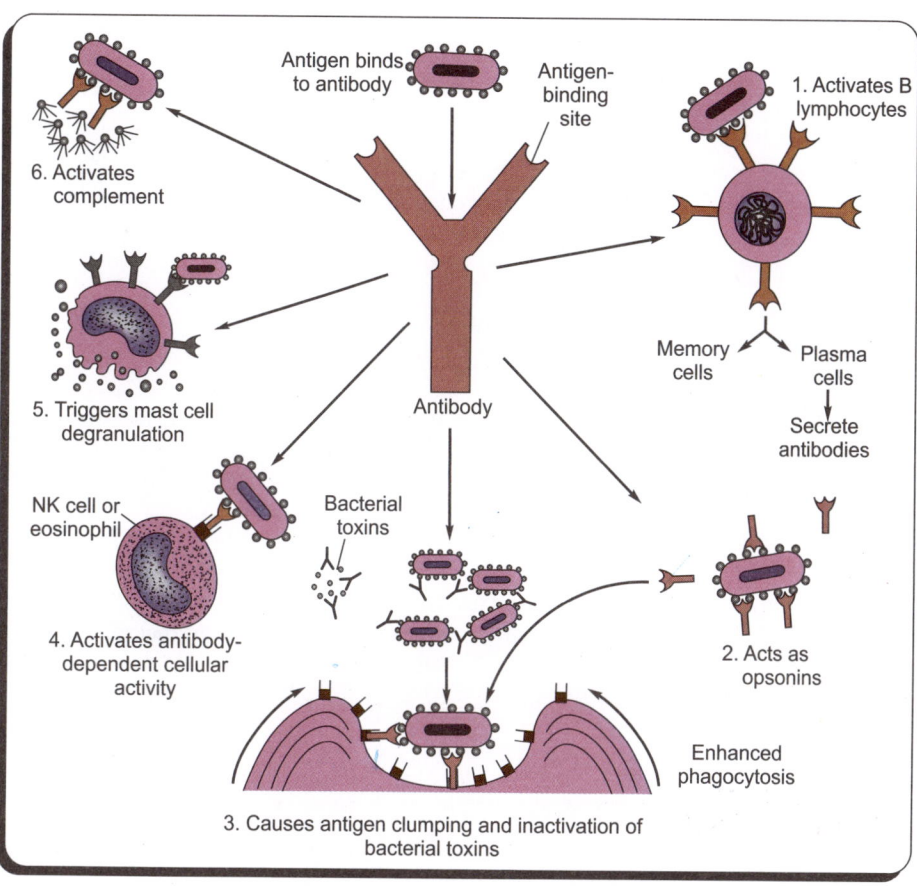

Figure 9.16 Actions of antibodies.

DISEASES ASSOCIATED WITH THE IMMUNE SYSTEM

HYPERSENSITIVITY (ALLERGY)

It is the exaggerated powerful immune response to an Ag (allergen). The allergen is usually harmless and is tolerated by most of the people but can induce an allergic reaction in the individual who is overly reactive to it.

Common allergens include certain foods (eggs, milk, peanuts), antibiotics (penicillins, tetracycline), cosmetics and vaccines (pertussis, typhoid).

There are four basic types of hypersensitivity reactions, which are as follows:

1. **Type I (anaphylactic reaction)**

  ❑ This is the most common hypersensitivity reaction and occurs in individuals who have inherited very high levels of immunoglobulin E (IgE).

  ❑ The anaphylactic reaction results from the interaction of allergen and IgE and causes the activation of mast cells and basophils. In response, mast cells and basophils release histamine, prostaglandins and leukotrienes, which cause vasodilation, increased smooth muscle contraction in the airway of lungs and increased vascular permeability. As a result, a person may experience inflammatory responses, profound bronchoconstriction and shock due to excessive vasodilation. The condition, if not controlled, can even lead to death.

2. **Type II (cytotoxic reaction)**: It is caused by Abs (IgM or IgG) directed against Ags on a person's body cells or tissue cells. These reactions may occur in incompatible blood transfusion reactions or in certain haemolytic diseases of the newborn.

3. **Type III (immune complex reaction)**
   - ❑ These reactions usually result from the Ag–Ab complexes that are not cleared efficiently from the blood by phagocytosis and eventually get deposited in the tissues (e.g. kidneys, skin, joints and the eye).
   - ❑ These deposited immune complexes result in inflammatory response and are responsible for conditions such as glomerulonephritis and rheumatoid arthritis (RA).

4. **Type IV (delayed hypersensitivity) reaction**
   - ❑ This reaction usually appears 12–72 h after allergen exposure. Type IV reaction occurs when Ag provokes the clonal expansion of T lymphocytes, and a large number of cytotoxic T cells are released to eliminate the Ag. Some of the new T cells may return to the site of allergen entry into the body and result in the production of γ-interferon and activation of macrophages and tumour necrosis factor (TNF).
   - ❑ This results in the inflammatory response and this type of reaction is quite common in incompatible skin graft.

AUTOIMMUNE DISEASES

Autoimmune diseases result when the body fails to recognize its own tissues and attacks the body's own cells.

Some important autoimmune diseases are as follows:

1. **Rheumatoid arthritis**: The body produces Abs against the synovial membrane, which leads to chronic inflammation of the joints, resulting in stiff, painful and swollen joints.

2. **Greave's disease**: The body produces Abs against thyroid cells, resulting in the stimulation of the gland and hyperthyroidism.

3. **Myasthenia gravis**: It is an autoimmune disorder that occurs due to the development of Abs directed against acetylcholine receptors in the skeletal muscles. The Abs bind to and block the acetylcholine receptors and eventually block the transmission of nerve impulse. This causes progressive and extensive muscle weakness.

ACQUIRED IMMUNODEFICIENCY SYNDROME (AIDS)

It is a condition caused by the human immunodeficiency virus (HIV) and results in the progressive destruction of immune system cells, especially T lymphocytes, monocytes, macrophages and some B lymphocytes. The progressive destruction of immune system cells causes the suppression of both Ab-mediated and cell-mediated immunity with the consequent development of widespread opportunistic infections.

Some severe opportunistic infections that occur due to AIDS include the following:

1. Pneumonia, caused by pneumocystis carinii.
2. Recurrent infection of the alimentary tract, resulting in nausea, diarrhoea and weight loss
3. Meningitis and encephalitis
4. Development of malignant tumours (e.g. lymphomas of lymph nodes)

OVERVIEW OF THE BODY'S DEFENCE MECHANISMS

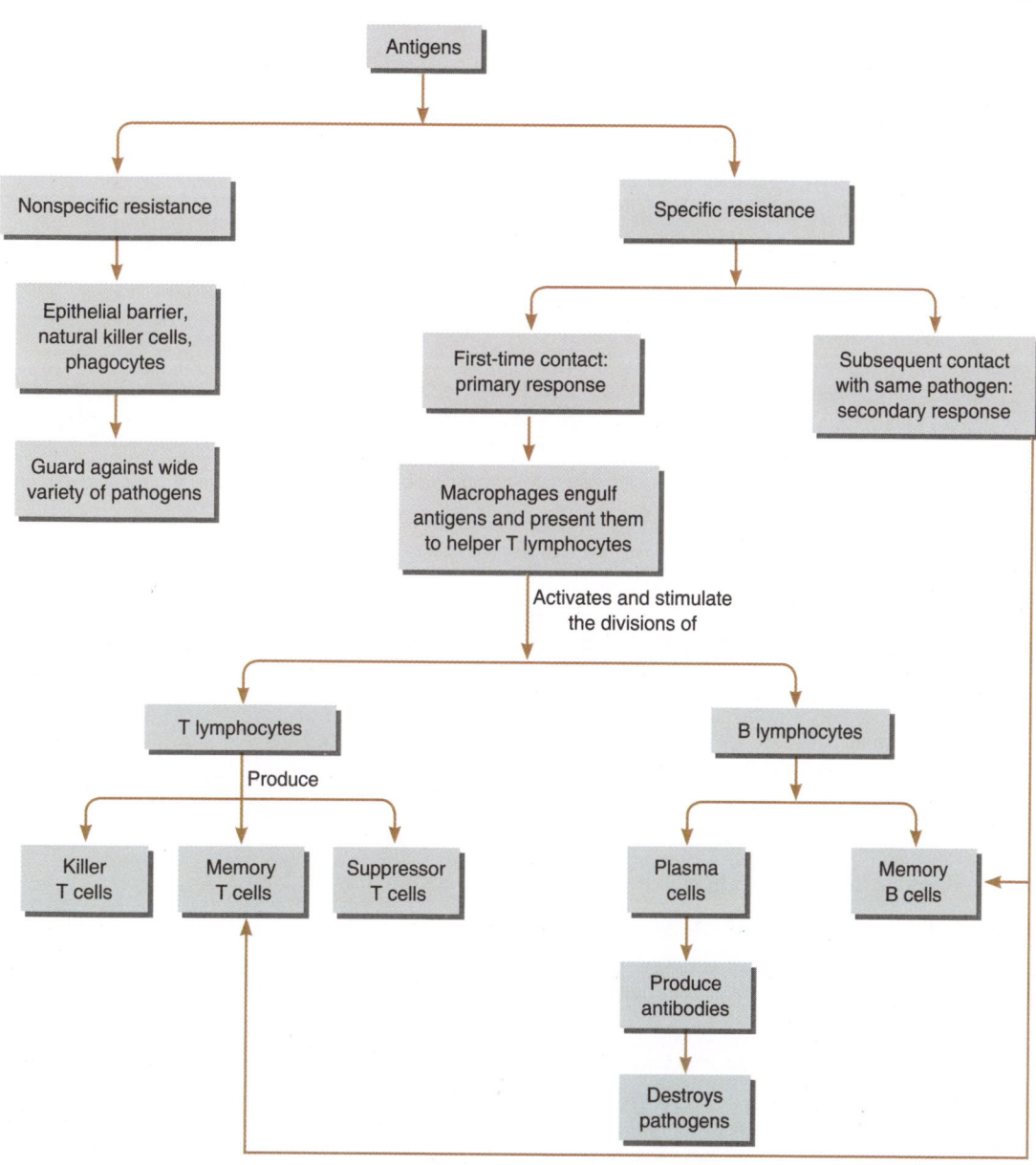

Ageing and the Immune System

❑ With age, the functional capacity of the immune system decreases. This is mainly due to decreased responsiveness of T lymphocytes towards antigens and decreased T lymphocytes production. B lymphocytes also become less responsive, which results in decreased production of antibodies in response to antigens.

❑ The elderly also tend to produce more antibodies against their body's own cells (autoantibodies), resulting in more susceptibility to autoimmune disorders. The decreased response of immune system towards cancer cells also makes the elderly more prone to many types of cancers.

❑ All these age-related changes in the immune system make the elderly more susceptible to infections.

Happiness and Health

❑ People who are happy, lively, calm or exhibit other positive emotions are less likely to become ill.

❑ Laughing lowers the levels of stress hormones and strengthens the immune system.

❑ Having 100–200 belly laughs a day is the equivalent of a high-impact workout, burning off up to 500 calories.

❑ When happy people contract a virus, or 'catch a cold', they report fewer symptoms' and it is also reported that people with strong positive attitudes about life are often able to overcome illness much quicker than people who harbour negative feelings.

❑ In addition, eating a balanced diet, regular exercise, adequate sleep and meditation have a positive effect on our health.

Review Questions

Long Answer Questions

1. Distinguish between specific and nonspecific defences against infection and describe some barriers to infection.

2. What kind of cells provides a second line of nonspecific defence if the mechanical and chemical barriers have been breached?

3. What are the two ways in which immunity can be acquired by the body?

4. Why is it important for the immune system to be able to discriminate 'self' from 'nonself' antigens?

5. What are the chemical characteristics of antibodies? Explain the various actions of antibodies.

6. What are the five main classes or isotypes of antibodies (immunoglobulins) produced by the immune system?

7. Identify the components of the immune system and describe cell-mediated immunity.

8. Describe the functions of the B and T lymphocytes.

9. Why do tissue transplant rejections occur in recipients?

10. What are autoimmune diseases? Discuss some examples of autoimmune diseases.

11. Differentiate between humoral and cell-mediated adaptive immunity.

12. Define an antibody. Using an appropriately labelled diagram, describe the structure of an antibody monomer. Indicate and label variable and constant regions, heavy and light chains.

13. Describe the specific roles of helper, regulatory and cytotoxic T cells in normal cell-mediated immunity.

Multiple Choice Questions

1. The immune system is involved in
   - (a) Destruction of abnormal or mutant cell types that arise within the body
   - (b) Allergic reactions
   - (c) Rejection of organ transplants
   - (d) All of the above

2. Active immunity is
   - (a) Borrowed from an active disease case
   - (b) Developed in direct response to a disease agent
   - (c) The product of borrowed antibodies
   - (d) Passive antibodies
   - (e) Passive immunity that is activated

3. In the cell-mediated immune response, T lymphocytes divide and secrete
   - (a) Antigens
   - (b) Plasminogens
   - (c) Collagens
   - (d) Cytokines

4. B lymphocytes are primarily involved in
   - (a) Humoral immunity
   - (b) Autoimmune disorders
   - (c) Graft rejection
   - (d) Cell-mediated immunity

5. Plasma cells are
   - (a) Responsible for specific immunity
   - (b) Derived from B cells
   - (c) Involved in the production of antibodies
   - (d) All of the above

6. Transfusing a person with blood plasma proteins from a person or animal that has been actively immunized against a specific antigen provides
   - (a) Active immunity
   - (b) Passive immunity
   - (c) Autoimmunity
   - (d) Anti-immunity

Chapter 9

7. Substances against which the body launches an immune response are called

   (a) Antibodies   (b) Antigens

   (c) Anticlines   (d) Agglutinins

8. The antibodies produced and secreted by B lymphocytes are soluble proteins called

   (a) Immunoglobulins

   (b) Immunosuppressants

   (c) Lymphokines

   (d) Histones

9. Which is the proper order of events in cell-mediated immunity?

   (a) Antigen enters tissue, macrophages engulf antigen, antigen presented to members of a clone of lymphocytes, sensitized T lymphocytes attack antigen-bearing agents

   (b) Antigen enters tissues, antigen passed to members of a clone of lymphocytes, lymphocytes sensitized, macrophages engulf antigen, T lymphocytes attack antigen-bearing agents

   (c) Antigen enters tissues, macrophages engulf antigen, antigen passed to members of a clone of lymphocytes, lymphocytes sensitized, B lymphocytes secrete antibodies that react with antigen-bearing agents

   (d) Antigen enters tissues, lymphocytes sensitized, antigen passed to members of a clone of lymphocytes, macrophages engulf antigen, T lymphocytes attack antigen-bearing agents

10. Which of the following is involved in the activation of a B cell?

   (a) Antigen

   (b) Helper T cell

   (c) Cytokine

   (d) All of the above

Match the Following

1. Helper T cells/inducer T cells	(a) Protects against bacteria and viruses by enhancing
2. Cytotoxic T cells/killer T cells	(b) Potently activates of the complement system
3. Suppressor T cells/regulatory T cells	(c) Production of cytokines and lymphokines
4. Memory T cells	(d) Destruction of infected body cells
5. IgA	(e) Suppress the activities of activated T cells and B cells
6. IgD	(f) Exist in the body for years, enabling it to respond quickly to any future infection
7. IgE	(g) Provides localized protection by preventing the Ags from crossing the epithelial membranes
8. IgG	(h) Important in B-cell activation
9. IgM	(i) Involved in allergic and hypersensitivity reactions

Chapter 9

State True or False

1. The polypeptide chains of antibodies have portions that are constant and portions that are variable.

2. It is the constant region that is responsible for binding with the antigen.

3. When antigenically stimulated, B lymphocytes proliferate and form plasma cells.

4. A person who encounters a pathogen and who has a primary immune response develops passive immunity.

5. There are five major types of immunoglobulins: IgG, IgA, IgD, IgL and IgE.

6. The interaction of antigen with antibody is highly specific.

7. Antigens are small lipid molecules that stimulate the immune response.

8. Passive immunity is the transfer of antibodies developed in one individual into the body of another.

9. T and B lymphocytes may cooperate in response to a particular antigen.

10. IgM crosses the placenta and provides a fetus with antibody protection.

10 The Respiratory System

STUDY OBJECTIVES

- ✓ To compare the structural and functional features of external and internal nose and describe the position and structure of the nasal cavities.
- ✓ To know the various functions of the nose.
- ✓ To illustrate the various anatomical regions of the pharynx and know the pattern of pharyngeal muscles.
- ✓ To know the functions of the pharynx.
- ✓ To illustrate the different laryngeal cartilages and know the various functions of the larynx.
- ✓ To illustrate the structure and functions of the trachea.
- ✓ To describe the position and functions of different air passages involved in gaseous exchange.
- ✓ To describe how respiration is carried out and explain how external and internal respiration takes place in lungs.

- ✓ To explain the anatomy of the lungs and define the role of lungs in the respiratory system.
- ✓ To explain the phases of respiration.
- ✓ To describe the various terms associated with volumes and capacities.
- ✓ To understand the various tests available to assess lung function and its significance.
- ✓ To understand the respiratory centre in the brain and to describe how the respiratory centre controls respiration.
- ✓ To know about artificial respiration and its significance in emergency.
- ✓ To know the various methods of artificial respiration.

INTRODUCTION

Respiratory system is essential to maintain homeostasis, which is achieved by the exchange of gases—oxygen (O_2) and carbon dioxide (CO_2). The oxygen present in the atmosphere enters the body through the respiratory system and is utilized in various metabolic reactions to release energy and carbon dioxide. The released carbon dioxide in tissue fluids produces acidic conditions and thus can be lethal to the cells. Hence, it is quickly eliminated out of the body into the atmosphere.

The respiratory system works efficiently in coordination with the cardiovascular system (CVS). The respiratory system accounts for the exchange of O_2 and CO_2 and the CVS for the transport of blood, which is responsible for the exchange of gases between lungs and cells of the body. If either of these systems malfunctions, the body cells will die due to deprivation of oxygen and accumulation of carbon dioxide.

❑ The trillions of cells of our body need a continuous supply of oxygen to carry out the various vital processes necessary for survival.

❑ The overall exchange of gases between the atmosphere, the blood and the cells is called *respiration*.

❑ The respiratory system consists of the organs that exchange these gases between the atmosphere and the blood.

The following organs constitute the respiratory system (Fig. 10.1):

1. Nose and nasal cavity
2. Pharynx
3. Larynx

DO YOU KNOW?

❑ The study of the respiratory system is known as *pulmonology*.

❑ The right lung is slightly larger than the left one.

❑ Hairs in the nose help clean the air we breathe besides warming it.

❑ The highest recorded sneeze speed is 165 km/h.

❑ The surface area of the lungs is roughly the same size as a tennis court.

❑ The capillaries in the lungs would extend 1600 km if placed end to end.

❑ We lose half a litre of water a day through breathing. This is the water vapour we see when we breathe onto glass.

❑ A person at rest usually breathes 12–15 times a minute.

❑ The breathing rate is faster in children and women than in men.

MEDICAL TERMINOLOGY

❑ **Adventitia**: It is the outermost layer composed of connective tissue with elastic and collagenous fibres of an artery or another structure.

❑ **Aneurysm**: It is a sac formed by localized dilatation of the wall of an artery, a vein or the heart.

❑ **Arytenoid cartilage**: It is one of the two pyramid-shaped cartilages of the larynx.

❑ **Brachiocephalic vein**: It is either of the two veins that drain blood from the head, neck and upper limbs and unite to form the superior vena cava.

❑ **Concha:** It is the structure that resembles a shell in shape.

❑ **Corniculate cartilage**: It is a nodule of cartilage at the apex of each arytenoid cartilage.

❑ **Cribriform plate:** It is the horizontal plate of the ethmoid bone that is perforated with foramina for the olfactory nerves.

❑ **Cricoid**: It is ring shaped.

❑ **Cricothyroid muscle:** It is one of the intrinsic muscles of the larynx.

❑ **Cuneiform cartilage**: It is either of a pair of cartilages, one on either side in the aryepiglottic fold.

❑ **Cyanosis**: It is a blue coloration of the skin and mucous membranes due to the presence of greater than 5 g/dL of deoxygenated haemoglobin in blood vessels near the skin surface.

❑ **Dyspnoea:** It is a condition of shortness of breath

❑ **Ethmoid**: It is the very thin bone structure of the nose, through which the ethmoid sinuses and other neural structures pass.

❑ **Goodpasture's syndrome**: It is an idiopathic autoimmune disorder most common in young white males, characterized by alveolar haemorrhage, lung infiltrates, renal failure due to rapidly progressive glomerulonephritis.

❑ **Granulomatous vasculitis:** It is disseminated visceral giant cell arteritis.

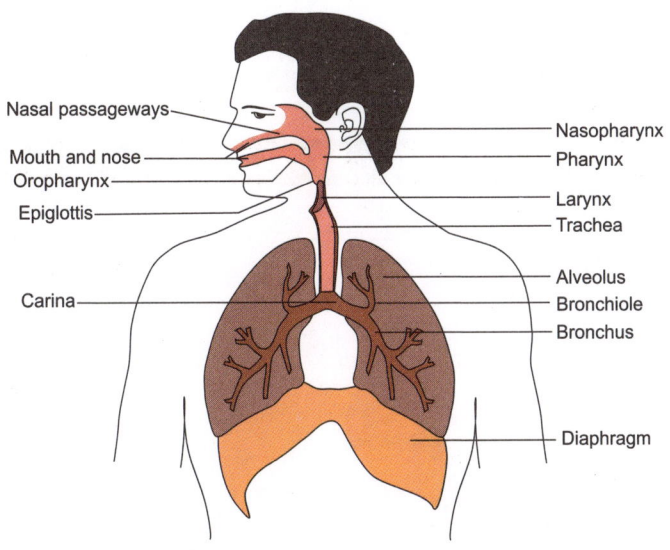

Figure 10.1 Overview of the respiratory system.

MEDICAL TERMINOLOGY

❑ **Hamulus**: It is a small hook-like projection or process as at the end of a bone.

❑ **Hyoid bone**: It is a horseshoe-shaped bone at the base of the tongue, just superior to the thyroid. cartilage.

❑ **Hypercapnia**: It is a condition where there is greater than the normal amount of carbon dioxide in the blood.

❑ **Hypoxaemia**: It is a condition where there is an abnormally low amount of oxygen in the blood.

❑ **Lamina propria**: It is a layer of connective tissue that lies just under the epithelium of the mucous membrane.

❑ **Maxilla**: It is the moustache bone formed by the fusion of two bones along the palatal fissure that forms the upper jaw.

❑ **Meatus**: It is an opening or a passage. Nasal meatus is one of the four portions (common, inferior, middle and superior) of the nasal cavity on either side of the septum.

❑ **Mediastinum**: It is a median septum or partition.

❑ **Pneumotachograph**: It is an apparatus for recording the rate of airflow to and from the lungs.

❑ **Pneumothorax**: It is a collection of air or gas in the chest or pleural space that causes part or all of a lung to collapse.

❑ **Pterygoid**: It pertains to a wing-like structure.

❑ **Pulmonary alveolar proteinosis:** It is an abnormal accumulation of surfactant within the alveoli, interfering with gas exchange.

❑ **Raphe**: It is a crease or ridge that divides an organ in half.

❑ **Sarcoidosis**: It is a disease characterized by the development of granuloma.

❑ **Sinus**: It is a sac or cavity in any organ or tissue.

❑ **Stylohyoid ligament**: It is the ligament attached to the tip of the styloid process of the temporal bone and to the lesser corner of the hyoid bone.

4. Trachea
5. Bronchi, bronchioles and alveoli
6. Lungs

ANATOMY OF THE RESPIRATORY SYSTEM

NOSE AND NASAL CAVITY

Nose is the first respiratory organ. It can be divided anatomically into the following:

❑ External nose
❑ Internal nose (Fig. 10.2)

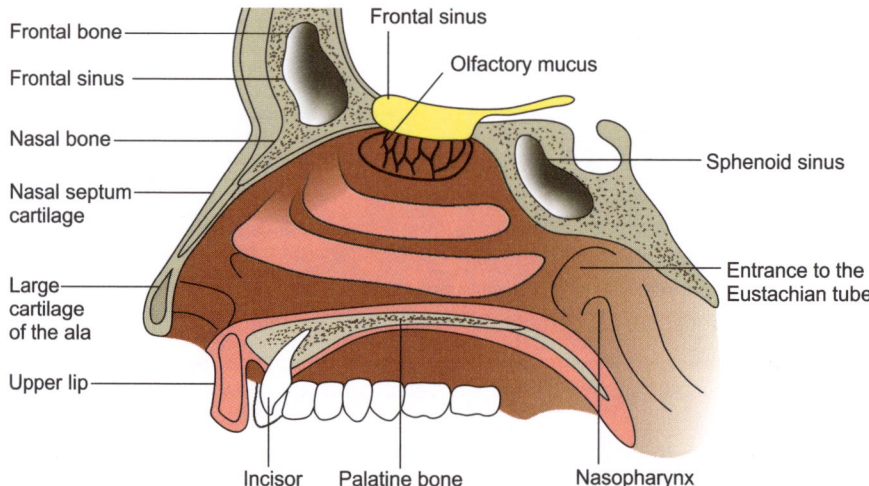

Figure 10.2 Anatomy of the nose.

External nose

It is the outer portion of the nose that appears on the face. It is formed by three bones: frontal, nasal and maxilla, and the hyaline cartilage, which consists of septal nasal cartilage, lateral nasal cartilage and alar cartilage.

❑ Skin and mucus membrane cover the hyaline cartilage.
❑ The external nose has two openings known as *nostrils* or *nares*. The anterior nares (that contain nasal hairs) open into the nasal cavity. The posterior nares open into the pharynx.

Internal nose

It is the inner large cavity present in the anterior portion of the skull. It merges posteriorly with the pharynx and anteriorly with the external nose.

❑ The **roof** of the internal nose is formed by ethmoid bone, nasal bone, sphenoid bone and frontal bone.

❏ The roof of the mouth consisting of hard and soft palates forms the floor of the internal nose. Palatine bones and maxilla form the hard palate and involuntary muscles constitute the soft palate.

❏ The lateral walls of the internal nose are composed of the following:

➤ Ethmoid bone

➤ Maxilla bones

➤ Lacrimal bones

➤ Palatine bones

➤ Inferior conchae

❏ The medial wall consists of the nasal septum, which divides the inner large cavity into two equal passages.

Lining of the nose

❏ The nose is lined with ciliated columnar epithelium containing mucus-secreting goblet cells. It serves as the opening for paranasal sinuses and nasolacrimal ducts.

❏ The paranasal sinuses are cavities in the bones of the face and the skull bones that contain air and provide a chamber of resonation for sound upon speaking or singing.

❏ Paranasal sinuses mainly include the following (Fig. 10.3):

➤ **Maxillary sinuses**: They open in the lateral walls of the internal nose.

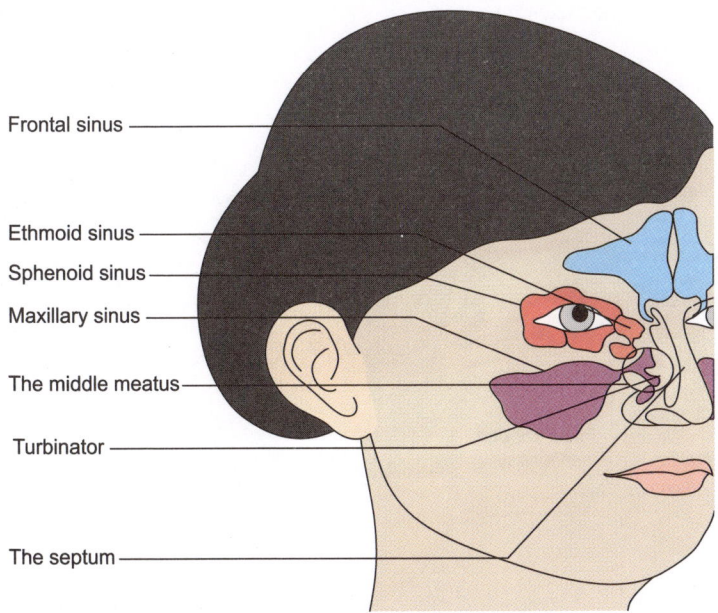

Frontal sinus

Ethmoid sinus
Sphenoid sinus
Maxillary sinus

The middle meatus

Turbinator

The septum

Figure 10.3 Sinuses and associated parts.

➤ **Frontal sinuses**: They open into the roof of the internal nose.

➤ **Sphenoidal sinuses**: They also open into the roof of the internal nose.

➤ **Ethmoid sinuses**: They open in the upper part of the lateral walls of the internal nose.

❏ The nasolacrimal ducts that serve to drain tears from the eyes extend from the nose (lateral wall of the internal nose) to the eye (conjunctiva).

The nasal cavity

It is the space in the internal nose. It is divided by the nasal septum into two equal parts.

❏ The anterior portion of the nasal septum consists of hyaline cartilage. The posterior portion of the nasal septum consists of vomer, perpendicular plate of the ethmoid bone, palatine bones and maxillae.

❏ The extension from each side of the lateral walls of the nasal cavity forms the following three shelf-like projections called *concha(e)* (Fig. 10.4):

➤ Superior nasal concha

➤ Middle nasal concha

➤ Inferior nasal concha

❏ These conchae further divide each part of the nasal cavity into three hollow passages called *meatuses*. They are as follows:

➤ Superior meatuses

➤ Middle meatuses

➤ Inferior meatuses

❏ The conchae and their cavities are lined with the mucus membrane. The surface area of the internal nose is increased by the meatuses.

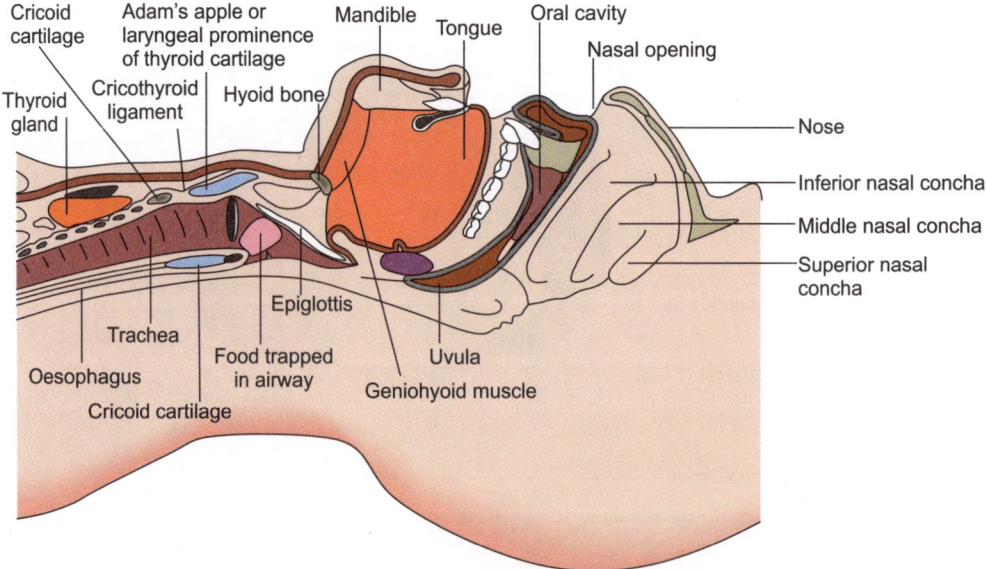

Figure 10.4 The upper respiratory tract.

Functions of the nose

The nose is a skilfully created part of the face that performs various functions, which can be divided as follows:

1. **Respiratory functions**
    (a) Breathing
    (b) Air conditioning
        ❑ Warming
        ❑ Humidification
    (c) Cleansing
2. **Nonrespiratory functions**
    (a) Smell/olfactory function
    (b) Voice

1. Respiratory functions

a. Breathing

The most important respiratory function of the nose is breathing. The two external openings, that is nares, allow the air to pass into and out of the body (act of breathing).

b. Air conditioning

As the nose acts as an interface between the internal and external environment, it performs some additional function concerned with the conditioning of the inspired air. It is achieved by humidification and warming.

Warming

Warming is an important function of the nose. It is attributed to blood vessels in the lining of the nasal mucosa. The warm blood flowing in these blood vessels provide warmth to the air.

Humidification

Humidification of the air in the nose is achieved after the inspired air comes into contact with the mucosa. It is followed subsequently by its saturation with water vapour.

c. Cleansing

The nostril hairs entrap the macroparticles, whereas the microparticles stick to the mucus. This refrains their entry and thus filters the air reaching into the lungs. Mucus performs two important functions: first it prevents drying and second it protects the epithelium from irritation. The cilia beat synchronously to thwart the mucus towards the throat where it can be expectorated out.

2. Nonrespiratory functions

a. Smell/olfactory function

Nose is the sense organ of smell (olfaction). Olfaction is detected by the olfactory receptors present on the cells called *olfactory receptor cells*. These receptors are clustered in large numbers (millions) in the superior conchae and the cribriform plate of the ethmoid bone (for more details, see the chapter Sense Organs).

b. Voice/speech

Nose plays a supportive role in speech. The resonation of air in the nose helps in providing the voice its peculiar sound. This is the reason why a person with stuffed nose sounds different from a normal person.

PHARYNX

Pharynx is a musculofacial funnel-shaped tube about 5.1 in. (about 12–15 cm long). It connects the nasal and oral cavities (head) to the larynx and oesophagus (the neck region) and serves as the common passageway for food and air.

It extends from the base of the skull and continues to the level of sixth vertebra.

The pharyngeal walls are attached anteriorly to the oral cavity, larynx and nasal cavity.

Based on this, pharynx can be *anatomically* divided into the following three regions (Fig. 10.5):

❑ Nasopharynx
❑ Oropharynx
❑ Laryngopharynx

1. Nasopharynx

❑ The nasopharynx lies at the back of the posterior conchae of the nasal cavity and above the level of the soft palate.
❑ The roof of the nasopharynx is formed by the inclining skull base and consists of sphenoid bone (posterior part) and occipital bone (basal part).

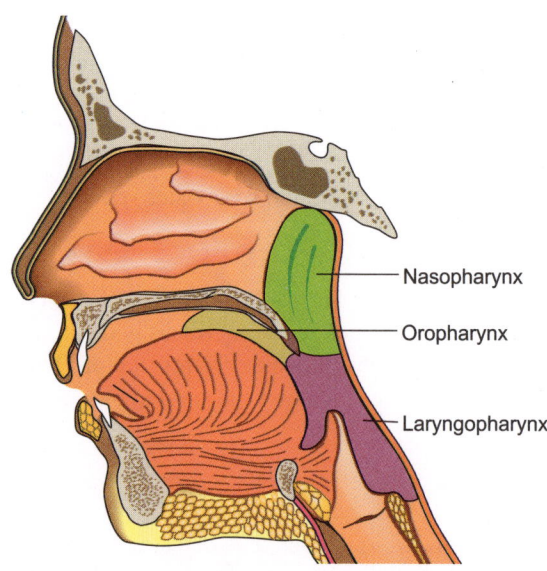

Figure 10.5 Anatomical divisions of the pharynx.

❏ The roof and lateral walls together form the hemispherical vault atop the pharyngeal cavity, which always remains open.
❏ The soft palate separates the nasopharynx from the oropharynx. The mucus membrane lines the soft palate.
❏ The lateral walls of the nasopharynx have the opening of pharyngotympanic (eustachian) tubes, two internal nares and the opening into oropharynx. The posterior wall houses the pharyngeal tonsils.

2. Oropharynx

❏ It lies posteriorly to the oral cavity, inferiorly to the soft palate and superiorly to the epiglottis (upper margin).
❏ The oropharynx has only one opening from the mouth.
❏ The oropharynx serves as the common passage for air, food and drink.

3. Laryngopharynx

❏ It extends from the oropharynx above to the oesophagus at the level of the sixth thoracic vertebrae.
❏ Anterior wall of the laryngopharynx has the opening of the laryngeal inlet. It consists of the posterior part of the larynx (Fig. 10.6).

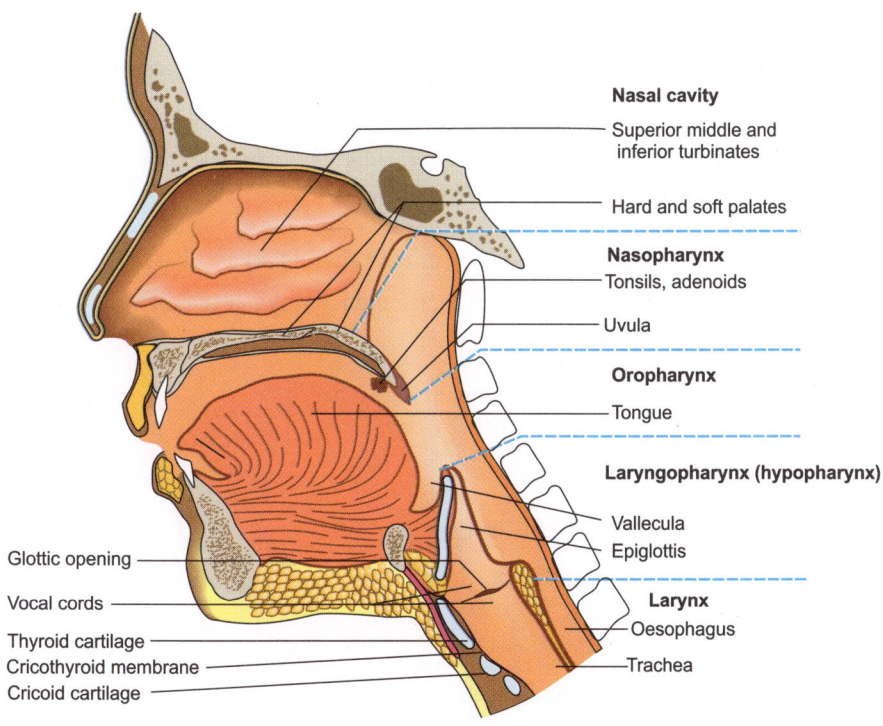

Figure 10.6 Anatomy of the pharynx and its associated parts.

Muscles

On the basis of the orientation of muscle fibre, the muscles of the pharynx can be categorized into:

❏ Constrictor muscles-mainly involved in constriction of pharynx
❏ Longitudinal muscles

Blood vessels

Arteries

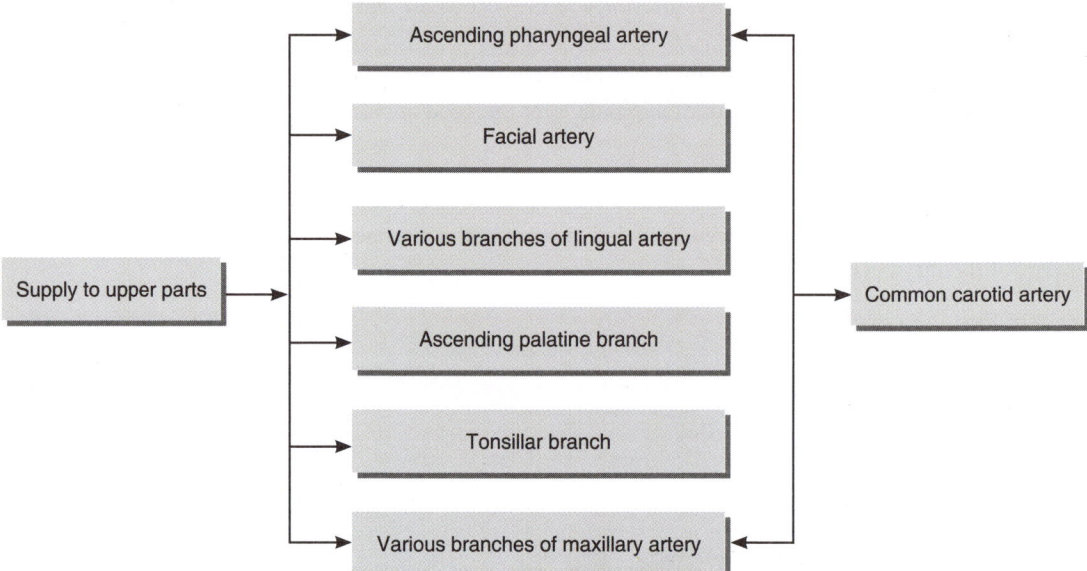

Supply to the lower part of the pharynx ⟶ inferior thyroid artery-pharyngeal branches.

Veins: Veins form the plexus, which flow into the facial and interjugular regions

Nervous supply

Parasympathetic supply ⟶ vagus glossopharyngeal nerve

Tissue layers

Pharynx is lined by the following three tissue layers:

❏ Mucus membrane
❏ Fibrous tissue
❏ Muscle tissue

Mucus membrane lining the nose continues in the nasopharynx. It is composed of ciliated columnar epithelium. Stratified squamous cells (tougher) form the mucus lining in the oropharynx and the laryngopharynx. It is continuous with the mucus lining of the oesophagus and mouth.

Fibrous tissue forms the middle layer. It is thick in the nasopharynx and becomes thin at the lower end.

Muscle tissue covers the pharynx. It is made of numerous involuntary constrictor muscles. It has an important role in deglutition (process of swallowing). As these muscles are involuntary in nature, deglutition is not under voluntary control.

Functions of the pharynx

It can be categorized into the following three main categories:

1. Digestive function
2. Respiratory function
3. Other functions
    (a) Taste
    (b) Hearing
    (c) Protection
    (d) Speech
    (e) Air conditioning

1. Digestive function

Pharynx is the organ that coordinates effectively both respiratory and digestive functions. It provides the common passageway to food and drink. It channels the food through the oropharynx and laryngeal parts without any obstruction.

The constrictor muscles present in the pharynx push the food down to the oesophagus seamlessly.

2. Respiratory function

Pharynx provides the passageway for air as well. When air enters from the nasal cavity, it passes to the nasopharynx and oropharynx. The failure of the pharynx may lead to respiratory problems.

3. Other functions

a. Taste

It is an additional function of the pharynx. The epithelium of the oral and pharyngeal parts of the larynx contains numerous olfactory nerve endings for taste.

b. Hearing

The two Eustachian tubes that open into the nasopharynx help balance the internal ear pressure. Thus, pharynx plays a role in hearing.

c. Protection

Pharynx plays a role in providing protection from infections. The tonsils (collection of lymphatic tissue) release antibodies in response to foreign substances (antigens). It is a part of the defence system of the body.

d. Speech

The pharynx provides a resonating chamber for the sound emanating from the larynx. Thus, it imparts a specific characteristic to the voice/sound.

e. Air conditioning

Pharynx humidifies and warms the inspired air.

Chapter 10

LARYNX

Larynx, also called the *voice box*, extends from cervical vertebrae 3 to 4 (C3–C6) in front of the laryngopharynx. It connects the laryngopharynx with the trachea.

Cartilages of larynx

The wall of larynx is composed of the following nine different pieces of cartilages (Fig. 10.7):

- ❏ Thyroid cartilage – 1
- ❏ Epiglottis – 1
- ❏ Cricoid – 1
- ❏ Arytenoids – 2
- ❏ Cuneiform – 2
- ❏ Corniculate – 2

All the nine cartilages are connected to one other by the intrinsic muscles of the larynx and to other structures by extrinsic muscles.

Thyroid cartilage: Thyroid cartilage is formed by the two flat pieces of hyaline cartilages. These pieces fuse together anteriorly to form the laryngeal prominence, popularly known as *Adam's apple*. It is present in both sexes, but at puberty it grows extensively in males under the influence of male sex hormones.

Epiglottis: Epiglottis is a leaf-shaped organ made of fibroelastic cartilage covered with stratified squamous epithelium. Inferiorly it is attached to the anterior portion of thyroid cartilage and hyoid

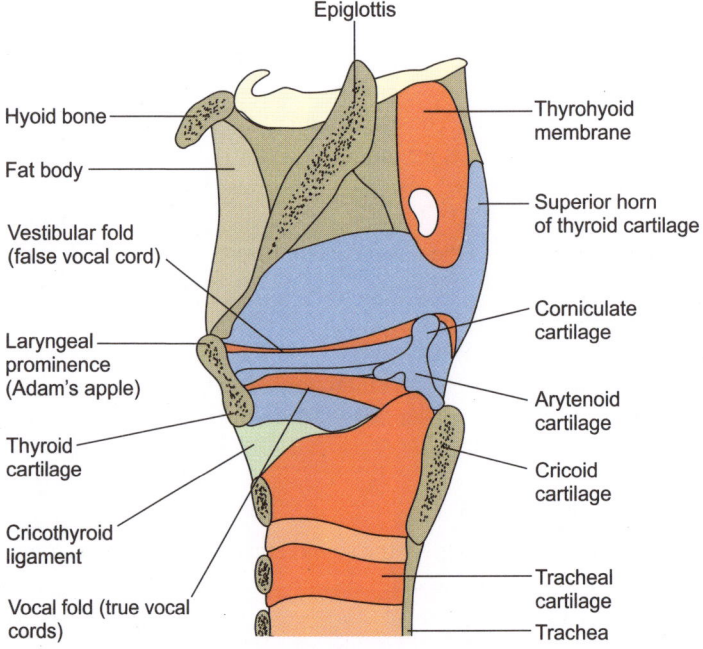

Figure 10.7 Cartilages of the larynx.

bone and superiorly it is unattached. It acts as a lid and closes the larynx during swallowing of food or drink.

Cricoid cartilage: Cricoid cartilage is a ring-shaped hyaline cartilage that forms the inferior wall of the larynx. It is joined with the first cartilage of trachea by the cricotracheal ligament and with the thyroid cartilage by the cricothyroid ligament. It is covered with ciliated columnar epithelium. The upper respiratory system ends at the cricoid cartilage of the larynx.

Arytenoid cartilages: The two arytenoid cartilages are the triangular-shaped hyaline cartilages that are positioned at the top of the cricoid cartilage. They form the posterior wall of the larynx. They are covered with ciliated columnar epithelium. They provide attachment to the vocal folds (true vocal cords). Arytenoid cartilages influence the change in position and tension of the true vocal cords.

Corniculate cartilages: These are the conical-shaped two small elastic cartilages present at the apices of the arytenoid cartilages.

Cuneiform cartilages: These are the club-shaped two fibroelastic cartilages present on the anterior side of the corniculate cartilages. They provide support to the vocal folds and epiglottis (lateral part).

Voice apparatus/voice organs

The following organs are responsible for sound/voice production (Fig. 10.8):

- ❑ Lips
- ❑ Tongue
- ❑ Teeth
- ❑ Hard palate
- ❑ Soft palate
- ❑ Uvula
- ❑ Ventricular folds (false vocal cords)
- ❑ Vocal folds (true vocal cords)
- ❑ Lungs

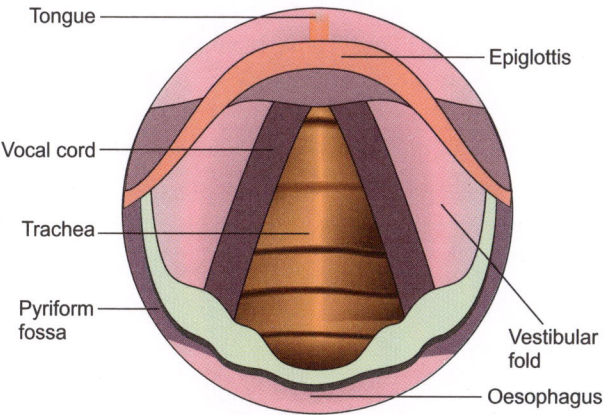

Figure 10.8 Vocal folds.

Note: Sound is not produced by the vibration of vocal cords as in the sound produced by vibrating the strings of a guitar. In fact, the changes taking place in air pressure, when a jet of air blows over through the vocal cords, produce sound.

Mechanism of voice production

The vocal cords are two pale folds of mucous membrane that extend from the inner wall of thyroid prominence anteriorly to the arytenoids cartilages posteriorly.

The intrinsic laryngeal muscles contract to bring the vocal folds together (adducted).

↓

Once the vocal folds are closed, the respiratory muscles and chest wall immediately increase the air pressure underneath the vocal folds.

↓

Finally, the pressure developing underneath the vocal folds surmounts the pressure holding them together.

↓

The air bursts out and seepages through the vocal folds (abducted).

↓

As the air quickly flows out through the vocal folds, the pressure underneath them gets decreased.

↓

This causes the vocal folds to come together again.

↓

Again the pressure underneath the vocal folds increases and the same process is repeated.

↓

Each time air passes through the vocal cords, rapid changes take place in air pressure.

↓

These changes in air pressure produce sounds used to make speech.

Blood supply

The vessels supplying blood to larynx are as follows (Fig. 10.9):

1. Superior laryngeal artery
2. Inferior laryngeal artery

The vessels draining out the blood from larynx are as follows:

1. Superior laryngeal vein
2. Inferior laryngeal vein

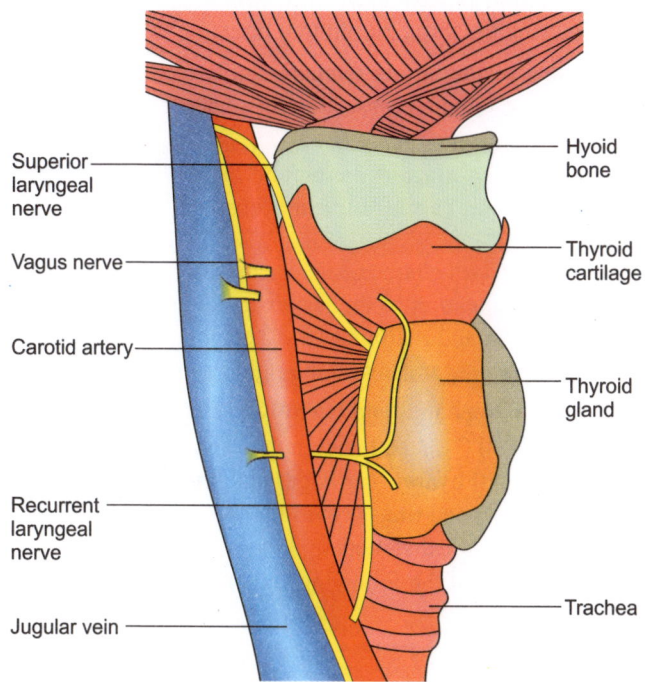

Superior laryngeal nerve

Vagus nerve

Carotid artery

Recurrent laryngeal nerve

Jugular vein

Hyoid bone

Thyroid cartilage

Thyroid gland

Trachea

Figure 10.9 Blood and nerve supply to the larynx.

Nerve supply

The larynx is innervated by two branches of vagus nerves:

1. Superior laryngeal nerve
   (a) External laryngeal nerve
   (b) Internal laryngeal nerve
2. Recurrent laryngeal nerve
   (a) Left recurrent laryngeal nerve
   (b) Right recurrent laryngeal nerve

Functions of larynx

1. **Sound production**: Larynx plays a vital role in the production of sound. The pitch of the voice depends on the tension and length of the vocal cords.

   In males, at puberty, the vocal cords become enlarged and thick. This is the reason why males have lower sound pitch than females.

2. **Voice/speech**: The sound produced by vocal cords is rigged by the tongue, cheek and lips, resulting in speech. The pitch of the voice depends on the length and tightness of the cords. Volume of the voice depends on the force with which the cords vibrate.

3. **Protection of bronchi and lungs**: A portion of the epiglottis can move freely up and down. During swallowing (deglutition), both the pharynx and the larynx rise up, causing the epiglottis to move

downwards and close the glottis (space between the vocal cords). The closing of larynx prevents food and liquids from entering the lower respiratory tract.

4. **Cleansing**: The inner lining of the larynx contains goblet cells that produce mucus. The mucus helps trap dust particles, which are not removed in the upper respiratory tract.

5. **Conditioning of air**: As air travels through the respiratory passage, its temperature and moisture content changes to maintain homeostasis.

TRACHEA

The trachea, or windpipe, is a continuation of the larynx and extends downwards to the right and left bronchi. It is a tract for passage of air and is around 10–12 cm long and 2–2.5 cm in diameter. It extends to the 5th thoracic vertebrae where it separates into the right and left bronchi (Fig. 10.10).

❑ Trachea lies posteriorly to the oesophagus and laterally to the lungs and thyroid gland.

❑ The trachea is composed of 16–20 C-shaped, incomplete and horizontal rings, positioned one above the other. The rings are made up of hyaline cartilages, and the incomplete portion of these rings lies towards the oesophagus. The C-shaped rings provide support to the walls of the trachea to prevent it from collapsing during inhalation or exhalation.

❑ The wall of the trachea is made up of the following layers (Fig. 10.11):

1. Mucosa
2. Submucosa

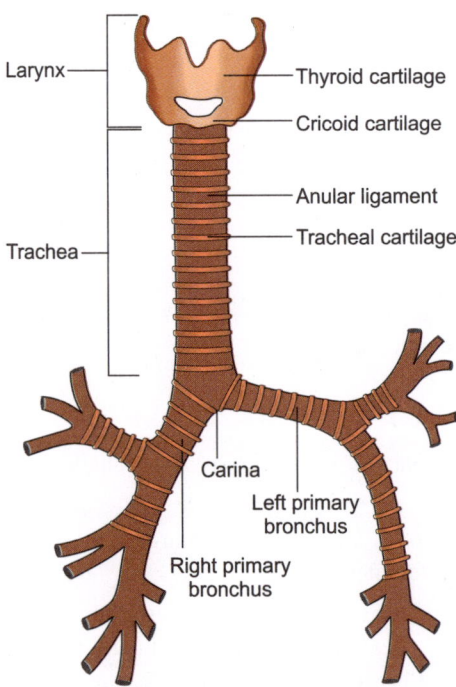

Figure 10.10 Anatomy of the trachea.

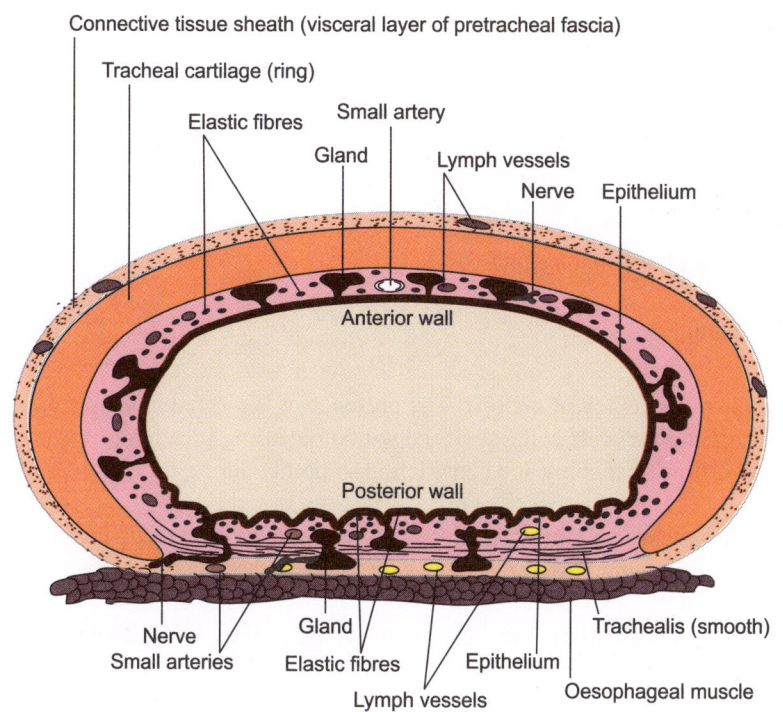

Connective tissue sheath (visceral layer of pretracheal fascia)

Tracheal cartilage (ring)

Elastic fibres   Small artery

Gland   Lymph vessels

Nerve   Epithelium

Anterior wall

Posterior wall

Nerve   Gland   Trachealis (smooth)
Small arteries   Elastic fibres   Epithelium
                    Lymph vessels   Oesophageal muscle

Figure 10.11 Cross-section of the trachea.

3. Hyaline cartilage
4. Adventitia

❏ The inner wall of the mucosal layer of the trachea is composed of ciliated columnar epithelium, consisting of goblet cells, and lamina propria, containing reticular and elastic fibres.

❏ The middle layer is the submucosal layer and the cartilaginous layer is arranged in a helical manner. The submucosal layer is made up of areolar tissue along with blood, lymph vessels and seromucous glands.

❏ The outer layer consists of a fibromuscular membrane made up of the trachealis muscle and elastic connective tissue that envelops the cartilages.

Blood supply

Arterial blood

The inferior thyroid and bronchial arteries mainly supply arterial blood.

Venous blood

The inferior thyroid veins drain venous blood into the brachiocephalic veins.

Nerve supply

Both the parasympathetic and sympathetic fibres supply the trachea. The recurrent laryngeal nerves and the vagus nerve form the parasympathetic supply, whereas the nerves from the sympathetic ganglia form the sympathetic supply.

Functions of trachea

1. Provides support and efficient airflow
2. Cleansing
3. Warming and humidification
4. Cough

1. **Provides support and efficient airflow**: The presence of C-shaped incomplete cartilaginous rings acts as a support and prevents collapse of the windpipe during breathing. It also helps prevent the obstruction of airflow by dilating and constricting smoothly during the act of swallowing and nerve stimulation.
2. **Cleansing**: The synchronous beating of the cilia present in the mucus membrane helps remove foreign particles from adhering to the mucus by pushing them upwards towards the larynx, after which it is swallowed or expectorated.
3. **Warming and humidification**: Trachea, along with the nose, tries to maintain air at the body temperature by providing efficient air conditioning (i.e. warming and humidifying).
4. **Cough**: Trachea contains nerve endings that are sensitive to irritant stimuli, which generate nerve impulses conducted by the vagus nerves to the respiratory centre in the brain. The reflex response from the brain results in deep inspiration followed by closure of the glottis, contraction of respiratory muscles and release of air under pressure, which pushes mucus and foreign particles out of the mouth.

BRONCHI, BRONCHIOLES AND ALVEOLI

Bronchi and bronchioles

The bronchi or bronchus (singular) is an airway passage in the respiratory tract, which conducts air into the lungs. The bronchi do not conduct any gaseous exchange.

The right bronchus is wider, shorter and more vertical compared with the left bronchus. The right bronchus is subdivided into three lobes, whereas the left bronchus is divided into two lobes (Fig. 10.10). The lobes are divided into segmental bronchi, also known as tertiary bronchi; each of the bronchus supplies a bronchopulmonary section, which is a division of a lung separated from the rest of the lung by a connective tissue septum. This allows the surgical removal of bronchopulmonary section without affecting other sections.

There are 10 sections per lung, but anatomical development causes several sectional bronchi in the left lung to fuse, causing 8 sections. The sectional bronchi divide into many primary bronchioles, which then divide into terminal bronchioles. The terminal bronchioles each give rise to many respiratory bronchioles, which further divide into 2–11 alveolar ducts. There are 5 or 6 alveolar sacs associated

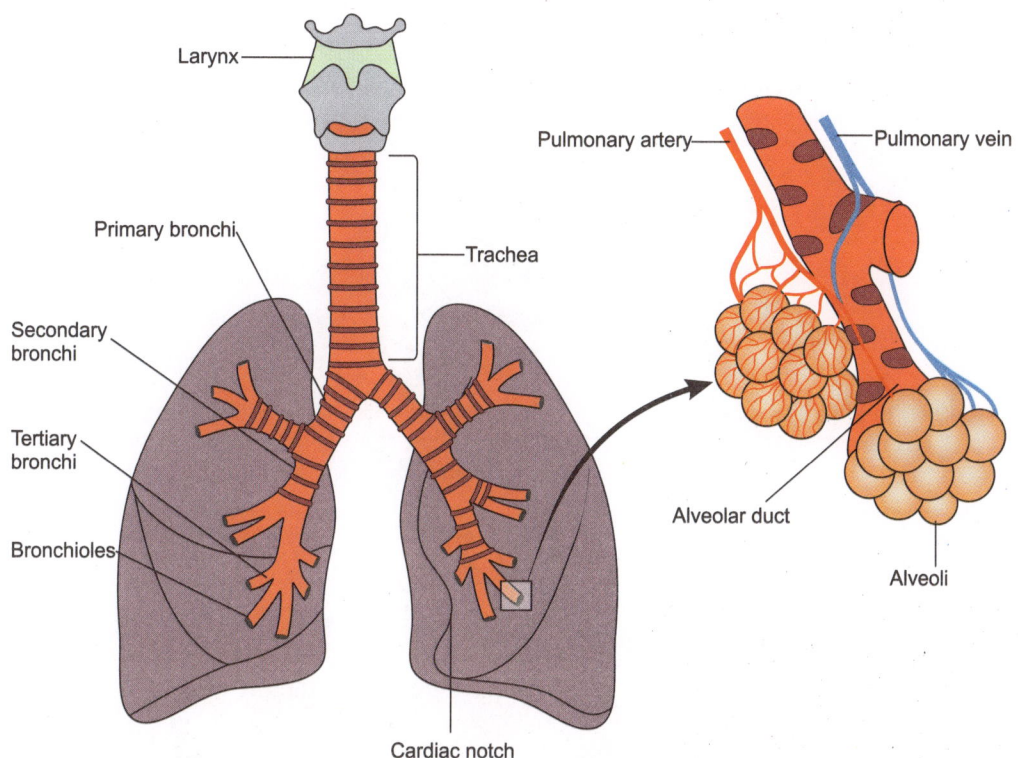

Figure 10.12 Bronchi, bronchioles and alveoli.

with each alveolar duct. The alveolus is the *basic anatomical unit of gas exchange* in the lung (Fig. 10.12).

Hyaline cartilage is associated with the bronchi, present as irregular rings in the larger bronchi and in the form of small plates and islands in the smaller bronchi. Smooth muscle is also present continuously around the bronchi. As the branching continues throughout the bronchial network, the amount of hyaline cartilage in the walls decreases until it is absent in the smallest bronchioles. As the cartilage decreases, the amount of smooth muscle increases. The mucous membrane also changes from ciliated pseudostratified columnar epithelium to simple cuboidal epithelium to simple squamous epithelium.

Alveoli

Alveoli (singular: *alveolus*) are the small air sacs in the lung where the exchange of gases takes place.

The paired human lungs contain about 600 million alveoli. The average diameter of adult alveolus is around 200–300 μm. Each alveolus is composed of the epithelial layers and the extracellular matrix surrounded by capillaries (Fig. 10.13).

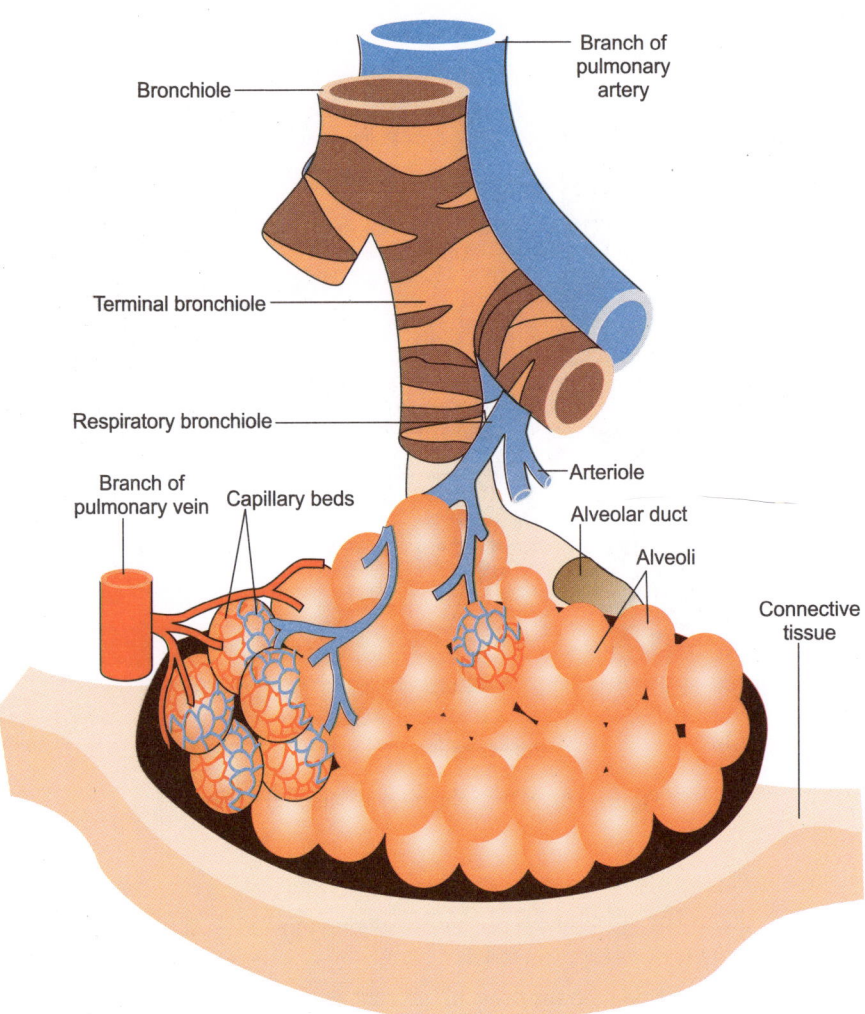

Figure 10.13 Blood supply to bronchioles and alveoli.

Alveolar cells are of the following three types:

Type I → squamous alveolar cells → form the alveolar wall structure

Type II → great alveolar cells → secrete pulmonary surfactant → to lower the surface tension of water → cause increased permeability of gaseous exchange

Type III → macrophages → kill/destroy foreign particles

During the exchange process, the blood containing carbon dioxide from all the body parts reaches the alveoli, releases carbon dioxide and takes up oxygen in the alveolar blood vessels to transport to all the body cells.

Alveoli are elastic in nature. As a person breathes in, the alveolar sacs fill up and inflate with air, whereas they spring back as a person breathes out to expel carbon dioxide.

LUNGS

Lungs are the vital organs of the respiratory system. There are two lungs, one lying on each side of the mediastinum in the thoracic cavity. They extend from the diaphragm to just superiorly to the clavicles and lie posteriorly and anteriorly against the ribs.

The lungs have the following surfaces: an apex, a base, a mediastinal surface and a costal surface.

- ❑ **Apex** is the narrow, rounded, superior portion of the lungs that rises into the base of the neck at the level of *3rd clavicle*.
- ❑ **Base** is a broad, concave, crescent-shaped inferior portion of the lungs that lies over the convex area of the diaphragm.
- ❑ **Costal surface** is a convex surface of the lungs that lies against the ribs. It is articulated with costal cartilages and intercostals muscles.
- ❑ **Mediastinal surface** is also known as medial surface. This concave surface consists of hilum at the level of 5th, 6th and 7th thoracic vertebra. It serves as a region through which the following enter and exit:
  - ➤ Bronchi
  - ➤ Pulmonary artery
  - ➤ Pulmonary vein
  - ➤ Bronchial artery
  - ➤ Bronchial vein
  - ➤ Nerves
- ❑ The left lung is smaller than the right lung as the heart occupies the space left to the midline.

Structure of the lungs

The lungs lying on each side of the mediastinum are separated by the heart, great vessels, trachea, right bronchi, left bronchi, oesophagus, lymph vessels, lymph nodes and nerves (Fig. 10.14).

Each lung is enclosed and protected by a closed sac of serous membrane called pleura. The pleura is a double-layered membrane. It consists of visceral pleura and parietal pleura.

The visceral pleura is the upper membrane that lines the wall of the thoracic cavity, whereas the parietal pleura is the inner membrane that covers the lung.

In between the two membranes of pleura, there is a cavity called the *pleural cavity* that contains a gliding thin fluid secreted by the two membranes. It lubricates and prevents friction between the two pleural membranes.

Interiorly, the lungs are composed of bronchi, bronchioles, alveoli, connective tissues, blood vessels and lymph vessels.

Both the lungs are divided into lobes. The right lung is carved into the following three different lobes: superior lobe, middle lobe and inferior lobe.

The left lung is carved into the following two different lobes: superior lobe and inferior lobe.

Each lobe consists of numerous lobules. Each lobule contains arteriole, venule and a branch from the terminal bronchiole and lymphatic vessels. Each lobule is enclosed in elastic cartilage tissue.

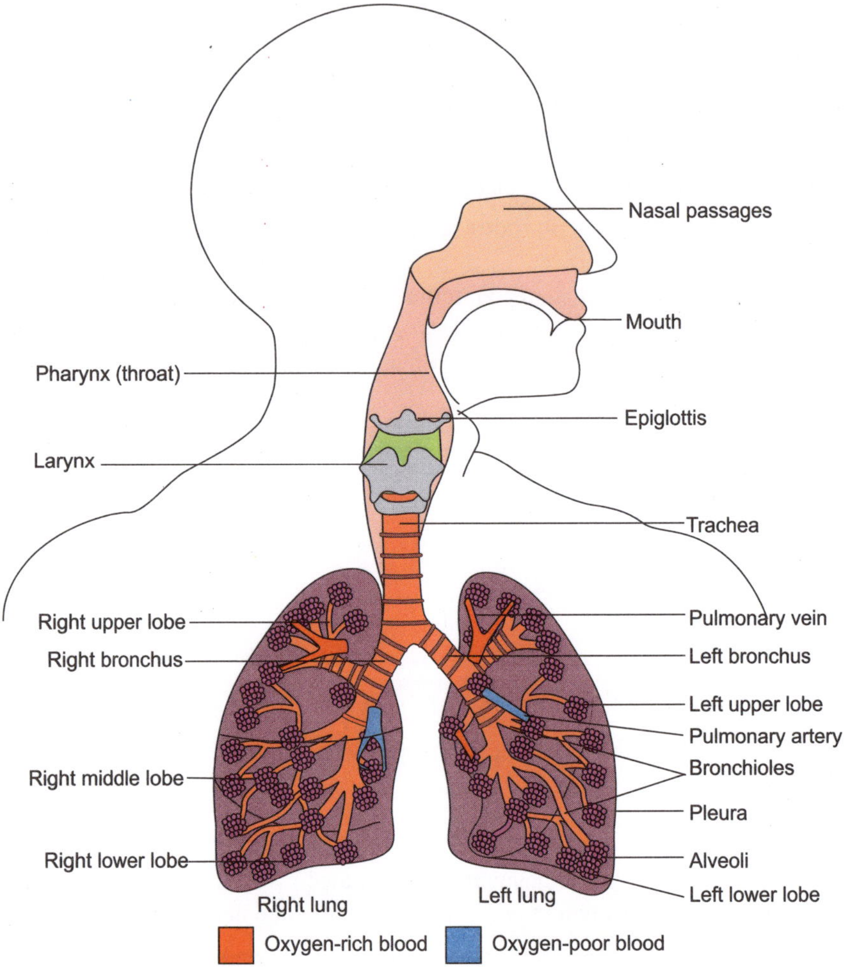

Nasal passages

Mouth

Pharynx (throat)

Epiglottis

Larynx

Trachea

Right upper lobe

Pulmonary vein

Right bronchus

Left bronchus

Left upper lobe

Pulmonary artery

Right middle lobe

Bronchioles

Pleura

Right lower lobe

Alveoli

Left lower lobe

Right lung

Left lung

Oxygen-rich blood

Oxygen-poor blood

Figure 10.14 Anatomical structure of lungs.

The terminal bronchioles further divide into respiratory bronchioles, which are microscopic branches; they in turn subdivide into various alveolar ducts.

Lung

↓

Lobes

↓

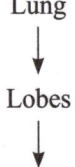

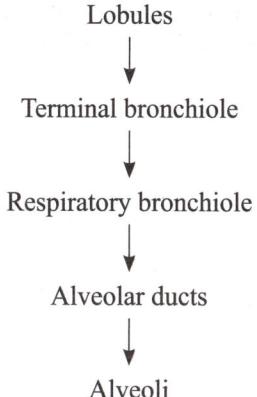

Lobules

↓

Terminal bronchiole

↓

Respiratory bronchiole

↓

Alveolar ducts

↓

Alveoli

Blood supply to lungs

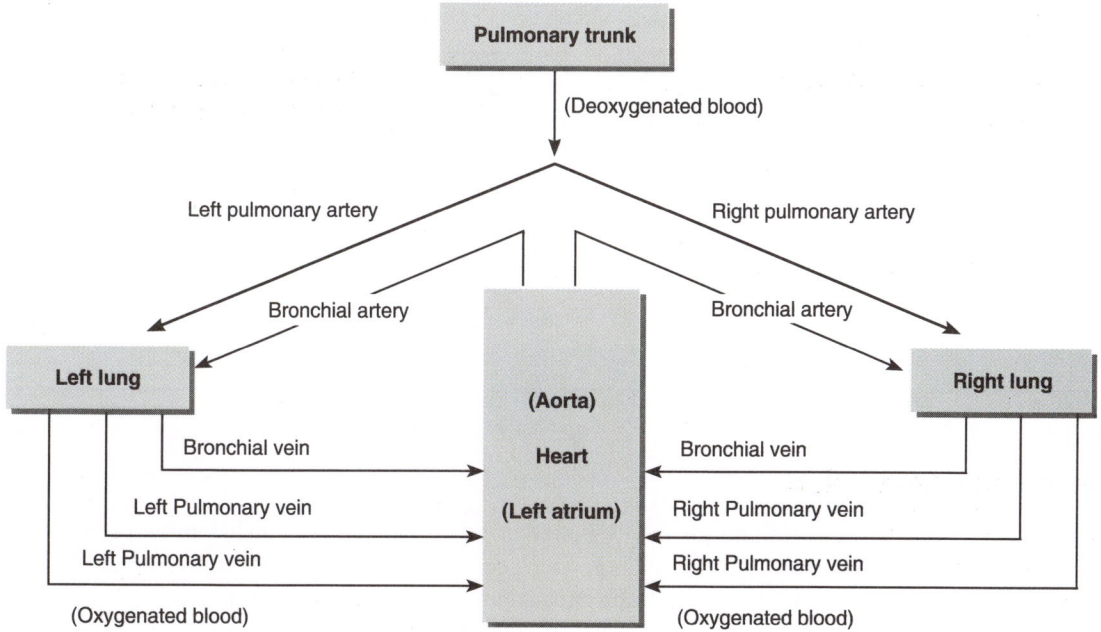

Functions of lungs

1. Support and efficient airflow
2. Cleansing
3. Warming and humidification
4. Cough

PHYSIOLOGY OF THE RESPIRATORY SYSTEM

BASIC STEPS IN RESPIRATION

In human physiology, respiration may be defined as the transport of oxygen from the atmospheric air to the cells within tissues and the transport of carbon dioxide in the opposite direction.

In human beings, respiration is carried out in the following four steps:

1. **Ventilation**: It is the movement of the enveloped air into and out of the alveoli.
2. **Pulmonary gas exchange**: It is the exchange of gases between the alveoli and the pulmonary capillaries.
3. **Gas transport**: It is the movement of gases within the pulmonary capillaries through the systemic circulation to the capillaries of various organs and then the movement of gases back to the lungs.
4. **Peripheral gas exchange**: It is the gaseous exchange between the tissue capillaries and the cells of these tissues.

Table 10.1 Oxygen consumption by the organs and muscles of the body

S. no.	Organ/muscle	Oxygen consumption (mL O_2/min per 100 g)
1.	Brain	3.0
2.	Skin	0.2
3.	Heart (at rest)	8.0
4.	Heart (during heavy exercise)	70.0
5.	Kidney	5.0
6.	Skeletal muscle (at rest)	1.0
7.	Skeletal muscle (during contraction)	50.0

Pulmonary ventilation

Pulmonary ventilation (or breathing) is the exchange of gases between the outside air and the alveoli of the lungs. Ventilation is mechanical in nature, which depends on the difference between the pressure of atmospheric air and that in the alveoli. Lung expansion and reduction in volume and inspiration and expiration of air are brought about by a dome-shaped sheet of muscle, the diaphragm, and the intercostal muscles.

Intercostal muscles

❑ There are 11 pairs of intercostals muscles that occupy the spaces between 12 pairs of ribs.
❑ The first rib is fixed. Therefore, when the intercostal muscles contract, they pull all the other ribs towards the first rib. Owing to the shape and size of the ribs, they move outwards when they are pulled upwards, thereby enlarging the thoracic cavity.

Diaphragm

❏ It is a dome-shaped muscular structure that separates the thoracic and abdominal cavities.

❏ The intercostal muscles and the diaphragm contract simultaneously, enlarging the thoracic cavity in all directions.

❏ A healthy adult person ventilates about 12–15 times per minute, but this rate changes with age, exercise, disease and other factors.

❏ Ventilation can be divided into the following classes:

1. *Minute ventilation*: It is the total volume of gas entering the lungs per minute from the outside.
2. *Alveolar ventilation*: It is the volume of gas that reaches the areas of lungs where gas exchange occurs per unit time.
3. *Dead space ventilation*: It is the volume of gas that always remains in the airways (trachea, bronchi, etc.) per unit time.

External and internal respiration

External respiration

❏ External respiration or pulmonary gas exchange is the diffusion of oxygen between the alveoli and the blood in pulmonary capillaries and the diffusion of carbon dioxide in the opposite direction.

❏ The medulla oblongata in the brain sends impulses to the central nervous system. The central nervous system relays it to the diaphragm, which pulls away from the lungs, allowing the lungs to expand. This is associated with the expansion of the trachea, sinuses and alveoli in the lungs.

❏ The alveolar wall is one-cell thick and is surrounded by many tiny capillaries through which beta haemoglobin containing carbon dioxide enters the lungs. This carbon dioxide is exchanged with oxygen in the lungs by diffusion. The oxygenated haemoglobin is called alpha haemoglobin.

❏ The slow flow of blood through the capillaries increases the time available for the gas exchange to occur.

❏ The oxygen and carbon dioxide concentrations when the blood leaves the capillaries remain in equilibrium with that of alveolar air.

Internal respiration

❏ Internal respiration or systemic gas exchange is the process by which the gases in the air that have already been drawn into the lungs by external respiration are exchanged with gases in the blood or tissues to remove carbon dioxide from the blood and replace it with oxygen. Thus, it is the exchange of gases by diffusion between blood capillaries and cells of the tissues (Fig. 10.15).

❏ Internal respiration is the gas exchange down the concentration gradient.

❏ The oxygen-containing alpha-haemoglobin cells diffuse through the veins and capillaries of organs, muscle cells and skin cells. When an oxygen molecule binds to an alpha cell's binding site, it interacts causing the iron molecule in the cell to change its shape, exposing a new binding site. Carbon dioxide molecule connects to these binding sites, breaking the bonds of the oxygen molecules. The body cells then take in oxygen molecules and the alpha cells turn into beta cells, which again return back to the lungs to continue the cycle.

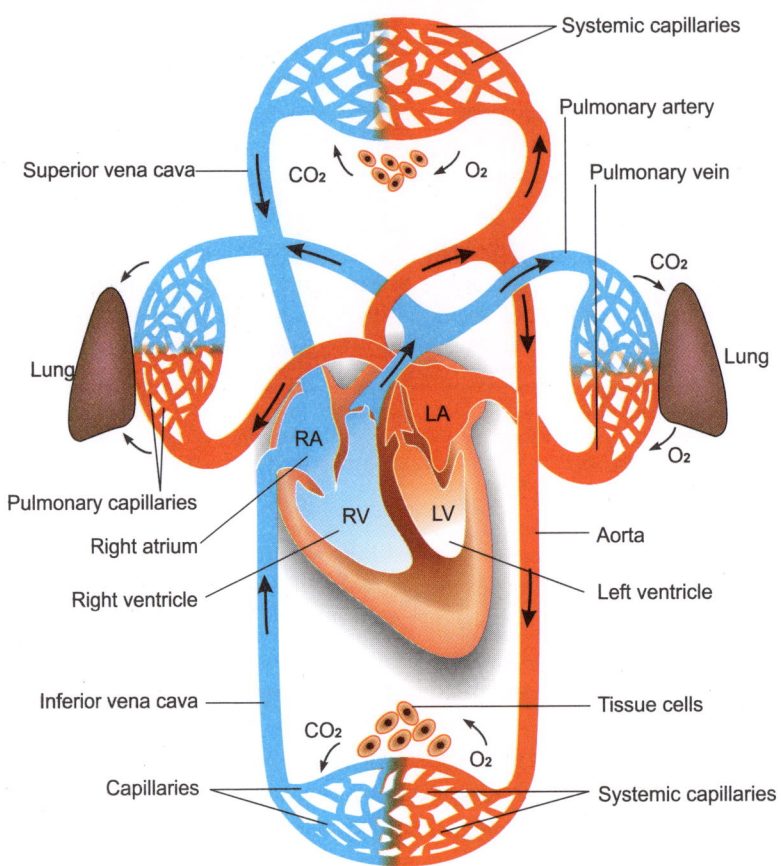

Figure 10.15 Gas exchange between the lungs and heart.

CYCLE OF RESPIRATION

A cycle of respiration occurs 12–18 times per minute and it consists of the following three phases: inspiration, expiration and pause.

The lungs can *ex*pand and contract by the following two ways:

1. By downward and upward movement of the diaphragm, to lengthen or shorten the chest cavity.
2. By upward and downward movement of the ribcage, to increase or decrease the diameter of the chest cavity.

Normal quiet breathing, that is eupnŏea, occurs mainly by the movement of the diaphragm.

Inspiration

❑ During inspiration, the intercostal muscles and diaphragm contract, which descends the diaphragm and raises the rib cage outwards.

❑ Thus, the volume of the thoracic cavity increases and the lung stretches.

❑ The intrapulmonary volume increases as well, which causes the intrapulmonary pressure to drop below the atmospheric pressure. The pressure within the alveoli and in the airways also reduces, so that air starts flowing into the lungs until the intrapulmonary pressure becomes equal to the atmospheric pressure.

❏ The process of inspiration requires energy for muscle contraction and thus it is an active process.

❏ At resting condition, inspiration lasts for about 2 s.

The process of inspiration can be divided into the following three parts:

1. **Compliance work/elastic work** is the expansion of the lungs against the lung and chest elastic forces.
2. **Tissue resistance work** is the work required to overcome the viscosity of the lungs and chest wall structures.
3. **Airway resistance work** is the work required to overcome resistance for movement of air into the lungs.

Expiration

❏ During expiration, the intercostal muscles relax, the diaphragm moves upward and the ribcage descends down (Fig. 10.16).

❏ The volume of the thoracic cavity decreases, thereby enabling the lungs and chest wall to recoil, and the intrapulmonary volume also decreases. This causes a rise in intrapulmonary pressure, and the air starts moving out of the lungs until the intrapulmonary pressure becomes equal to the atmospheric pressure.

❏ During heavy breathing, the elastic recoil of the lungs is not enough to cause necessary expiration; this required force is provided by the contraction of the abdominal muscles.

❏ Expiration is thus a passive process caused by elastic recoil of the lungs and chest wall. Therefore, under resting conditions, the respiratory muscles work to cause inspiration and not expiration.

❏ At resting condition, expiration lasts for about 3 s.

After expiration, a pause or gap is maintained until the new respiratory cycle starts.

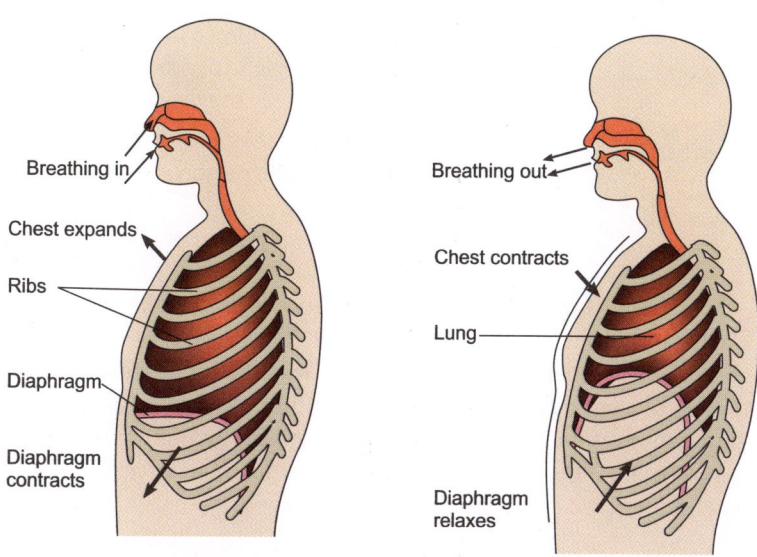

Figure 10.16 Inspiration (breathing in) and expiration (breathing out).

LUNG VOLUMES AND CAPACITIES

Pulmonary function tests are useful to assess the functional status of the respiratory system both in physiological and in pathological conditions.

The pulmonary function tests include the evaluation of lung volumes and lung capacities.

Lung volumes can be measured directly by various methods while lung capacities can only be deduced from lung volumes (Fig. 10.17).

Usually, a normal healthy human breathes around 12–15 times per minute. An adult healthy human male has a total lung capacity of about 6 L of air, but the total amount is not used during normal breathing.

In mammals, the mechanism of breathing is known as *tidal breathing*, which represents the volume of air that is inhaled and exhaled in normal, resting breathing.

At the end of a forced respiration, the air within the lung can be divided into four parts or lung volumes, the summation of which is equal to the maximum volume of the lungs up to which it can be expanded. The significance of each of these volumes is given in Table 10.2.

Table 10.2 Components of lung volume

Measurement	Value (male/female)	Description
Tidal volume (V_t)	500/390 mL	It is the amount of air that is breathed in and out of the lungs during each cycle of breathing.
Residual volume (RV)	1.2/0.93 L	It is the volume of air left in the lungs after a maximal forced exhalation (it always remains in the lungs and cannot be expired out).
Expiratory reserve volume (ERV)	1.2/0.9 L	It is the maximum amount of air that can be expelled from the lungs during maximal expiration. (After a normal breath, the lungs contain the residual volume and the expiratory reserve volume. If a person then exhales maximum, only the residual volume of 1.2 L remains).
Inspiratory reserve volume (IRV)	3.0/2.3 L	It is the extra volume of air that can be inspired over and above the normal tidal volume when a person inspires with total force.

V_t is the tidal volume.

Note: A person who lives in high altitude or mountain region will have a higher lung capacity than one who is born and brought up in the sea level. This is due to the lower partial pressure of oxygen at high altitudes because of which oxygen less readily diffuses into the bloodstream. The diffusing capacity of the body increases in high altitudes to process more air. A person may develop a condition called *altitude sickness* when somebody living at sea level travels to high-altitude locations. It is because the lungs cannot take in sufficient oxygen but they remove adequate quantity of carbon dioxide.

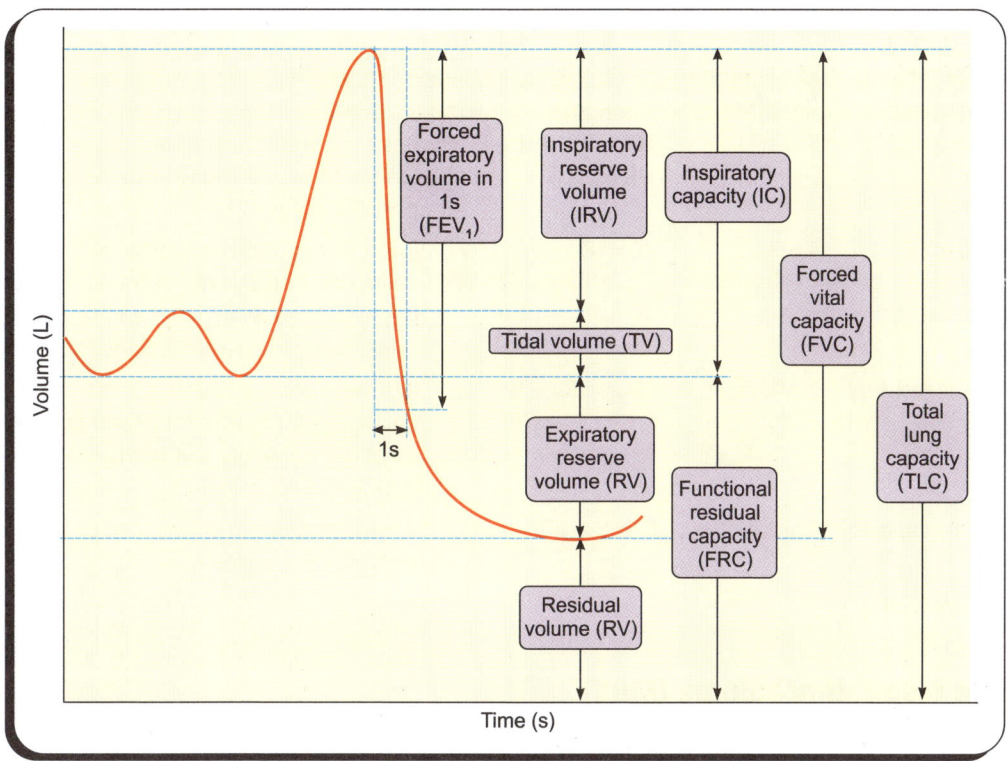

Figure 10.17 Lung volumes and capacities.

In describing the events in pulmonary cycle, it is sometimes required to consider two or more of the volumes together. Such combinations are called *lung capacities*.

The important lung capacities are described in Table 10.3.

Forced vital capacity (FVC) can be expressed as a series of volumes in specific time intervals. The amount of air exhaled in the first second of the FVC manoeuvre is known as the *forced expiratory volume in the first second of expiration* (FEV_1). It can provide information on obstruction of the airways as it is measured over a definite time interval.

FEV_1 depends on the amount of air in the lung and the effort given during exhalation and it is decreased by a diminution in TLC or due to less effort.

Another way to measure obstruction is to express it in a ratio of FEV_1/FVC. It does not depend on the person's size and TLC, and thus can be specifically used to measure obstruction of the respiratory tract. Usually, this ratio is around $\geq 75\%$ and a value less than 75% indicates obstruction.

These values vary with the age and height of the person and also have significant ethnic and racial variations. The tidal volume, vital capacity, inspiratory capacity and expiratory reserve volume can be measured with a spirometer. These are the basic parts of a ventilatory pulmonary function tests.

Chapter 10

Table 10.3 Different lung capacities

Measurement	Value (male/female)	Calculation	Description
Total lung capacity (TLC)	5.8/4.7 L	TLC = IRV + V_t + ERV + RV	It is the maximum volume to which the lungs can be expanded with the most possible effort.
Vital capacity (VC)	4.6/3.6 L	VC = IRV + V_t + ERV	It is the maximum volume of air that can be moved into and out of the lungs. When it is measured on a forced expiration, it is called the *forced vital capacity* (FVC).
Functional residual capacity (FRC)	2.4/1.9 L	FRC = ERV + RV	It is the amount of air that is left in the air passages and alveoli at the end of normal quiet breathing (it stays in the lungs during normal breathing).
Inspiratory capacity (IC)	3.5/2.7 L	IC = V_t + IRV	It is the amount of air that can be inspired with maximum effort.

V_t is the tidal volume.

Minute respiratory volume (MRV)

❏ It is the total volume of air inhaled and exhaled each minute.
❏ It is equal to the tidal volume multiplied by the respiratory rate per minute. The normal tidal volume is around 500 mL, and the normal respiratory rate is about 12 breaths per min. Hence, the minute respiratory volume is around 6 L/min approximately.
❏ A human being can stay alive for a short time with a minute respiratory volume of 1.5 L/min and a respiratory rate of around 3–4 breaths per minute.

Dead space

❏ It is the volume of the respiratory system that does not participate in gaseous exchange, which is approximately 300 mL in normal lungs.
❏ **Anatomic dead space**: It is the volume of the conducting airways with air that does not participate in gaseous exchange, and it equals to around 150 mL.
❏ **Physiological dead space**: It is the volume of the lung that does not participate in gaseous exchange. In normal lungs it is the same as the anatomic dead space (150 mL); however, it may be greater in lung disorders.

Alveolar ventilation

❏ The aim of pulmonary ventilation is to renew the air in the gas exchange areas of the lungs, where air is in proximity to the pulmonary blood, which includes the alveoli, alveolar sacs, alveolar ducts and bronchioles.
❏ The rate at which new and fresh air reaches these areas is called *alveolar ventilation*. In other words, it is the volume of air that moves into and out of the alveoli per minute.

❑ It is a major factor in determining the concentration of oxygen and carbon dioxide in the alveoli.

❑ Thus, mathematically it can be represented by the following equation:

$$V_a = F(V_t - V_d)$$

where V_a is the alveolar ventilation per minute, F the frequency of respiration per minute, V_t the tidal volume and V_d the volume of physiologic dead space

If the normal tidal volume is 500 mL, physiologic dead space volume is 150 mL and respiratory rate is 12 breaths per minute, then alveolar ventilation equals $12 \times (500 - 150)$, that is, 4200 mL/min.

PULMONARY FUNCTION TESTS

Pulmonary function tests are a set of procedures used to determine the efficiency of lungs in terms of its intake and release of air and the way they exchange gases like oxygen between the atmosphere and the body's circulation.

The tests can measure the cause of shortness of breath and help confirm lung disorders such as asthma, bronchitis or emphysema. The tests can also be performed before any lung surgery to ensure the person would not have a reduced lung capacity.

Purpose of pulmonary function tests

Pulmonary function tests are carried out for the following:

1. To evaluate signs and symptoms of lung disease (e.g. dyspnoea, cough, wheezing, cyanosis, hypoxaemia, hypercapnia).
2. To measure the current stage of the disease and to evaluate its progress.
3. To assess how a patient is responding to different treatments.
4. To screen the people who are at risk of pulmonary disease like smokers or people with occupational exposure to toxic substances.
5. To determine the patient's condition before surgery to assess the risk of respiratory complications after surgery.
6. To determine how much a patient's airways have narrowed due to disorders.

Precautions: Pulmonary function tests are contraindicated in patients without any symptoms, or who have had a recent heart attack or who have certain types of other cardiovascular diseases.

Components of pulmonary function tests

❑ Spirometry
❑ Diffusing capacity (DLCO)
❑ Residual volume, total lung capacity

Spirometry

❑ Spirometry (the measuring of breath) measures the mechanical function of the lung, chest wall and respiratory muscles by determining the total volume of air exhaled from a full lung (total lung capacity) as compared to an empty lung (residual volume).

❑ It is measured by a simple instrument called spirometer.

❑ It is useful for generating pneumotachographs, which can be helpful in evaluating conditions such as dyspnoea, pulmonary fibrosis, asthma, chronic obstructive pulmonary disease (COPD), cystic fibrosis and also operative risks.

Chapter 10

- ❏ Relative contraindications for spirometry testing include pneumothorax, angina pectoris, myocardial infarction, thoracic and abdominal aneurysms, eye surgery or patients with a history of syncope.
- ❏ Spirometry is a convenient noninvasive procedure that requires the patient to inhale deeply, after all air has been expelled out. This manoeuvre is followed by a rapid exhalation to exhaust all the air from the lungs.
- ❏ In spirometry, the common parameters evaluated include vital capacity (VC); forced vital capacity (FVC); forced expiratory volume (FEV) at time intervals of 0.5, 1.0, 2.0 and 3.0 s; forced expiratory flow 25–75% (FEF 25–75) and maximal voluntary ventilation (MVV) (Fig. 10.18).
- ❏ Results can be given in raw data (litres, litres per second), and the percentage is used to predict for the patients of similar characteristics based on height, age, sex and weight.

Some terms associated with spirometry tests

- ❏ **FEV1/FVC ratio (FEV1%)**: It is the ratio of FEV1 to FVC, and in healthy adults it is usually around 75–80%. In obstructive diseases such as asthma, COPD and chronic bronchitis, the value is reduced, while in restrictive diseases such as pulmonary fibrosis, the value may be normal or increased.
- ❏ **Forced expiratory flow (FEF) 25–75% or 25–50%**: It is the average speed of air that is expelled out of the lung during the middle portion of the expiration. It is expressed in litres per second and indicates the condition in the lower respiratory tract. It also acts as an early warning sign of airway disease and in diseases such as asthma, the value will be reduced.
- ❏ **Forced inspiratory flow (FIF) 25–75% or 25–50%**: It is similar to FEF 25–75% or 25–50% and its measurement is taken during inspiration.

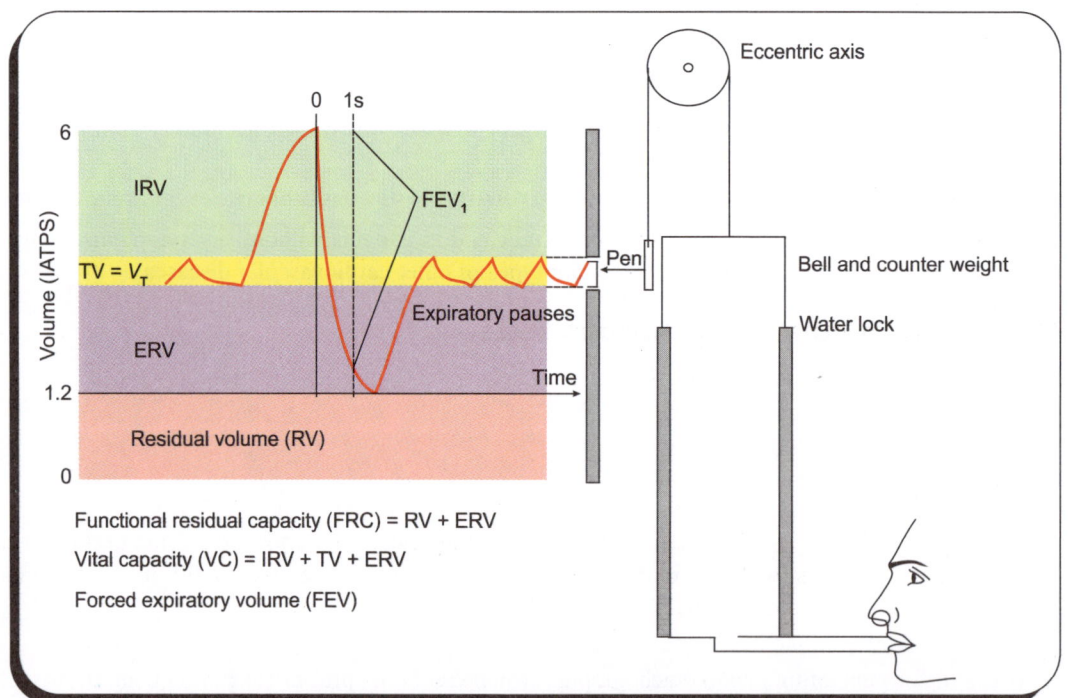

Figure 10.18 Spirometry graph.

- **Peak expiratory flow (PEF)**: It is the maximum speed of air achieved during the maximally forced expiration after full inspiration.
- **Maximum voluntary ventilation (MVV)**: It is an evaluation of the maximum amount of air that can be inhaled and exhaled per minute, expressed in litres per minute.

Table 10.4 Patterns of lung function in obstructive and restrictive lung diseases

Parameters	Asthma	COPD	Parenchymal disease
FVC	No or In	No or In	De
FEV1	De	De	De
FEV1/FVC	<75%	<75%	≥75%
TLC	No or In	No or In	De
RV/TLC	No or In	No or In	No
Airway resistance	In	In	No
DLCO	No	De	De

No = Normal; In = Increased; De = Decreased

Diffusing capacity (DLCO)

- DLCO is a measure of the ability of the lungs to transfer gas. It is the amount of carbon monoxide uptake from a single inspiration in a specified time (generally 10 s).
- The gas used to test the diffusing capacity must be more soluble in blood than in lung tissue. Also, the gas must ardently bind to haemoglobin. As carbon monoxide meets these requirements, it is most preferred for DLCO evaluation.
- The value is decreased in conditions that:
  - ➤ Minimize the ability of blood to bind to the diffusing gas such as anaemia.
  - ➤ Decrease the surface area of the alveolar-capillary membrane such as emphysema and pulmonary embolism.
  - ➤ Alter the cell membrane permeability such as pulmonary fibrosis.

Residual volume and total lung capacity

- The residual volume, and thus the total lung capacity, cannot be measured by spirometry.
- They are measured by specific tests in which an inert gas like helium is breathed in or to sit in an airtight place in which the pressure is measured as the person breathes. These measurements are called *static lung volumes*.
- For obstructive lung diseases, measurement of these two parameters can provide evidence on air trapping and hyperinflation.
- For restrictive diseases, the total lung capacity can confirm the degree of restriction.

BREATHING PATTERNS AND MODIFIED RESPIRATORY MOVEMENTS

Eupnoea (Greek; *eu*: well and *noia*: breath) is a term in the human respiratory system for normal, good and unlaboured breathing. It is also known as *quiet breathing* or *resting respiration*. It may consist of shallow and deep breathing, in which expiration employs the recoil of the lungs.

Chapter 10

In other conditions, *apnoea* is transient cessation of respiration, while *dyspnoea* is laboured respiration.

There are two main types of breathing: *costal* (meaning 'of the ribs') or chest breathing, and *diaphragmatic,* abdominal or belly breathing. Only when a person breathes forcefully or in maximum, a third type is used, called clavicular breathing.

Costal breathing or chest breathing

❑ Costal breathing is characterized by an outwards, upwards movement of the chest wall.
❑ In chest breathing, the expansion is centred at the midpoint and thus it aerates mostly the midportion of the lung.
❑ Chest breathing requires more effort in lifting the ribcage, and thus the body has to work harder to achieve the same blood gas mixing as with diaphragmatic breathing.
❑ Chest breathing is useful during exercise but it is inappropriate for normal, day-to-day activity. Since this breathing is associated with fight or flight response of an individual, it may be linked to symptoms of arousal like tension and anxiety. In chest breathing, the breath is generally shallow and jerky, resulting in unsteadiness of the mind.

Diaphragmatic breathing

❑ The principal muscle involved in diaphragmatic or abdominal breathing is the diaphragm, a dome-shaped sheet of muscle that separates the chest cavity from the abdomen.
❑ It is a type of breathing carried out by breathing deep into one's lungs using the diaphragm rather than by using the rib cage.
❑ When a person breathes in, the diaphragm contracts and pushes downwards, causing the abdominal muscles to relax and rise. This causes the lungs to expand and create a partial vacuum, which allows air to be drawn in. When breathing out, the diaphragm relaxes, the abdominal muscles contract and air is expelled.
❑ Of the two major types of breathing, diaphragmatic breathing is more efficient because greater expansion and ventilation occur in the lower part of the lung where blood perfusion is the highest.
❑ Diaphragmatic breathing in association with physical and mental relaxation can reduce high blood pressure, anxiety disorders and stuttering. It promotes a natural, even movement of breath, which provides strength to the nervous system and relaxes the body.

Clavicular breathing

❑ This type of breathing is significant only when maximum air or oxygen is required. The name is derived from the two collar bones or clavicles, which are pulled up slightly at the end of maximum inhalation, expanding the top of lungs.
❑ This type of breathing is usually seen in patients with asthma or chronic bronchitis.

Respiration is also associated with human emotions such as laughing, crying, sobbing and sighing. It can be used to remove foreign matter from the lower part of the airways through coughing and sneezing. All these modified respiratory movements are reflexes, but some of them can be controlled voluntarily. The modified respiratory movements include the following:

1. **Sneezing**: It is the spasmodic contraction of the muscles that helps expel air forcefully through the nose and mouth. Its function is to expel mucus containing foreign particles or external stimulants and thus clean the nasal cavity. During sneezing, the uvula and soft palate lowers down while the

back of the tongue elevates to partially close the mouth passage so that the air ejected out from the lungs can be expelled from the nose.

2. **Coughing**: It is an act of sudden and sometimes repetitively occurring reflex, which is useful in clearing the breathing passages from foreign particles, irritants, secretions and microbial organisms. Coughing may occur voluntarily or involuntarily and consists of three phases: a long and deep inhalation, a strong exhalation against a closed glottis and a violent release of air following opening of the glottis through the upper respiratory passages, which is generally accompanied by a distinct sound.

3. **Yawning**: It is a reflex and deep simultaneous inhalation of air and stretching of the eardrums, followed by exhalation of breath. It causes depression of the mandible and is usually associated with tiredness, boredom, stress and lack of stimulation. The cause for yawning is unknown.

4. **Sighing**: It is a long and deep inhalation simultaneously followed by a short, audible and forceful exhalation of air arising from emotional changes and tiredness.

5. **Crying**: It is a secretomotor phenomenon characterized by the shedding of tears from the lacrimal gland, without any irritation of the ocular parts. It is an emotional state in humans where an inhalation is usually followed by short convulsive exhalations during which the glottis remains open.

6. **Sobbing**: It is a convulsive gasping while weeping aloud so that a series of convulsive inhalations is followed by a single relatively long exhalation.

7. **Laughing**: It is an audible expression or feeling of joy and happiness, and includes the same basic movements as crying. Anatomically, it is caused when the epiglottis constricts the larynx. It may start from a joke, tickling sensation or other external stimuli.

8. **Hiccupping**: It is an involuntary spasmodic contraction of the diaphragm that usually repeats several times in a minute. It produces a sharp 'hic' sound on inhalation, when a sudden rush of air into the lungs causes the closure of the epiglottis. It may be caused by central and peripheral nervous system disorders, and it is known in medical terminology as *synchronous diaphragmatic flutter (SDF)* or *singultus*.

9. **Valsalva manoeuvre**: It is a forced exhalation against a closed rima glottidis, during periods of straining, by closing one's mouth and pinching one's nose shut. It has four phases of physiological response: initial rise in blood pressure, reduction in venous return and compensation to the heart, release of pressure on the chest and return of cardiac output.

TRANSPORT OF OXYGEN AND CARBON DIOXIDE IN THE BLOODSTREAM

Composition of air

Alveolar air

The composition of atmospheric air and alveolar air differs from each other. Alveolar air contains higher concentration of carbon dioxide and less oxygen and is saturated with water vapour. External respiration, that is gas exchange between the alveoli and the blood stream, does not depend on the respiratory cycle, as it is a continuous process. During each inspiration, only some of the alveolar gases are exchanged.

Expired air

Expired air consists mainly of oxygen, carbon dioxide, nitrogen and water vapour. It is a mixture of alveolar air and atmospheric air. Its composition at sea level is given in Table 10.5.

Table 10.5 Composition of atmospheric air, alveolar air and expired air

Gas	Atmospheric air (%)	Alveolar air (%)	Expired air (%)
Oxygen	20.85	13.55	16.0
Nitrogen and rare gases	78.61	74.85	78.0
Carbon dioxide	0.04	5.35	4.0
Water vapour	0.50	6.25	Saturated

Transport of oxygen and carbon dioxide in the blood is required for internal respiration.

Oxygen transport

❑ Haemoglobin, having the molecular weight of 68,000, is made from 4 haemes (porphyrin ring containing iron) and a globin (a protein).
❑ Oxygen gets bound to the iron for transport, and since each iron atom can bind one oxygen molecule, haemoglobin can carry one, two, three or four oxygen molecules.
❑ Thus, oxygen is carried in the blood in chemical combination with haemoglobin as oxyhaemoglobin (98% of blood oxygen) and also in the dissolved state in the water of plasma and blood cells (2% of blood oxygen).
❑ Oxygen and haemoglobin bind together in a reversible reaction to form oxyhaemoglobin as shown below:

$$Hb + O_2 \leftrightarrow Hb - O_2$$

where Hb is the reduced haemoglobin and Hb - O_2 the oxyhaemoglobin

❑ Oxyhaemoglobin is an unstable compound that dissociates to release oxygen under conditions such as increase in carbon dioxide content of tissue fluid, increase in temperature and presence of 2,3-diphosphoglycerate in red blood cells.
❑ In normal tissues, increase in carbon dioxide production and heat leads to increase in release of oxygen, which helps in supplying oxygen to tissues when required.
❑ The difference in pH (7.4) of arterial blood and venous blood (7.3) can also cause release of oxygen from haemoglobin.
❑ Normal human blood contains around 15–16 g haemoglobin per 100 mL and 1 g of haemoglobin can carry about 1.35 mL of oxygen. Therefore, a saturated arterial blood will contain around 20 mL of oxygen per 100 mL. The amount of oxygen in the blood compared to the carrying capacity of haemoglobin is called oxygen saturation, and it is expressed as a percentage. It is directly proportional to the partial pressure of oxygen.

Carbon dioxide transport

❑ The amount of carbon dioxide in the blood is associated with the acid–base balance of the body fluids. Under normal conditions, an average of 4 mL of the carbon dioxide is transported from the tissues to the lungs in each 100 mL of blood.
❑ A very small portion of the carbon dioxide is transported in the dissolved state to the lungs. Only around 0.3 mL of carbon dioxide is transported in the dissolved form by 100 mL of blood flow, which is around 7% of the total carbon dioxide transported.

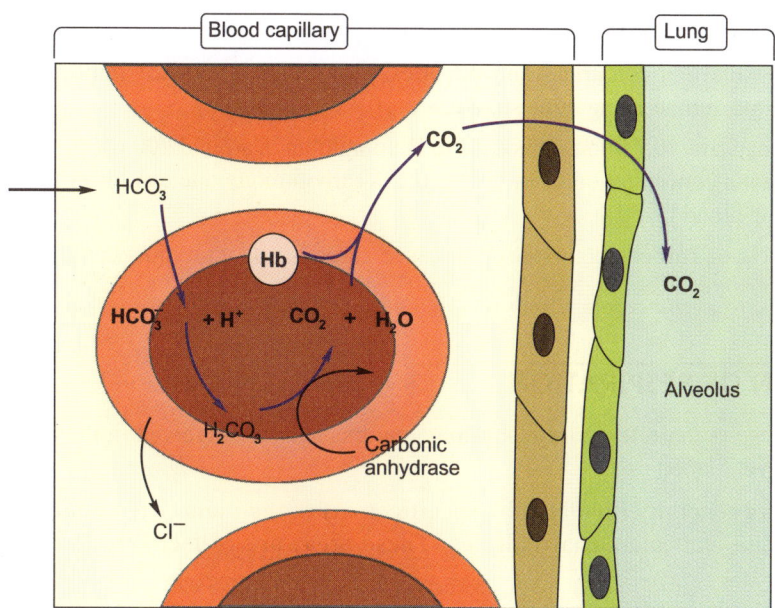

Figure 10.19 Exchange of carbon dioxide in the blood.

❑ The majority of carbon dioxide is transported in the form of bicarbonate ions. The CO_2 dissolved in the blood reacts with water to form carbonic acid, and this reaction is catalysed by the enzyme carbonic anhydrase that is present in the red blood cells.

❑ The reaction occurs very rapidly, which allows CO_2 to react with the red blood cells before the blood leaves the tissue capillaries. The carbonic acid formed is very unstable and thus dissociates into hydrogen and bicarbonate ions. These hydrogen ions then combine with the haemoglobin in the red blood cells, whereas the bicarbonate ions diffuse from the red blood cells into the plasma (Fig. 10.19).

$$CO_2 + H_2O \leftrightarrow H_2CO_3 \leftrightarrow H^+ + HCO_3^-$$

❑ In plasma, sodium chloride is present in a large quantity, which dissociates into sodium and chloride ions. When the negatively charged bicarbonate ions move out of red blood cells into the plasma, the negatively charged chloride ions move into the red blood cell to maintain the electrolyte equilibrium. This phenomenon is called *chloride shift*.

❑ This reversible combination of carbon dioxide with water in the red blood cells under the presence of carbonic anhydrase accounts for 70% of the CO_2 transported from the tissues to the lungs.

❑ Carbon dioxide also reacts directly with amine radicals of the haemoglobin to form carbaminohaemoglobin. It is a reversible reaction.

$$Hb + CO_2 \leftrightarrow Hb - CO_2$$

❑ Normally about 1.5 mL of CO_2 is transported in each 100 mL of blood from the peripheral tissues to the lungs in the form of carbaminohaemoglobin (i.e. around 30% of the total quantity transported). This reaction is slower than the reaction of CO_2 with water inside the red blood cells.

Chapter 10

Carbon monoxide poisoning

❏ Carbon monoxide is a colourless and odourless gas found in exhaust fumes and pollution from automobiles, gas furnaces, cigarette smoke, etc.

❏ The binding capacity of carbon monoxide to haemoglobin is around 200 times stronger than that of oxygen, so that a concentration of as low as 0.1% carbon monoxide can lower the oxygen-carrying capacity of the blood by 50%.

❏ Elevated levels of carbon monoxide may cause carbon monoxide poisoning, which can be fatal sometimes.

REGULATION OF RESPIRATION

Regulation of respiration refers to the physiological mechanisms involved in the control of breathing and pulmonary ventilation.

Respiration is generally regulated by specific areas of the brain that stimulate the contraction of the diaphragm and intercostal muscles. These areas are collectively termed as respiratory centres.

The respiratory centres control the rate and force of respiration and include the following:

1. **Medullary inspiratory centre** (medulla oblongata) includes the following two groups:

   (a) *Ventral respiratory group/expiratory centre* regulates exhalation. The stimulation of this centre causes contraction of expiratory muscles and expiration.

   (b) *Dorsal respiratory group/inspiratory centre* regulates inspiration. Stimulation of this centre causes contraction of inspiratory muscles and prolonged inspiration (Fig. 10.20).

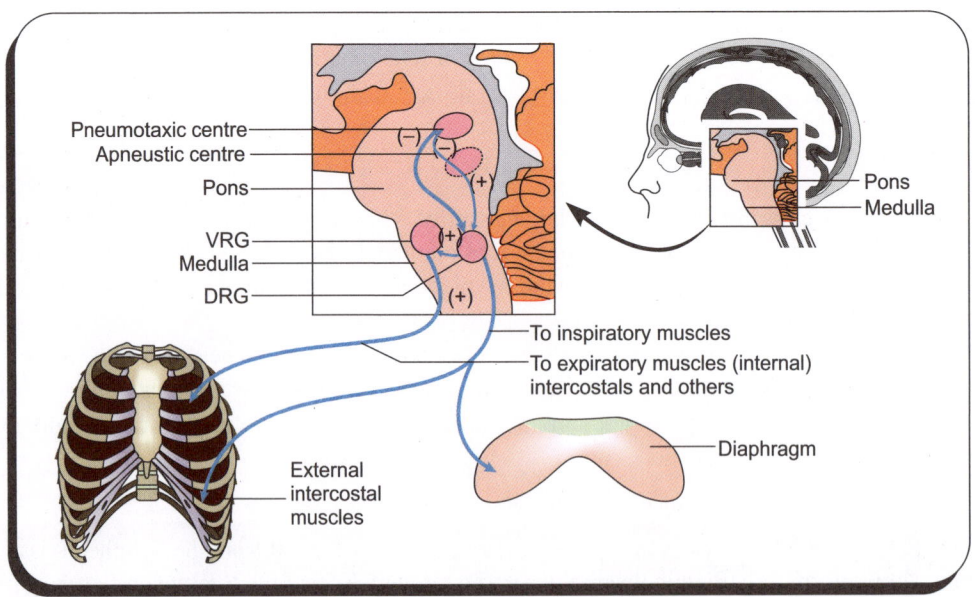

Figure 10.20 Control of respiration.

2. **Pons** includes the following two groups:
   (a) *Pneumotaxic centre* regulates the activity of inspiratory centre by sending inhibitory impulses to the inspiratory area. It also increases the rate of respiration by reducing the duration of inspiration.
   (b) *Apneustic centre* sends stimulatory impulses to the inspiratory area to accelerate the depth of inspiration. It is also responsible to increase the duration of inspiration.

Factors affecting respiratory centres

The respiratory centres regulate the respiratory movements, by receiving the impulses from various sources that include the following:

1. **Central chemoreceptors**
   - ❑ These are the receptors present in the brain that responds to the changes in chemical constituents of blood.
   - ❑ They are situated in the medulla oblongata near the inspiratory centre and are in close contact with the blood and cerebrospinal fluid.
   - ❑ When the carbon dioxide level increases in blood, it easily crosses the blood–brain barrier and enters the cerebrospinal fluid. There, the carbon dioxide molecules combine with water to form carbonic acid, which immediately dissociates into hydrogen ion and bicarbonate ion. The hydrogen ions decrease the pH of the fluid that stimulates the chemoreceptors. In response to this acidic pH, the chemoreceptors send stimulatory impulses to the inspiratory centre, causing increased rate and force of breathing.
   - ❑ In this way, the excess carbon dioxide is washed out and then the respiration is brought back to normal.

2. **Peripheral chemoreceptors**
   - ❑ These receptors are located in the walls of the aortic arch and carotid arteries. They detect variations of oxygen, carbon dioxide and pH in the arterial blood. An increase in pH and CO_2 and a decrease in O_2 cause the stimulation of these receptors, which then send the impulses to the respiratory centre.
   - ❑ The respiratory centre then stimulates the inspiratory centre that leads to increase in the rate and force of respiration.

3. **Mechanoreceptors or stretch receptors**
   - ❑ These are the receptors present in the walls of bronchi and bronchioles that respond to the stretching of the lung tissues. They get activated when the lungs expand to their maximum limit. The impulses from the lungs due to the stretching bring about a respiratory reflex called *Hering–Breuer reflex*.
   - ❑ During inspiration, when the lung stretches, these receptors get stimulated and hence produce impulses. The impulses produced are carried to the respiratory centre. The respiratory centre then gives the reflex response, that is it inhibits the inspiratory centre that terminates inspiration and allows expiration to begin.
   - ❑ This reflex response is protective as it restricts the inspiration and limits the overstretching of lung tissues and is termed as the *Hering–Breuer reflex*.
   - ❑ It also mediates the reflex responses of respiratory tract constriction, hyperventilation and coughing. The receptors in the upper airway are related to reflex responses like sneezing, coughing, and hiccups. The spinal cord reflex responses include the activation of respiratory muscles as compensation, hypoventilation and an increase in breathing rate and volume.

Chapter 10

ARTIFICIAL RESPIRATION

Artificial respiration is any measure or an act of simulating respiration that causes air to flow in and out of a person's lungs when natural breathing is insufficient or ceases as in respiratory paralysis, drowning, choking, opiate overdose, electric shock or inhalation of gas.

There are natural methods for performing artificial respiration, like blowing air into a person's mouth when performing cardiopulmonary resuscitation (CPR), and also hand-operated or mechanical ways to provide the needed breaths if the person is not breathing on his own or inadequately, making it an essential life-saving skill for first aid.

Respiration can be performed by an artificial lung (usually in respiratory paralysis), a pulmotor or other types of mechanical respirators, such as a resuscitator and tank respirator.

The method of manual insufflations has proved to be more efficient than the mechanical manipulation of the patient's chest or arms. The method of manual insufflations is known as the *expired air resuscitation (EAR)*, *mouth-to-mouth resuscitation* or *rescue breathing*.

Lack of breathing or inadequate breathing may cause the brain cells to deteriorate quickly as the body does not receive enough oxygen. The brain cells have to rely on a constant oxygen supply to stay alive. In these circumstances, artificial respiration is vital as it can prevent brain cell death by providing supply of oxygen.

The most widely taught and accepted technique is mouth-to-mouth or sometimes mouth-to-nose method of artificial respiration.

In the mouth-to-mouth method, air is expelled from the rescuer's lungs directly into the victim's mouth (Fig. 10.21). The technique is direct and the effectiveness can be visually determined by the rescuer. The following steps can be performed for rescue breathing,:

Sweep out any foreign material from the mouth by hand

↓

Place the victim on his back with the head tilted backwards and the chin pointing upwards

↓

Pinch the nostril, seal the mouth and exhale directly into the victim's mouth

↓

If there is no exchange of air, check the position of the head. If there is still no exchange, turn the victim on his/her side and rap between the shoulder blades to dislodge any foreign matter that may block the airways

↓

The reviver shall stop blowing when the victim's chest expands and head turns away, and feel for a pulse on the victim's neck

↓

Continue breathing into the subject until natural breathing resumes or until professional help arrives

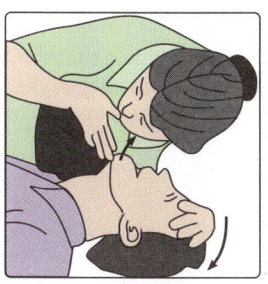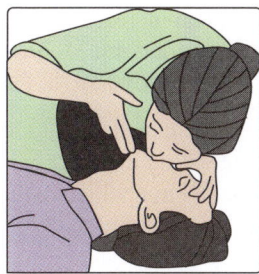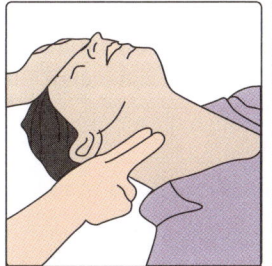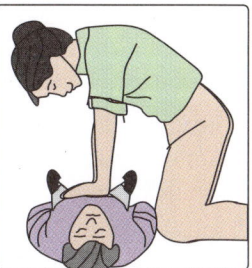

Figure 10.21 Artificial respiration.

Rescue breathing should continue at a normal breathing pace of about 12–15 times per minute, until the victim is fully able to breathe on his/her own. A close watch must be kept as relapses are common.

Most training organizations recommend the use of a protective barrier between rescuer and patient in methods involving mouth to patient to minimize cross-infection risk. Barriers that are popular include pocket masks and face shields.

For short-term mechanical ventilation, tracheal intubation may be used. In this process, a tube is inserted through the nose or mouth and advanced into the trachea. Tubes with inflatable cuffs provide protection against leakage and aspiration. The tubes may cause coughing and pain; therefore, they are generally used in unconscious or anaesthetized patients during surgery. Simultaneous use of oxygen therapy may greatly increase the efficiency of artificial respiration.

DISORDERS OF THE RESPIRATORY SYSTEM

Disorders of the upper respiratory tract

Infectious and inflammatory disorders

Infections of the upper respiratory tract (URIs) are common acute illnesses caused by microorganisms (mostly viruses and bacteria) in the nose, nasal cavity, larynx and pharynx. URIs are very common in the general population. They may be mild and self-limiting. They show a seasonal variation and rarely cause death but may act as a gateway to other serious infections.

The mucosa that lines the upper airway gets invaded by the microbes. More than 200 different viruses have been found to be responsible for URIs, with rhinovirus, coronavirus, adenovirus, enterovirus, and so on being some of the common viruses. Bacteria may also be responsible for URIs, such as *Streptococcus* in pharyngitis.

Transmission of bacteria and viruses may occur when a person exposed to pathogens touches the nose or mouth by hand or by inhaling droplets from an infected person who coughs or sneezes. Inflammation of the mucosa causes increased secretions from the glands, watery discharge, and thereby sneezing and coughing, which helps in spreading the infection.

Common cold and influenza (flu)

Common cold is one of the most common URIs caused majorly by rhinovirus and coronavirus.

Common cold occurs by seasonal variation and causes an increased mucus production (runny nose), swelling of nose linings (making it difficult to breath and congestion), nose irritation (sneezing), sore throat, watery eyes, chills, headache and cough.

The virus may transfer through the air or by direct physical contact with hands and so on. There is no cure for common cold, and antibiotics are not useful in treating it. Increased fluid intake is necessary to prevent dehydration, and abstaining from smoking is one of the palliative measures.

Influenza is a contagious viral infection that occurs mainly in the winter season. It is caused by influenza virus, which is of three types: A, B and C. Influenza types A and B are responsible for causing epidemics of respiratory illness, whereas type C does not cause any illness at all.

The virus continuously undergoes mutation or changes, making people remain susceptible to infection throughout their lives. The infection mainly spreads by airborne transmission. Some of the common symptoms of flu include high fever, muscle aches and pains, headache, nonproductive cough, stuffy nose, sore throat and nausea.

To prevent influenza types A and B in healthy children and adults, nasal spray vaccines are available. Also, antiviral drugs like oseltamivir and zanamivir are available to prevent flu in children. People generally recover from influenza within a week, but exhaustion and tiredness may last for more than 3 weeks.

Sinusitis

Sinusitis is an infection of the sinuses situated near the nasal passage, usually occurring after a common cold or an allergic inflammation. The conditions may be acute, subacute or chronic, with high recurrence rates.

In sinusitis, the opening of the paranasal sinuses gets blocked due to inflammation, the nasal tissue swells and mucus production increases. Sinusitis may also occur due to structural abnormalities of the nose, enlarged adenoids, swimming, foreign matter sticking in the nose, cleft palate, and so on.

The bacteria that cause sinusitis include *Streptococcus pneumoniae*, *Haemophilus influenzae* and *Moraxella catarrhalis*.

The symptoms of sinusitis that depend on the age of the person include runny nose, cough, eye swelling, headaches, fever, sore throat and drip in the throat from the nose.

Sinusitis may be treated using antibiotics, nasal decongestants, nasal spray, humidifier, performing sinus surgery, and so on.

Tonsillitis and pharyngitis

Tonsillitis and pharyngitis are mainly infections of the throat. The inflammation of the tonsils is called *tonsillitis,* whereas that of the throat is known as *pharyngitis*. Infections of both the throat and the tonsil may occur in a single person as well. They are most commonly seen in children below age 10 years.

Viruses like adenovirus, influenza virus, herpes simplex virus; bacteria such as *Streptococcus*, *Neisseria gonorrhoeae*, *Haemophilus influenzae type B*; and also fungi and parasites are mainly responsible for causing infection in the throat.

Severe infection of the tonsils may lead to suppuration and discharge of pus. Swelling ultimately subsides in acute cases but recurrent inflammation may cause fibrosis and permanent enlargement of the tonsils. When the tonsils are inflamed it is known as *adenoids* and they bulge out. Temporary enlargement of the tonsils protects the nasal and pharyngeal mucosal layers against infection but chronic infections can make them fibrotic and obstruct the airways, mainly in children.

The onset of symptoms may be quick or slow, depending on the cause of the infection. Symptoms may include sore throat, nasal discharge, fever (due to release of endotoxins), headache, nausea, painful swallowing, foul breath and decrease in appetite.

For treatment, antibiotics may be used if the infection is bacterial; antiviral agents can be used for viral cases; and analgesics, increased fluid intake and throat lozenges can be recommended.

Laryngitis and laryngotracheitis

Laryngitis is the inflammation of the larynx, whereas laryngotracheitis is the inflammation of the larynx, trachea and subglottic area of the airways. The condition may be acute or chronic (for smokers) depending on exposure to dust particles, pollution, and so on. It usually occurs in children below 1 year but may affect people of any age, and depends on seasonal variation (usually occurs in winter).

The infection is mainly caused by viruses like paramyxoviruses type 1, 2 or 3, influenza viruses and respiratory syncytial virus. Other uncommon viruses include adenovirus, rhinovirus and enterovirus. Bacterial causes of laryngitis are much less common and include group A *Streptococcus*, *Corynebacterium diphtheriae*, *Mycoplasma pneumoniae* and *Haemophilus influenzae*.

It has nasopharyngeal symptoms like dysphagia, throat pain, hoarseness of voice, dry cough, emesis, pain in the ribcage, dyspnoea, fever and myalgia. Worsening conditions in children may cause cyanosis and ultimately respiratory failure.

Corticosteroids and anti-inflammatory drugs may be used to treat this disorder.

Croup

Croup is a disease occurring most commonly in children in which the area around the larynx and the trachea gets swollen, causing problems in breathing.

The disease is caused by various viruses such as parainfluenza virus, adenovirus, respiratory syncytial virus and influenza virus.

The infection starts in the upper respiratory tract and then spreads gradually into the voice box and trachea.

The most common symptoms of croup include congested and runny nose, cough, laryngitis, fever and sometimes stridor. The symptoms worsen at night but shows improvement within a week.

Immediate treatments based on medications include breathing treatments to open up the airways, parenteral doses of medications to decrease the swelling of airways and also steroids. Increased fluid intake, analgesics and humidifiers may be used for supportive care at home.

Stridor

Stridor is the occurrence of a high-pitched sound usually during inspiration caused by the obstruction or narrowing of a child's upper respiratory tract. The characteristic sound depends on the location of the obstruction in the airways. Generally stridor occurs in children due to their short and narrow upper airways.

Some of the most common reasons for stridor in children include the following factors:

1. Congenital causes such as subglottic stenosis, subglottic haemangioma and laryngomalacia.
2. Infections such as croup, epiglottitis, bronchitis and tonsillitis.

3. Traumatic causes such as presence of foreign bodies in the airways and fracture in the neck.

Stridor may be treated by medications through the oral and parenteral routes and through surgery.

Epiglottitis

Epiglottitis is a life-threatening and acute infection that spreads through the upper airways.

It is caused by the bacteria *Haemophilus influenzae type B (HIB)* and group A haemolytic *Streptococcus*. The condition results in inflammation and swelling of the epiglottis. The disease usually occurs in children below 10 years but may also occur in adults. The disease can occur at any time without seasonal variation. Breathing problems are common including stridor, which may gradually worsen, leading to airway obstruction and resulting in a medical emergency.

Some of the common symptoms of epiglottitis include fever, drooling, sore throat, dysphagia (pain during swelling), dry or no cough, dysphonia (loss of voice) and respiratory distress.

Vaccines are available for the treatment of epiglottitis caused by the bacteria. HIB vaccine is recommended for infants below 2 years . Since epiglottitis is a medical emergency, immediate care is required to prevent airway occlusion, along with close monitoring and assistance in breathing. Antibiotics must be given intravenously and intravenous fluids and steroids must be administered to reduce swelling of the airways.

Allergic rhinitis

Rhinitis is an allergic reaction that causes the release of histamine and other mediators of inflammation from the mast cell granules and basophils when airborne irritants or stimulants (pollen grains, dust mites, mould) come in contact with the nose. Rhinitis may be seasonal or perennial in nature.

In allergic rhinitis, immediate type of hypersensitivity develops to allergens such as pollen grains and it causes inflammation of the nasal mucosa and conjunctiva. This type of antigen–antibody reaction is mediated by the IgE antibodies produced by B-lymphocytes. Histamine release causes vasodilation, increased capillary permeability, swelling of tissues and excessive secretion by glands.

Symptoms of allergic rhinitis include sneezing, runny nose, congestion, discomfort in the eyes, throat, snoring, nasal discharge, ear infections and nose bleeding.

Allergic rhinitis may be treated by using drugs such as anti-histaminics, anti-inflammatory agents, corticosteroids and nasal decongestants, and also by avoiding allergens, dusty areas and pet animals.

Diphtheria

Diphtheria is an infection of the upper respiratory tract caused by the anaerobic Gram-positive bacterium *Corynebacterium diphtheriae.* It is a contagious disease, which can spread by direct physical contact or by air through infected persons. It mainly affects the tonsils, pharynx and/or the nasal cavity.

Diphtheria has largely been eradicated from the developed countries by vaccination. The DPT (diphtheria–pertussis–tetanus) vaccine has been recommended for school-going children.

The onset of diphtheria is gradual and symptoms include nausea, vomiting, chills, fever, sore throat, fatigue and problems in swallowing. The long-term effects of diphtheria include fast heart rate, low blood pressure, peripheral neuropathy and skin diseases.

In patients with acute diphtheria, diphtheria antitoxin may be given based on clinical diagnosis. Antibiotics such as erythromycin (oral or parenteral), procaine penicillin G (intramuscular) and rifampin can be administered to eradicate the microorganism and prevent its transmission.

Tumours

Benign tumours may occur in the nasal septum. Malignant tumours may occur rarely in the nose, sinuses, nasopharynx and larynx.

Laryngeal cancer

Cancers of the larynx are squamous cell carcinomas as they originate from the squamous cells present in the laryngeal epithelium. Laryngeal cancers mainly affect the glottis, while subglottic and supraglottic tumours are rare. Laryngeal cancer may spread directly to other structures by metastasis. It can spread to the lymph nodes and the lungs.

Smoking and chronic consumption of alcohol are the main risk factors for laryngeal cancer. Also, people with a history of head and neck cancer are at higher risk.

Symptoms of cancer include hoarseness of voice, lump in the neck, sore throat, cough, stridor and ear pain.

Chest X-rays, CT and MRI scans, laryngoscopy, biopsy and nasal endoscopy may be used to diagnose the disease.

Treatment mainly depends on the type and stage of tumour. Chemotherapy, radiation therapy and surgery are the main options for treatment.

Disorders of the bronchi

Acute bronchitis

Acute bronchitis is an infection of bronchi or bronchioles. Usually respiratory syncytial virus, parainfluenza virus, rhinovirus, coronavirus, influenza virus and adenovirus are the viral causes of acute bronchitis. Bacterial causes include *Streptococcus pneumoniae*, *Haemophilus influenzae*, fungi such as *Candida albicans* and *Cryptococcus neoformans*. It can also occur due to environmental irritants, air pollution and tobacco smoke.

Symptoms of acute bronchitis include dry cough, dyspnoea, wheezing, fever, myalgia, hoarseness of voice, chest pain and fatigue.

For treatment of this disorder, inhaled bronchodilators, cough suppressants, inhaled corticosteroids, antibiotics such as azithromycin, macrolides, and fluoroquinolones may be used singly or in combination.

Chronic bronchitis

Chronic bronchitis is a disease characterized by excessive bronchial mucus secretion along with productive cough on most days for more than 3 months a year and which continues for 2 or more consecutive years. It occurs mainly in chronic cigarette smokers and owing to exposure to environmental pollutants.

Mucus-secreting glands get hypertrophied with excessive mucus secretion, which is accompanied by hyperplasia of smooth muscles and bronchial hyperresponsiveness. Oedema and reduction in the number of cilia also occur. The excess mucus production causes narrowing of airways, hampering the ciliary function.

Dyspnoea, wheezing, pulmonary hypertension, breathlessness and productive cough are the main symptoms. The bronchus gets gradually replaced by fibrotic tissue. This may be accompanied by respiratory failure, and hypoxaemia and hypercapnia may develop in severe cases.

Bronchiectasis

Bronchiectasis is a chronic inflammatory or infectious disease in which multiple dilatations of bronchi and bronchioles occur, accompanied by pustular discharge. It usually affects people of middle age. The bronchi may get obstructed by pus, mucus and inflammatory exudates, resulting in the collapse of alveoli close to this blockage. The pressure of inspired air leads to dilatation. Severe coughing to remove the sputum may cause an increase in pressure in the blocked area, causing further dilatation.

Bronchiectasis may be caused by obstruction of bronchioles; recurrent pulmonary infections such as pulmonary abscess, tuberculosis, measles; genetic disorders such as alpha-1 antitrypsin deficiency and cystic fibrosis; and inhalation of toxic chemicals.

Symptoms include productive cough with thick and copious sputum, wheezing, dyspnoea, fatigue, cyanosis and weight loss. Progressive lung fibrosis may lead to hypoxia, pulmonary hypertension and heart failure.

It can be diagnosed by sputum tests, chest X-ray, pulmonary function tests and bronchoscopy.

Bronchiolitis obliterans

Bronchiolitis obliterans is an inflammatory obstructive disease of the bronchioles caused by bronchial exudates and fibrous granulation tissue. The obstruction of bronchioles is triggered by injury to the bronchial epithelium.

The causes of this disease include exposure to toxic chemicals, bone marrow or lung transplantation, pneumonitis, viral respiratory infections and rheumatoid arthritis.

Symptoms include nonproductive cough, wheezing and dyspnoea.

Chest X-ray can be used to diagnose the disease.

Asthma

Asthma is a disorder characterized by airway inflammation, hypersensitivity to various environmental stimuli and obstruction of the airways. It may be reversible spontaneously with or without treatment.

Asthma affects around 5–8% of the US population, being more common in children and in the winter season. Airway obstruction occurs due to various reasons such as smooth muscle spasms in the walls of bronchi and bronchioles, oedema of the airways, increased mucus secretion and damage to the airway epithelium.

The common allergens or triggering agents in asthma include pollen grains, dust mites, moulds, specific food, cold air, cigarette smoke, exercise and emotional changes.

In severe cases of asthma, inflammation, fibrosis, oedema and necrosis of bronchial epithelial cells occur. Chemical mediators such as prostaglandins, leukotrienes, histamine and thromboxane can be used for treatment.

There are two types of asthma based on the symptoms and people affected: extrinsic or atopic asthma and intrinsic asthma.

Extrinsic asthma generally affects children and young people who show hypersensitivity reactions to foreign substances such as pollen grains and feather pillows. The exacerbation of attacks tends to decrease with age.

Intrinsic asthma usually occurs in adults with no history of childhood allergic reactions. It is associated with the inflammation of the upper respiratory tract.

Symptoms of asthma include breathing difficulties or breathlessness, coughing, wheezing, chest discomfort, fatigue, anxiety and tachycardia.

The drugs used for the treatment of asthma include inhaled and systemic corticosteroids, beta-adrenergic receptor agonists and leukotriene receptor blockers.

Disorders of the lungs

Tuberculosis

Tuberculosis (TB) is a chronic bacterial infection that generally infects the lungs; however, other organs may also be involved.

It is primarily an airborne disease that occurs in the following three stages:

1. **Exposure**: It occurs when a person comes in physical contact or is exposed to another person who has TB.
2. **TB infection**: It is a latent stage where a person has TB bacteria in the body but shows no signs or symptoms of the disease.
3. **TB infection**: It occurs when the person shows signs and symptoms of the disease with a positive skin test and a positive chest X-ray.

The bacterium causing TB is *Mycobacterium tuberculosis*. Not all people infected with *M. tuberculosis* develop active TB. TB affects people of all ages, races, both genders with impaired immune systems.

The common symptoms for TB include persistent cough, fatigue, loss of appetite, weight loss, fever, blood in cough and night perspiration.

Treatment options for TB include hospitalization and medications such as isoniazid, ethambutol, rifampin and streptomycin. World Health Organization's DOT (direct observation therapy) treatment may last for months.

Pulmonary emphysema

Emphysema is a chronic lung disorder in which the alveoli may be destroyed, narrowed, collapsed, stretched and overinflated. Overinflation of the alveoli may occur as a result of breakdown of the alveolar wall, decreasing the respiratory capacity and causing breathlessness. Damage to the alveoli is irreversible and creates 'holes' in the lung tissues.

Emphysema develops gradually. The lung has a set of elastic fibres that allows the lungs to expand and contract. Emphysema occurs when a chemical imbalance causes destruction of the elastic fibres. Chemical imbalance may occur due to smoking, exposure to air pollutants, smoke fumes and dust and a rare inherited disorder alpha-1 antitrypsin deficiency syndrome.

Symptoms of pulmonary emphysema include shortness of breath, cough, fatigue, anxiety, weight loss, sleep disturbance and chest pain.

Emphysema can be detected by pulmonary function tests (spirometry), blood tests, chest X-ray, sputum analysis and electrocardiogram.

Treatment options include quitting smoking, antibiotics, bronchodilators, exercise, oxygen supplementation, lung surgery and lung transplantation.

Pneumothorax

Pneumothorax is the condition in which air gets filled in the pleural cavities. It may be due to surgical opening of the chest or the result of gunshot wound and may cause the lungs to collapse.

Treatment normally includes evacuation of air from the pleural cavity by inserting a chest tube.

Pleurisy

Pleurisy is the inflammation of the pleural membrane. It may cause pain in early stages, and if the condition persists, it may result in accumulation of fluid in the pleural space.

Pneumonia

Pneumonia is an infection of lungs caused by bacteria, virus or chemical irritants. It is a severe infection in which the alveoli get filled with pus and other liquid. Lobar pneumonia may affect one or more lobes of the lungs, whereas bronchial pneumonia affects several parts throughout both lungs.

The main types of pneumonia include the following:

1. **Bacterial pneumonia** is caused by various bacteria such as *Streptococcus pneumoniae*. It can affect people of all ages but those who are prone include alcoholics, debilitated persons, postoperative patients and persons with viral infections and weakened immune systems.
   The symptoms of bacterial pneumonia include chills, chest pain, cough with mucus, fever, perspiration, rapid pulse, high breathing rate, chattering teeth and delirium.
2. **Viral pneumonia** is caused by a number of viruses and accounts for half of the cases of pneumonia. The early symptoms of pneumonia are the same as those of bacterial pneumonia, but gradually increasing breathlessness and worsening of the cough may occur.
3. **Mycoplasma pneumonia** has different symptoms. It is caused by mycoplasmas, a microorganism with the characteristics of both viruses and bacteria. They usually cause a mild pneumonia that can affect people of all ages. Symptoms include severe cough with production of mucus.

Treatment may include antibiotics for bacterial pneumonia and mycoplasma pneumonia, and there is no effective treatment for viral pneumonia, which is generally cured on its own. Cough suppressants and oxygen therapy may be useful in most of the cases.

Pulmonary embolism

Pulmonary embolism is a severe and life-threatening condition caused by the blocking of pulmonary artery by foreign matter such as blood clot or thrombus, fatty deposits and tumour.

Conditions that may predispose to pulmonary embolism include heart disease, COPD, surgery, cancer, paralysis, ageing and sickle cell disease.

Signs and symptoms of pulmonary embolism include chest pain, cough mixed with blood-streaked sputum, dyspnoea, excessive perspiration, shock, cyanosis, anxiety and loss of consciousness.

The immediate treatment of pulmonary embolism includes anticoagulant therapy to dissolve the clot and reinstate the blood flow. Oxygen therapy and sedatives are given to reduce the symptoms and surgery may also be performed to remove the emboli or thrombus.

Interstitial lung diseases (pulmonary fibrosis)

Interstitial lung disease (ILD) includes more than 170 lung disorders, which may be chronic, nonmalignant and noninfectious in nature. ILD is so named because the interstitium, the tissue between the air sacs of the lungs, is affected by fibrosis or scarring.

The symptoms and progression of these diseases vary from person to person, but they all begin with inflammation.

The types of these diseases include the following:

1. **Bronchiolitis**: It is the inflammation of the bronchioles.
2. **Alveolitis**: It is the inflammation of the air sacs.
3. **Vasculitis**: It is the inflammation of the lung capillaries.

More than 70% of ILDs are diagnosed as pneumoconiosis, a drug-induced disease, or hypersensitivity pneumonitis. In ILD, the lung is affected in the following ways:

1. Lung tissue gets damaged.
2. The walls of the alveoli become inflamed.
3. Scarring occurs in the interstitium.

Fibrosis results in irreversible loss of the tissue's ability to breathe and carry oxygen. Air sacs, as well as the lung tissue surrounding it and the capillaries, get destroyed by the formation of scar tissue. The disease may have a gradual or a progressive deterioration. The condition may remain same for a long time or may change quickly. On progression, the lung tissue becomes thick and stiff and breathing becomes difficult.

The common symptoms of ILD which may vary widely include shortness of breath, fatigue, loss of appetite, weight loss, dry cough, chest pain, laboured breathing and lung haemorrhage.

ILD is caused by various environmental pollutants and sarcoidosis, certain drugs, radiation, collagen diseases and family history.

Its occurrence can be diagnosed by lung function tests, blood tests, X-ray, computerized axial tomography (CAT) scan, bronchoscopy, bronchoalveolar lavage and lung biopsy.

Treatment of ILD includes oral medications (including corticosteroids, influenza vaccine, pneumonia vaccine), oxygen therapy and lung transplantation.

Primary pulmonary hypertension

Pulmonary hypertension is a disorder in which the blood pressure in the pulmonary artery increases much above the normal levels.

The specific cause of pulmonary tension is unknown. The blood vessels that are sensitive to certain internal or external factors may constrict when exposed to these factors. A genetic factor, an immune system factor or sensitivity to chemicals or drugs may also be responsible.

The common symptoms of pulmonary hypertension include fatigue, breathing difficulty, dizziness, syncope, oedema in the ankles and legs, cyanosis, chest pain, fast pulse and palpitations. In advanced stages of the disease, the patient becomes unable to perform activities, has symptoms even while at rest and becomes bedridden.

Treatment for pulmonary hypertension includes drugs such as anticoagulants, diuretics, calcium channel blockers, oxygen therapy and lung transplantation.

Chapter 10

Severe acute respiratory syndrome

Severe acute respiratory syndrome (SARS) is a respiratory disease caused by the virus SARS coronavirus. It caused a near pandemic in the year 2002–2003, with around 8000 known infected cases and 770 deaths worldwide. It rapidly infected individuals in more than 35 countries around the world. Mortality rate is around 50% for people over 60 years but low in young people.

Initial symptoms of SARS are flu-like and include high fever, myalgia, lethargy, gastric problems, cough, sore throat, shortness of breath and other nonspecific symptoms.

The causative organism coronaviruses are enveloped RNA viruses that are pathogens for mammals and birds. These viruses can cause respiratory tract infections in humans, livestock and pet animals.

SARS is a viral disease; hence, antibiotics are ineffective. Usually, supportive treatment with antipyretic drugs, oxygen therapy and ventilator support is provided. Corticosteroids and the antiviral drug ribavirin have proved promising in therapy and have been widely used. A SARS vaccine has also been developed by China.

Lung cancer

Lung cancer generally starts in the lining of the bronchi but can also begin in other areas such as the trachea, bronchioles or alveoli. Mostly, lung cancers are carcinomas and develop over a period of many years. More than 90% of lung cancers belong to a class called *bronchogenic carcinoma*.

Lung cancers can be divided into the following two types:

1. **Nonsmall cell lung cancer**: There are three types of this cancer based on the type of cells in the tumour, which include the following:
   (a) *Squamous cell carcinoma or epidermoid carcinoma* is the most common type of lung cancer in men, which usually begins in the bronchi but spreads slowly.
   (b) *Adenocarcinoma* generally begins on the outer edges of the lungs and the lining of the bronchi. It mostly affects women and in those who have never smoked.
   (c) *Large cell carcinomas* are a group of cancers with large, abnormal-shaped cells, which generally begin in the outer edges of the lungs.
2. **Small cell lung cancer**: It is also called as oat cell cancer based on the cell shape, grows rapidly and spreads quickly to other organs.

Lung cancer usually does not show symptoms at first, but become present once the tumour starts growing. Some of the common symptoms include cough, chest pain, shortness of breath, recurrent lung infections such as pneumonia, blood with sputum, hoarseness of voice, swelling of the face and neck, pain in the shoulder, arm, hand, fever, fatigue and headache. Some symptoms may be caused by substances made by cancer cells, known as *paraneoplastic syndrome*.

The risk factors for lung cancer include smoking tobacco, marijuana, recurring inflammation from tuberculosis, asbestos exposure, industrial grade talc, radioactive ores, arsenic, coal products, mustard gas, radon, family history of lung cancer, air pollution and vitamin deficiency.

Surgery, radiation therapy and chemotherapy are the possible options for treatment of lung cancer. Surgery can be carried out in three ways: segmental or wedge resection (to remove a small part of a lung), lobectomy (removal of an entire lobe of a lung) and pneumonectomy (removal of an entire lung).

OVERVIEW OF THE RESPIRATORY SYSTEM

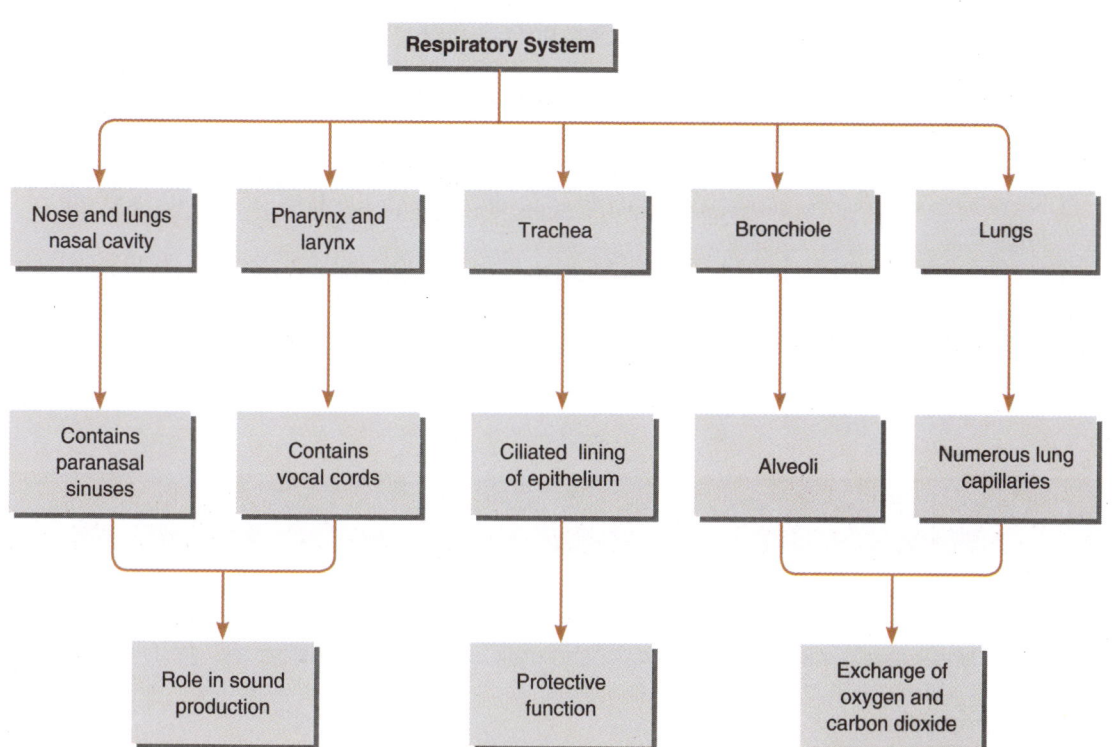

Effects of Smoking

❏ Irritants in the smoke destroy cilia that are present on the lining of the respiratory system. Without cilia, the epithelium cannot clear the passageway of mucus and debris, which makes it an ideal environment for the growth of microorganisms, leading to respiratory infections.

❏ The irritants in smoke cause increased mucus secretion and swelling of the mucosal lining, which triggers the cough reflex, resulting in a condition called as *smoker's cough*.

❏ Nicotine constricts the bronchioles that lead to decrease in the flow of air into and out of lungs.

❏ Carbon monoxide present in the smoke binds to haemoglobin and reduces its oxygen-carrying capacity.

❏ The major adverse effects of smoking on the respiratory system include lung cancer, chronic bronchitis and emphysema.

Embryonic Development of the Respiratory System

❏ During the 4th week of development, the respiratory system begins as an outgrowth of the foregut just anterior to the pharynx, which is called *respiratory diverticulum or lung bud*. It is lined by the endoderm, which further develops into epithelial lining of the larynx consisting of epithelium and glands of trachea, bronchi and alveoli. It is surrounded by mesoderm, which gives rise to connective tissue, cartilage and smooth muscles.

❏ The distal end of the respiratory diverticulum elongates to form a globular tracheal bud, which forms the trachea. The tracheal bud then divides into bronchial buds, which further develop with the bronchi.

❏ Respiratory bronchioles take around 24 weeks for development.

❏ Lung tissue becomes highly vascular and respiratory bronchioles, alveolar ducts and some alveoli develop during 16–26 weeks of pregnancy.

❏ The various primitive alveoli that develop from 26 weeks to birth consist of the following:
    1. Type 1 alveolar cells
    2. Type 2 surfactant-producing cells that lower the surface tension of alveolar fluid and thus reduce the tendency of collapsing of alveoli on exhalation.
    3. Blood capillaries also develop.

❏ Mature alveoli develop within 30 weeks. One-sixth of the full complement of alveoli develops before birth and the rest develops after birth.

❏ When the lungs develop, they acquire their pleural sacs. The space between the pleural layer—that is visceral pleura and the parietal pleura, which is developed from mesoderm—is called pleural cavity.

❏ During development of the fetus, the aspiration of fluid into the lungs occurs in the fetus due to their breathing movements. This fluid contains a mixture of amniotic fluid, mucus from bronchial glands and surfactant.

Ageing and the Respiratory System

❏ With advancing age, the tissues of the respiratory tract become less elastic and more rigid, which result in decrease in the lung capacity. This decrease reaches up to 35% by the age of 70.

❏ The levels of oxygen-carrying capacity by the blood and the exchange of gases across the respiratory membranes of the alveoli decrease as we age. Moreover, the ciliary action of the epithelial lining the respiratory tract reduces, which results in the accumulation of mucus inside the respiratory tract.

❏ All these age-related factors make the elderly much more susceptible to bronchitis, pneumonia, emphysema and other respiratory infections.

Exercise and the Respiratory System

❏ The respiratory and cardiovascular systems undergo various adjustments in response to the intensity and duration of exercise.

❏ During maximal exercise, the oxygen-diffusing capacity increases threefold to meet the increased oxygen demand.

❏ The gradual increase in the intensity of exercise increases the depth of pulmonary ventilation, which is followed by the increased breathing rate and increased frequency of breathing.

❏ These changes in respiration occur in response to the impulses from chemoreceptors and proprioceptors that stimulate the respiratory centre and increase the depth and frequency of respiration with exercise.

HOW TO KEEP YOUR RESPIRATORY SYSTEM HEALTHY

1. Do not smoke cigarettes
2. Exercise daily to the point of being out of breath and do activities such as swimming or playing badminton
3. Try holding your breath as long as possible to expand your lungs—do this every 3–5 h
4. Maintain a balanced diet
5. Get a yearly medical check-up of your respiratory system

Review Questions

Long Answer Questions

1. Describe the three functions performed by the internal structures of the nose.
2. Discuss the three parts of pharynx and its functions.
3. Describe the various movements of the thoracic cage and lungs during respiration.
4. Explain the transport of oxygen and carbon dioxide in blood.
5. Discuss the various lung volumes and lung capacities.
6. Discuss the anatomy of nose and nasal cavity.
7. Explain the functions of pharynx.
8. Discuss in detail the regulation of respiration.
9. Explain the cycle of respiration.
10. Discuss the anatomy and physiology of lungs.

Short Notes

1. Artificial respiration
2. Nonrespiratory functions of the respiratory tract
3. Transport of oxygen in blood
4. Nervous regulation of respiration
5. External respiration
6. Chemoreceptors
7. Respiratory centres
8. Hypercapnia
9. Baroreceptors
10. Internal respiration
11. Hypoxia
12. Dyspnoea
13. Fetal respiration
14. Internal respiration
15. Apnoea

Multiple Choice Questions

1. What is the respiratory system?
   - (a) The body's breathing system
   - (b) The body's system of nerves
   - (c) The body's food-processing system
   - (d) The body's blood-transporting system

2. Air can enter the body and travel to the lungs
   - (a) Through the mouth and the nose
   - (b) Through the oesophagus and gullet
   - (c) Through the windpipe and the pores
   - (d) Through the nose and the nervous system

3. What is the purpose of the little hair inside the nose?
   - (a) To fight disease
   - (b) They serve no purpose
   - (c) To keep dust out of the lungs
   - (d) To tickle the nose and cause sneezing

4. What is another name for the windpipe?
   - (a) Lungs
   - (b) Larynx
   - (c) Trachea
   - (d) Oesophagus

5. What happens to the windpipe or trachea, before it reaches the lungs?
   - (a) It branches in two directions
   - (b) It branches in three directions
   - (c) It vibrates and creates sounds
   - (d) It closes up so that no oxygen can escape

6. What important activity takes place in the lungs?
   - (a) Food is digested
   - (b) Liquid waste is filtered from the blood
   - (c) Oxygen is exchanged for carbon dioxide
   - (d) The trachea is exchanged for the larynx

7. Oxygen moves from the lungs into the bloodstream through
   - (a) Nerve fibres
   - (b) A large artery in the heart
   - (c) Small blood vessels in the lungs
   - (d) A tube in the lungs called the jugular vein

8. Which organ is made up of air-carrying tubes and tiny sacs?
   - (a) The brain
   - (b) The lungs
   - (c) The stomach
   - (d) The diaphragm

9. What body structure protects the lungs from outside harm?
   - (a) Cartilage
   - (b) Tiny sacs
   - (c) The rib cage
   - (d) The diaphragm

10. The lowermost portion of the pharynx is
    - (a) Oropharynx
    - (b) Nasopharynx
    - (c) Laryngopharynx
    - (d) Pharyngeal tonsils

Chapter 10

11. The volume of air that can be exhaled during forced breathing in addition to tidal volume is
    (a) Residual volume
    (b) Expiratory reserve volume
    (c) Vital capacity
    (d) Total lung capacity

12. What portion of the regulatory centres that control breathing is located in the pons and promotes inspiration?
    (a) Apneustic area
    (b) Pneumotaxic area
    (c) Rhythmicity centre
    (d) Aortic and carotid bodies

13. What is the function of the pleurae?
    (a) To compartmentalize, protect and lubricate the lungs
    (b) To serve as a passageway and for the continued cleansing of air
    (c) To produce mucus
    (d) To lighten the skull

14. The lower end of the larynx is formed by which cartilage?
    (a) Thyroid
    (b) Cricoid
    (c) Arytenoid
    (d) Cuneiform

15. What is the force that causes air to flow into the lungs during inspiration and out of the lungs during expiration?
    (a) Muscle contraction
    (b) Surface tension
    (c) Diaphragm movements
    (d) Atmospheric pressure

Match the Following

Column A

1. Eustachian tubes
2. Fauces
3. Serous membrane that surrounds the lungs
4. Vestibular folds
5. Simple squamous epithelial cells that form a continuous lining of the alveolar wall; sites of gas exchange
6. Adam's apple
7. Alveoli
8. Normal quite breathing
9. Secondary bronchi

Column B

(a) Pleura
(b) Alveoli
(c) Eupnoea
(d) Apnoea
(e) Costal breathing
(f) Hypoxia
(g) Diaphragmatic breathing
(h) Hypercapnia
(i) Breathing

10. Absence of breathing
11. Ventilation
12. Shallow, chest breathing
13. Tertiary bronchi
14. Deep abdominal breathing
15. Trachea
16. Epiglottis
17. Deficiency of oxygen at the tissue level
18. Above-normal partial pressure of carbon dioxide
19. Tertiary bronchi

(j) Segmental bronchi
(k) Opening from mouth
(l) Cricoid cartilage
(m) False vocal cords
(n) Lobar bronchi
(o) Auditory/nasopharynx
(p) Surface for respiration
(q) True vocal cords
(r) Thyroid cartilage
(s) Blocks glottis during swallowing
(t) Windpipe

Careers in Pulmonology

✓ Respiratory therapists are allied health specialists who are responsible for the treatment of acute or chronic dysfunction of the cardiopulmonary system.

✓ In hospitals and rehabilitation centres, there are three different respiratory therapist careers – outpatient care, acute care and teaching.

✓ Pulmonologists are physicians who specialize in the diagnosis and treatment of diseases of the lungs.

✓ Thoracic surgeons are physician specialists who are concerned with diseases and disorders of the thoracic area.

The Cardiovascular System

CHAPTER OUTLINE

STUDY OBJECTIVES

✓ To describe the position of the heart within the thorax and structure of the heart.

✓ To describe the various layers of the wall of the heart.

✓ To explain the different chambers of the heart and the valves in the heart.

✓ To explain the circulation of blood through the heart and the blood vessels of the body.

✓ To describe the fetal circulation and the circulation of blood through the lungs.

✓ To understand the conducting system of the heart and the pathway of conduction of impulse through the heart.

✓ To understand the different stages of the cardiac cycle and discuss the various heart sounds produced during the different stages of the cardiac cycle.

✓ To know about electrocardiogram (ECG) and ECG machine, various waves of ECG and the significance of ECG.

✓ To know the physiological and pathological variations of blood pressure and explore the various factors that maintain blood pressure.

✓ To discuss cardiac output and the regulation of cardiac output.

✓ To discuss heart rate and know the physiological and pathological variations of heart rate.

✓ To give a brief idea about the various disorders of the cardiovascular system.

INTRODUCTION

The cardiovascular system comprises the heart and numerous blood vessels. The heart is the muscular pump that forces blood through a system of blood vessels that includes various arteries, veins and capillaries. The heart is a unique organ as it undergoes rhythmic changes (i.e. contracting, taking rest and immediately again contracting), and this process continues for the entire lifetime. These rhythmic changes of pumping the blood continuously keep us alive and healthy.

From the moment it begins beating until the moment it stops, the human heart works tirelessly.

❏ The major function of the cardiovascular system is to supply life-supporting oxygen, nutrients and other essential substances to the tissues of the body and to remove carbon dioxide and metabolic end products from the tissues.

❏ This exchange of nutrients and waste products is mediated through capillaries, which are the thinnest blood vessels.

❏ The cardiovascular system plays a vital role in coordinating and integrating various systems of the body.

ANATOMY AND PHYSIOLOGY OF THE HEART

The heart is a roughly cone-shaped hollow muscular organ, about the size of a closed fist. It is approximately 12 cm (5 inch) long and 9 cm (3.5 inch) wide at its broadest point and about 6 cm (2.5 inch) thick (Fig. 11.1).

It weighs about 225 gm in women and 310 gm in men.

DO YOU KNOW

❏ The study of cardiovascular system is known as *cardiology*.

❏ If we strung together all the veins, arteries and capillaries, they could circle the globe two and a half times. There are more than 60,000 miles of blood vessels in an adult body.

❏ The sound of a heartbeat is actually the sound of the heart valves closing as the blood is pushed through the heart chambers.

❏ An average heart beats about 30 million times in a year and two and a half billion times in an average lifetime. An average adult heart pumps about 4000 gallons of blood a day.

❏ It takes about 20 s for a red blood cell to circulate the whole body.

❏ Oxygenated blood appears red, whereas deoxygenated blood appears blue.

❏ There are 10 major places to check the pulse: superficial temporal artery, common carotid artery, facial artery (head and neck), axillary artery, brachial artery, radial artery (arm), femoral artery, popliteal artery, dorsalis pedis artery and posterior tibial artery (leg and foot).

MEDICAL TERMINOLOGY

❏ **Anastomoses**: Many parts of the body receive blood from branches of more than one artery that are usually connected to each other. These connections are called *anastomoses* and they provide alternate routes for blood to reach a particular organ.

❏ **Anterior**: It means situated before or towards the front.

❏ **Aortic stenosis**: It is abnormal narrowing of the aortic valve that restricts blood from moving from the left ventricle into the aorta.

❏ **Articulation**: It is a joint or juncture between bones or cartilages in the skeleton of a vertebrate.

❏ **Coronary ischaemia**: It is a medical term for not having enough blood through the coronary arteries.

❏ **Depolarization**: It is to become partially or wholly unpolarized.

❏ **Endothelium**: It is an epithelium of mesodermal origin composed of a single layer of thin flattened cells that line the internal body cavities and the lumens of vessels.

❏ **Involuntary**: This means it is not subject to control of the will.

❏ **Mediastinum**: It is the space in the chest between the pleural sacs of the lungs that contain all the tissues and organs of the chest, except for the lungs and pleura.

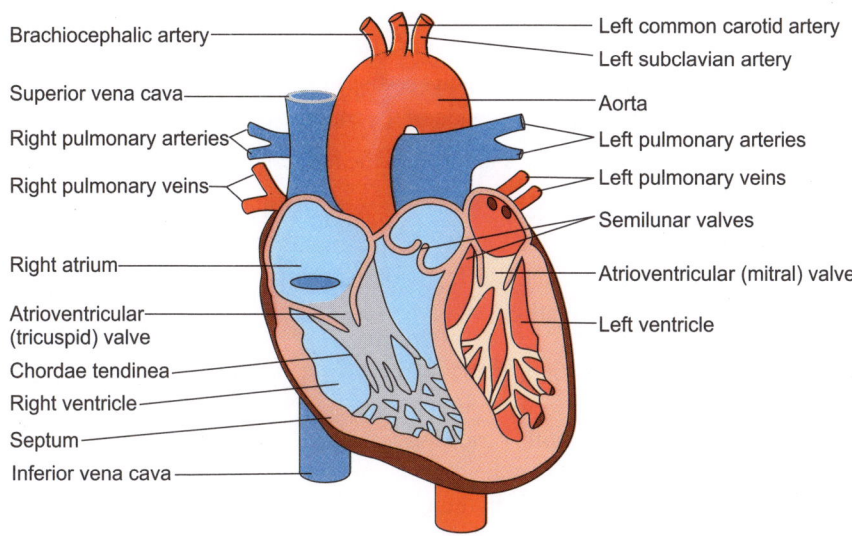

Brachiocephalic artery

Superior vena cava

Right pulmonary arteries

Right pulmonary veins

Right atrium

Atrioventricular (tricuspid) valve

Chordae tendinea

Right ventricle

Septum

Inferior vena cava

Left common carotid artery

Left subclavian artery

Aorta

Left pulmonary arteries

Left pulmonary veins

Semilunar valves

Atrioventricular (mitral) valve

Left ventricle

Figure 11.1 Schematic diagram of the human heart.

MEDICAL TERMINOLOGY

- ❏ **Mitral regurgitation**: It is disorder of the heart in which the mitral valve does not close properly when the heart pumps out blood.
- ❏ **Myocardial infarction**: It is the interruption of blood supply to part of the heart, causing some heart cells to die.
- ❏ **Pacemaker**: It is a group of cells or a body part (as the sinus node of the heart) that serves to establish and maintain a rhythmic activity.
- ❏ **Patent ductus arteriosus**: It is congenital disorder in heart wherein a neonate's ductus arteriosus fails to close after birth.
- ❏ **Phonocardiogram**: This instrument is used to record the heart sounds graphically by placing an electronic sound transducer over the chest and connecting it to a recording device like polygraph. This instrument can be used to record all the four heart sounds.
- ❏ **Plateau**: It is to reach a level, period or condition of stability.
- ❏ **Posterior**: It means situated behind.
- ❏ **Regurgitate**: The term indicates 'to become thrown or poured back'.
- ❏ **Repolarization**: It is the restoration of the difference in charge between the inside and outside of the cell membrane following depolarization.
- ❏ **Rheumatic fever**: It is a childhood disease that may damage the heart valves or the outer lining of the heart.
- ❏ **Striated**: It is to mark with striations.
- ❏ **Turbulence**: It is unstable flow of a liquid or gas.

POSITION

The heart is positioned in the thoracic cavity, between the lungs in the mediastinum. The position of heart is oblique, that is slightly more to the left side of the midline of the body (Fig. 11.2).

The apex of the heart is anterior, inferior and towards the left, whereas the base is superior, posterior and towards the right.

The heart is demarcated by the following:

❑ A point 9 cm to the left of the midsternal line (apex of the heart).
❑ The seventh right sternocostal articulation.

LOCATION

The surface of the heart is associated with various organs from different positions. The inferior side, that is the apex of the heart, rests mostly on the diaphragm, whereas the superior side, that is the base, is linked with the great blood vessels, that is the aorta, superior vena cava, pulmonary arteries and pulmonary veins.

The anterior surface of the heart is protected by the sternum, ribs and intercostals muscles, whereas the posterior surface is associated with the oesophagus, trachea, inferior vena cava and thoracic vertebrae.

The lungs are present on the sides of the heart, that is on the lateral position of the heart surface.

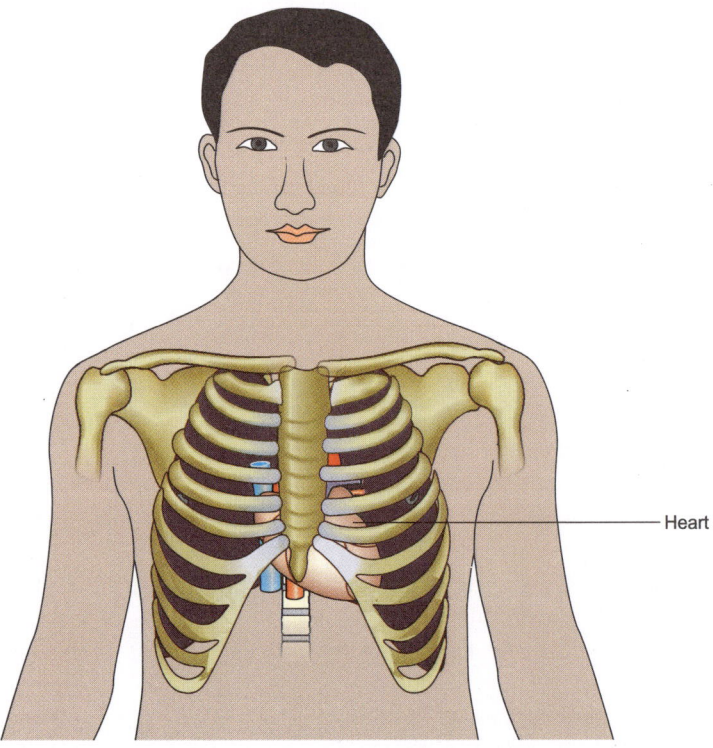

— Heart

Figure 11.2 Position of the heart.

STRUCTURE

Layers of wall of the heart

The heart is made up of the following three layers of tissues:

1. Outer pericardium
2. Middle myocardium
3. Inner endocardium

1. Pericardium (Fig. 11.3)

❑ It is the outer covering that surrounds and protects the heart.
❑ Pericardium is made up of two layers: the outer fibrous layer and the inner serous layer.
❑ The outer fibrous layer is tough, inelastic and of fibrous nature, which helps in protecting the heart from overstretching. This layer continues as tunica adventitia of the large blood vessels and is attached with the diaphragm below.
❑ The inner serous layer is a thin delicate membrane made of two layers, namely the outer parietal layer and the inner visceral layer. The outer parietal layer lines the fibrous layer of the pericardium and the inner visceral layer is attached tightly to the surface of the heart. The visceral layer is also called the *epicardium*.
❑ Both the layers of the serous membrane are made up of flattened epithelial cells that secrete a thin film of serous fluid between the parietal and visceral layers. This serous fluid is called *pericardial fluid* and the space where it is present between the parietal and visceral layers is called the *pericardial cavity*.
❑ The pericardial fluid reduces the friction between the membranes and allows smooth movement of the heart when it expands and contracts during a cardiac cycle.
❑ In healthy condition, the two layers of serous membrane lie very close to each other with only a thin film of pericardial fluid between them.

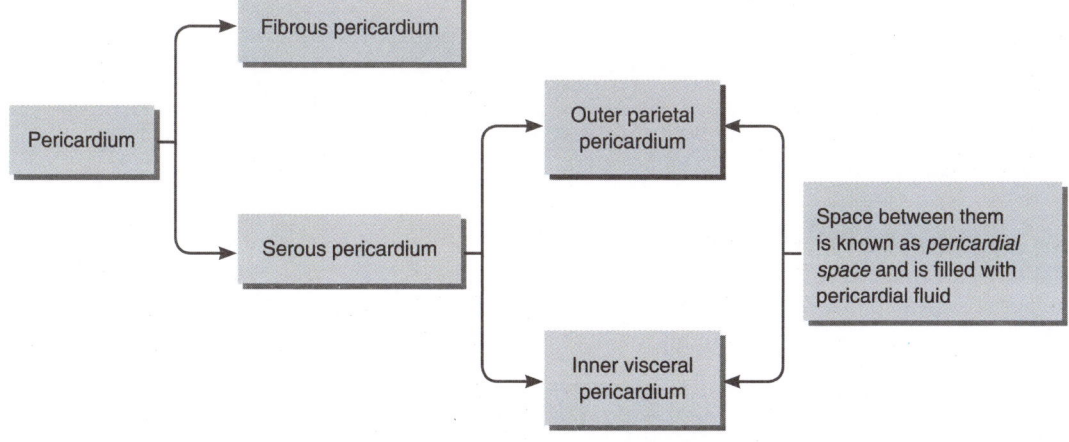

Figure 11.3 Structure of pericardium.

Chapter 11

2. Myocardium

❑ This is the middle layer of the wall of the heart present underneath the epicardium (Fig. 11.4).

❑ The myocardium is composed of *cardiac muscle tissue* and makes up the bulk of the heart.

❑ The cardiac muscle fibres are involuntary, striated and branched. Each fibre has a nucleus, which lies in the centre of the cell. The branches of cardiac muscle fibres join together with the branches of the adjacent or neighbouring fibres. The point of the union of the branches or the joint is called the *intercalated disc*, which forms tight junctions as the membrane of both the muscle fibres fuse together tightly.

❑ Microscopically, these intercalated discs can be seen as thicker and darker lines between different fibres and give the appearance of being a sheet of muscle.

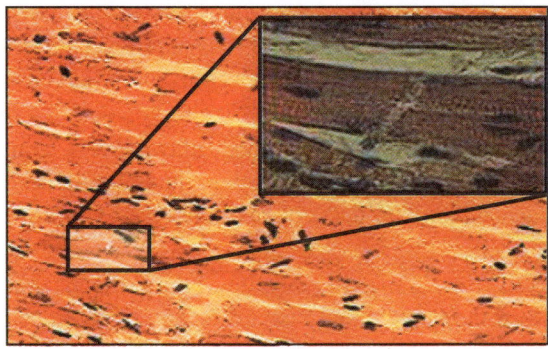

Figure 11.4 Cardiac muscle fibres.

❑ The intercalated discs play an important role during contraction of the muscle because when the impulse is initiated, it spreads rapidly from one fibre to another and facilitates the pulling of muscle fibres with one another. Thus, the sheet arrangement of the myocardium enables the atria and ventricles to contract in a coordinated manner.

3. Endocardium

❑ This is the third and innermost layer of the heart wall.

❑ It is a thin, smooth and glistening layer of endothelium that overlies a thin layer of connective tissue. It acts as a lining for the myocardium and also covers the chambers and valves of the heart.

❑ The endocardium continues as the endothelium of the blood vessels.

The chambers of the heart

The heart is divided into four chambers. The two superior/upper chambers are known as *right atrium* and *left atrium*, whereas the two inferior/lower chambers are called the *right ventricle* and *left ventricle* (Fig. 11.5).

The right and left sides of the heart are separated from one another by a fibrous septum so that blood cannot cross from one side to the other. The septum between the two atria is called the *interatrial septum*, whereas that between ventricle is the *interventricle septum*.

Each atrium has a pouch-like structure on its anterior surface called an *auricle*, named due to its similarity with the ear of a dog. The auricle slightly increases the capacity of the atrium and thereby makes space for a greater volume of blood.

The surface of the heart also comprises a series of grooves called *sulci* that contain a varying amount of fat and coronary blood vessels. Each sulcus divides the myocardium into separate muscle masses. The deep coronary sulcus separates the atria from ventricles. The anterior interventricular sulcus and the posterior interventricular sulcus separate the right and left ventricles from one another at the anterior and posterior surfaces, respectively.

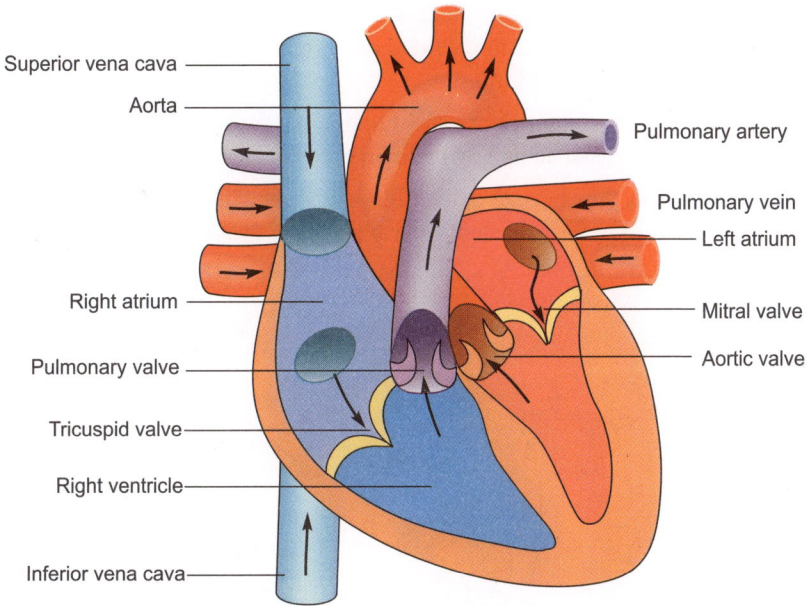

Figure 11.5 The chambers of the heart.

The right atrium receives venous (deoxygenated) blood from all parts of the body except the lungs. It receives the blood through the following three veins:

1. **Superior vena cava**, also known as the *anterior vena cava*, that returns the venous blood from the upper parts of the body, the head, neck and arms.
2. **Inferior vena cava**, also known as the *posterior vena cava*, that brings the blood from the lower parts of body, the legs and abdomen.
3. **Coronary sinus** that drains the blood from most of the vessels that supply to the heart.

The blood in right atrium is then squeezed into the right ventricle.

The right ventricle then pumps the blood into the pulmonary artery, which further splits into the right and left pulmonary arteries after leaving the heart. These arteries carry the venous (deoxygenated) blood to the lungs where the blood releases carbon dioxide and picks up oxygen. The oxygenated blood then returns to the heart via four pulmonary veins that empty into the left atrium.

This is the only exception in the body where artery carries venous blood and veins carry oxygenated blood.

The blood from the left atrium is then passed into the left ventricle (Fig. 11.6).

The right atrium and left atrium are separated by the interatrial septum, present between them. A prominent feature of this septum is an oval depression called fossa ovalis, which is the remnant of foramen ovale. The foramen ovale is an opening in the interatrial septum of the fetal heart that normally closes soon after birth.

The left ventricle pumps the arterial blood into systemic aorta. From here, the oxygenated blood goes to the coronary arteries (which supply to the heart), the arch of aorta and descending aorta. The branches of arch of aorta and descending aorta transport oxygenated blood to all parts of the body.

Note: During fetal life, a blood vessel called ductus arteriosus diverts blood from the pulmonary artery into the aorta, so that only a small amount of blood enters the nonfunctioning fetal lungs. The ductus arteriosus normally closes shortly after birth.

The thickness and size of the chamber vary according to the functioning of each chamber, that is the amount of blood received and distance up to which the blood must be pumped.

The atria are thin-walled as they have to deliver blood into the adjacent ventricles, whereas the walls of ventricles are thicker as they have to pump the blood to a greater distance. The thickness of the

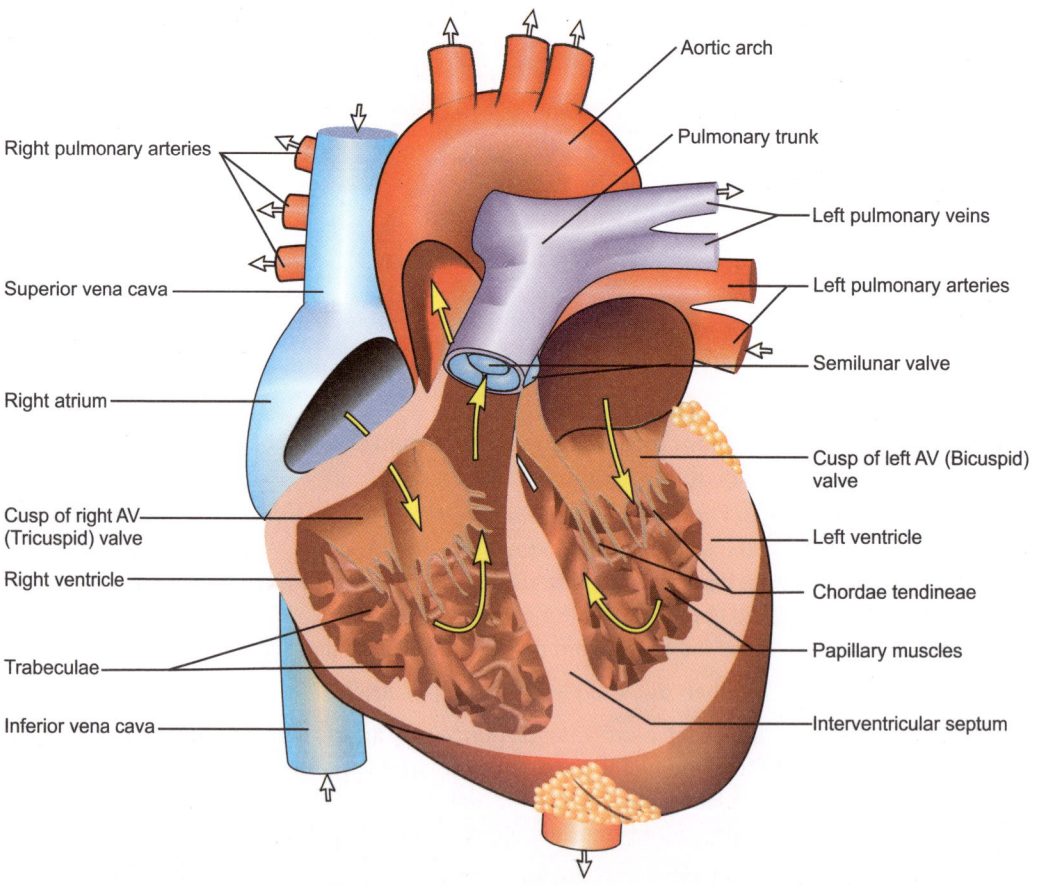

Figure 11.6 The structure of the heart.

walls of two ventricles also varies. The left ventricle wall is thicker than the right ventricle as the right ventricle pumps blood into the nearby lungs, whereas the left ventricle pumps blood to all parts of the body. Thus, the left ventricle works harder than the right ventricle to maintain the same rate of blood flow.

Valves of the heart

The valves of the heart permit the flow of blood in only one direction. The valves open to let the blood flow through and close to prevent backflow of blood into the pumping chamber.

There are four valves in the human heart: two atrioventricular valves (AV valves) and two semilunar valves (Fig. 11.7).

AV valves

The AV valves separate the atrium (the upper chamber) and the ventricle (the lower chamber).

The valve between right atrium and right ventricle is called the *tricuspid valve* as it consists of three flaps/cusps. The AV valve between the left atrium and left ventricle is known as the *bicuspid or mitral valve* as it has two flaps/cusps. These flaps are made of double folds of endocardium, which is strengthened by a little fibrous tissue. The cusps of these AV valves are connected to tendon-like cords, the *chordate tendinae*, which in turn are connected to small conical projections called *papillary muscles* located on the inner surface of the ventricles.

The papillary muscles play an important role in closure of the cusps, thus preventing the backflow of blood from ventricles to atria during contraction.

The valves between the atria and ventricles open and close in response to the pressure changes as the heart contracts and relaxes.

When the ventricles are relaxed, the pressure in the atria is more than that in the ventricles. The increased pressure of atria opens the AV valves and allows the blood to move from atria to ventricles.

When the ventricles contract, the pressure in the ventricles becomes more than that in the atria. The increased pressure in the ventricles closes the AV valves and prevents the backflow of blood.

If AV valves are damaged, blood may regurgitate into the atria when the ventricles contract.

Semilunar valves

The semilunar valves are present at the opening of systemic aorta and pulmonary artery and are known as *aortic valve* and *pulmonary valve*, respectively. These are called *semilunar valves* due to their half-moon shape.

Both these semilunar valves have similar structure and each one has three flaps that allow the blood to flow only in one direction.

The semilunar valves open when pressure in the ventricles is more than that in the arteries, which allows the movement of blood from the ventricles into the pulmonary artery and systemic aorta.

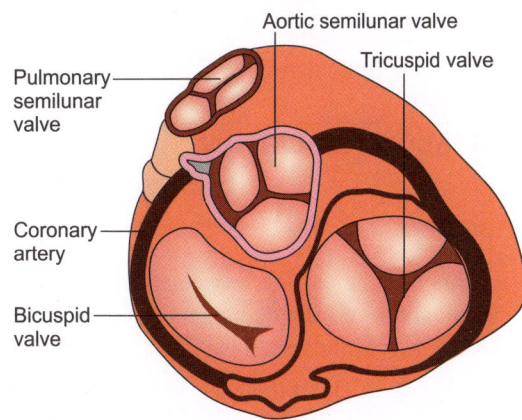

Figure 11.7 The atrioventricular and semilunar valves.

When the ventricles relax, blood starts flowing back towards the heart. This backflowing of blood causes the semilunar valves to close tightly, thus allowing the blood to move only in one direction.

FLOW OF BLOOD THROUGH THE HEART

The deoxygenated (venous) blood returns from the lower and upper portions of the body through the superior and inferior vena cava, respectively, and these veins empty their contents into the right atrium.

The blood then passes via the right AV valve (tricuspid valve) into the right ventricle, and from there it is pumped through the pulmonary semilunar valve (tricuspid valve) into the pulmonary artery by contraction of the right ventricle.

After leaving the heart, the pulmonary artery divides into the left and right pulmonary arteries, which carry the venous blood to the left and right lungs, respectively. In the lung alveoli, the exchange of gases takes place, that is blood looses carbon dioxide and picks up oxygen.

The oxygenated blood then returns to the left atrium through four pulmonary veins, two from each lung.

When the left atrium contracts, the blood is pushed through the left AV valve (bicuspid valve/mitral valve) into the left ventricle.

The left ventricle with its thick muscular walls then contracts and pumps the blood through the aortic semilunar valve (tricuspid) into the aorta, which then caries the blood throughout the body (see Fig. 11.6).

The contraction and relaxation of chambers of the heart follows a particular pattern in which both atria undergo contraction simultaneously and, at the same time, the two ventricles relax. This is followed by the simultaneous contraction of both ventricles while the two atria relax at that time. Then, all the chambers rest before the new cycle of contraction and relaxation begins again.

BLOOD CIRCULATION

The blood circulates continuously throughout the body and the circulation of blood can be described in the following two processes:

1. Systemic circulation
2. Pulmonary circulation

SYSTEMIC CIRCULATION

Systemic circulation includes the pathway through which blood is circulated to different parts of the body.

In this circulation, the oxygenated blood is pumped through the aortic semilunar valve into the systemic aorta and the deoxygenated blood is returned to the right atrium of the heart through the superior and inferior vena cava from all parts of the body (Fig. 11.8).

The left ventricle of the heart is the pump for ejection of oxygenated blood into the aorta. From the aorta, the blood is distributed into separate smaller arteries that carry it to all the organs throughout the body except the lungs. In systemic tissues, arteries divide into smaller diameter arterioles, which are

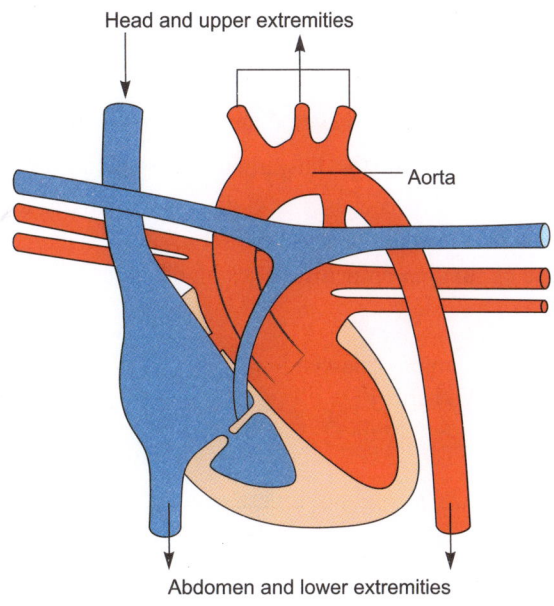

Head and upper extremities

Aorta

Abdomen and lower extremities

Figure 11.8 Systemic circulation.

(Deoxygenated blood looks dark, thus veins depicted in blue colour)
(Oxygenated blood looks bright red, thus arteries shown in red colour)

further branched into various capillaries. The capillary walls are permeable to various substances and thus they are responsible for the exchange of various substances between blood and the tissues.

After exchange of nutrients and gases across the thin capillary walls, the blood enters the venules, which carry the deoxygenated blood away from the tissues and merge to form smaller veins, which are further merged in larger veins. These larger veins ultimately join with the vena cava and the blood flows back to the right atrium.

Various arteries that branch from the aorta and supply blood to various organs of the body have been summarized as follows:

1. Aorta starts from the upper part of the left ventricle and after passing upwards for a short way, it arches backwards and to the left. This portion of the aorta is called the arch of aorta.

Just above the Arch of Aorta near the level of aortic valve, the aorta branches into right and left coronary arteries, which supply arterial blood to the heart. The circulation of blood through the heart via coronary arteries and veins is called *coronary (cardiac) circulation* (Fig. 11.9).

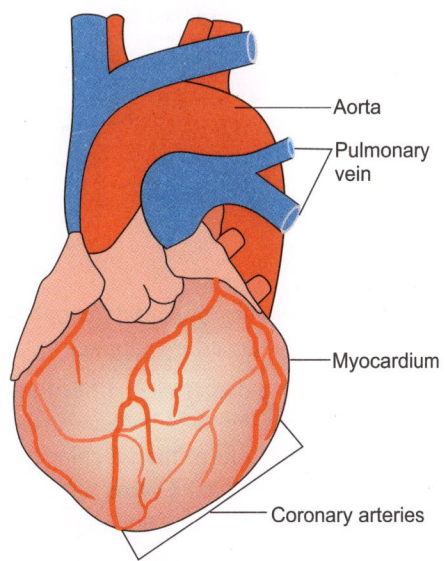

Aorta

Pulmonary vein

Myocardium

Coronary arteries

Figure 11.9 Coronary circulation.

❑ The coronary arteries receive about 5% of the blood pumped from the heart, which highlights the importance of the heart in the various functions of the body.

❑ The myocardium contains many anastomoses that connect the branches of different coronary arteries; thus, they provide sufficient arterial blood even if any coronary artery is partially blocked.

The left coronary artery divides into the left anterior descending (LAD) artery and circumflex branch.

LAD (also known as the *anterior interventricular branch*) supplies oxygenated blood to the walls of both ventricles, whereas the circumflex branch supplies blood to the walls of the left ventricle and the left atrium.

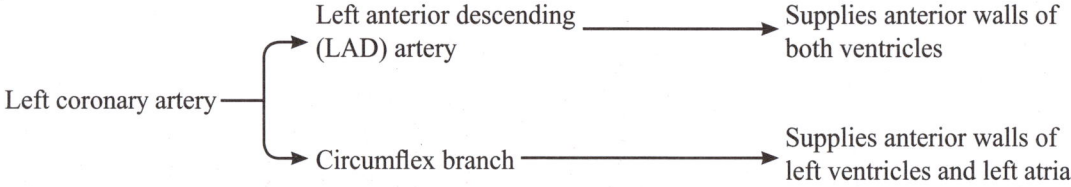

The right coronary artery divides into the posterior interventricular branch and the marginal branch.

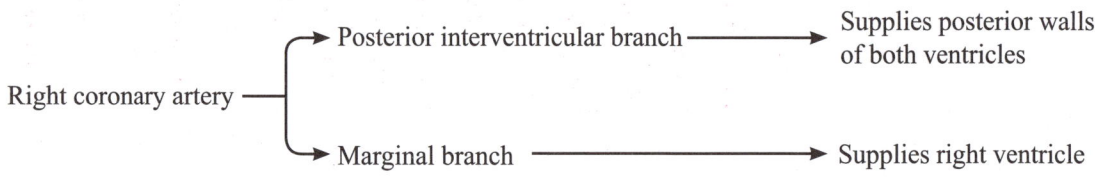

After supplying the oxygenated blood through coronary arteries and exchanging oxygen and nutrients in the heart muscle, the deoxygenated blood drains into the cardiac veins. The cardiac veins further carry blood towards the coronary sinus; from this, the venous blood is emptied into the right atrium.

The arch of aorta divides into three main branches as follows:

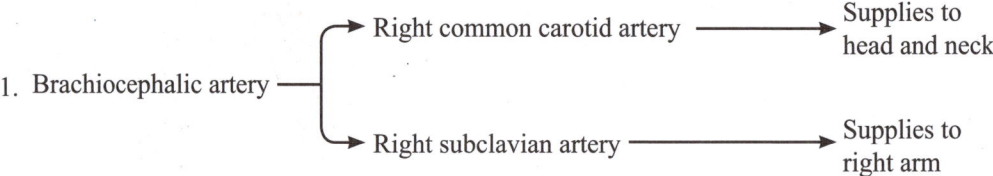

2. Left common carotid artery supplies to head and neck
3. Left subclavian artery supplies to left arm

The venous blood from the head and neck is returned to the jugular vein, which unites with the subclavian veins. The subclavian vein drains blood from the upper limbs. The jugular vein and subclavian vein both unite to form the brachiocephalic vein, which is situated on each side of the neck. The left and right brachiocephalic veins further join to form the superior vena cava, which drains all the venous blood from the head, neck and upper limbs into the right atrium of the heart.

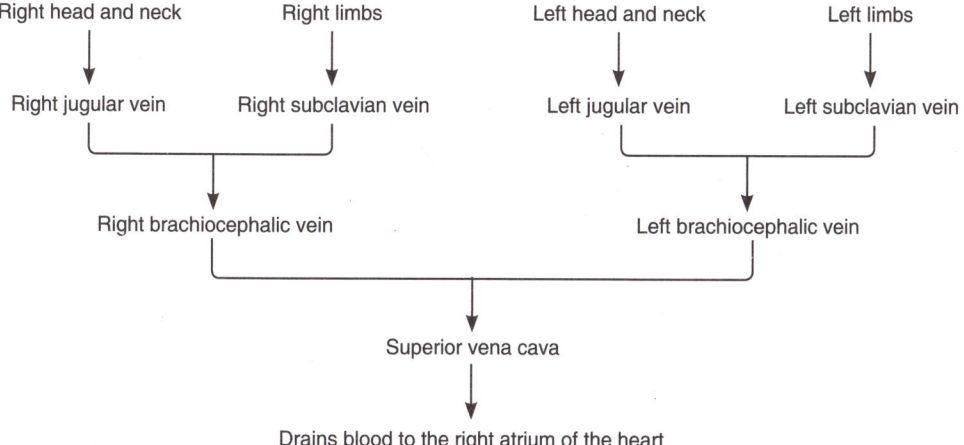

2. The arch of aorta then descends through the thoracic cavity behind the heart and at this level it is termed as the thoracic aorta (Fig. 11.10).

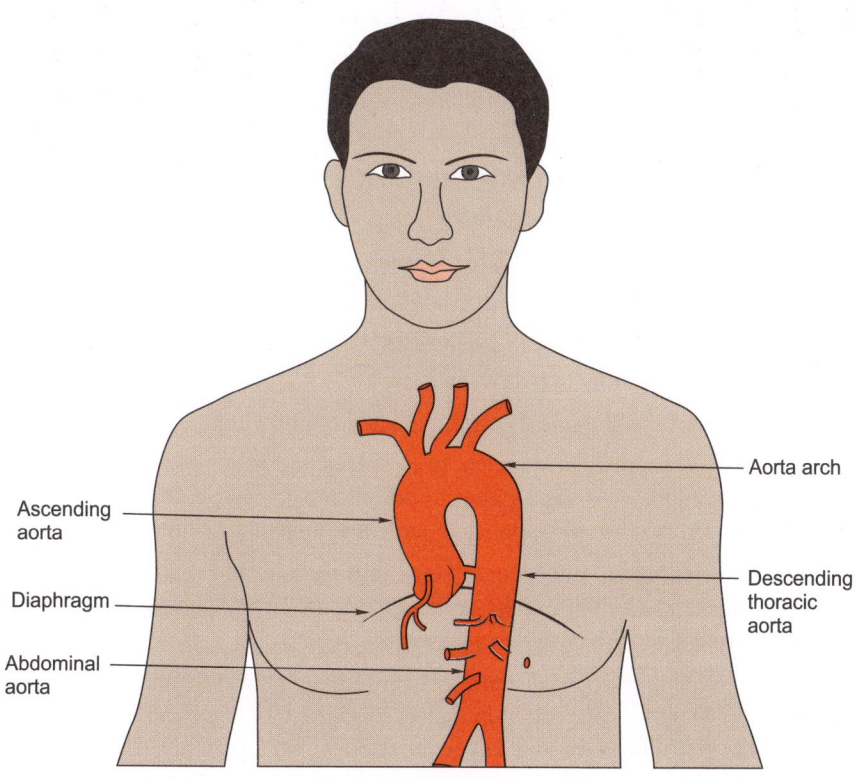

Figure 11.10 The arch of aorta, thoracic aorta and abdominal aorta.

The thoracic aorta divides into many branches, which supply to the organs present within the thoracic cavity. The following are the various branches of the thoracic aorta:

1. Bronchial arteries ⟶ Supply to bronchial lungs
2. Oesophageal arteries ⟶ Supply to oesophagus
3. Intercostal arteries ⟶ Supply to ribs and tissues of thorax

The venous blood from the organs in the thoracic cavity is drained into the azygos vein and hemiazygous vein.

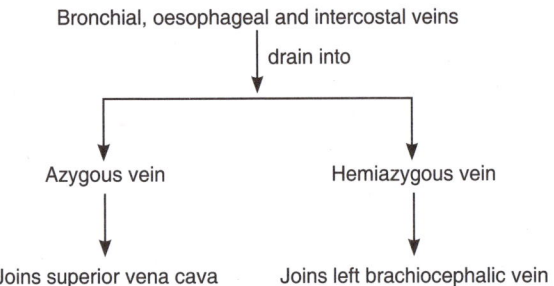

3. At the level of twelfth thoracic vertebrae, the aorta passes downwards in the abdominal cavity behind the diaphragm and is known as *abdominal aorta* at this level.

The abdominal aorta is the continuation of thoracic aorta. The abdominal aorta divides into various paired and unpaired branches.

The paired branches of the abdominal aorta include the following:

1. Phrenic artery ⟶ supplies to diaphragm
2. Renal artery ⟶ supplies to kidney
   The renal artery further branches to form suprarenal arteries, which supply blood to adrenal glands.
3. Testicular arteries ⟶ supply to testes in males
4. Ovarian arteries ⟶ supply to ovaries in females

The unpaired branches of the abdominal aorta include the following:

1. Coeliac artery ⟶ supplies to stomach, liver, spleen and pancreas
2. Superior mesenteric artery ⟶ supplies to intestine
3. Inferior mesenteric artery ⟶ supplies to large intestine and rectum

Paired testicular, ovarian, renal and adrenal veins join the inferior vena cava to drain the impure blood. The blood from the remaining organs in the abdominal cavity passes through the liver via the portal circulation before entering the inferior vena cava.

Thus, it can be noted that the aorta is described according to its location and it divides into numerous branches throughout its length. Some of the branches are paired, that is there is the same name for the right and left branches (e.g. the right and left renal arteries, which supply the kidneys), while some branches are unpaired (e.g. coeliac artery, which supplies pancreas and spleen).

Portal circulation

In portal circulation, the venous blood from splenic vein (spleen), mesenteric vein, gastric vein (stomach) and cystic vein (gallbladder) passes to the liver via the portal vein. In this way, blood with a high concentration of nutrients, which are absorbed from the stomach and intestine, first goes to the liver, where it undergoes certain modifications in the concentration of nutrients. The portal vein thus passes to the liver before entering the inferior vena cava.

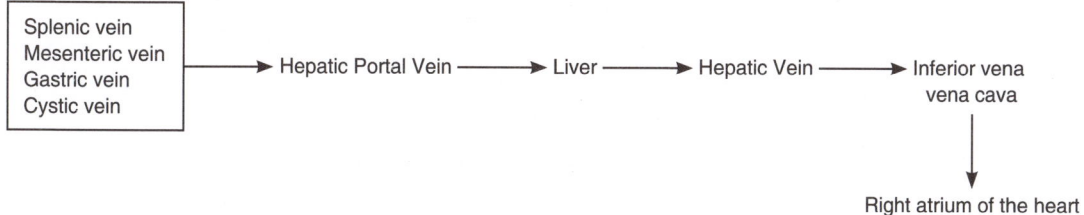

4. At the level of fourth lumbar vertebrae, the abdominal aorta further branches into the right and left iliac arteries.

Each iliac artery further divides into the internal and external iliac arteries.

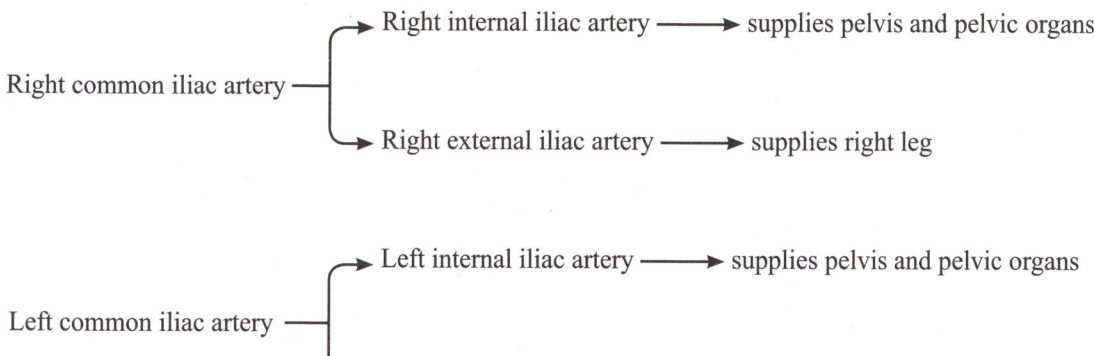

The external and internal iliac veins join to form the common iliac vein, which drains the blood directly into the inferior vena cava.

PULMONARY CIRCULATION

Pulmonary circulation includes the circulation of blood from the right ventricle of the heart to the lungs and the returning back of blood to the left atrium of the heart.

In this circulation, the deoxygenated blood in the right ventricle is pumped through the pulmonary semilunar valve into the pulmonary artery. The pulmonary artery, after leaving the heart, divides into the right and left pulmonary arteries, which carry blood to the right and left lungs, respectively. Within the

Chapter 11

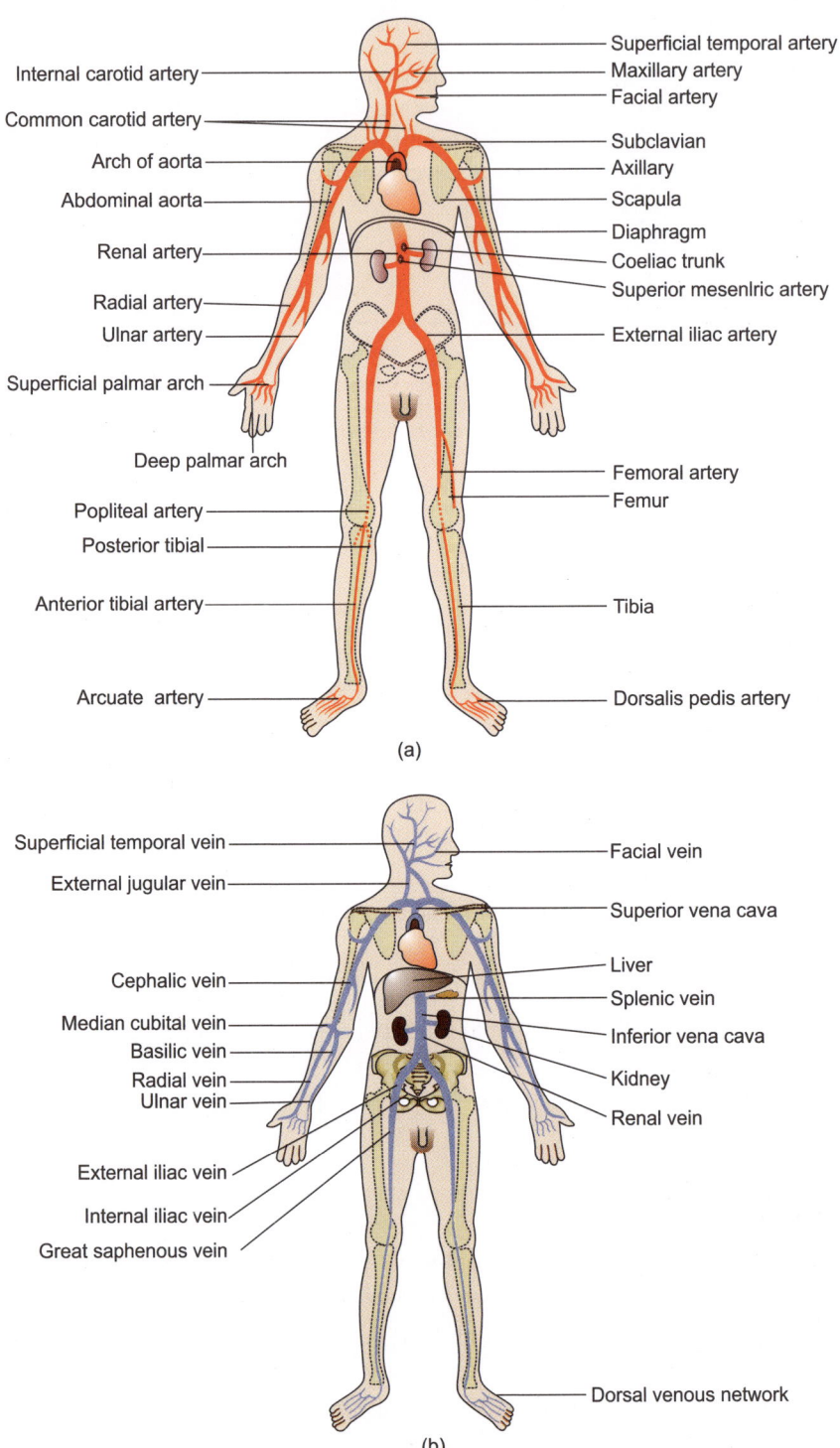

Internal carotid artery
Common carotid artery
Arch of aorta
Abdominal aorta
Renal artery
Radial artery
Ulnar artery
Superficial palmar arch
Deep palmar arch
Popliteal artery
Posterior tibial
Anterior tibial artery
Arcuate artery

Superficial temporal artery
Maxillary artery
Facial artery
Subclavian
Axillary
Scapula
Diaphragm
Coeliac trunk
Superior mesenlric artery
External iliac artery
Femoral artery
Femur
Tibia
Dorsalis pedis artery

(a)

Superficial temporal vein
External jugular vein
Cephalic vein
Median cubital vein
Basilic vein
Radial vein
Ulnar vein
External iliac vein
Internal iliac vein
Great saphenous vein

Facial vein
Superior vena cava
Liver
Splenic vein
Inferior vena cava
Kidney
Renal vein
Dorsal venous network

(b)

Figure 11.11 Systemic circulation: (a) Arteries; (b) Veins.

lungs, these arteries divide and subdivide into smaller arterioles and capillaries. In pulmonary capillaries, the blood loses its carbon dioxide and picks up oxygen (Fig. 11.12).

The pulmonary capillaries, which now contain freshly oxygenated blood, join up and eventually form two pulmonary veins. These four pulmonary veins (two from each lung) then return the oxygenated blood to the left atrium of the heart, which is further pumped into the left ventricle and then during ventricular systole the blood is forced into the aorta and circulated throughout the body.

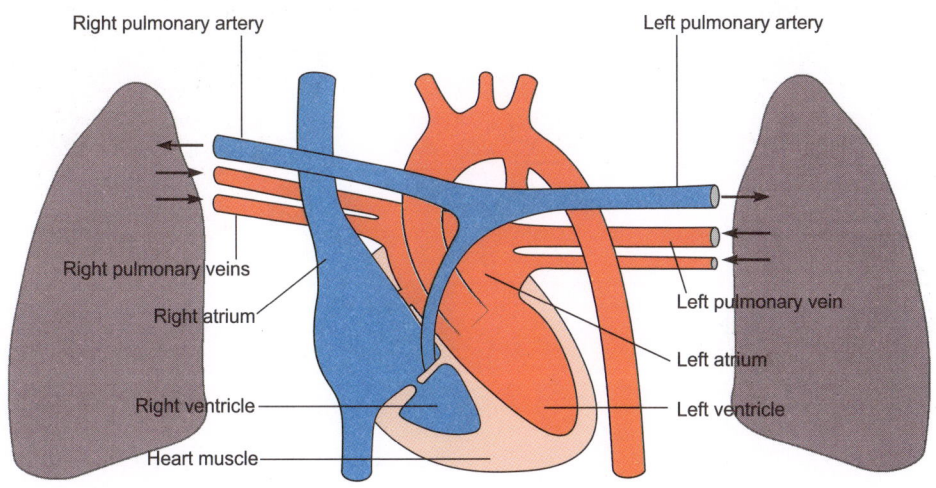

Figure 11.12 Pulmonary circulation.

FETAL CIRCULATION

Fetal circulation is the circulation of blood in the fetus that provides oxygen and nutrients to its tissues and removes carbon dioxide and other wastes.

This is the pathway of blood that is present only between the developing fetus and its mother since many organs in the fetus do not start functioning till birth, such as lungs, gastrointestinal system and kidneys. Therefore, certain modifications are present in the route of blood flow in fetal circulation, which helps meet prenatal requirements.

The unique modifications in the fetal circulation include special structures like:

1. **Placenta**: It is the structure that forms inside the mother's uterus and attaches to the umbilicus (navel) of the fetus. It enables the exchange of materials between fetal and maternal circulation by diffusion.
2. **Two umbilical arteries**: These are the branches of internal iliac arteries that carry the deoxygenated blood from the fetus to the placenta, where the fetal blood picks up oxygen and nutrients and eliminates carbon dioxide and wastes.
3. **Umbilical vein**: It returns the oxygenated blood back to the fetus.
   The only blood vessel that carries fully oxygenated blood is the umbilical vein (Fig. 11.13).

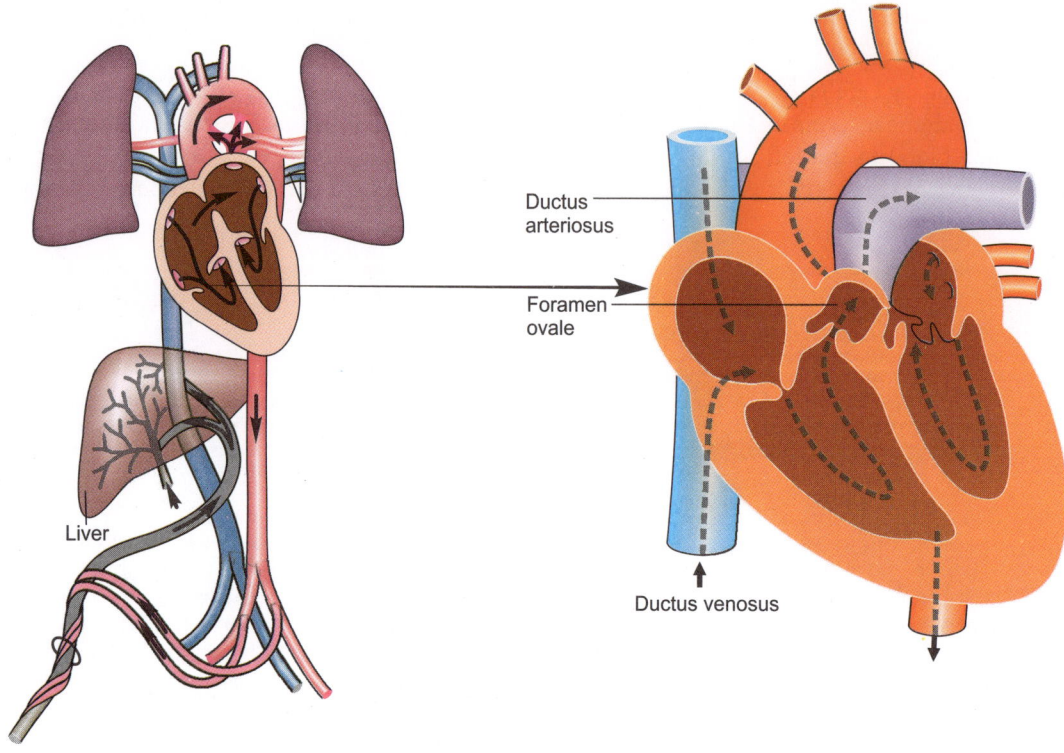

Figure 11.13 Fetal circulation.

4. **Ductus venosus**: This is a branch of umbilical vein that drains most of the oxygenated blood into the inferior vena cava. The deoxygenated blood in the inferior vena cava mixes with the oxygenated blood from ductus venosus and this mixed blood then enters the right atrium.
5. **Foramen ovale**: This is a small opening present in the septum between the right and left atria. It allows blood to flow between the right and left atria so that most of the blood bypasses the nonfunctional fetal lungs.
6. **Ductus arteriosus**: It is a small vessel that connects the pulmonary artery with the aorta. In this way, most of the blood bypasses the fetal lungs and the blood in the aorta is carried to all fetal tissues through systemic circulation.

After birth, when the lungs, kidney and gastrointestinal tract start functioning, the following changes occur in blood circulation:

1. When the lungs start functioning ⟶ Blood from lungs enters the left atrium, which increases pressure in the left atrium ⟶ causes closure of foramen ovale and prevents blood flow between right atrium and left atrium. The fossa ovalis is formed, which is a depression in the septum where the foramen ovale closes.
2. Blood entering right atrium ⟶ diverted towards right ventricle due to closure of foramen ovale ⟶ right ventricle pumps blood into pulmonary artery ⟶ which causes vasoconstriction and closure of ductus arteriosus.

3. The placenta is expelled after birth ⟶ placental circulation stops ⟶ thus, umbilical vein, ductus venosus and umbilical arteries collapse

If these changes do not take place after birth, they become congenital abnormalities.

CARDIAC CONDUCTION SYSTEM

The heart has an inherent regulating system that generates and distributes electrical impulses over the heart to stimulate the cardiac muscle, causing coordinated and rhythmic contractions. This intrinsic system is called the *cardiac conduction system* and the source of this electrical activity is a network of specialized cardiac muscle fibres called *autorhythmic fibres*.

These autorhythmic fibres are self-excitable and they automatically stimulate the cardiac muscle to contract without the need for any external stimulation. Actually, they continue to stimulate the heart to contract even after it is removed from the body.

Only 1% of the cardiac muscle fibres become autorhythmic fibres during development of the embryo. The autorhythmic fibres are small groups of specialized neuromuscular cells in the cardiac muscles and have the following two important functions:

1. They act as pacemaker and initiate the impulse that causes contraction of the heart.
2. They form a network of specialized cardiac muscle fibres, that is the conduction system that conducts the impulse, causing coordinated and synchronized contractions, which makes the heart an effective pump.

The cardiac impulses pass through the conduction system in the following sequence:

1. Cardiac excitation begins at the *sinoatrial node*, also known as the *SA node* or *pacemaker of the heart*. This SA node is a small mass of specialized cells located in the wall of the right atrium near the opening of the superior vena cava. It normally initiates the impulses more rapidly than other groups of neuromuscular cells and sets the pace for the heart rate. Once an impulse is initiated by the SA node, the impulse spreads over both atria, causing them to contract simultaneously.
2. After causing atrial contractions, the impulse that was initiated by the SA node reaches the *atrioventricular node (AV node)*, which is a small mass of neuromuscular tissue located in the wall of the atrial septum near the AV valves. The AV node conducts the impulse further towards the ventricles.
   The AV node also has a secondary pacemaker function, which it performs only when the SA node is not functioning properly or impulses are not getting transmitted from the atria. However, the AV node generates impulses at a slower rate compared with the SA node.
3. From the AV node, the impulse enters the *atrioventricular bundle (AV bundle)*, also known as the *bundle of His*. The AV bundle is a mass of specialized fibres that originate from the AV node and it is the only site where impulses can be conducted from atria to the ventricles. (Otherwise, the fibrous portion of the heart acts as an insulator between atria and ventricles.)
4. The AV bundle branches and continues down towards both sides of the septum as the *right and left bundle branches;* thus, it distributes the impulse over the ventricles.
5. Finally, the right and left bundle branches further break up into fine fibres called *Purkinje fibres*. The actual contraction of the ventricles is stimulated by these purkinje fibres, which push the blood upwards toward the semilunar valves into the pulmonary artery and the aorta (Fig. 11.14).

The auto rhythmic fibres in the SA node initiate an impulse 100 times/min.

Chapter 11

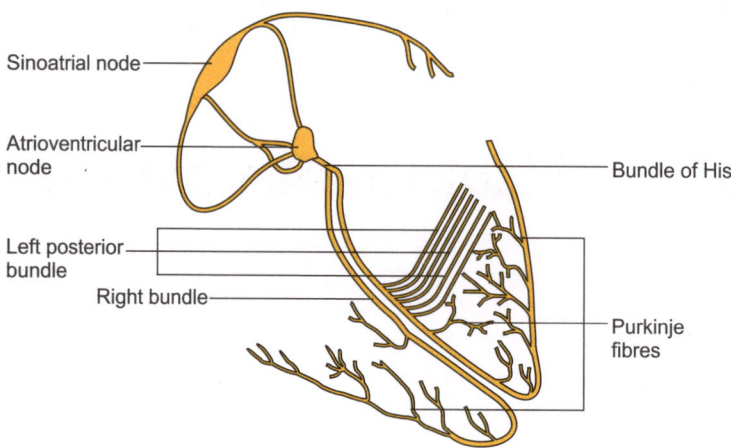

Figure 11.14 Cardiac conduction system.

The heart is also influenced by the nerve impulses from the autonomic nervous system (ANS). These consist of parasympathetic and sympathetic nerve impulses and their actions are antagonistic. Parasympathetic stimulation reduces the rate of impulse production and decreases the force of heart beat. Conversely, sympathetic stimulation increases the rate and force of the heart beat.

ACTION POTENTIAL IN CARDIAC MUSCLE

The electrical activity that takes place in the cardiac muscle is called *action potential*. Duration of the action potential in cardiac muscle is 0.25–0.35 s approximately.

The action potential in a single cardiac muscle fibre occurs in the following four phases (Fig. 11.15):

1. Phase 0: A rapid depolarization
2. Phase 1: Initial repolarization
3. Phase 2: Plateau phase
4. Phase 3: Final repolarization

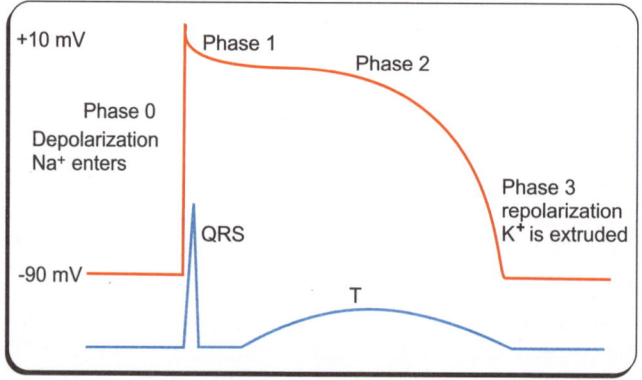

Figure 11.15 Action potential in the cardiac muscle.

1. **Depolarization**
   - ❑ This phase is very rapid and lasts for about 2 ms. The rapid depolarization is due to the rapid opening of voltage-gated fast Na$^+$ channels and the rapid influx of sodium ions.
   - ❑ These sodium channels are referred to as 'fast' as they open very rapidly in response to an impulse.

2. **Initial repolarization**: This phase occurs just before the plateau phase due to the opening of K$^+$ channels and efflux of a small number of K$^+$ ions for a very short time. Simultaneously, fast Na$^+$ channels close and slow Na$^+$ channels open, causing slow influx of a small number of Na$^+$ ions.

3. **Plateau phase**
   - ❑ The plateau phase is the phase of maintained depolarization.
   - ❑ This phase occurs due to the opening of voltage-gated slow Ca$^+$ channels. These channels open for a longer time, which causes the influx of a larger number of Ca ions from the interstitial fluid into the cytosol. The increased Ca$^+$ concentration in the cytosol ultimately causes contraction.
   - ❑ This phase lasts for about 0.25 s.

4. **Repolarization**
   - ❑ It is a slow process and lasts for about 0.05–0.08 s.
   - ❑ This phase starts at the end of the plateau phase when the voltage-gated K$^+$ channels open. This causes the efflux of a large number of K$^+$ ions out of the cardiac muscle fibres and this continues till the end of the repolarization phase.

THE CARDIAC CYCLE

The function of the heart is to ensure the constant circulation of blood throughout the body; to achieve this, the different chambers of the heart undergo various changes during each heart beat. These changes are repeated during every heart beat in a cyclic manner.

Thus, the cardiac cycle can be defined as the succession of all the coordinated events that take place during every heart beat. During each heartbeat or cardiac cycle, the two atria contract simultaneously while the two ventricles relax, which is followed by the contraction of both the ventricles and relaxation of the atria. The period of contraction is called *systole* and the phase of relaxation is termed as *diastole*.

STAGES OF CARDIAC CYCLE

When the heart beats at the normal rate of 72 times/min, the duration of each cardiac cycle is about 0.8 s. The duration of systole is 0.27 s and that of diastole is 0.53 s.

The various stages of cardiac cycle include:

1. Atrial systole: Atrial systole, that is the contraction of the atria, lasts for about 0.1 s. This phase is also called the *last rapid filling phase* and is considered as the last phase of ventricular diastole (relaxation).

During this phase, the atria contracts and exerts pressure on the blood present within the atria. This pressure forces the blood through the open AV valves into the relaxing ventricles. In this phase, the AV valves (bicuspid and tricuspid) are open and the semilunar valves (aortic and pulmonary) are closed (Fig. 11.16).

The atrial systole pushes around 52 mL of blood into the ventricles, which already contain approximately 105 mL of blood. Thus, at the end of the atrial systole (or ventricular diastole), each ventricle contains about 130 mL of blood and this blood volume is called *end-diastolic volume (EDV)*.

2. Ventricular systole: This phase occurs in the following two stages:

(a) *Isometric contraction or isovolumetric contraction* (Fig. 11.17).

❑ This phase lasts for 0.05 s. As the ventricular systole begins, pressure rises in the ventricles, which forces the AV valves to close and prevents the backflow of blood into the atria. The semilunar valves are already closed.

❑ In this phase, the ventricles contract but there is no change in the volume of ventricles or length of cardiac muscle fibres in the ventricles. Hence, this phase is referred to as *isometric* (same length) or *isovolumetric* (same volume) *contraction phase*.

❑ Continued contraction of the ventricles sharply increases the pressure inside the ventricles. When pressure in the ventricles increases above the pressure in the pulmonary artery and aorta, the semilunar valves of the pulmonary artery and aorta open, which leads to the ejection of blood into these vessels.

(b) *Ejection period* (Fig. 11.18)

❑ The ejection period lasts for about 0.25 s.

❑ In this phase the ventricles contract and semilunar valves open, leading to the ejection of blood from both the ventricles. The left ventricle ejects about 70 mL of blood into the aorta and the right ventricle ejects the same volume of blood into the pulmonary artery.

❑ The volume of blood (about 60 mL) remaining in each ventricle at the end of ventricular systole is termed as *end-systole volume (ESV)*.

❑ Stroke volume, that is, the volume of blood that is ejected per beat from each ventricle, can be calculated as follows:

SV = End diastolic volume – End systolic volume

= 130 mL – 60 mL = 70 mL

The isometric contraction and ejection phase together form the ventricular systole phase. Hence, the duration of the ventricular systole (VS) phase is the sum of the duration of both the phases, that is isometric contraction (IC) and ejection phase (EP).

Duration of VS phase = IC + EP

= 0.05 + 0.25 s = 0.3 s

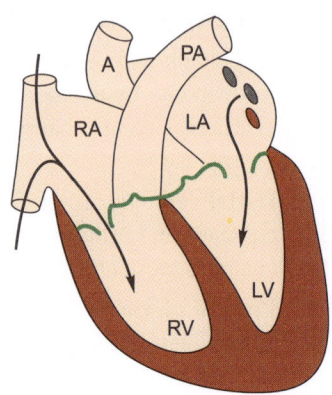

Figure 11.16 Atrial systole.

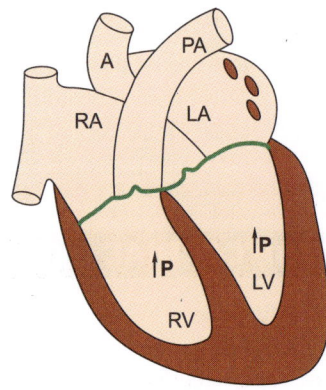

Figure 11.17 Isovolumetric contraction.

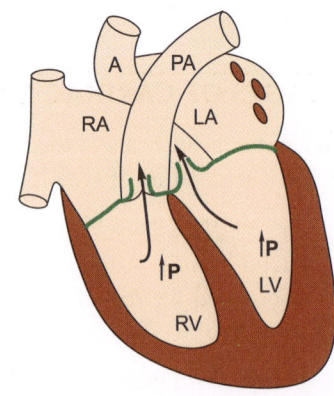

Figure 11.18 Ejection period.

3. Relaxation period: During the relaxation period, both atria and ventricles are relaxed (Fig. 11.19).

Due to the ejection of blood, the pressure in the aorta and pulmonary artery increases and the pressure in the ventricles decreases. When the pressure in the ventricles decreases below that in the aorta and pulmonary artery, the semilunar valves close. This phase indicates end of the systole and beginning of diastole and is termed as the *ventricular diastole phase* and this phase lasts for 0.04 s.

After the semilunar valves close, the blood volume in the ventricles does not change because in this phase, all the valves of the heart are closed. This is the *period of isovolumetric relaxation,* which lasts for 0.08 s.

As the ventricles continue to relax, the pressure in the ventricles falls quickly. When the pressure in the ventricles become less than the pressure in the atria, the AV valves open and filling of the ventricles begins.

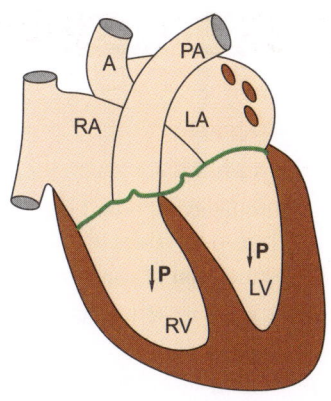

Figure 11.19 Isovolumetric relaxation phase.

In the isovolumetric relaxation phase, when all the valves are closed and both atria and ventricles are relaxing, the right atria is being filled with the blood through the superior vena cava and inferior vena cava and the left atria through the pulmonary veins.

Thus, opening of the AV valves indicates the beginning of the ventricular filling phase.

The filling of the ventricles (Fig. 11.20) occurs in the following two phases:

1. *Rapid filling phase*
   The blood accumulates in both atria during atrial diastole. When AV valves are opened, there is a sudden rush of blood into the ventricles and major part (70%) of ventricular filling occurs. This phase is called the *rapid filling phase,* which lasts for 0.11 s.

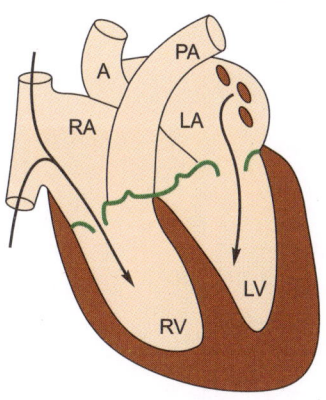

Figure 11.20 Filling phase.

2. *Slow filling phase*
   After the sudden rush of blood, the filling of ventricles becomes slow; thus, this phase is called the *slow filling phase*. This phase lasts for 0.19 s.

Thus, the relaxation period (RP) includes ventricular diastole (VD), isovolumetric relaxation (IR) and ventricular filling (VF) phases.

RP = VD + IR + VF phases

= VD + IR + (fast filling + slow filling) phases

= 0.04 + 0.08 + (0.11 + 0.19)

= 0.4 s

4. Atrial systole: After the slow filling phase, the atria contract and the cycle is repeated again.

HEART SOUNDS

The various events during each cardiac cycle produce some sounds in the heart, which are called *heart sounds*.

Heart sounds are generally produced due to the following:

1. Turbulence of blood in the heart due to its movement in various chambers of the heart.
2. Closure of valves
3. Contraction of cardiac muscle

The process of listening to sounds within the body is called *auscultation* and it is usually done by using a stethoscope. The heart sounds can also be recorded graphically using a phonocardiogram (Fig. 11.21).

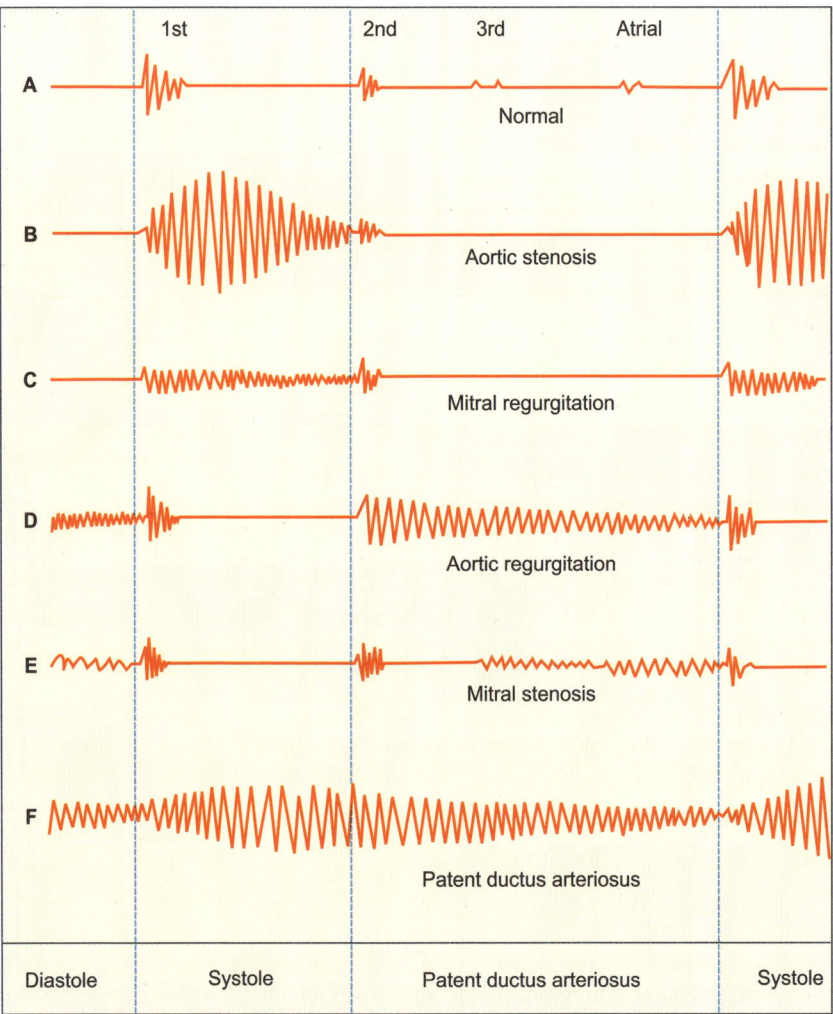

Figure 11.21 Phonocardiograms from normal and abnormal heart sounds.

DIFFERENT HEART SOUNDS

Four heart sounds are generated during each cardiac cycle and each heart sound corresponds to a particular event in the cardiac cycle.

The first and second heart sounds are more prominent and can be described as LUBB and DUBB sounds. These two heart sounds can be heard using the stethoscope.

The third heart sound is a mild sound and can be heard only by using a microphone. The fourth sound is inaudible and can only be recorded graphically by a phonocardiogram.

1. **First heart sound**: The first sound, LUBB, is louder and longer than the second sound. This sound is produced at the beginning of ventricular systole due to the simultaneous closure of both the AV valves.
2. **Second heart sound**: The second sound, DUBB, is softer and shorter than the second sound. This sound is produced at the beginning of ventricular diastole due to the simultaneous closure of both the semilunar valves, that is the aorta and pulmonary valves.
   Both these heart sounds can be easily heard using a stethoscope.
3. **Third heart sound**: The third heart sound normally is not loud enough to be heard and can be heard only using a microphone. This sound is produced due to the turbulent movement of blood during the rapid ventricular filling period of the cardiac cycle.
4. **Fourth heart sound**: The fourth heart sound is inaudible and can only be recorded graphically using a phonocardiogram. This sound is produced due to turbulent movement of the blood and contraction of atrial muscles during the atrial contraction phase of the cardiac cycle.
   Table 11.1 mentions the different heart sounds.

Table 11.1 Summary of the heart sounds

Heart sounds	Phase of cardiac cycle	Causes	Characteristics
First	Beginning of ventricular systole	Closure of both AV valves	• Louder and longer • Resembles the word LUBB
Second	Beginning of ventricular diastole	Closure of both semilunar valves	• Shorter and softer • Resembles the word DUBB
Third	Rapid ventricular filling	Rushing of blood into ventricles	Heard by microphone
Fourth	Atrial contraction	Blood turbulence and contraction of atrial muscle	• Inaudible • Recorded by phonocardiogram

IMPORTANCE OF HEART SOUNDS

They can be used as an important tool for diagnostic purposes in clinical practice because the heart sounds are altered in the case of cardiac diseases.

A summary of these alterations is described in Figure 11.21.

ELECTROCARDIOGRAM

The electrical activity within the heart generates small electric currents that can be detected by attaching electrodes to the surface of the body. The recording of these electrical activities of the heart is called an *electrocardiogram (ECG)*. It is the summed electrical activity of all the cardiac muscle fibres during each heartbeat.

Electrocardiograph is the instrument used to record the electrical activities of the heart and this technique is called *electrocardiography* (Fig. 11.22).

This technique was discovered by Dutch physiologist Willem Einthoven, who is known as the *father of ECG*.

ELECTROCARDIOGRAPH OR ECG MACHINE

This instrument amplifies the electrical signals from the heart and records them on a moving strip of paper. The markings (lines) on this paper are called *ECG grid*.

The ECG is recorded by placing electrodes on the arms and legs (limb leads) and at six positions on the chest (chest leads). These electrodes connect the surface of the body with the ECG machine and record the ECG by amplifying the heart's electrical activity.

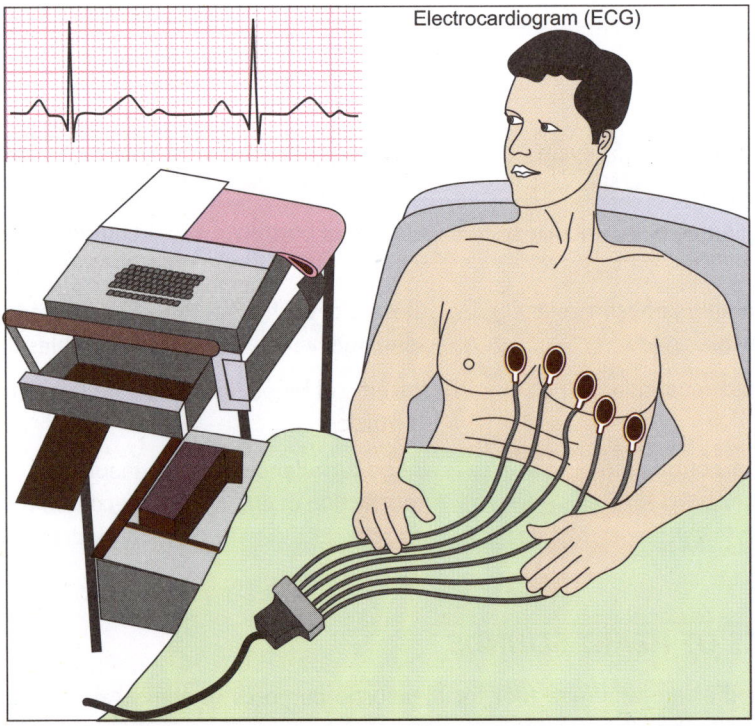

Electrocardiogram (ECG)

Figure 11.22 ECG machine.

The normal ECG tracing shows five waves, which have been named as P, Q, R, S and T (Fig. 11.23).

1. **P wave**
   - ❏ It is the first wave in ECG and is a small upward deflection on the ECG.
   - ❏ This wave arises when the impulse from the SA node spreads throughout both the atria.
   - ❏ The P wave represents atrial depolarization or contraction of the atrial muscle.

2. **QRS complex**
   - ❏ This second wave continues as a large, upright, triangular wave and ends as a downward wave.
   - ❏ QRS complex is obtained due to the depolarization of the ventricles. This complex represents the rapid spread of impulse from the AV node through the AV bundle and purkinje fibres, thus resulting in the spread of electrical excitation in the ventricles.
   - ❏ Q wave is due to the depolarization of the basal portion of the interventricular septum.
   - ❏ R wave is due to the depolarization of the apical portion of the interventricular septum and ventricular muscle.
   - ❏ S wave is due to the depolarization of the basal portion of ventricular muscle.
   - ❏ The ventricles start contracting shortly after the QRS complex begins.

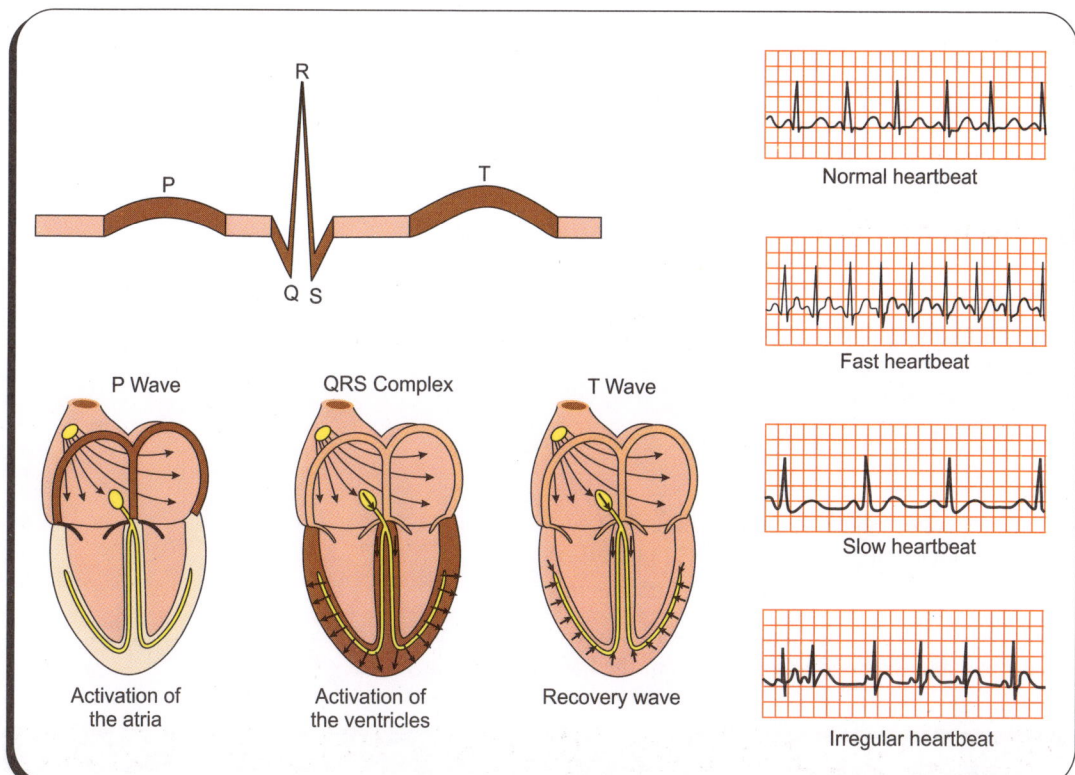

Figure 11.23 Electrocardiograph.

3. **T wave**
   - ❑ It represents the relaxation of the ventricular muscle or ventricular repolarization.
   - ❑ This wave is a dome-shaped upward deflection and it occurs just before the ventricles start relaxing.
   - ❑ ECG analysis also involves the examination of the time spans between waves, which are called *intervals and segments of ECG.*

The various intervals and segments of ECG include:

1. **P–Q interval**
   - ❑ It is the interval between the beginning of the P wave and the onset of the Q wave.
   - ❑ It is the time required for an impulse to travel from the SA node to the ventricles through the atrial muscle and the AV node. Thus, this interval signifies atrial depolarization and conduction of impulse through the AV node.
   - ❑ The lengthening of P–Q interval signifies coronary artery disease or rheumatic fever.

2. **Q–T interval**
   - ❑ It is the interval between the start of the QRS complex and the end of T wave; that is it is the time from the beginning of ventricular depolarization till the end of ventricular repolarization.
   - ❑ The Q–T interval lengthening signifies myocardial damage, coronary ischaemia and conduction abnormalities.

3. **S–T segment**
   - ❑ It is the time interval between the end of S wave and the start of T wave.
   - ❑ It represents the time when the ventricular fibres are fully contracted or depolarized.
   - ❑ The elevation of the S–T segment indicates myocardial infarction and its depression indicates myocardial ischaemia.

Significance of ECG

ECG is a very important technique to determine the following:

1. Abnormalities in the conduction pathway
2. Enlargement of the heart
3. Damage to the heart

The size of ECG waves can also indicate abnormality.

For example:

1. Larger P wave indicates atrial enlargement.
2. Larger Q wave indicates myocardial infarction.
3. Larger R wave indicates ventricular enlargement.

Thus, by examining the pattern of waves and time interval between various segments, the state of myocardium and the conduction system of the heart can be analyzed.

BLOOD PRESSURE

Blood pressure (BP) is the force or pressure exerted by the blood on the walls of blood vessels.

BP is generated by contraction of the ventricles and it is the highest in aorta and large arteries. As the distance from the left ventricle increases, the blood pressure falls progressively. This is proved by the fact that blood pressure is the lowest in venules and veins because they are the farthest from the left ventricle. Therefore, generally the term *blood pressure* refers to *arterial blood pressure*.

It is very important to maintain BP within normal limits; if it becomes too high, it may lead to rupture of blood vessels and if it falls very low, then there would be inadequate blood supply to various organs of the body.

Normal BP during resting condition in young adults is 120 mm Hg during systole (contraction) and 80 mm Hg during diastole (relaxation).

Arterial BP is expressed by the following four different terms:

1. **Systolic BP**: This is the maximum pressure exerted in the arteries when the blood is pushed into the aorta after contraction of the left ventricle. In adults, it is about 120 mm Hg.
2. **Diastolic BP**: This is the minimum pressure in the arteries during diastole (relaxation) of heart. In adults, it is about 80 mm Hg.
3. **Pulse pressure**: This is the difference between systolic and diastolic BP. Normally it is about 40 mm Hg.
4. **Mean Arterial BP (MABP)**: This is the average pressure in the arteries. It is calculated as follows:

    MABP = Diastolic BP + 1/3 (Systolic BP – Diastolic BP)

    = Diastolic BP + 1/3 (Pulse pressure)

VARIATIONS IN BP

The variations in BP can be physiological and pathological.

Physiological variations occur with change in normal day-to-day conditions and they are normalized by the regulatory mechanisms in the body. Pathological variations in BP indicate some diseases.

1. **Physiological variation**
   (a) *Age*: Arterial BP increases with age.
   (b) *Sex*: In females, BP is lower than that in males till menopause. After menopause, both males and females of the same age have equal BP.
   (c) *Meals*: BP normally increases for a few hours after meals and BP is more in obese compared with lean persons.
   (d) *Emotional conditions*: During emotional conditions like excitement, fear and anxiety, BP increases.
   (e) *Exercise*: After moderate exercise, systolic pressure increases but there is no effect on diastolic BP.

    After severe exercise, the systolic pressure rises but diastolic BP decreases due to decrease in peripheral resistance after severe exercise.

2. **Pathological variation**
   (a) *Hypertension*: It is the persistent increase in BP. A person is said to be hypertensive if systolic pressure is greater than 150 mm Hg and diastolic pressure is greater than 90 mm Hg.
   (b) *Hypotension*: It is the persistent decrease in BP. A person is said to be hypotensive if systolic pressure is less than 100 mm Hg and diastolic pressure is less than 50 mm Hg.

Chapter 11

DETERMINANTS OF BP—FACTORS THAT MAINTAIN BP (Fig. 11.24)

BP is determined by mainly cardiac output (CO) and peripheral resistance and a change in either of these parameters tends to alter BP.

1. **CO**
   - ❏ CO is the amount of blood pumped from each ventricle.
   - ❏ Blood pressure is directly proportional to CO.
   - ❏ BP ∝ CO (directly proportional)
   - ❏ CO depends on blood volume. As the blood volume increases, CO also increases and therefore BP increases.
   - ❏ Also, CO is determined by stroke volume and heart rate.
   - ❏ Stroke volume is the amount of blood pumped out by each ventricle during each beat.
   - ❏ CO can be calculated as follows:
   - ❏ CO = Stroke volume × heart rate
   - ❏ Thus, increased stroke volume leads to increased CO, which leads to increase in BP.

2. **Peripheral resistance**
   - ❏ Peripheral resistance (PR) is the opposition or resistance to the blood flow due to friction between blood and walls of blood vessels.
   - ❏ BP is directly proportional to PR.
   - ❏ BP ∝ PR.

PR depends on the following three factors:

1. **Diameter of blood vessels**
   - ❏ The smaller the diameter of blood vessels, the greater the resistance or opposition to the blood flow.
   - ❏ Therefore, diameter of blood vessels α 1/BP (inversely proportional).
   - ❏ Vasoconstriction constricts the arterioles, which increases the resistance and thus increases BP.

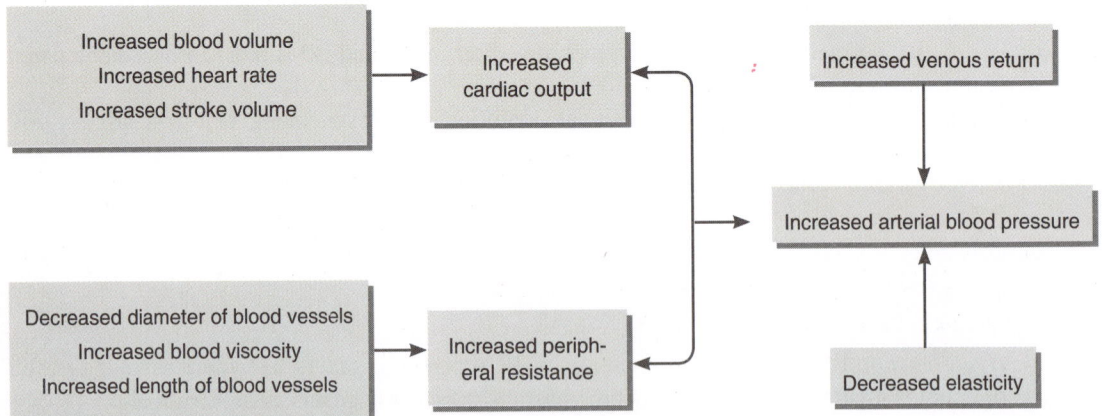

Figure 11.24 Factors that affect blood pressure.

2. **Viscosity of blood**
   - ❏ The viscosity (or thickness) of blood depends on the ratio of red blood cells to plasma (fluid) volume.
   - ❏ Increased viscosity of blood, like in polycythaemia, increases the resistance and thus tends to increase BP.
   - ❏ Therefore, BP ∝ viscosity of blood (directly proportional).
   - ❏ Decreased viscosity of blood, as in anaemia or haemorrhage, decreases resistance and hence decreases BP.

3. **Length of blood vessel**
   - ❏ Resistance to blood flow ∝ length of blood vessel (directly proportional).
   - ❏ The more the length of blood vessel, more would be resistance to blood flow, which increases BP. For example: Obese people have additional blood vessels in the adipose tissue and hence they often suffer from hypertension.

Other factors that maintain BP include

1. **Venous return**
   - ❏ Venous return is the volume of blood flowing back to the heart through veins and the pressure generated by the contraction of the left ventricle of the heart is responsible for the venous return.
   - ❏ BP ∝ venous return (directly proportional).
   - ❏ Therefore, if venous return is more ⟶ Filling of ventricles increases

$$\downarrow$$

Increased BP ⟵ Increased CO

2. **Elasticity of blood vessels**
   - ❏ BP ∝ 1/Elasticity of blood vessels (inversely proportional)
   - ❏ Blood vessels can maintain BP due to their elastic property, that is the presence of elastic tissues in the tunica media of blood vessels.
   - ❏ Aging (which replaces the elastic tissue by inelastic fibrous tissue) and arteriosclerosis (hardening of blood vessels due to deposition of cholesterol and fatty acids) reduce the elastic property of blood vessels and thus tends to increase BP.

REGULATION OF BP

The body regulates BP within normal limits by three regulatory mechanisms in the body. Some of the mechanisms allow rapid adjustment of BP to cope with the sudden changes, whereas others act slowly and provide long-term regulation of BP.

The regulatory mechanisms that regulate BP include:

1. Nervous mechanism or short-term BP regulation
2. Renal mechanism or long-term BP regulation
3. Hormonal mechanism

Chapter 11

I. Nervous mechanism or short-term regulation of BP

The nervous regulation to maintain BP quickly brings BP to normal limits and operates only for a short period. Hence, it is called *short-term regulation.*

The nervous system regulates BP through the *vasomotor system*, which comprises three components: Vasomotor centre (VC), vasoconstrictor fibres and vasodilator fibres.

1. **Vasomotor centre**
   - ❑ This is also called *cardiovascular centre* (CVC), which is present in medulla oblongata and pons of the brain stem. The CVC is a collection of interconnected neurons that help regulate heart rate and stroke volume.
   - ❑ The VC controls the diameter of blood vessels by causing vasoconstriction (through vasoconstrictor centre) or vasodilation (through vasodilator centre).
   - ❑ The vasoconstrictor centre sends impulses to blood vessels through sympathetic vasoconstrictor fibres, which, when stimulated, cause constriction of blood vessels and thereby increases BP.
   - ❑ The vasodilator centre suppresses the vasoconstrictor centre and causes vasodilation, which leads to decrease in BP. The impulses from this centre are passed through the vagus nerve (parasympathetic nerve fibres).

2. **Vasoconstrictor fibres**
   - ❑ These are the nerve fibres that cause constriction of blood vessels, leading to increased BP
   - ❑ These nerve fibres belong to the sympathetic division of ANS and cause vasoconstriction by the release of neurotransmitter adrenaline (Adr).

3. **Vasodilator fibres**
   - ❑ These nerve fibres cause dilation of blood vessels, thus decreasing BP.
   - ❑ These nerve fibres mainly belong to the parasympathetic division of ANS and cause vasodilation by the release of neurotransmitter acetylcholine (ACh).

Mechanism of regulation of BP

The VC or CVC of the vasomotor system receives, integrates and coordinates the inputs from the following:

1. Baroreceptors (pressure receptors)
2. Chemoreceptors
3. Higher centres in the brain

1. **Baroreceptors**
   - ❑ These are the receptors that produce response to change in BP. They are situated in the aorta (arch of aorta) and carotid sinuses (i.e. internal carotid artery).
   - ❑ A rise in BP in the aorta or carotid sinus stimulates baroreceptors, which in turn send the impulses to VC. The VC responds by activating the vasodilator centre. The vasodilator centre suppresses the vasoconstrictor centre and increases the impulses through the vasodilator (parasympathetic) fibres, which release the neurotransmitter Ach and cause dilation of blood vessels, thus leading to decreased BP.

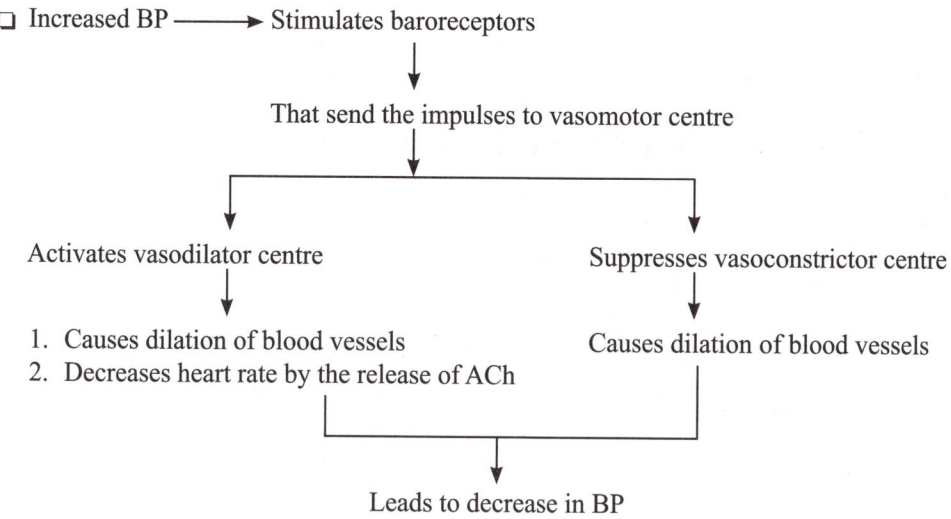

❑ Increased BP ⟶ Stimulates baroreceptors

That send the impulses to vasomotor centre

Activates vasodilator centre   Suppresses vasoconstrictor centre

1. Causes dilation of blood vessels   Causes dilation of blood vessels
2. Decreases heart rate by the release of ACh

Leads to decrease in BP

❑ The fall in blood pressure causes inactivation of baroreceptors that decreases the discharge of impulses towards the VC. In response, the VC decreases parasympathetic stimulation and increases sympathetic stimulation by activating the vasoconstrictor centre, thereby causing increased BP.

2. **Chemoreceptors**
   ❑ These receptors produce response to changes in the chemical constituents of blood.
   ❑ They are located close to the baroreceptors of the carotid sinus and the arch of aorta in small structures called *carotid bodies* and *aortic bodies,* respectively. They detect the changes in the blood level of oxygen, carbon dioxide and hydrogen ions as these receptors are very sensitive to lack of oxygen, excess of carbon-dioxide and hydrogen ion concentration in blood.

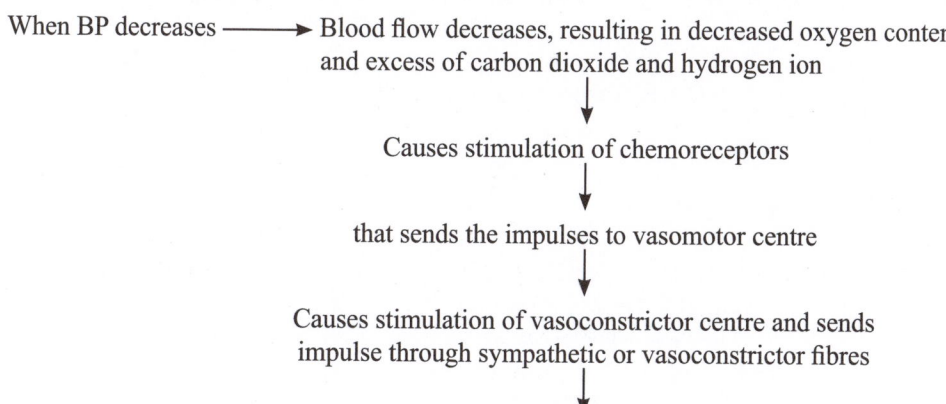

When BP decreases ⟶ Blood flow decreases, resulting in decreased oxygen content and excess of carbon dioxide and hydrogen ion

Causes stimulation of chemoreceptors

that sends the impulses to vasomotor centre

Causes stimulation of vasoconstrictor centre and sends impulse through sympathetic or vasoconstrictor fibres

Leads to increased BP

3. **Higher centres in the brain:** The VC is also controlled by impulses from two higher centres in the brain, which are as follows:
   Cerebral cortex: During emotional states such as fear, anxiety, pain and anger, the cerebral cortex sends impulses to the VC, which gets activated. The VC then stimulates the vasoconstrictor fibres and increases BP.

Hypothalamus: Stimulation of the anterior hypothalamus causes vasoconstriction and thus increases BP.

Stimulation of the posterior hypothalamus causes vasodilation and thus decreases BP.

II Renal mechanism or long-term regulation of BP

The kidneys play an important role in the long-term regulation of blood pressure and continue to regulate even when neural regulation is not able to regulate blood pressure. Hence, renal mechanism is also called *long-term regulation*.

The kidneys regulate BP in the following two ways:

1. Renin–angiotensin–aldosterone system (RAAS)
2. Action of antidiuretic hormone (ADH)

1. **Renin–angiotensin–aldosterone system**

When blood pressure decreases

↓

Blood flow to kidney is decreased

↓

That stimulates juxtaglomerular cells in the kidney to release renin hormone

↓

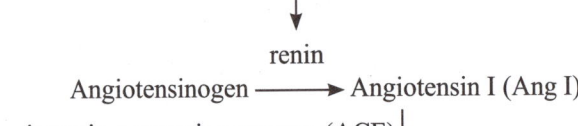

Angiotensinogen $\xrightarrow{\text{renin}}$ Angiotensin I (Ang I)

Angiotensin-converting enzyme (ACE) ↓

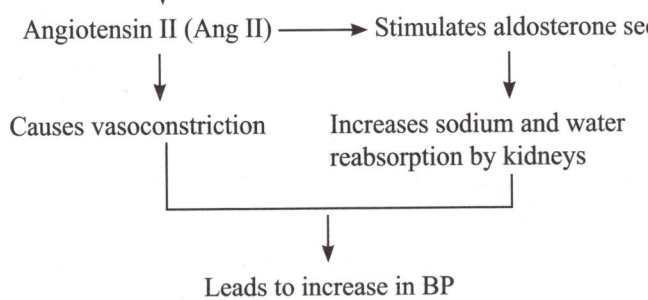

Angiotensin II (Ang II) ⟶ Stimulates aldosterone secretion

↓   ↓

Causes vasoconstriction   Increases sodium and water
                           reabsorption by kidneys

↓

Leads to increase in BP

2. **ADH action**

When BP decreases

↓

ADH is released from the posterior pituitary

↓

Which causes vasoconstriction and also increases ECF volume

↓

Leading to increase in BP

III Hormonal mechanism

Various hormones are involved in the regulation of blood pressure, which are as follows:

1. **Adrenaline**: It is released from the adrenal medulla and increases CO by increasing the rate and force of contractions. Also, it causes vasoconstriction, thereby increasing BP.
2. **Thyroxine**: It increases blood volume and force of contraction of the heart. Hence, it increases CO and thereby increases BP.
3. **Aldosterone**: It causes sodium and water retention, thus increasing ECF volume and blood volume; therefore, it causes increase in BP.
4. **Angiotensin II**: Angiotensin II causes vasoconstriction and also causes sodium and water retention.
5. **Atrial natriuretic peptide (ANP)**: It is released from the atrial cells of the heart and leads to decrease in BP by causing vasodilation and promoting loss of sodium and water.
6. **Acetylcholine**: It causes vasodilation and thus decreases BP.

Some local substances also regulate BP by vasoconstriction and vasodilation. They include the following:

1. **Local vasoconstrictors**: For example endothelins, thromboxane.
2. **Local vasodilators**: For example endothelium-derived relaxing factor (EDRF).

CARDIAC OUTPUT

❏ CO is the amount of blood pumped from each ventricle

CO = Stroke volume × Heart rate

(mL/min) (mL/beat) (beats/min)

where stroke volume is the volume of blood ejected out by each ventricle during each beat.

❏ In a healthy adult in resting condition, stroke volume is approximately 70 mL, and if the heart rate is 72/min, CO would be 5 L/min.

❏ CO is the most important factor in the cardiovascular system because the rate of blood flow through different parts of the body depends on CO.

The liver receives maximum amount (30%) of blood pumped by the heart, and the heart, which pumps blood to all other organs, receives the least amount (5%) of blood.

❏ **Cardiac Reserve**: This is the maximum amount of blood that can be pumped out of the heart above the normal value. In other words, it is the difference between a person's maximum CO and CO at rest. The average person has a cardiac reserve 4–5 times the value at rest. It plays a very important role in increasing the CO during exercise when increased blood supply is required to meet the increased tissue requirement of oxygen and nutrients.

VARIATIONS IN CO

The variations can be either physiological or pathological.

1. **Physiological variations**
   (a) *Age*: In children, it is less due to reduced blood volume.
   (b) *Emotional conditions*: Emotions such as anxiety, fear, pain and excitement increases CO.
   (c) *Exercise*: CO is increased with exercise due to increased heart rate and force of contraction.

(d) *High altitude*: CO is increased at high altitude because of decreased oxygen, adrenaline is released, which increases CO.

(e) *Pregnancy*: CO increases by 45–50% during the later months of pregnancy.

2. **Pathological variations**

CO is increased during:

(a) Fever

(b) Anaemia (due to hypoxia)

(c) Hyperthyroidism (due to increased basal metabolic rate)

CO is decreased during:

(a) Hypothyroidism (due to decreased basal metabolic rate)

(b) Cardiac disorders like

   ❏ Incomplete heart block (defective pumping)

   ❏ Atrial fibrillation (decreased filling)

   ❏ Congestive heart failure (weak contractions)

REGULATION OF CO

As CO = Stroke volume × Heart rate

CO can be regulated by regulating the stroke volume and heart rate.

I. Regulation of stroke volume

Stroke volume is the volume of blood ejected out by each ventricle during each beat.

The following three factors regulate stroke volume:

1. Preload
2. Force of contraction
3. Afterload

1. Preload

❏ Preload (i.e. the degree of stretch on the heart before it contracts) depends on the amount of blood returning to the heart through the superior and inferior vena cava (venous return).

❏ Also, the amount of blood pumped out by the heart depends on the amount of blood in the ventricles at the end of diastole (i.e. ventricular end diastolic volume [VEDV]).

❏ In other words, preload α VEDV, that is increased preload (stress) is due to the increase in end diastolic volume (EDV), and the greater is the EDV, the higher will be the force of contraction.

❏ Thus, it can be noted that EDV depends on the following two factors:

1. Venous return: It is the amount of blood returning to the right ventricle.
2. Duration of ventricular diastole

When heart rate increases ⟶ Duration of diastole decreases

⟱

Decreases EDV ⟵ That decreases filling time

2. **Force of contraction**

❏ As discussed previously, the force of contraction depends on EDV.

Hence, increased EDV increases stretch (preload) on the heart

↓

Increased length of cardiac muscle fibres

↓

That increases force of contraction

❏ This can be compared to the stretching of a rubber band, that is the more the rubber band is stretched, the more forcefully it will snap back.

❏ The substances that increase the force of contraction are called *positive inotropic agents* and those that decrease the force of contraction are called *negative inotropic agents*.

❏ Examples of positive inotropic agents include adrenaline, increased Ca^+ level in interstitial fluid and digitalis drug.

❏ Negative inotropic agents include Ca^+ channel blockers, increased K^+ level in interstitial fluid and anoxia.

3. **Afterload**: At the end of the isometric contraction period, high pressure in the ventricles causes the blood to push the semilunar valve to open, which leads to ejection of blood into the aorta and pulmonary artery. The pressure in the aorta and pulmonary artery that must be overcome before a semilunar valve can open is termed as *afterload*.

Increased afterload (due to atherosclerosis)

↓

Decreases stroke volume

↓

Therefore, more blood remains in the ventricles at the end of systole

II Regulation of heart rate

The heart rate determines CO. If the heart rate increases, CO increases, and vice versa (Fig. 11.25).

Heart rate is regulated by the nervous mechanism of ANS, which regulates through the release of hormones from the adrenal medulla.

The nervous mechanism for the regulation of heart rate includes the following three components:
1. Vasomotor centre (VC)
2. Motor (efferent) nerve fibres to the heart
3. Sensory (afferent) nerve fibres from the heart

1. Vasomotor centre (VC)

❏ It is also called *cardiovascular centre* (CVC) and this centre regulates both BP and heart rate.

- As discussed in the section Nervous Regulation of Blood Pressure, the VC comprises the vasoconstrictor area and the vasodilator area.
- The vasoconstrictor area sends impulses through sympathetic nerve fibres and thus causes vasoconstriction and increased heart rate.
- The vasodilator area causes dilation of blood vessels and stimulation of this causes decreased heart rate.
- The VC receives impulses from different sources in the body, which include the following:
    1. Impulses from higher centres such as the cerebral cortex and hypothalamus.
    2. Baroreceptors, which respond to changes in the pressure.
    3. Chemoreceptors, which respond to changes in chemical constituents of blood.
- The VC sends the output through sympathetic and parasympathetic nerves.

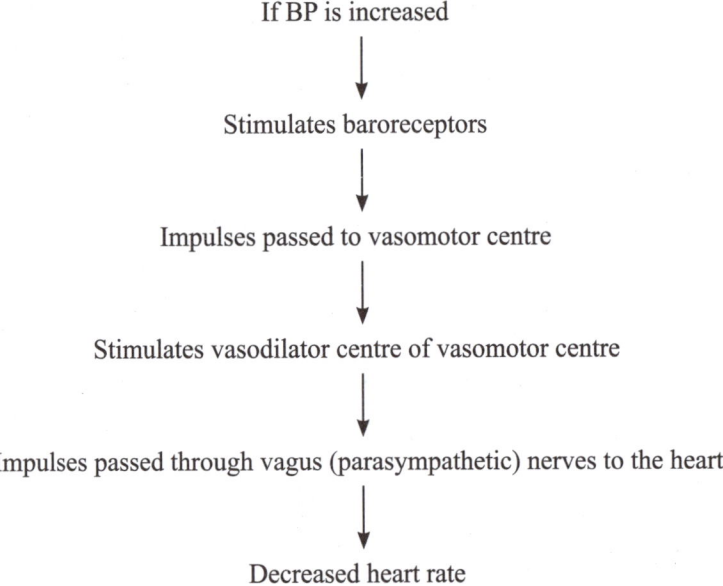

If BP is increased

↓

Stimulates baroreceptors

↓

Impulses passed to vasomotor centre

↓

Stimulates vasodilator centre of vasomotor centre

↓

Impulses passed through vagus (parasympathetic) nerves to the heart

↓

Decreased heart rate

- Thus, vasomotor centre plays the main role in regulating heart rate and it regulates by sending the impulse through sympathetic (cardioaccelerator) or parasympathetic (cardioinhibitory) nerve fibres.

2. Motor (efferent) fibres to the heart

- The heart receives efferent nerves from both the divisions, that is parasympathetic and sympathetic fibres of ANS
- Stimulation of parasympathetic (vagus) nerve causes reduction in heart rate and decreased force of contraction. Thus, they are also called cardioinhibitory nerves.
- Stimulation of sympathetic nerves increases heart rate and force of ventricular contraction. This increase is due to the release of neurotransmitter adrenaline and these nerves are called *cardiac accelerator nerves*.

3. Sensory (afferent) nerve fibres from the heart

These nerve fibres carry sensation of stretch and pain from the heart to the brain.

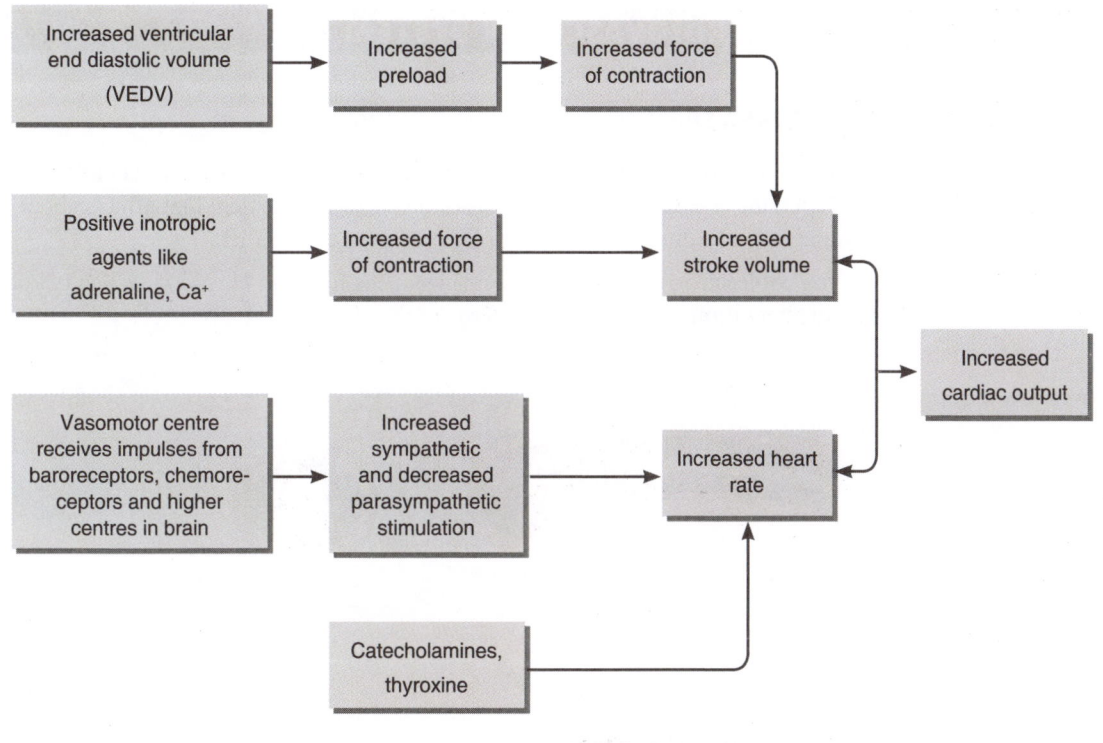

Figure 11.25 Regulation of heart rate.

HEART RATE

❑ Normal heart rate is 72/min.
❑ Heart rate is maintained at normal level constantly with the help of regulatory mechanisms in the body.
❑ Heart rate may show certain physiological variations such as the following:

1. **Posture**: Heart rate fastens when the person is upright than when lying down.
2. **Exercise**: With exercise heart rate increases.
3. **Emotional state**: Emotional states such as excitement, fear and anxiety increase heart rate.
4. **Gender**: Heart rate is faster in women than in men.
5. **Age**: Heart rate is more rapid in babies and small children compared with adults. A newborn has a resting heart rate of over 120 beats/min.
6. **Temperature**: Heart rate rises and falls with body temperature.

REGULATION OF HEART RATE

This topic has been discussed in the section Regulation of CO (refer to page no. 431 for details).

DISORDERS OF THE CARDIOVASCULAR SYSTEM

CORONARY ARTERY DISEASE

Coronary artery disease (CAD), also called *coronary heart disease* or *atherosclerosis*, is a condition in which plaque builds up inside the coronary arteries. It is a serious medical problem that affects about 8 million people annually and is the leading cause of death for both men and women.

Plaque is made up of fat, cholesterol, calcium and other substances found in the blood. When plaque builds up in the arteries, the condition is called *atherosclerosis* (Fig. 11.26).

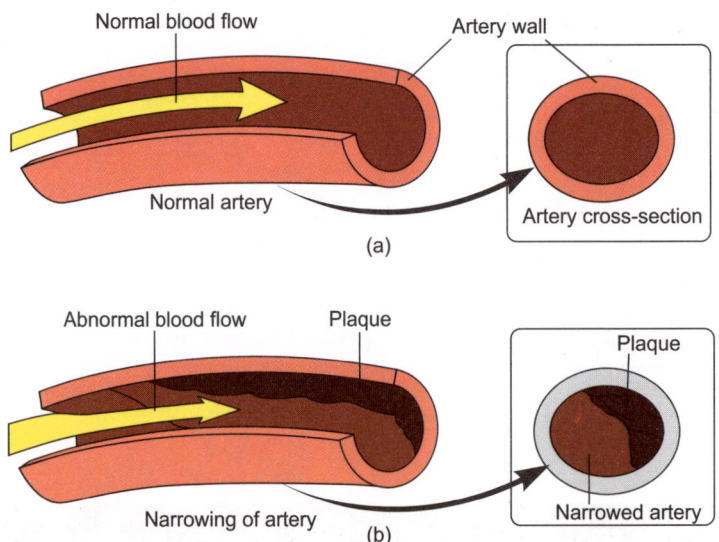

Figure 11.26 (a) Normal artery; (b) Abnormal artery with deposited plaque.

Plaque narrows the arteries and thus causes reduction of blood flow to the heart muscle. Gradually, the narrowing of arteries may also cause the formation of blood clots, which can partially or completely block the blood flow.

This condition may lead to several other complications of the heart as follows:

1. **Angina**: It is chest pain or discomfort that occurs when enough oxygen-rich blood is not flowing to an area of myocardium. It may feel like pressure or squeezing in the chest and the pain may also occur in the shoulders, arms, neck, jaw or back.
2. **Heart attack**: It occurs when the blood flow to an area of myocardium gets completely blocked. This prevents oxygen-rich blood from reaching that area of the heart muscle and causes it to die (Fig. 11.27).
3. CAD can also cause weakening of heart muscle gradually and lead to heart failure and arrhythmia. Heart failure is a condition in which the heart cannot pump enough blood throughout the body. Arrhythmias are problems with the speed or rhythm of heartbeat.

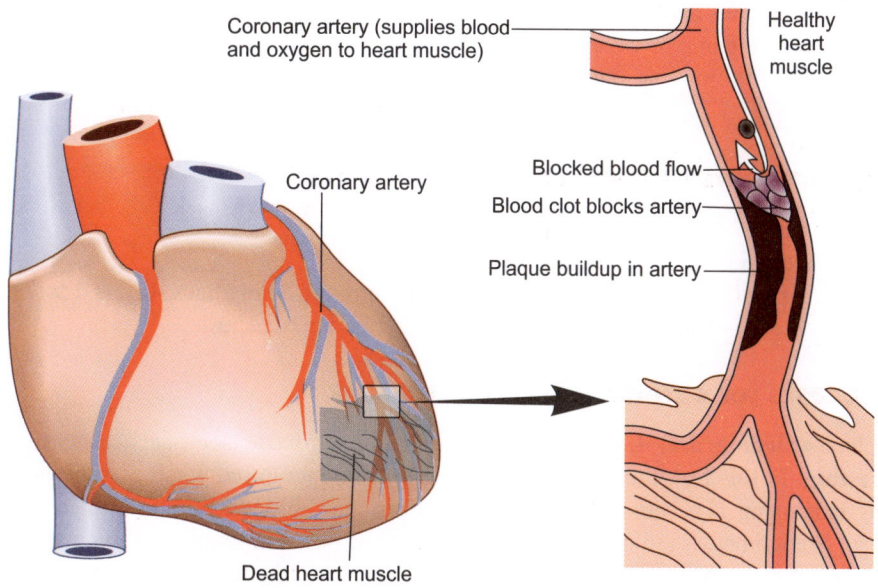

Coronary artery (supplies blood and oxygen to heart muscle)

Coronary artery

Healthy heart muscle

Blocked blood flow

Blood clot blocks artery

Plaque buildup in artery

Dead heart muscle

Figure 11.27 (a) Dead heart muscle; (b) Plaqued artery.

Major risk factors of coronary artery disease

1. **High cholesterol levels**: This includes high LDL cholesterol (bad cholesterol) and low HDL cholesterol (good cholesterol).
2. **High blood pressure**: Blood pressure is considered high if it stays at or above 140/90 mm Hg over a period of time.
3. **Smoking**: This can damage blood vessels and can raise cholesterol levels and blood pressure. Smoking also does not allow enough oxygen to reach the tissues in the body.
4. **Diabetes**: This is a disease in which the blood sugar level in the body is high because the body does not make enough insulin or does not use its insulin properly.
5. **Overweight or obesity**: Overweight is the extra body weight from muscle, bone, fat and/or water, whereas obesity is the high amount of extra body fat.
6. **Metabolic syndrome**: *Metabolic syndrome* is the term designated for a group of risk factors linked to overweight and obesity that increases the risk for heart disease and other health problems such as diabetes and stroke.
7. **Lack of physical activity**: Lack of activity can worsen other risk factors for CAD.
8. **Age**: As we get older, the risk for CAD increases.
   (a) In men, the risk for CAD increases after age 45.
   (b) In women, the risk for CAD risk increases after age 55.
9. **Family history of heart disease**.
10. **Sleep apnoea**: Sleep apnoea is a disorder in which breathing stops or gets very shallow while sleeping. Untreated sleep apnoea can increase the risk of high blood pressure, diabetes, and even a heart attack or stroke.

11. **Stress**: Research shows that the most common 'trigger' for a heart attack is an emotionally upsetting event, particularly the one involving anger.
12. **Alcohol**: Heavy drinking can damage the heart muscle and worsen other risk factors for heart disease.

Signs and symptoms of coronary artery disease

1. Shortness of breath
2. Angina, that is chest pain or discomfort
3. Sometimes, CAD can be diagnosed only by the symptoms of a heart attack, that is discomfort in the centre of the chest or arrhythmia, that is a fluttering feeling in the chest.

Diagnostic tests for coronary artery disease

1. **ECG (Electrocardiogram)**: It is a test that detects and records the electrical activity of the heart.
2. **Stress testing**: In this test, the functioning of the heart is monitored when placed under physical stress by exercising. The abnormal changes in heart rate, blood pressure or heart rhythm are monitored. Sometimes, a radioactive dye, sound waves, positron emission tomography (PET) or cardiac magnetic resonance imaging (MRI) is also used to take pictures of the heart when it is working and when it is at rest.
3. **Chest X-ray**: This can reveal any signs of heart failure.
4. **Blood tests**: They determine the level of fats, cholesterol and sugar in blood.
5. **Coronary angiography**: This test uses dye and special X-rays to detect blood flow through the coronary arteries.

Treatment for coronary artery disease

1. Lifestyle changes, that is increased physical activity, losing weight, eating healthy diet and to quit smoking.
2. Medicines may include anticoagulants, aspirin and other antiplatelet medicines, ACE inhibitors, beta blockers, calcium channel blockers, nitroglycerin, glycoprotein IIb-IIIa, statins, fish oil and other supplements high in omega-3 fatty acids.
3. Medical procedures include:
   (a) **Angioplasty**: It is done to open blocked or narrowed coronary arteries. During angioplasty, a thin tube with a balloon or other device on the end is threaded through a blood vessel to the narrowed or blocked coronary artery. Once in place, the balloon is inflated to push the plaque outward against the wall of the artery. This widens the artery and restores the flow of blood.
   (b) Sometimes a small mesh tube called *stent* is placed in the artery to keep it open after angioplasty.
   (c) **Coronary artery bypass grafting (CABG)**: Arteries or veins from other areas in the body are used to bypass (i.e. go around) the narrowed coronary arteries. CABG can improve blood flow to the heart, relieve chest pain and possibly prevent a heart attack.

CONGESTIVE HEART FAILURE

Congestive heart failure (CHF) is defined as the inability of the heart to supply sufficient blood flow to meet the body's needs. It is a common, disabling and potentially deadly condition.

Heart failure can be right sided or left sided or both. The right ventricle fails when the pressure developed within it by contraction is less than the force needed to push the blood through the lungs, whereas left ventricular failure occurs when the pressure developed in the left ventricle by contraction is less than the pressure in the aorta and the ventricle is not able to pump out all the blood that it receives.

Common causes of heart failure include myocardial infarction (heart attacks), ischaemic heart disease, hypertension, valvular heart disease and cardiomyopathy.

Various symptoms of heart failure are shortness of breath (which gets worse when lying flat, called orthopnoea), fatigue, cough, fluid accumulation (swollen legs, feet and ankles), lung congestion, heart enlargement and exercise intolerance.

Treatment commonly consists of lifestyle measures (such as decreased salt intake) and medications (such as diuretics, digitalis, ACE inhibitors and nitrates). Sometimes, surgery is needed to ameliorate the symptoms.

CARDIAC MURMURS

These are the abnormal heart sounds produced because of the changed pattern of blood flow or turbulent blood flow. A murmur is usually present when there is a heart valve problem and it can be heard using a stethoscope.

They can be caused by a heart attack, high blood pressure, rheumatic fever, pregnancy, fever, thyrotoxicosis (overactive thyroid gland) or anaemia.

There are two main types of heart murmurs: diastolic and systolic. Diastolic murmur occurs after the second heart sound, whereas systolic murmur occurs between the first and second heart sounds and is produced during systole.

Cardiac murmurs occur when a valve does not work properly. If a valve does not open completely (*stenosis*), less amount of blood can move through the smaller opening. If a valve does not close tightly or completely (*insufficiency* or *regurgitation*), blood may leak backward. These problems can cause the heart to work harder to pump the same amount of blood or blood may back up in the lungs or body.

PERICARDITIS

Pericarditis is an inflammation of the pericardium (the fibrous sac surrounding the heart).

The following may be the causes of pericarditis:

1. Infection, due to viral, bacterial, or fungal infection.
   (a) The common viral pathogens include coxsackievirus, cytomegalovirus, herpesvirus and HIV.
   (b) *Pneumococcus* or tuberculous pericarditis is the most common bacterial forms.
   (c) Fungal pericarditis is usually due to histoplasmosis, *Aspergillus*, *Candida* and *Coccidioides*.
2. Immunologic conditions including systemic lupus erythematosus or rheumatic fever.
3. Trauma to the heart, for example puncture, resulting in infection or inflammation.
4. Side effect of some medications, for example isoniazid, cyclosporine and hydralazine.
5. Postpericardiotomy syndrome.
6. Idiopathic: No identifiable aetiology.

The treatment in pericarditis includes mainly nonsteroidal anti-inflammatory drugs. Severe conditions may require antibiotics, steroids, colchicine and, in rare cases, surgery.

Chapter 11

MYOCARDITIS

Myocarditis is inflammation of the myocardium that is caused by infection of the heart muscle by virus or some immune diseases (such as systemic lupus).

The various symptoms of myocarditis include pain in the chest, fever, fatigue, joint pain and breathlessness. When myocarditis is more serious, it leads to weakening of the heart muscle and can cause heart failure or heart rhythm irregularities.

Treatment measures mainly involve alleviating heart failure (salt restriction, ACE inhibitors, beta blockers, etc.) and heart rhythm abnormalities. Other medications include corticosteroids such as methylprednisolone, prednisone and medrol.

ENDOCARDITIS

Endocarditis is inflammation of the inside lining of the heart chambers and heart valves (endocardium).

Risk factors for developing endocarditis include weakened valves, prior valve surgery, bacterial or fungal infections, congenital heart disease, intravenous drug use or rheumatic fever.

The symptoms of endocarditis include excessive sweating, fatigue, fever, chills, abnormal urine colour, muscle pain, shortness of breath, swelling of feet, legs and abdomen, weakness and weight loss.

The diagnostic tests for endocarditis include echocardiogram, erythrocyte sedimentation rate (ESR), chest X-ray, blood culture and echocardiogram.

Treatment includes long-term antibiotic therapy to remove the bacteria. Surgery to replace the heart valve is usually needed when the person develops heart failure or there are symptoms of stroke.

ISCHAEMIC HEART DISEASE

Ischaemia in the heart mainly occurs due to the formation of plaque, which may cause narrowing or occlusion of a coronary artery.

The complications due to ischaemia depend on the size of coronary artery involved and on the extent of plaque deposition, that is whether the artery is narrowed or completely blocked.

Narrowing of a coronary artery leads to angina pectoris, whereas obstruction leads to myocardial infarction.

1. Angina pectoris

❑ It is the condition of severe pain that occurs due to narrowing of the coronary artery, which is unable to meet the heart's requirements.

❑ The pain occurs mostly occurs during extra physical effort as the narrowed coronary artery is unable to meet the increased CO.

❑ The pain may start as a tightness or squeezing sensation in the chest and may spread to the neck, chain or down the left arm towards the elbow.

❑ In the early stages of angina, the chest pain stops when the CO returns to normal level, that is resting condition, but as the condition worsens, pain continues in resting states also.

2. Myocardial infarction

❏ Myocardial infarction (MI) is the complete obstruction to blood flow in a coronary artery that may lead to death of an area of cardiac muscle tissue.

❏ The damage due to MI is permanent as the cardiac muscle cannot regenerate, and thus the dead muscle is replaced with nonfunctional fibrous tissue.

❏ MI is usually accompanied by severe chest pain that may continue even in resting conditions.

❏ The most common cause of MI is atheromatous plaque and the extent of myocardial damage depends on the size of blood vessel and the site of infarct. An infarct can also damage the conduction system of the heart and may cause sudden death.

❏ The treatment for MI mainly involves the use of a thrombolytic (clot-dissolving) agent such as streptokinase in combination with an anticoagulant drug such as heparin. In emergency conditions, coronary angioplasty or coronary artery bypass grafting can also be performed.

CARDIAC ARRHYTHMIA

Cardiac arrhythmia is the disorder of rhythm or heart rate and is the result of abnormal generation or conduction of impulses. The heart may beat irregularly, too fast or very slow.

The symptoms of cardiac arrhythmia include chest pain, shortness of breath, dizziness and fainting.

The causes of arrhythmia include the factors that stimulate the heart such as stress, caffeine and alcohol and the other risk factors include congenital defect, coronary artery disease, myocardial infarction and valvular diseases.

The different categories of arrhythmia include:

1. Bradycardia: It refers to slow heart rate (below 60 beats/min).
2. Tachycardia: It refers rapid heart rate (above 100 beats/min).
3. Fibrillation: It refers to rapid, irregular heartbeats.
4. Supraventricular or atrial arrhythmia: It originates in the atria.
5. Ventricular arrhythmia: It originates in ventricles.

The treatment includes the use of anti-arrhythmic drugs such as verapamil, diltiazem, atenolol and a device called as defibrillator. Nowadays, automatic implantable cardioverter defibrillators are also available that can be an effective emergency treatment for cardiac arrest.

CONGENITAL ABNORMALITIES

These are the abnormalities present in the heart and blood vessels at birth and these may be due to intrauterine developmental errors or due to failure of the heart to adapt to the extrauterine life.

Many such defects are not serious and thus there are no symptoms but others are life threatening and must be surgically repaired.

The congenital abnormalities include:

1. Patent ductus arteriosus (Fig. 11.28)

❏ Before birth, the ductus arteriosus (i.e. a temporary vessel that joins the aorta and pulmonary artery) allows blood from the pulmonary artery to directly pass to the aorta. This process bypasses the pulmonary circulation as fetal lungs are non-functional.

Chapter 11

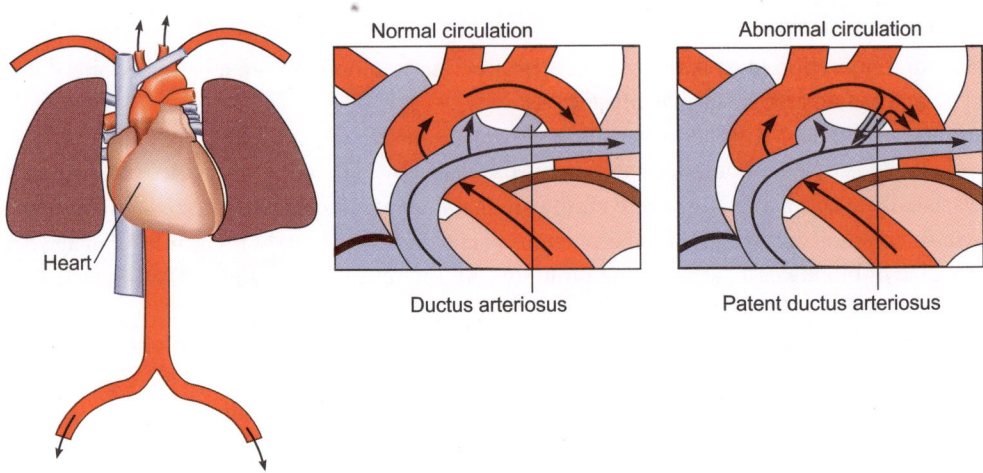

Figure 11.28 (a) Normal heart; (b) Patent ductus arteriosus.

❏ At birth, when the lungs start functioning, the ductus arteriosus should close completely. If it remains open or patent, aortic blood regurgitates into the lower pressure pulmonary artery and increases the volume of blood in pulmonary circulation. This leads to pulmonary congestion and, eventually, cardiac failure.

❏ The treatment includes the use of medications such as aspirin but in severe cases, surgery is required.

2. Coarctation of the aorta (Fig. 11.29)

❏ Coarctation is the condition when a segment of the aorta is very narrow and thus it reduces the flow of oxygenated blood to the body.

❏ The reduced blood flow forces the ventricles to work hard, which ultimately leads to the development of high blood pressure.

❏ The most common site of coarctation is between the left subclavian artery and ductus arteriosus.

❏ Treatment usually involves surgical removal of the area of obstruction.

3. Septal defect

❏ This is commonly called as *hole in the heart* and can be described as an opening in the septum that separates the left and right sides of the heart.

❏ Before birth, most of the oxygenated blood from the placenta enters the left atrium from the right atrium through a valve-like opening called as foramen ovale, thus bypassing the nonfunctional fetal lungs.

❏ After birth, when the lungs start functioning, this valve closes and later, the closure becomes permanent due to fibrosis.

❏ When the fetal foramen ovale between the two atria fails to close after birth, the condition is called *atrial septal defect* (Fig. 11.30). In severe cases, this may cause hypertrophy of the myocardium and eventually lead to heart failure.

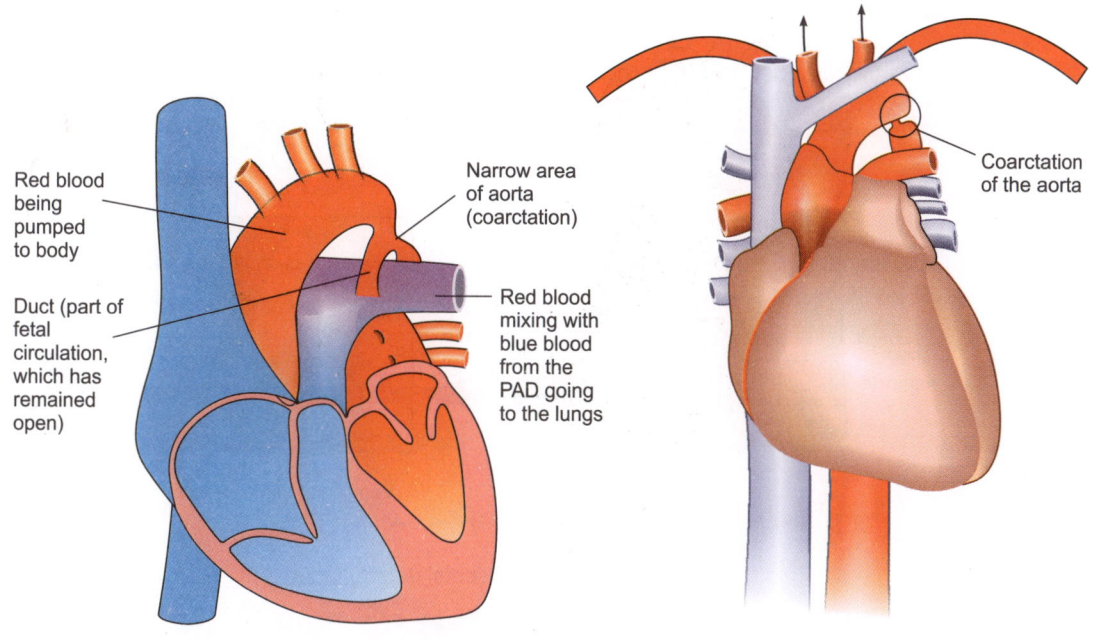

Red blood being pumped to body

Duct (part of fetal circulation, which has remained open)

Narrow area of aorta (coarctation)

Red blood mixing with blue blood from the PAD going to the lungs

Coarctation of the aorta

Figure 11.29 Coarctation of aorta.

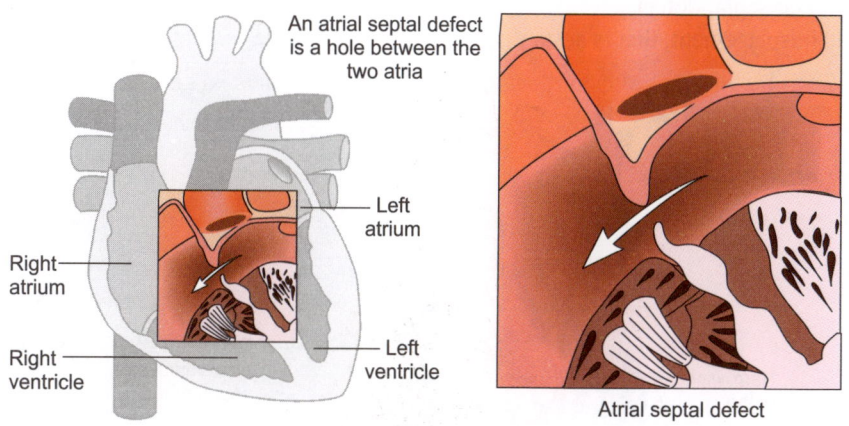

An atrial septal defect is a hole between the two atria

Left atrium

Right atrium

Right ventricle

Left ventricle

Atrial septal defect

Figure 11.30 Atrial septal defect.

❑ *Ventricular septal defect* is the condition when there is incomplete development of the interventricular septum (Fig. 11.31).

❑ The treatment of both atrial and ventricular septal defects usually involves surgical intervention.

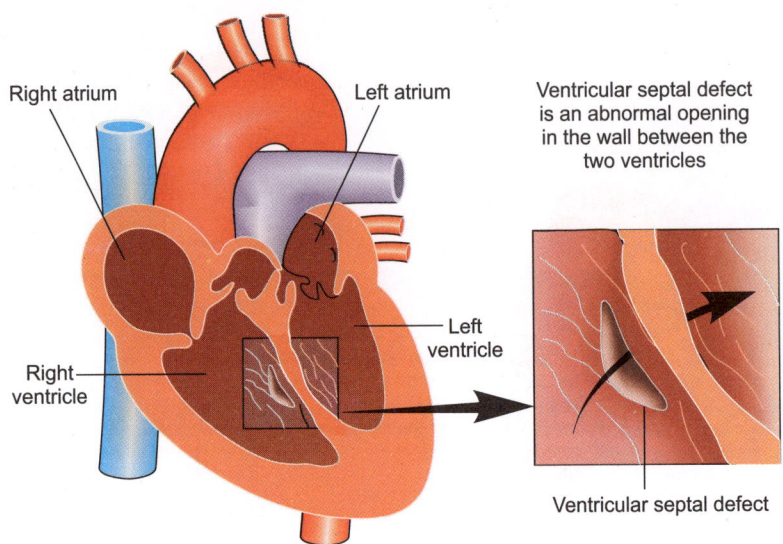

Figure 11.31 Ventricular septal defect.

4. Fallot's tetralogy

❑ This condition is a characteristic combination of the following four congenital cardiac abnormalities (Fig. 11.32):

1. Ventricular septal defect
2. Aortic misplacement, that is aorta displaced to the right side

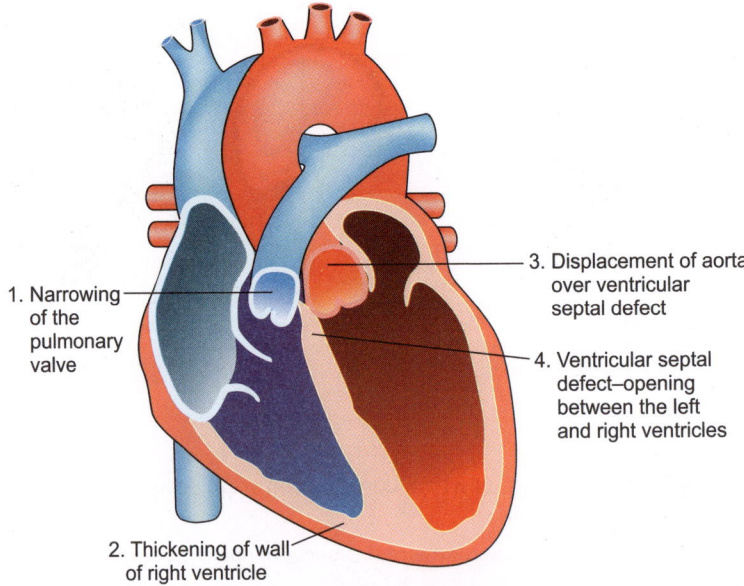

Figure 11.32 Fallot's tetralogy: four abnormalities that result in insufficiently oxygenated blood pumped to the body.

3. Stenosis of pulmonary artery
4. Enlargement of right ventricle

❏ This condition causes cyanosis (bluish discoloration), growth retardation and exercise intolerance in babies and young children. In infants, this condition is referred to as *blue baby*.

❏ The treatment involves mainly surgical repair.

RHEUMATIC HEART DISEASE

This condition usually occurs in young children due to infection with streptococcus bacterium.

The bacterium produces a toxin that triggers an immune response that can damage or destroy the heart valves. This condition is called *rheumatic fever* and it causes inflammation of the endocardium of the heart.

Although rheumatic fever may weaken the entire wall of the heart, most often it damages the mitral and aortic valves.

Treatment mainly includes antibiotic regimen.

HYPERTENSION

Hypertension, that is persistently high blood pressure, is the most common disorder affecting the heart and blood vessels and is the major cause of heart failure (Fig. 11.33).

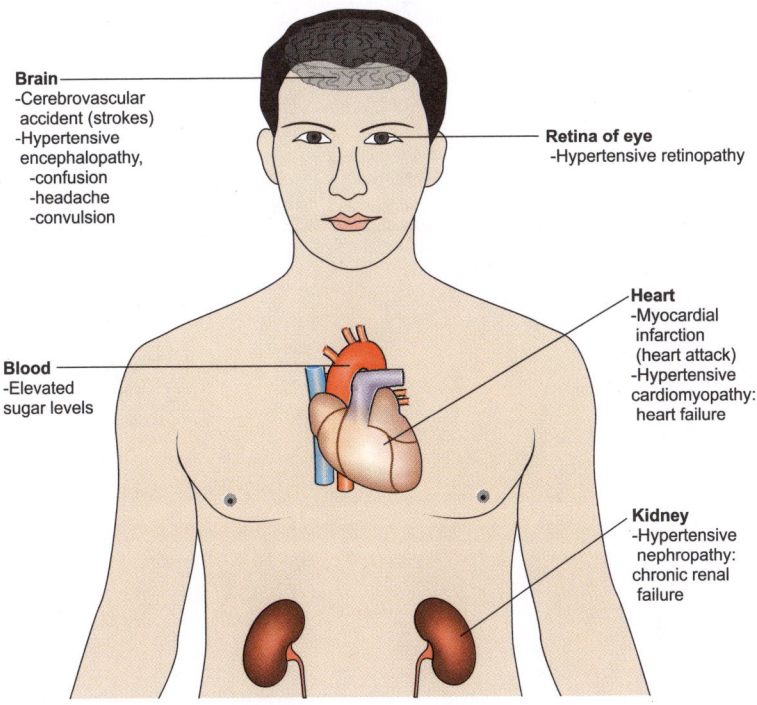

Figure 11.33 Complications of hypertension.

The following are the various causes of hypertension:

1. Hypersecretion of aldosterone increases sodium and water reabsorption by kidneys and thus increases the volume of body fluids.
2. Hypersecretion of adrenaline that increases heart rate and force of contraction.
3. Obstruction of blood flow to kidneys

The various complications due to hypertension have been described in Figure 11.30.

Treatment involves use of diuretics, ACE inhibitors, beta blockers and vasodilators.

OVERVIEW OF THE CARDIOVASCULAR SYSTEM

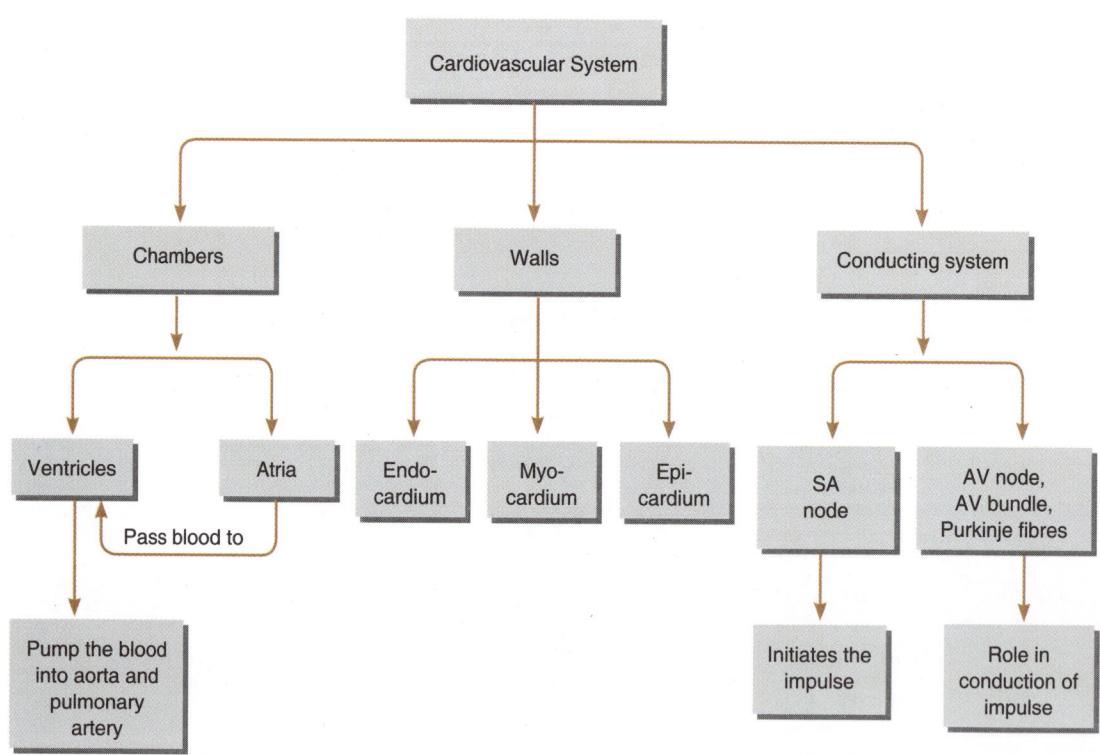

Embryonic Development of the Cardiovascular System

❏ The heart is the first functional organ in an embryo. During the first few weeks after conception, the fetal heart occupies most of the fetus midsection. The heart size to body size ratio is nine times greater in the fetus than in the infant. During those first few weeks, the fetal heart lies high in the chest. Soon, it moves down to occupy its position in the chest cavity.

❏ *Before the end of the 3rd week of gestation*: The heart begins its development from cardiogenic mesoderm. The heart precursor cells form a pair of tubes called *endothelial tubes* that differentiate into endocardium (that lines the heart chamber and valves) and myocardium (forms cardiac muscle).

❏ *Migration of heart precursor cells*: The heart precursor cells migrate towards the midline and fuse into a single heart tube, referred to as the *primitive heart tube*. This primitive heart tube develops into five distinct regions:

  1. Truncus arteriosus: It develop into pulmonary artery and ascending aorta.
  2. Bulbus cordis: It develops into right ventricle.
  3. Ventricle: It gives rise to the left ventricle.
  4. Atrium: It develops into left and right atria.
  5. Sinus venosus: It forms coronary sinus and SA node.

❏ Initially, the two atria partly separate and when their separation is complete, the ventricles begin to separate. Interatrial septum develops at the 7th week of gestation. Just after that, interventricular septum develops.

❏ Contraction of the heart starts by day 22.

❏ The atrioventricular (AV) valves are formed between the fifth and 8th week of gestation, which is followed by the formation of semilunar valves.

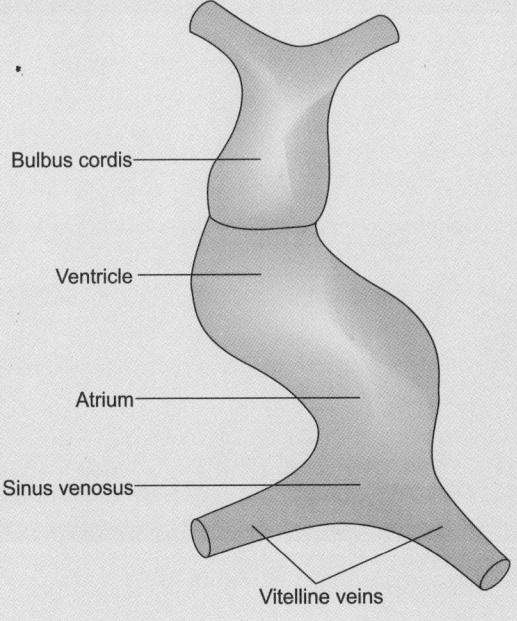

Bulbus cordis

Ventricle

Atrium

Sinus venosus

Vitelline veins

Chapter 11

Ageing and the Cardiovascular System

❏ Ageing is associated with various changes in the cardiovascular system such as
  1. Decreased elasticity of the aorta
  2. Enlargement of left ventricle
  3. Loss of cardiac muscular strength
  4. Narrowing of aortic and mitral valve
  5. Increased blood pressure
  6. Decline in cardiac output
❏ There is a gradual decrease in the heart rate with age. This decrease leads to various changes in cardiac muscles such as
  1. Decreased Ca^+ transport
  2. Increased rate of ATP breakdown
  3. Decreased aerobic metabolism
  4. Decreased effect of sympathetic hormones on heart rate
❏ All these age-related factors make the elderly much more susceptible to coronary artery disease, congestive heart failure, arrhythmia and atherosclerosis.

Exercise and the Cardiovascular System

❏ The respiratory and cardiovascular systems undergo various adjustments in response to the intensity and duration of exercise.
❏ The heart rate increases during exercise and the increase is up to 180 beats/min in moderate exercise and can reach up to 240–260 beats/min in severe exercise.
❏ The increase in cardiac output with exercise is directly proportional to increase in the amount of oxygen consumed. Cardiac output can increase up to 20 L/min in moderate exercise and 35 L/min in severe exercise.
❏ During maximal exercise, the cardiac output increases due to increase in heart rate and stroke volume.
❏ The gradual increase in the intensity of exercise increases the systolic blood pressure due to increase in heart rate and stroke volume.

HOW TO KEEP YOUR CARDIOVASCULAR SYSTEM HEALTHY

1. Do not smoke cigarettes.
2. Exercise regularly to control weight.
3. Maintain a balanced diet that should include whole grain cereals, fruits and legumes.
4. Avoid excessive intake of sugar and salt.
5. Get a yearly medical check-up of your heart.
6. Fresh black or red grapes juice prevents heart attacks and averts pain and palpitations.
7. Have plenty of rest as it relaxes the body, mind and spirit.

Review Questions

Long Answer Questions

1. Define cardiac cycle. Describe the various events of a cardiac cycle.
2. Define electrocardiogram. Describe the waves, segments and intervals of normal ECG. Add a note on ECG leads.
3. Give the definitions, normal values and variations of cardiac output. Explain the factors regulating cardiac output.
4. Give an account of regulation of cardiac function.
5. Describe the innervation of the heart and the regulation of heart rate.
6. Define arterial blood pressure. Describe the nervous regulation of arterial blood pressure. Write a note on regulation of vasomotor tone.
7. Explain blood flow through the heart, naming the major blood vessels entering and exiting the heart, the chambers and valves.
8. Describe the systemic and pulmonary blood circulation routes.
9. Explain how the conduction system of the heart functions and what factors may affect its rate.

Short Notes

1. Pacemaker
2. Conducting system in the heart
3. Isometric contraction phase
4. Heart sounds
5. Phonocardiogram
6. Cardiac murmurs
7. Waves of normal ECG
8. Venous return
9. Nerve supply to the heart
10. Baroreceptors
11. Velocity of blood flow
12. Determinants of arterial blood pressure
13. Vasomotor centre
14. Renal regulation of blood pressure
15. Vasoconstrictor and vasodilator substances
16. Hypertension
17. Myocardial infarction
18. Angina pectoris
19. Fetal circulation
20. Patent ductus arteriosus

Chapter 11

Multiple Choice Questions

1. Which of the following is correct regarding hypertension?
   - (a) 80% of cases have no clear underlying cause
   - (b) Chronic renal disease is the commonest secondary cause
   - (c) It is the commonest cause of spontaneous subarachnoid haemorrhage
   - (d) Atherosclerosis in arterioles is accelerated

2. Which of the following is correct regarding acute myocardial infarction?
   - (a) The underlying pathology is rupture of an unstable atherosclerotic plaque with formation of an occlusive thrombus
   - (b) Blockage of the left anterior descending artery causes infarction of the lateral wall of the left ventricle
   - (c) Sudden death is usually due to the onset of ventricular tachycardia
   - (d) Ventricular aneurysm formation is a possible short-term complication

3. Which of the following is correct regarding infectious endocarditis?
   - (a) The infection always arises on a heart valve
   - (b) Most patients present with symptoms of heart failure due to valve destruction
   - (c) Acute endocarditis is a destructive infection usually caused by *Streptococcus viridans*
   - (d) Subacute endocarditis is usually associated with a structural abnormality of the heart

4. Which of the following is correct regarding chronic left ventricular failure?
   - (a) Most cases are due to diastolic failure
   - (b) The average prognosis from diagnosis is 10 years
   - (c) Most cases are due to coronary artery atherosclerosis
   - (d) Electrocardiography is useful to assess ejection fraction

5. Which vein in the body carries oxygenated blood?
   - (a) Pulmonary vein
   - (b) Jugular vein
   - (c) Subclavian vein
   - (d) Inferior vena cava

6. Which of the following is correct regarding atherosclerosis?
   - (a) Atherosclerotic plaques are thought to develop in response to persistent endothelial cell injury
   - (b) In a developing atherosclerotic plaque, vascular smooth muscle cells migrate from the adventitia into the media where they secrete collagen
   - (c) Larger atherosclerotic plaques are more prone to rupture
   - (d) An acute coronary syndrome is an example of inducible ischaemia caused by a stable atherosclerotic plaque

7. Which of the following is correct regarding primary cardiomyopathies?
   - (a) They are common causes of cardiac failure
   - (b) Coronary artery angiography must be performed before a diagnosis of dilated cardiomyopathy can be made
   - (c) Hypertrophic cardiomyopathy typically presents with sudden death
   - (d) Arrhythmogenic right ventricular cardiomyopathy is associated with fatty replacement of the right ventricle.

Match the Following

1.	Parietal pericardium	(a)	Pacemaker
2.	Bicuspid valve	(b)	Mitral valve
3.	Auricle	(c)	Visceral pericardium
4.	Trabeculae carneae	(d)	Right AV valves
5.	SA node	(e)	Pericardial sac
6.	Chordae tendinae	(f)	Contraction phase
7.	Purkinje fibres	(g)	Bundle of His
8.	Systole	(h)	Folds of myocardium
9.	Tricuspid valve	(i)	Adrenaline
10.	Sympathetic neurotransmitter	(j)	Aortic valve

Careers in Cardiology

✓ Cardiologists are physicians who are specialized in the diagnosis and treatment of the disorders of the heart.

✓ Cardiac surgeon has more training and is more experienced in the diagnosis and treatment of heart disorders.

✓ Cardiovascular technologists are health professionals who perform diagnostic examinations on the patients for peripheral vascular studies and cardiology.

✓ Electrocardiographic technicians are health specialists who record the electrical impulse of the heart. They operate and maintain electrocardiographic (ECG) equipment and provide the recorded ECG and data on heart performance to the physician.

✓ Cardiac sonographers are health professionals who are trained in cardiovascular technology. They take the pictures of a patient's heart by using ultrasound technology. These pictures are used for diagnosis by cardiologists.

Chapter 11

12 The Digestive System

CHAPTER OUTLINE

- Components of the Digestive System
- Layers of the Digestive System
- Neuronal Control of the Gastrointestinal Tract—the Enteric Nervous System
- Blood Circulation of the Digestive System—Splanchnic Circulation
- Components of the Gastrointestinal Tract (Anatomy and Physiology)
- Accessory Organs
- Digestion and Absorption of Nutrients in the Gastrointestinal tract
- Diseases of the Digestive System

STUDY OBJECTIVES

- ✓ To describe the various components of the digestive system.
- ✓ To understand the neuronal control of the digestive system, i.e. the enteric nervous system.
- ✓ To understand the flow of blood in the digestive system, i.e. splanchnic circulation.
- ✓ To explain the anatomical structure and physiology of the different parts of the gastrointestinal tract.
- ✓ To study the anatomical structure and functions of the accessory organs.
- ✓ To study the digestion and absorption of carbohydrates, proteins and vitamins in the digestive system.

INTRODUCTION

To maintain good health we need food, the main source of chemical energy. Often, the food we eat consists of large molecules and cannot be used by our body cells. This is where the digestive system has a role to play (digestion = *dis*: apart; *gerere*: to carry).

Digestive system breaks down the food into smaller molecules that can be easily taken up by the cells and are processed to form the body structure and also are used to derive energy for various metabolic processes.

It resembles a tube that starts from the mouth, runs through the thorax and abdomen and ends at the anus (Fig. 12.1). It primarily performs the following functions:

- ❑ **Ingestion**: It is the consumption of food substances.
- ❑ **Propulsion**: It is the movement of food contents.
- ❑ **Mixing**: It is the churning of food.
- ❑ **Digestion**: It is the mechanical and chemical breakdown of food.

❑ **Absorption**: It is the passage of digested food into the blood and lymph.

❑ **Elimination**: It is the removal of unwanted substances from the body.

Each of these functions is explained in detail later in the chapter.

COMPONENTS OF THE DIGESTIVE SYSTEM

The following two components form the digestive system (Fig. 12.2):

❑ Alimentary canal/gastrointestinal (GI) tract
❑ Accessory organs

DO YOU KNOW

❑ Every day nine quarts of digested food, liquids and digestive juices flow through the digestive system, but only two pints are lost as faeces.

❑ Muscles contract in waves to move the food down the oesophagus. This means that food would get to a person's stomach, even if they were standing on their head.

❑ The average male will eat about 50 tons of food during his lifetime to sustain a weight of 150 pounds.

❑ Within the colon, a typical person harbours more than 400 distinct species of bacteria.

❑ In the mouth, food is either cooled or warmed to a more suitable temperature.

❑ The liver performs more than 500 functions.

❑ A full-grown horse's coiled up intestine is 89-ft long.

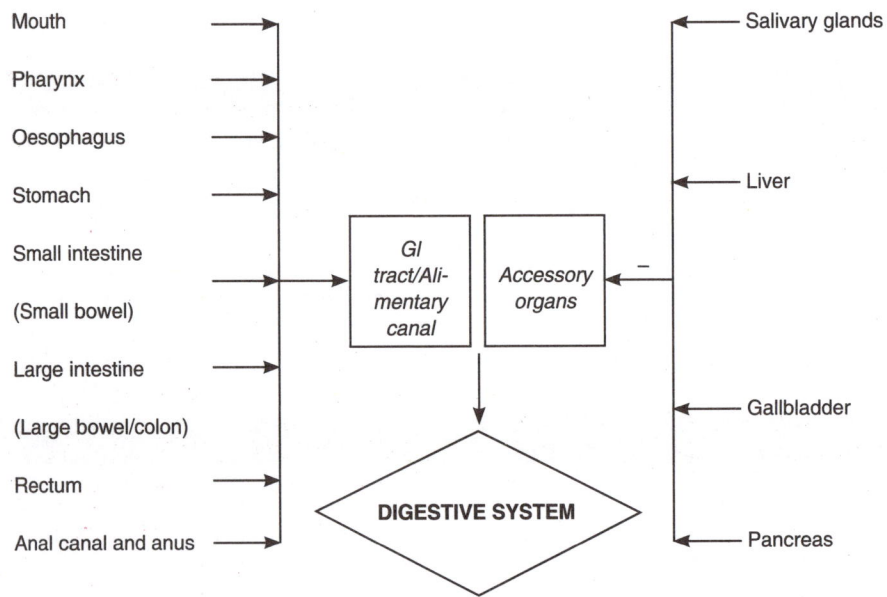

Figure 12.1 Components of the digestive system.

MEDICAL TERMINOLOGY

❑ **Distension**: It is the enlargement or ballooning effect.
❑ **Faeces**: It is the waste product from an animal's digestive tract expelled through the anus during defecation.

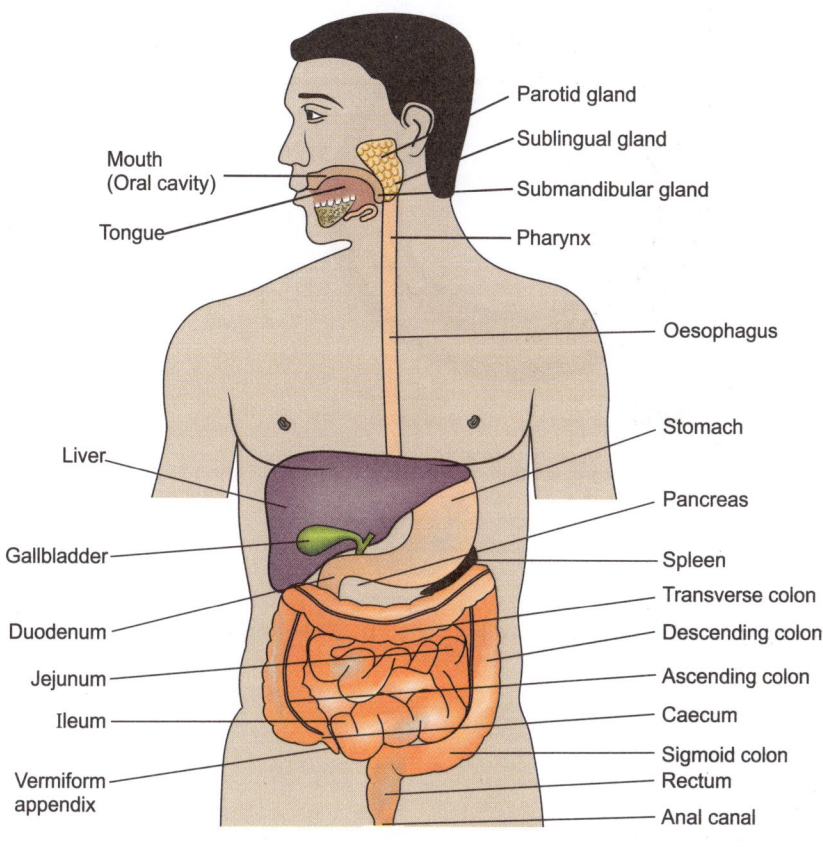

Figure 12.2 Overview of the digestive system.

LAYERS OF THE DIGESTIVE SYSTEM

The wall in the GI tract is formed by four different layers. The layers include the following:

❑ Mucosa
❑ Submucosa
❑ Muscularis (muscle layer)
❑ Adventitia/serosa/peritoneum

The typical cross section of the intestinal wall depicting the four different layers is shown in Figure 12.3.

MEDICAL TERMINOLOGY

❑ **Peristalsis**: It is the radially symmetrical contraction of muscles that propagates in a wave down the muscular tube.
❑ **Tonsil**: It is the lymph glands that destroy the harmful bacteria and prevent infection in the digestive tract.

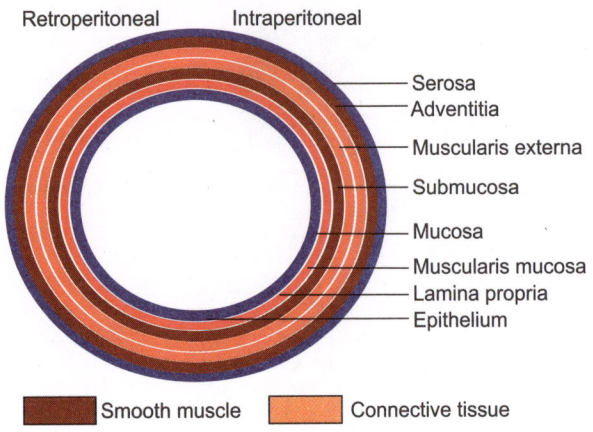

Figure 12.3 Cross section of the intestinal wall showing four layers.

MUCOSA

Mucosa forms the inner lining of the alimentary canal. It can be further divided into three sublayers:

❏ Epithelial layer
❏ Lamina propria
❏ Muscularis mucosa

Epithelial layer

This is the mucosal layer that has direct access to the contents in the lumen of the GI tract (Fig. 12.4).

Different types of epithelium cells covering different parts of GI tract are summarized in Table 12.1.

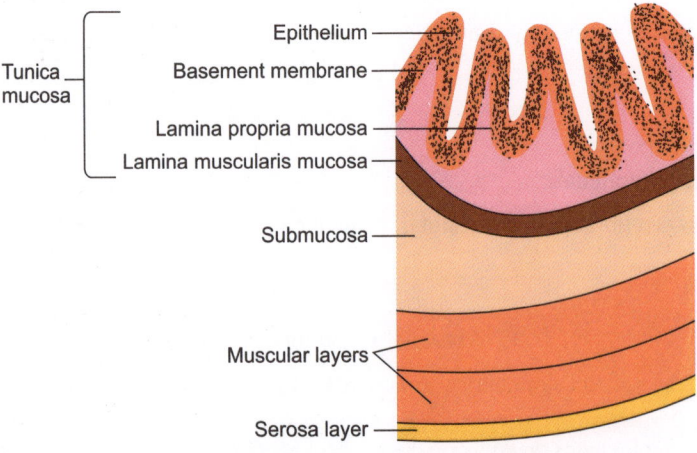

Figure 12.4 Epithelium and other layers of mucosa.

Table 12.1 Types of epithelium in the mucosa of digestive system

Parts of GI tract	Types of epithelium	Function
Stomach Small intestine Large intestine	Simple columnar epithelium	Absorption and secretion
Mouth Pharynx Oesophagus Posterior anus	Squamous epithelium	Protective function

Lamina propria

❑ It connects the epithelium to muscularis mucosa.
❑ It is composed of loose connective tissues.
❑ It contains the following blood vessels:
   ➤ Lymph vessels
   ➤ Mucosa-associated lymphoid tissue (MALT)
   ➤ Solitary lymphatic nodules

Muscularis mucosa

It is the thin layer present outside the lamina propria that permits enfolding of the mucosa membrane of the stomach and small intestine.

This increases the surface area for the digestion and absorption of the food.

SUBMUCOSA

The layer present between the mucosa and the muscularis is called *submucosa*.

It contains the following:
❑ Blood vessels
   ➤ Arteriole
   ➤ Venules
   ➤ Capillaries
❑ Lymphatic vessels
   ➤ Lymphatic tissues
❑ Submucosal plexus (also known as *Meissner's plexus*)
   ➤ Neuronal network present in submucosa

MUSCULARIS/MUSCLE LAYER

Muscularis binds submucosa and serosa.

It is composed of the following:

☐ Skeletal muscle
☐ Smooth muscle

  ➤ Circular smooth muscle (CSM) fibres—inner layer
  ➤ Longitudinal smooth muscle (LSM) fibres—outer layer

It contains myenteric plexus, an extensive neural network.

The types of muscularis forming the different parts of the GI tract are summarized in Table 12.2.

Table 12.2 Types of muscularis

Parts of GI tract	Types of muscularis	Function
Mouth Pharynx Half of oesophagus Anal sphincter (posterior anus)	Skeletal muscle	To assist in voluntary swallowing To exercise voluntary control on defecation Contraction of anus
Stomach Small intestine Large intestine	CSM and LSM	Breaking, mixing and propulsion of bolus of food

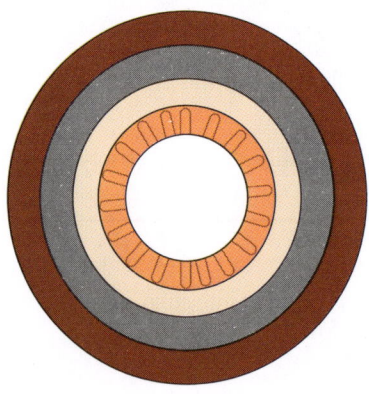

Figure 12.5 Longitudinal smooth muscle.

ADVENTITIA/SEROSA/PERITONEUM

It is the outer covering of the GI tract and is the largest serous membrane of the body.

It is the serous membrane composed of the following:

☐ Loose connective tissue
☐ Simple squamous epithelium

It can be subdivided into the following two layers:

➤ Parietal layer
➤ Visceral layer

The former covers the abdominal wall, whereas the latter covers the visceral organs present in the abdominopelvic region, hence called *visceral layer*.

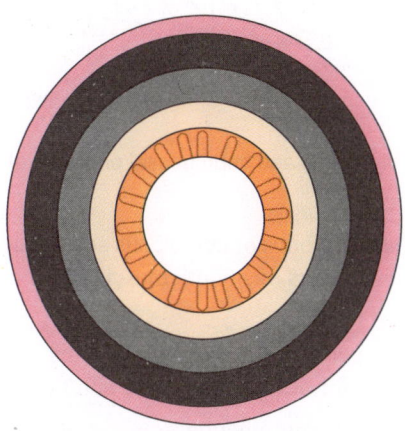

Figure 12.6 Serosa layer.

NEURONAL CONTROL OF THE GI TRACT — THE ENTERIC NERVOUS SYSTEM

The GI tract possesses an integral nervous system called the *enteric nervous system (ENS)*.

It functions independently, hence known as gut's brain/second/little brain, although its activities are limited to the GI tract.

Beginning in the oesophagus, it extends all the way to the anus to control and integrate the physiological condition of the alimentary tract, gut motility, exchange of fluid between the gut and its lumen, and local blood flow.

It contains about 100–500 millions neurons, which are principally of the following two types:

❏ Sensory neurons (primary afferent neurons)
❏ Motor neurons (primary efferent neurons)

The neurons in the ENS are mainly organized into two plexuses (i.e. the network of interconnected neurons):

❏ Meissner's plexus (also known as *submucosal plexus*)
❏ Auerbach's plexus (also known as *myenteric plexus*)

Meissner's plexus consists of small groups of nerve cells and connecting nerve fibre bundles in the submucosa, forming an extensive network from the anterior oesophagus to the anterior anal sphincter.

It serves a controlling function within the inner wall of each small section of the intestine by regulating the movements of the GI tract.

Chapter 12

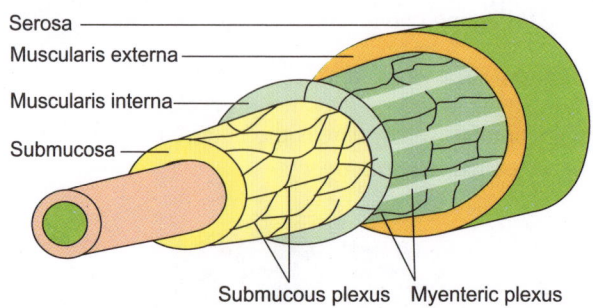

Fig 12.7 Myenteric and submucosal plexuses of the ENS.

Auerbach's plexus consists of small groups of nerve cells and connecting nerve fibre bundles present between the circular and longitudinal layers of smooth muscle fibres of the stomach and small and large intestines.

Similar to Meissner's plexus, Auerbach's plexus also forms an extensive network that extends throughout the GI tract from the anterior oesophagus to the anterior anal sphincter (Fig. 12.7).

On stimulation, it performs the following functions:

❑ It increases the tone of the gut wall.
❑ It causes an increase in intensity of the rhythmical contractions in the gut.
❑ It causes rapid peristaltic movements by increasing speed.
❑ It increases the secretions in the GI tract.

Note:

❑ Despite the ENS functioning on its own, it is regulated by parasympathetic and sympathetic part of the nervous system.

❑ Parasympathetic input is supplied by vagus nerve fibres and the sacral spinal cord. Its stimulation results in increased secretion and motility of the GI tract.

❑ While the sympathetic input to ENS is supplied by nerves from the thoracic and lumbar region (upper) of the spinal cord, their stimulation results in decreased secretion and motility in the GI tract.

BLOOD CIRCULATION OF THE DIGESTIVE SYSTEM— SPLANCHNIC CIRCULATION

The blood vessels in the digestive system form an extensive system called *splanchnic circulation*.

Mesenteric arteries, both superior and inferior, supply blood to the small intestine and colon. The stomach is supplied by the coeliac artery (Fig. 12.8).

Arteries in the gut subdivide into smaller branches, which spread in both directions of the gut. They spread in such a way that their tips meet on the side of the gut wall opposite to the attachment of the mesentery.

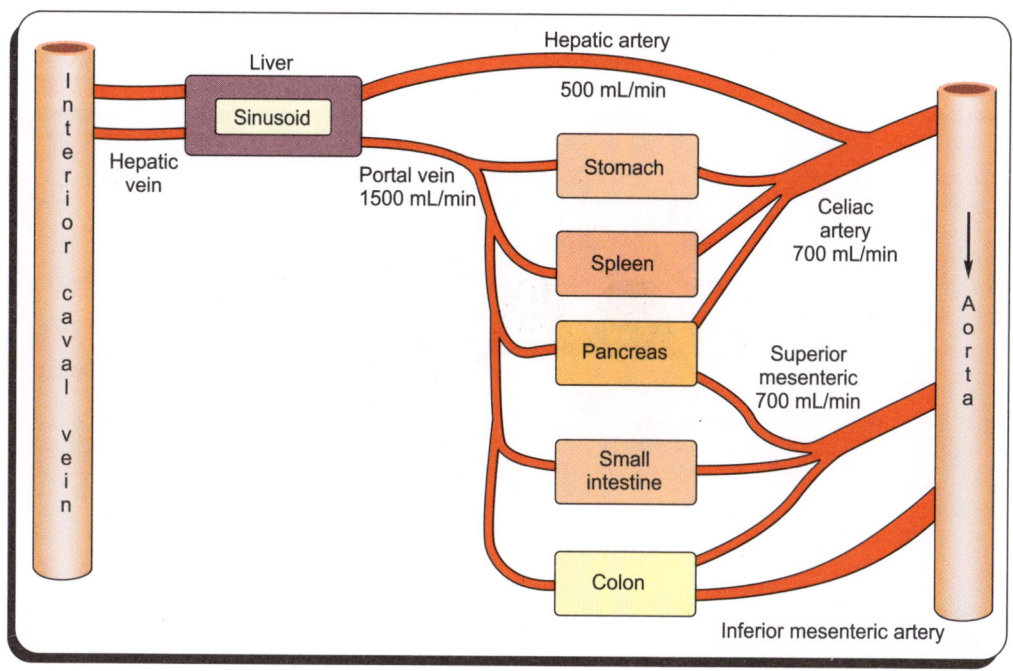

Figure 12.8 Splanchnic circulation.

They subdivide into much smaller branches to provide blood supply to muscle bundles, villi of the intestine and submucosal vessels below the epithelial layer.

After leaving the gut, spleen and pancreas, the blood flows to the liver through the hepatic portal vein. It courses through hepatic sinusoids and then to the vena cava through the hepatic portal vein to enter the general body blood circulation.

The reticuloendothelial cells lining the hepatic sinusoids act as a barrier against the harmful agents that can enter the blood circulation through the GI tract.

COMPONENTS OF THE GASTROINTESTINAL TRACT (ANATOMY AND PHYSIOLOGY)

MOUTH

Anatomical structure of the mouth

Also known as oral or buccal cavity, the mouth is formed by the following (Fig. 12.9):
- Lips
- Cheeks
- Palate—hard and soft
- Tongue

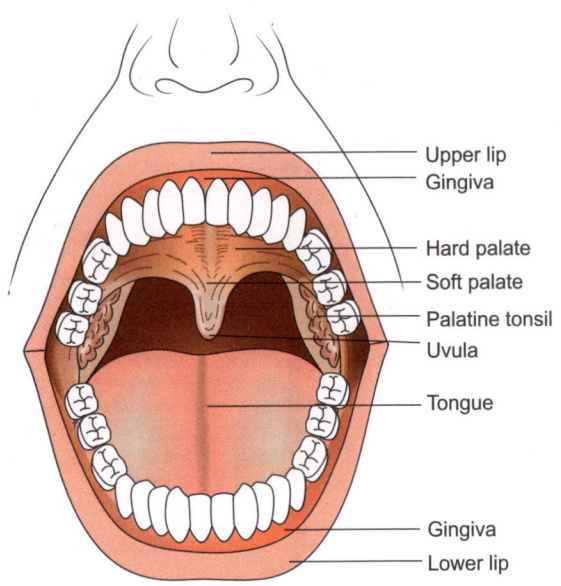

Figure 12.9 Overview of the oral cavity.

Lips or labia

❑ Lips form the opening of the oral cavity.
❑ They are made of muscles called orbicularis.
❑ Externally, lips are covered by skin.
❑ Internally, they are lined with the mucous membrane.
❑ The upper and lower lips are attached to their corresponding gums by the superior and inferior labial frenulum (folds of mucous membrane), respectively.

Cheeks

❑ Cheeks form the lateral walls of the mouth.
❑ They are covered externally by the skin and are internally lined with the mucous membrane.
❑ The mucous membrane of the oral cavity is composed of stratified squamous epithelial cells containing small mucus-secreting glands.
❑ In between the gums and cheeks, there lies a space called *vestibule*, and the remaining portion (i.e. the space between gums and teeth till the pharynx) is called *mouth/oral/buccal cavity proper*.

Palate

❑ Palate forms the roof of the mouth and is divided into the anterior hard palate and the posterior soft palate.
❑ The hard palate is formed by maxillae and palatine bones and it serves as a bony partition between the oral and nasal cavities.
❑ The soft palate is muscular and merges with the pharynx at the sides.
❑ From the centre of soft palate, a small, conical muscular fold hangs down called *uvula*.
❑ Along with soft palate, uvula assists in swallowing by closing the nasopharynx. Thus during swallowing, food (solid/liquid) is prevented to enter the nasal cavity.

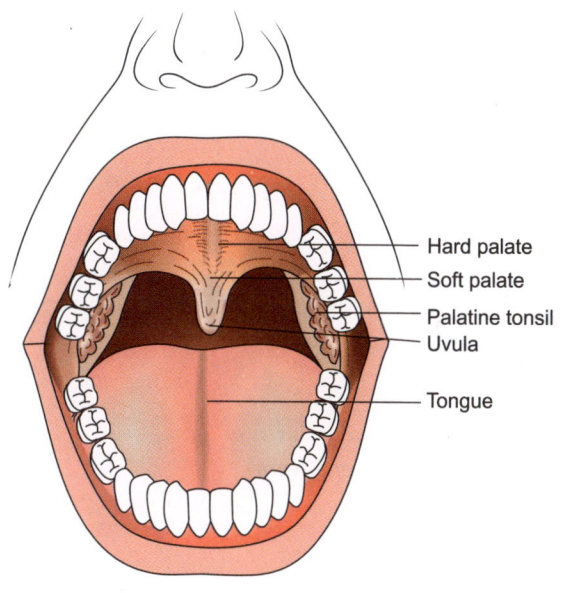

Figure 12.10 Hard palate, soft palate and uvula.

❏ The centre of the uvula gives rise to four muscular folds that run down laterally to the soft palate. The two folds lying anterior are called *palatoglossal arch.* They extend to the sides of the tongue. The other two muscular folds lying posterior are called *palatopharyngeal arch.* They extend to the lateral sides of the pharynx.

Tongue

❏ Tongue is a voluntary muscular structure that forms the floor of the mouth.
❏ It is made of stratified squamous epithelium cells.
❏ It can be divided into two symmetrical halves and each side contains two types of muscles: extrinsic muscles and intrinsic muscles.
❏ The types of extrinsic and intrinsic muscles and their function are summarized in Table 12.3.

Table 12.3 Types of extrinsic and intrinsic muscles

Types of muscles	Function

Extrinsic
  Hyoglossus
  Genioglossus
  Styloglossus
	Movement of tongue
	Aid in chewing the food

Intrinsic
  Transverse linguae
  Vertical linguae
  Longitudinal superior
  Longitudinal inferior
	Change the shape and size of tongue to assist in:
	Speaking
	Swallowing

❏ The tongue is attached by its base to the hyoid bone and by a fold of the mucous membrane called *frenulum* to the floor of the mouth.
❏ The superior portion of the tongue contains numerous little projections called *papillae* that contain nerve endings, often referred to as taste buds.
❏ There are primarily three types of papillae:
  ➤ Fungiform papillae
  ➤ Filiform papillae
  ➤ Vallate papillae
❏ Fungiform papillae are present at the tip of the tongue. Filliform papillae are present between the fungiform and vallate papillae. Vallate papillae are present towards the base of tongue (Fig. 12.11).

Blood and nerve supply to the tongue

❏ Arterial, an external carotid artery (lingual branch)
❏ Venous, a branch of interjugular vein (lingual vein)
❏ Nerve supply
  ➤ Mandibular nerves (lingual branch)
  ➤ Hypoglossal nerve (XII cranial nerve)
  ➤ Glossopharyngeal nerve (VII cranial nerve)
  ➤ Facial nerve (IX cranial nerve)

Functions of the tongue

❏ Mastication—chewing
❏ Deglutition—swallowing
❏ Role in speech
❏ Taste sensation

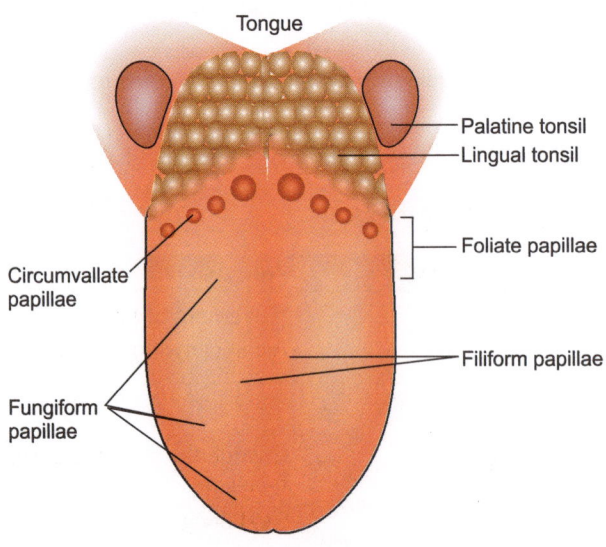

Figure 12.11 Tongue and its papillae.

Teeth

❏ The teeth are accessory digestive organs embedded in the sockets of the alveolar processes of the mandible and maxillae.

❏ **Structure of tooth**: Externally, a tooth can be divided into three parts: crown, neck and root.
  ➤ *Crown* is the upper, visible part protruding from the gingivae (gums).
  ➤ *Neck* is the slightly constricted part of the tooth where crown meets the root.
  ➤ *Root* is the part that is embedded in the socket. It can be 1, 2 or 3 in number. Larger teeth like molars have more than one root.

❏ Internally, a tooth consists of dentine, composed of calcified connective tissue that contains calcium. This connective tissue gives the tooth its basic shape and rigidity.

❏ Enamel covers the dentine of the crown. It is composed of calcium salts—calcium carbonate and calcium phosphate. It serves the protective function during wear and tear of chewing and acid contact. Both dentine and enamel are harder than bones.

❏ The root of the tooth is covered by a substance called *cementum* that attaches the root of tooth to the socket.

❏ The space enclosed in dentine at the centre of the tooth is called *pulp cavity* that comprises blood vessels, lymph vessels and nerves (Fig. 12.12).

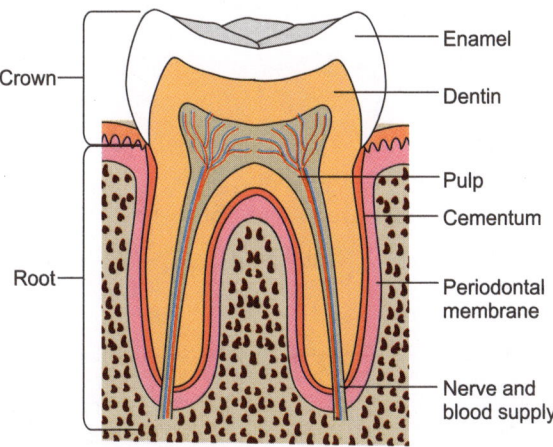

Figure 12.12 Structure of tooth.

Blood and nerve supply

❏ **Arterial**: Maxillary arteries (branches)
❏ **Venous**: Numerous veins that pour into internal jugular vein.
❏ **Nerves**: Branches of trigeminal nerves (V cranial nerve)

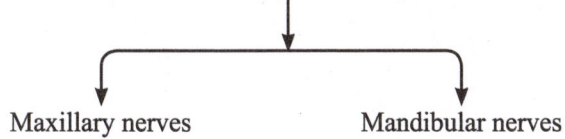

Types of teeth

Humans have the following four types of teeth (Fig. 12.13):

1. Molars
2. Premolars
3. Canine
4. Incisors

❏ They have two types of dentitions: deciduous and permanent.
❏ At the age of 10, almost all the deciduous (milk) teeth are replaced by permanent teeth.
❏ The number of teeth in the two types of dentitions are summarized in Table 12.4.

Table 12.4 Number of teeth in two different types of dentitions

Side of jaw	Types of teeth	Types of dentitions			
		Deciduous		Permanent	
		Upper jaw	Lower jaw	Upper jaw	Lower jaw
Left side	Molars	2	2	3	3
	Premolars	–	–	2	2
	Canines	1	1	1	1
	Incisors	2	2	2	2
Right side	Incisors	2	2	2	2
	Canines	1	1	1	1
	Premolars	–	–	2	2
	Molars	2	2	3	3
		Total =10	Total =10	Total =16	Total =16
		Total = **20**		Total = **32**	

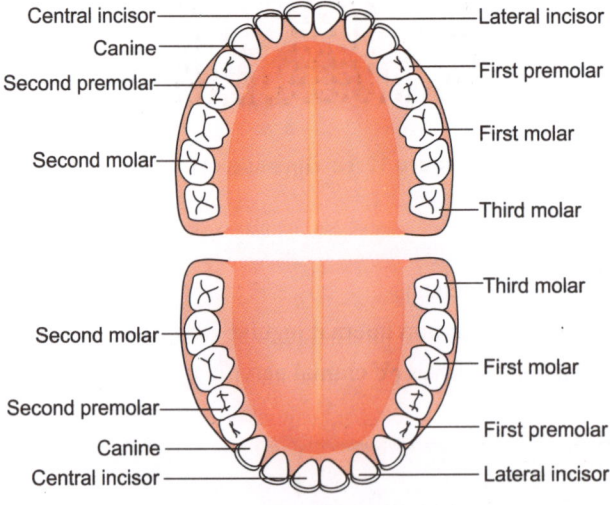

Central incisor — Lateral incisor
Canine — First premolar
Second premolar — First molar
Second molar — Third molar

Third molar
Second molar — First molar
Second premolar — First premolar
Canine — Lateral incisor
Central incisor

Figure 12.13 Types of teeth.

Physiology of the oral cavity

The food is ingested into the body through the oral cavity. This process is called *ingestion*.

The ingestion of food is followed by:

❏ Mastication or chewing
❏ Deglutition or swallowing (discussed in detail in the section Physiology of Pharynx)

Mastication

❏ This is the mechanical digestion of food that results from chewing and it is done by the teeth perfectly designed for this purpose.
❏ In this process, the food is manipulated by the tongue, broken down by teeth and then mixed with saliva, which results in the formation of a soft, flexible and easily swallowable mass of food called the *bolus*.
❏ The process of chewing, initiated by the chewing reflex, includes the following steps:

The reflex for the inhibition of the muscles of chewing is initiated by the presence of bolus of food in the oral cavity.

↓

This results in the lowering/dropping of the lower jaw.

↓

The lowering of the jaw causes the stretch reflex of its muscles and results in rebound contraction.

↓

As a result the jaw is closed, leading to the closure of teeth.

↓

The teeth closure causes the compression of the food bolus against the mouth, which once again leads to inhibition of the muscles of jaw, lowers jaw and stretches it up again (rebound contraction).

↓

This cycle is repeated again and again unless the food is masticated completely and ready to swallow.

Importance of mastication

❏ It is important for grinding the food into smaller particles.
❏ It increases the rate of digestion by increasing the surface area of the food particles.
❏ It is useful in breaking the outer membrane of indigestible cellulose present in most fruits and vegetables (uncooked), thus resulting in better digestion.

PHARYNX

Anatomical structure of the pharynx

The anatomical structure of the pharynx has been discussed previously in detail in the chapter Respiratory System.

Chapter 12

Physiology

Deglutition

After the process of chewing in mouth, the masticated food is propelled into the stomach through the process called *deglutition* or *swallowing*.

The process of swallowing occurs in the following three different stages:

❏ Voluntary stage
❏ First involuntary stage/pharyngeal stage
❏ Second involuntary stage/oesophageal stage

Voluntary stage

❏ It is a stage that is under our own conscious control, hence called voluntary stage.
❏ In this stage, the masticated food is voluntarily pushed down towards the pharynx.
❏ Tongue assists in the rolling of the food posterior into the pharynx by its upward and backward movement against the soft palate of the buccal cavity.

First involuntary stage/pharyngeal stage

❏ This stage does not last for more than 2 s.
❏ In this stage, the food bolus in the pharynx is pushed into the upper part of the oesophagus.
❏ This stage includes the following steps:

The soft palate moves up.

↓

The trachea shuts down.

↓

The upper part of the oesophagus opens up.

↓

A quick peristaltic wave arises from the pharynx.

↓

It pushes the food bolus in the pharynx down to the upper part of the oesophagus.

The second involuntary stage/oesophageal stage is discussed in the section Physiology of Oesophagus.

OESOPHAGUS

Anatomical structure of oesophagus

Oesophagus is the tubular organ (long tube about 25 cm in length and 2 cm in diameter) of the GI tract.

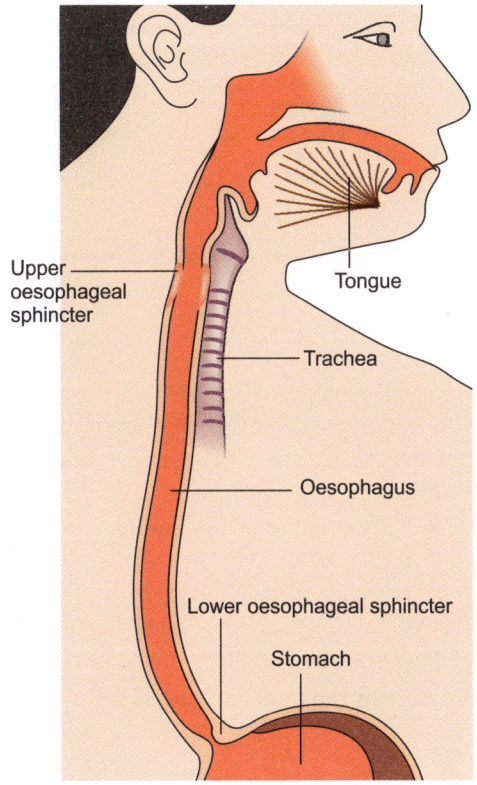

Figure 12.14 Oesophagus.

It is in continuation with the pharynx and passes through the diaphragm to open into the stomach. Just before opening into the stomach, it bends slightly upwards. This upward bent is supposed to prevent the backflow (regurgitation) of gastric contents into the oesophagus.

The tissue layers forming the oesophagus have been discussed previously in this chapter. For more details see the section Layers of the Digestive System.

The upper and lower ends of the oesophagus are guarded by two sphincters (Fig. 12.14):

❏ Upper oesophageal sphincter (cricopharyngeal sphincter)
❏ Lower oesophageal sphincter (cardiac sphincter)
❏ Upper sphincter serves to prevent the entry of air in the oesophagus during respiration. It also prevents aspiration of the oesophageal contents.
❏ Lower sphincter prevents the reflux of the gastric contents into the oesophagus (aberrant conditions being the exceptional case).

Blood and nerve supply

Arterial

Oesophageal arteries ——————(supply to)——————→ Thoracic region of oesophagus (from aorta)

Inferior phrenic arteries
Celiac artery (left gastric branch) } ——————(supply to)——————→ Abdominal region of oesophagus

Venous

Azygos and hemiazygos veins ——————(drain off)——————→ Thoracic region of oesophagus

Left gastric vein ——————(drain off)——————→ Abdominal region of oesophagus

Nerve supply

Vagus nerve supplies the parasympathetic innervations.

Sympathetic and parasympathetic both end in the myenteric and submucosal plexuses.

Physiology

Second involuntary stage/oesophageal stage

This stage begins when the bolus enters the oesophagus. In this stage, food in the pharynx is rapidly conducted to the stomach, primarily by the specific organized movements of oesophagus, hence also called the *oesophageal stage*.

It is mainly carried out through peristaltic movements (i.e. the coordinated contraction and relaxation of the longitudinal and circular muscle of the oesophagus) (Fig. 12.15).

The two oesophageal peristaltic movements that propel the bolus are:

❑ Primary peristaltic movements
❑ Secondary peristaltic movements

The peristaltic movements, initiated in the pharynx, continue in the oesophagus as the primary peristaltic movements. The time taken by the peristaltic wave to pass the bolus from the pharynx to the oesophagus to the stomach is only 8–10 s. As the bolus approaches the end of oesophagus, the lower oesophageal sphincter relaxes and the bolus moves into the stomach.

The secondary peristaltic waves come into act when the primary peristaltic wave fails to descend the food from the pharynx down to the stomach.

These waves are initiated due to distension of oesophagus caused by the food retained in stomach through the stimulation of central neural circuits of the myenteric plexus.

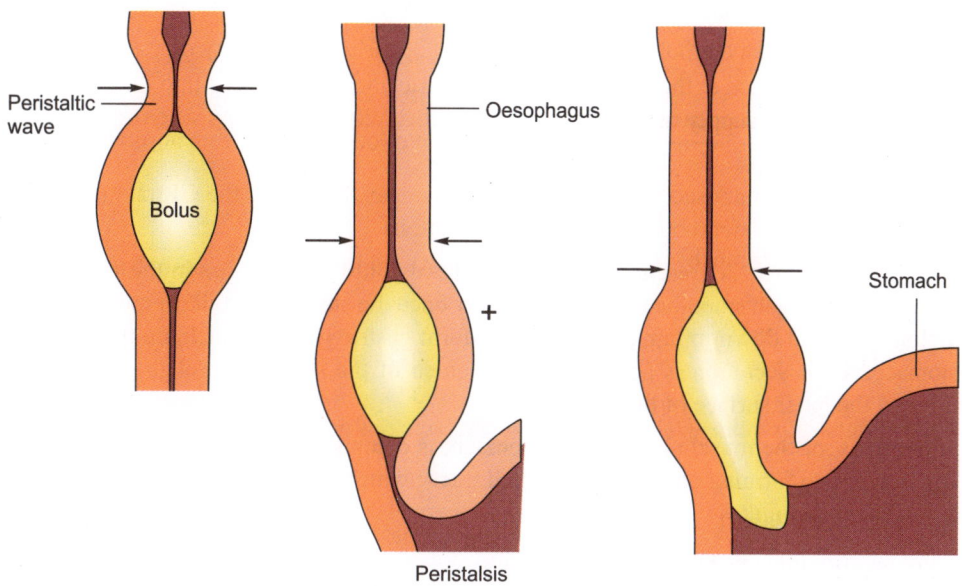

Figure 12.15 Oesophageal peristaltic movement.

STOMACH

Anatomical structure of stomach

Stomach is the J-shaped organ of the GI tract anatomically located in the epigastric, umbilical and left hypochondriac region of the abdomen. Its volume is 50 mL when empty and it can expand to accommodate 1–1.5 L of solids and liquids under normal conditions.

It is continuous with the oesophagus at the cardiac sphincter and with the duodenum at the pyloric sphincter. The large convex border of the stomach is called the *greater curvature* and the small concave border is called the *lesser curvature* of the stomach.

The stomach can be divided into the following four regions:

❑ Cardiac
❑ Fundus
❑ Body
❑ Pylorus

The region around the opening of the oesophagus forms the cardiac. The region that forms superior portion of stomach, left to cardiac, is the fundus. The middle large region, inferior to the fundus and extending to the pylorus forms the body. The pylorus is the region that connects the stomach with the duodenum (small intestine). This is slightly elevated at an acute angle.

Pylorus can be subdivided into two regions: pylorus antrum and pylorus canal.

❑ The pylorus antrum attaches to the body of the stomach.
❑ The pylorus canal forms the way through which chyme (bolus + gastric juice) runs directly into the duodenum.

The two muscular sphincters in the stomach are as follows:

❏ Cardiac sphincter (situated around the cardiac end): It opens towards cavity of the stomach.

❏ Pyloric sphincter (situated at the distal end of the pyloric antrum): It opens into the duodenum. This sphincter is relaxed and open when the stomach is inactive but it closes when food is present in stomach.

The stomach wall is composed of the same tissue layers as the rest of the GI tract (see the section Layers of the Digestive System) but with some modifications.

Mucosa of the stomach is present in the form of large folds called *rugae* in the empty or resting condition. However, rugae smoothen up and disappear once the stomach is full. In mucosa, the cells of the epithelium descend down to lamina propria and form gastric glands, which are the secretory cells of the stomach. Their secretion is poured into the lumen of the stomach through gastric pits (small depressions on the inner surface of the stomach).

The muscularis, or the muscle layer of the stomach, is composed of three layers of smooth muscle fibres (in place of two forming other parts of the GI tract), which are as follows (Fig. 12.16):

❏ Oblique layer (inner layer)

❏ Circular layer (middle layer)

❏ Longitudinal layer (outer layer)

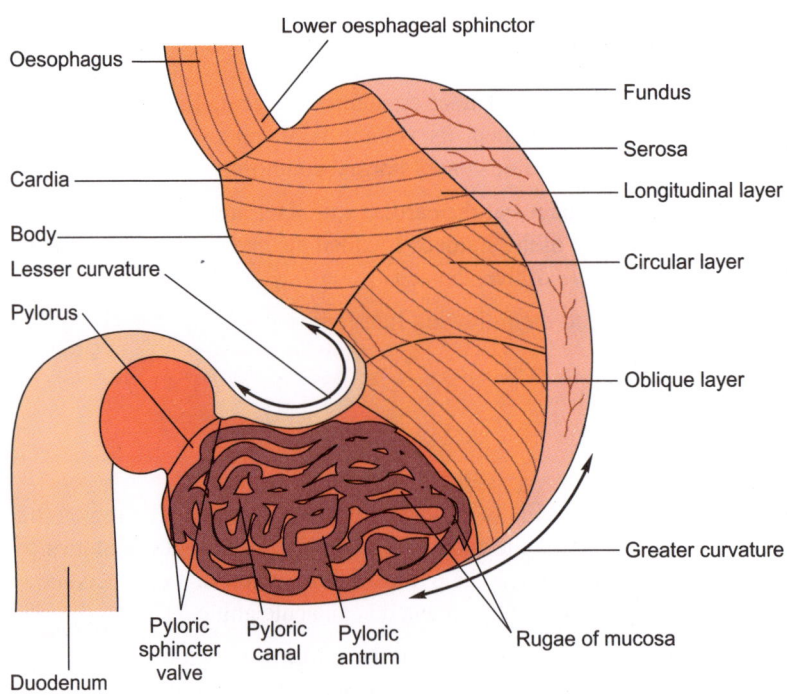

Figure 12.16 Stomach.

The pattern of smooth muscle fibres in stomach facilitates the following:
- ❏ Increased churning of food to form chyme
- ❏ Rapid peristaltic movements

Blood and nerve supply

See the sections Splanchnic Circulation and Neural Control of the Digestive System for more details.

The gastric gland is formed by the three types of cells that secrete their products into the stomach lumen. The three types of secreting cells are as follows:

1. **Chief cells**: They mainly secrete pepsinogen (the principal gastric enzyme) and gastrin (stimulates gastric activity).
2. **Parietal cells**: They secrete hydrochloric acid, which activates the pepsinogen to become pepsin (enzyme for protein breakdown).
3. **Mucous neck cells**: They secrete mucous.

Details of these cells have been summarized in Table 12.5.

The secretions of these gastric glands are collectively referred to as gastric juice. About 2 L of gastric juice is secreted daily by these specialized gastric glands.

Table 12.5 Types of cells forming gastric gland

Types of cells	Location	Secretion
Parietal cells (oxyntic cells)	Body and fundus of stomach	Water Intrinsic factor for vit. B_{12} absorption Hydrochloric acid Mucous Salts
Mucous neck cells	Surface of stomach	Mucous
Peptic cells (chief cells)	Antrum of stomach	Pepsinogen Gastric lipase Mucus Gastrin (secreted by G cells of peptic cells)

Physiology

Functions of gastric juice

1. **Digestive function**: The enzymes of the gastric juice play a major role in the digestion of proteins (e.g. pepsin and renin).
2. **Haemopoietic function**: The intrinsic factor in the gastric juice is necessary for the absorption of vitamin B_{12} from the gut into blood and this factor is very important for erythropoiesis.
3. **Protective function**: The mucus present in the gastric juice protects the wall of the stomach from mechanical injury as well as from hydrochloric acid.
4. **Hydrochloric acid**: It has bacteriolytic action and provides the acidic environment for the action of enzymes.

Chapter 12

Phases of gastric secretion

The secretion of gastric juice occurs when the food is taken in the mouth and it reaches its maximum level about 1 h after a meal.

There are three phases of gastric secretion, as follows:

- ❏ Cephalic phase
- ❏ Gastric phase
- ❏ Intestinal phase

Cephalic phase

- ❏ This phase is solely under nervous control. In this phase, the secretion of gastric juice occurs before food reaches the stomach. The impulses for gastric secretion are sent from the head; hence, this phase is called the *cephalic phase*.
- ❏ When the food is placed in the mouth, afferent impulses arise from taste buds and reach the appetite centre in amygdala and hypothalamus. From here, the efferent impulses pass through the vagus nerves that stimulate the gastric secretion by the release of acetylcholine.
- ❏ The smell, sight, taste or thought of food also stimulates gastric secretion by sending the impulses to the cerebral cortex that further activates the vagus nerves and increases the secretions. Thus, when the vagus nerves are cut (vagotomy), this phase of gastric secretion stops.
- ❏ Almost 20% of gastric acid is secreted in this phase.

Gastric phase

- ❏ This phase of gastric secretion occurs when the food enters the stomach.
- ❏ The presence of the food in stomach stimulates the following:
  - ➤ **Vagal reflexes**: It is the release of acetylcholine, leading to increased gastric secretion.
  - ➤ **Local reflexes of the ENS**: They further stimulate the gastric glands to release gastric secretions.
  - ➤ **Gastrin secretion**: It stimulates the gastric glands to produce more gastric juice.
- ❏ All these lead to about 70% of gastric acid secretion.

Intestinal phase

- ❏ This occurs when the chyme (bolus + gastric secretions) reaches the duodenum.
- ❏ In this phase, initially the gastric secretion increases, but later it is inhibited. Initially, when the chyme enters the duodenum (intestine), immediately the gastrin is secreted by intestinal mucosa that transports to stomach by blood. The gastrin then acts on the gastric glands of stomach and increases gastric secretion. Later, there is complete stoppage of secretion of gastric juice due to the release of hormones such as gastric inhibitory peptide (GIP), vasoactive intestinal polypeptide (VIP) and secretin in small intestine.

Mechanism of gastric acid (HCl) secretion

The hydrochloric acid secretion is an active process that takes place in the parietal cells of the stomach.

The mechanism of gastric acid secretion is explained in Figure 12.17.

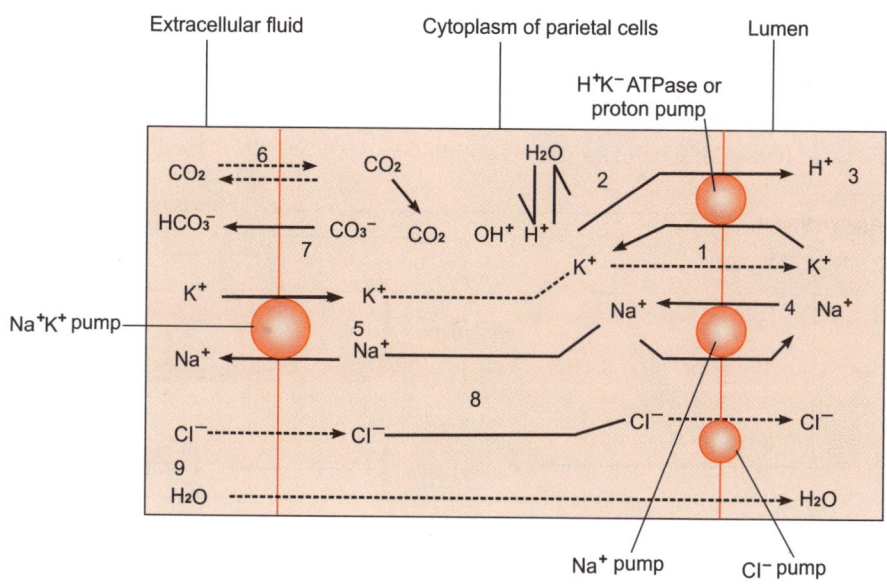

Figure 12.17 Mechanism of gastric acid secretion.

The mechanism of gastric secretion is as follows:

1. Potassium ions are absorbed from the cytoplasm of parietal cells into lumen of canaliculi.
2. Water dissociates to form hydroxyl and hydrogen ions.
3. The potassium ions are exchanged with hydrogen ions through active transport by the proton pump ($H^+ K^+$ ATPase).
4. Sodium ions are actively absorbed in the cytoplasm through the sodium pump.
5. Sodium ions in the cytoplasm are actively exchanged with potassium ions by the Na^+–K^+ pump.
6. Carbon dioxide from the blood stream reacts with hydroxyl ions to form HCO_3^- (carbonic acid) in the presence of the enzyme carbonic anhydrase.
7. HCO_3^- is transported to extracellular fluid (ECF).
8. Chloride ions are absorbed from the ECF in the cytoplasm and actively transported into lumen by the chloride pump and react with H^+ to form HCl, with Na^+ to form NaCl and K^+ to form KCl.
9. Water from the ECF is absorbed in the lumen by osmosis.

Regulation of gastric secretion

Stimulation

The secretion of gastric juice is stimulated by the following:

❑ Neurotransmitters: acetylcholine and histamine
❑ Hormone: gastrin

The stimulation of gastric acid is explained in Figure 12.18.

Chapter 12

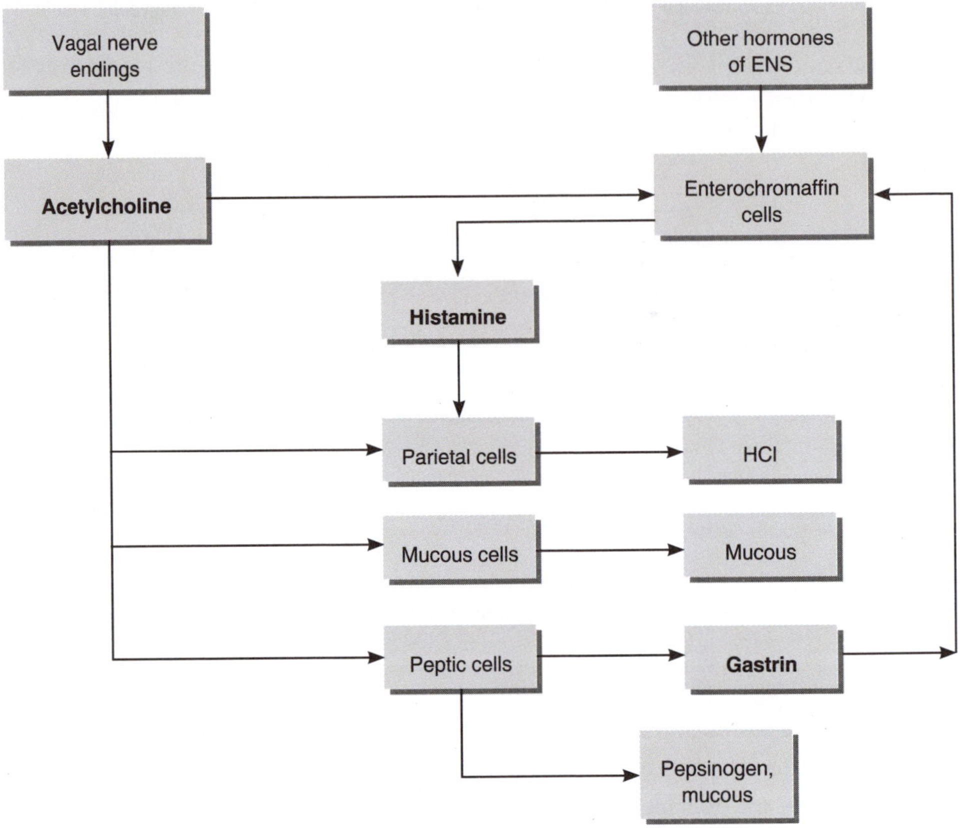

```
┌──────────────┐                              ┌──────────────┐
│ Vagal nerve  │                              │Other hormones│
│  endings     │                              │   of ENS     │
└──────┬───────┘                              └──────┬───────┘
       │                                             │
       ▼                                             ▼
┌──────────────┐                              ┌──────────────┐
│ Acetylcholine│─────────────────────────────▶│Enterochromaffin◀─┐
└──────┬───────┘                              │    cells     │   │
       │          ┌──────────────┐            └──────────────┘   │
       │          │  Histamine   │                               │
       │          └──────┬───────┘                               │
       ├──────────▶┌──────────────┐        ┌──────────┐          │
       │           │ Parietal cells│──────▶│   HCl    │          │
       │           └──────────────┘        └──────────┘          │
       ├──────────▶┌──────────────┐        ┌──────────┐          │
       │           │ Mucous cells │──────▶│  Mucous  │          │
       │           └──────────────┘        └──────────┘          │
       └──────────▶┌──────────────┐        ┌──────────┐          │
                   │ Peptic cells │──────▶│ Gastrin  │──────────┘
                   └──────┬───────┘        └──────────┘
                          ▼
                   ┌──────────────┐
                   │ Pepsinogen,  │
                   │   mucous     │
                   └──────────────┘
```

Figure 12.18 Stimulation of the gastric secretion.

Inhibition

The mechanism by which gastric secretion is inhibited is depicted in (Fig. 12.19).

Secretion of pepsinogen, other enzymes and intrinsic factor

❏ The peptic/chief cells secrete pepsinogen. After coming in contact with HCl and previously formed pepsin, it gets converted into its active form pepsin.

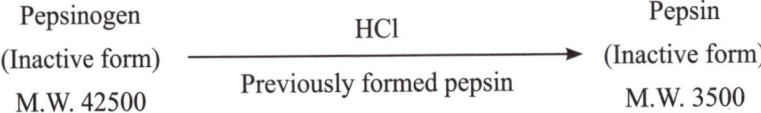

Pepsinogen (Inactive form) M.W. 42500 $\xrightarrow[\text{Previously formed pepsin}]{\text{HCl}}$ Pepsin (Inactive form) M.W. 3500

❏ Pepsin is a proteolytic enzyme. It causes the digestion of proteins in the stomach and works at an optimum pH of 1.8–3.4.

❏ The other enzymes secreted are as follows:
  ➤ Gastric amylases (cause digestion of starch)
  ➤ Gastric lipases (cause digestion of tributyrin)
  ➤ Gelatinases (act on gelatin)

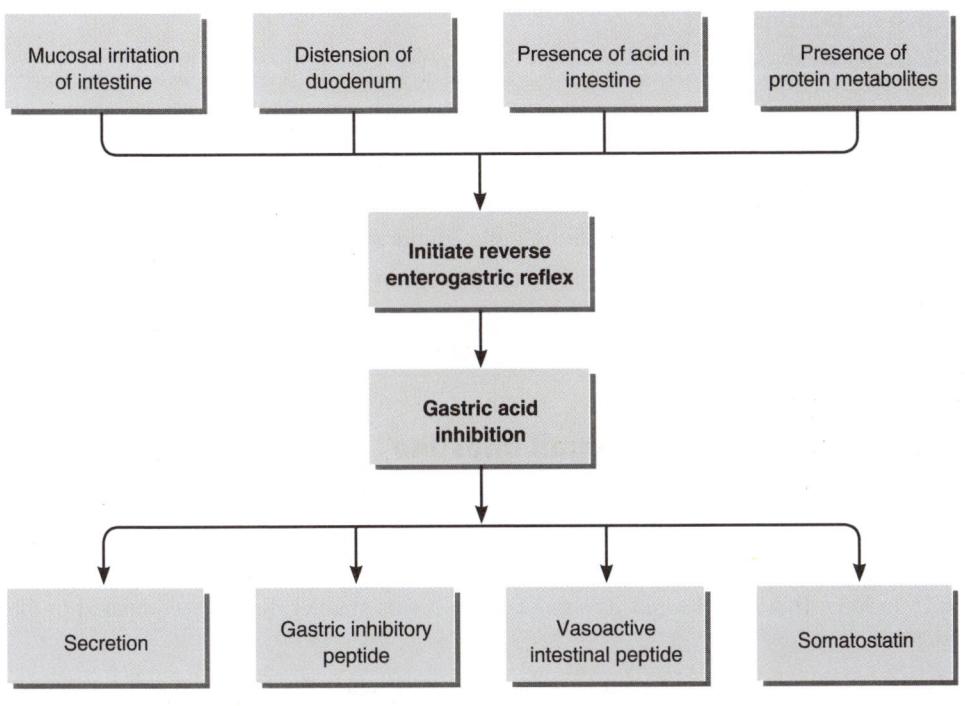

Figure 12.19 Inhibition of gastric acid secretion.

❑ The secretion of intrinsic factor by the parietal cells carries a significant importance. It is required for the absorption of vitamin B_{12}, the absence of which may not cause maturation of RBCs and can lead to manifestations like pernicious anaemia.

Functions of the stomach

The stomach performs the following main functions:

1. **Storage function**
   ❑ The stomach serves the storage function. It acts as a reservoir of food.
   ❑ It supplies small quantities of food to the duodenum for digestion and absorption at regular intervals.
   ❑ The ingestion of food causes a reduction in the tone of the muscular wall of the stomach, which accommodates a greater quantity of food. The tone of the wall of the stomach is controlled through vagal reflex by the brain stem.

2. **Mixing function**
   ❑ The stomach serves as the mixing chamber. It causes mixing of the food.
   ❑ The mixing is carried out by the mixing waves (peristaltic movements).
   ❑ When the food enters the stomach, it gives rise to weak mixing waves that originate in the centre of the body of the stomach every 15–20 s and cause the mixing of the food.

Chapter 12

3. **Propulsion function**
   - ❑ When the weak mixing waves progress down to the antrum, they turn into intense and powerful antral contractions.
   - ❑ These contractions propel the contents of the stomach into the duodenum and result in the emptying of the stomach called *gastric emptying*.

4. **Formation of chyme**: The mixing of food with the gastric secretions in the stomach results in the formation of chyme, which is a semifluid, milky, dilute mixture that passes into the duodenum.

5. **Haemopoietic function**: The intrinsic factor present in the gastric juice is very essential for the production of RBCs.

SMALL INTESTINE

Anatomical structure of the small intestine

Small intestine is the part of the GI tract where most of the digestion (chemical and mechanical) occurs along with the absorption of the nutrients.

It starts from the pyloric sphincter and leads into the large intestine at the ileocaecal sphincter. It is about 6.25 m long. It is called *small intestine* because of its smaller diameter compared to that of the large intestine.

It is located at the centre and inferior portion of the abdomen in the form of a coil surrounded by the large intestine.

The small intestine comprises the following three main parts (Fig. 12.20):

❑ Duodenum
❑ Jejunum
❑ Ileum

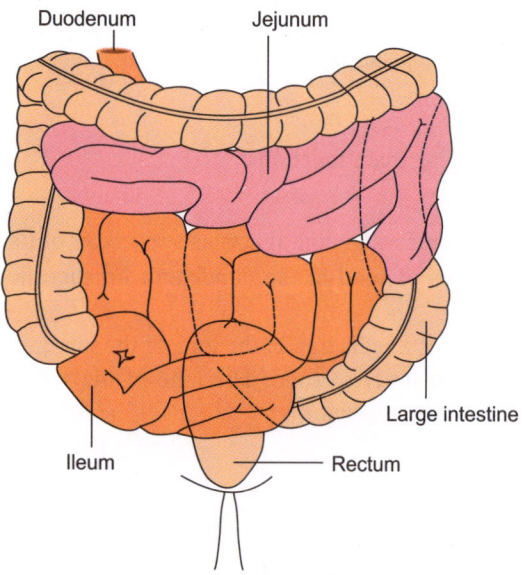

Figure 12.20 Small intestine and its parts.

Duodenum

❑ It is the first part of the intestine that begins at the pyloric sphincter of the stomach and is continuous with the jejunum.

❑ The secretions from the pancreas and gallbladder come directly into the duodenum through a common pathway called *hepatopancreatic ampulla* and this opening into the duodenum is guarded by hepatopancreatic sphincter (of Oddi) formed of smooth muscles.

Jejunum

❑ It forms the middle part of the small intestine and is longer than the duodenum (about 2 m in length).

Ileum

❑ It is the last part of the small intestine and is in continuation with the jejunum.

❑ It is the longest part of the small intestine (about 3 m in length).

❑ It ends at the ileocaecal valve that guards the entry of chyme into the caecum and thus prevents regurgitation.

❑ The wall of the small intestine is composed of the same tissue layers as the rest of the GI tract (see the section Layers of the Digestive System), but with certain modifications.

❑ The cells that form the epithelium of the mucosal layer of the small intestine along with their digestive functions are summarized in Table 12.6.

Table 12.6 Cells of the intestinal epithelium

Types of cells	Digestive functions
Absorptive cells	Digest and absorb the nutrients
Goblet cells	Secrete mucous
Paneth cells	Secrete lysozyme
S cells	Secrete secretin
CCK cells	Secrete cholecystokinin
K cells	Secrete glucose-dependent insulinotropic peptide (GIP)
Crypts of Lieberkuhn	Secrete intestinal juice or succus entericus
Brunner's gland	Secrete alkaline mucus

❑ There are certain special structural features of the small intestine that enable the process of digestion and absorption. These structural features include circular folds, villi and microvilli of the intestine.

Circular folds

❑ These are the permanent folds of the mucosal and submucosal layers of the small intestine and these folds do not disappear even when the small intestine is distended (unlike rugae of the stomach).

❑ They are present all over the duodenum, jejunum and middle part of the ileum.

❑ The function of circular folds is to increase the surface area of the small intestine to increase absorption.

Chapter 12

Villi (singular: villus)

❑ These are the finger-like projections present on the mucosal epithelium.

❑ These serve to increase the surface area of the epithelium to a great extent and thus help in digestion and absorption.

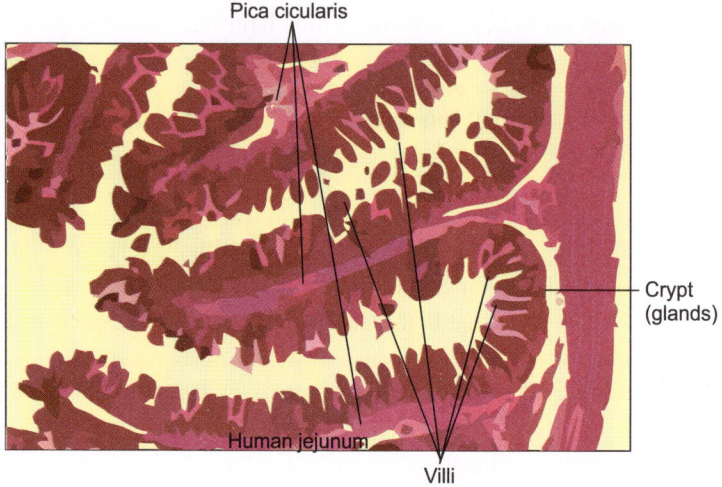

Figure 12.21 Microscopic structure of villi.

❑ Each villus comprises arterioles, venules, blood capillaries and lymph capillaries (lacteal). The nutrients absorbed by the epithelial cells covering the villus pass through the wall of blood or lymph capillary to enter the blood stream or lymph (Fig. 12.22).

❑ The villi are lined by columnar cells, called *enterocytes*, which give rise to many projections called *microvilli*.

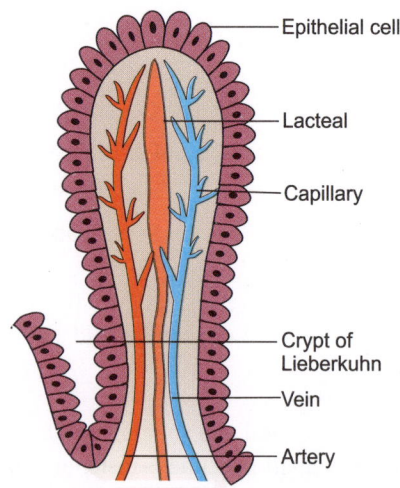

Figure 12.22 Blood vessels in villus.

Microvilli

- ❏ These are also called *brush border* of the small intestine.
- ❏ These are present in very large numbers and about 200 million microvilli are estimated to be present per square millimetre of the small intestine.
- ❏ These are very small in size, about 1 μm, and their function is to increase the surface area of the small intestine to facilitate absorption (Fig. 12.23).

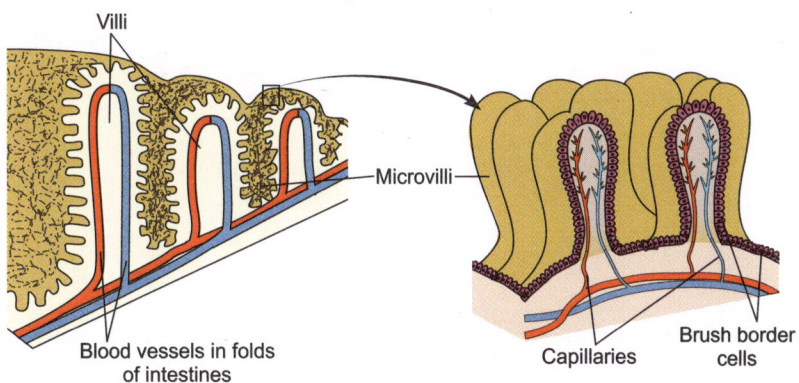

Figure 12.23 Microvilli.

Physiology

Mechanical digestion

There are two types of movements of the small intestine that carry out digestion in the small intestine mechanically:
- ❏ Mixing contractions (segmentations)
- ❏ Propulsive movements

Mixing contractions (segmentations)

These divide the small intestine into various segments.

The presence of chyme in the small intestine causes the distension that initiates the mixing contractions. The alternate contraction and relaxation results in the mixing of the chyme. This also brings the chyme in contact with mucosa for absorption (Fig. 12.24).

The frequency of these segmentation contractions is about 12/min in all parts of the small intestine.

Propulsive movements

These movements occur in all parts of the small intestine. The chyme is propelled towards the anus due to peristalsis wave at the rate of about 10 mm/min. Because of such a slow rate, the chyme from the duodenum takes about 3–5 h to reach the caecum.

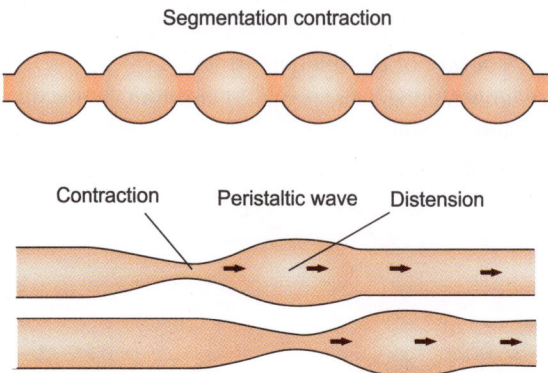

Figure 12.24 Mixing contractions (segmentations).

Chemical digestion

With the help of various enzymes present in the intestinal juice, pancreatic and gallbladder secretions, brush border enzymes, the chemical digestion of carbohydrates, proteins and fats occurs in small intestine.

The enzymes present in the intestinal juice (succus entericus) include the following:

❏ **Carbohydrate-digesting enzymes**: α-dextrinase, maltase, sucrase and lactase
❏ **Protein-digesting enzymes**: Peptidases (dipeptidase and aminopeptidase)
❏ **Nucleotide-digesting enzymes**: Nucleosidases and phosphatases

Note: The crypts of Lieberkuhn or intestinal glands are simple tubular glands present below villi and they secrete about 1500 mL of intestinal juice (succus entericus) daily.

This has been discussed in the section Digestion and Absorption of Nutrients in the GI Tract.

Intestinal juice plays a vital role in the digestion of food and the mucus protects the intestinal wall from acidic chyme, thereby preventing from intestinal ulcers.

The secretion of intestinal juice is regulated by the following neural and hormonal mechanisms:
1. **Neural regulation**
   ❏ Stimulation of parasympathetic nerves, which increases secretion.
   ❏ Stimulation of sympathetic nerves, which decreases secretion.
2. **Hormonal regulation**
   ❏ The intestinal mucosa secretes secretin and cholecystokinin when chyme enters the small intestine and these hormones promote intestinal secretion.

Functions of the small intestine

The small intestine performs the following main functions:
1. **Mechanical function**: The mixing movements of the small intestine help in the thorough mixing of the chyme with the digestive juices (intestinal, pancreatic and bile juice).

2. **Secretory function**: The small intestine secretes the intestinal juice (succus entericus) as well as certain hormones such as secretin.

3. **Digestive function**: The digestion of various food substances commences in the small intestine and this is carried out by various enzymes present in the intestinal juice.

4. **Absorptive function**: The presence of villi and microvilli in the mucosa greatly increases the surface area, and thus facilitates the absorptive function of the small intestine.

LARGE INTESTINE

Anatomical structure of the large intestine

Large intestine forms the last part of the GI tract and is located in the abdominal cavity surrounding the small intestine. It is about 5 ft in length and 2.5 in. in diameter.

The major functions of the large intestine include the completion of absorption, the production and absorption of certain vitamins and the formation and expulsion of faeces.

It starts from the ileocaecal sphincter and ends at the anus.

It is subdivided into the following four principal regions (Fig. 12.25):

1. Caecum
2. Colon
3. Rectum
4. Anal canal

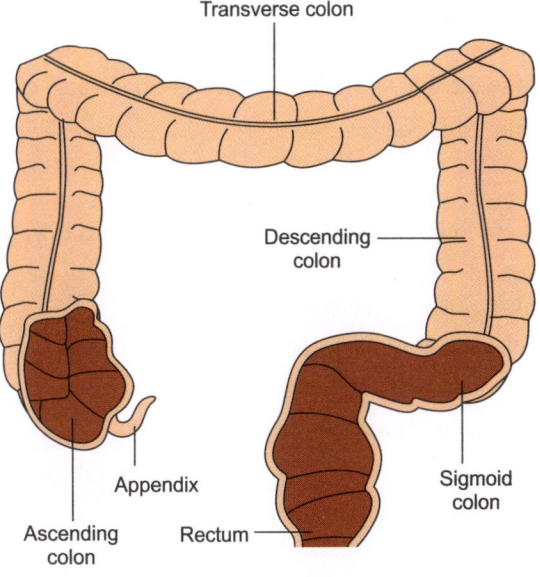

Figure 12.25 Large intestine.

Caecum

It begins at the point where ileum ends and this point of junction of ileum (small intestine) and caecum (large intestine) is guarded by ileocaecal sphincter. This sphincter allows the material to pass from the small intestine to the large intestine.

A long, coiled tube called as vermiform appendix or appendix is attached to the closed end of the caecum and it contains numerous lymphoid tissues.

Colon

The caecum merges with the long tube called the *colon*.

The colon can be subdivided into the following four parts:

1. Ascending colon
2. Transverse colon
3. Descending colon
4. Sigmoid colon

Ascending colon ascends up towards the liver and takes a sharp acute turn to its left at the right colonic (hepatic) flexure to become the transverse colon.

Transverse colon goes across the abdominal cavity towards the spleen, where it takes sharp acute turn downwards at the left colonic (splenic) flexure to form the descending colon.

Descending colon descends downward on the left side of the abdominal cavity to turn towards the pelvis.

After it enters the pelvis, it forms the sigmoid colon and this continues downwards to become the rectum.

Rectum

Rectum starts where the sigmoid colon terminates and it ends in the anal canal.

It lies anterior to the sacrum and coccyx.

Anal canal

The anal canal is about 2–4 cm long, starts from the rectum and runs towards the exterior to terminate at the anus.

It is guarded by the following two sphincters:

❏ Internal anal sphincter (made of smooth muscles—involuntary)
❏ External anal sphincter (made of skeletal muscles—voluntary)

During defecation, these sphincters open up to pass out faeces.

Wall of the large intestine is formed by all the four layers of the GI tract, with certain modifications.

❏ The absorptive and goblet cells are present in the epithelium of the mucosa mainly to absorb water and secrete mucus.
❏ The external longitudinal muscles of muscularis are thick and form longitudinal strips called *tenia coli*. Both longitudinal and circular muscle contractions aid the movement of faecal matter in the large intestine.

Physiology

The chief functions of the large intestine are to absorb water and electrolytes and store the faecal matter until defecation.

Mechanical digestion

The two movements of colon basically concerned with its functions are as follows:
- Haustrations
- Mass movements

Haustrations—the mixing movements

The constriction of tenia coli of the longitudinal muscles along with the inner circular muscles cause the unstimulated portion of the colon to bulge. This appears like a pouch called *haustra*.

These haustrations almost occlude the lumen of the colon to push the faecal matter from the caecum to the transverse colon.

These are very sluggish movements; therefore, it takes about 7–15 h for the chyme to move from the caecum to the transverse colon.

Mass movements

These are the modified types of peristalsis that take over the propulsion of food from the transverse colon to the sigmoid colon.

These movements push the mass of the faeces into the rectum, resulting in defecation.

These movements persist for 10–30 min and occur mostly 1–3 times each day.

Chemical digestion

The glands in the large intestine secrete juice that mainly contains mucus. This juice does not contain any enzyme. The mucus lubricates the mucosa of the large intestine, thus facilitating the movement of bowel.

In addition, the large intestine is heavily colonized by certain types of bacteria that are harmless and perform the following functions:

1. The bacteria ferment any remaining carbohydrates and release hydrogen, carbon dioxide and methane gases. These gases cause flatus (gas) in the colon, termed *flatulence* when it is excessive.
2. The bacteria produce three important vitamins that are absorbed in the colon: vitamin K required for clotting, biotin required for glucose metabolism and vitamin B_5 required to make certain hormones and neurotransmitters. These bacteria also decompose bilirubin to simpler pigments, including stercobilin that gives faeces their brown colour.

Defecation

The passage of faeces from the anus or the voiding of faeces is called *defecation*.

The mass movements force the contents of the sigmoid colon into the rectum and causes distension of the rectal wall. This distension stimulates stretch receptors and initiates the defecation reflex, which causes the desire for defecation.

In infants, defecation occurs involuntarily but with age (second or third year of life) the ability to override the defecation reflex is developed.

Defecation reflex

The distension of the rectum due to the faeces, forced into it by the mass movements, causes the initiation of defecation reflex (intrinsic defecation reflex) (Fig. 12.26).

The process of defecation involves the contraction of rectum and relaxation of internal and external sphincters.

The distension of the rectum spreads different signals through myenteric plexus of the ENS and initiates peristalsis in the descending colon, sigmoid colon and rectum.

As a result, the two anal sphincters are relaxed and open up to facilitate defecation.

The parasympathetic reflex, through the parasympathetic nerves in the pelvic region, strengthens this intrinsic defecation reflex mediated by the ENS to cause defecation.

When defecation is voluntarily postponed, the need to defecate tends to fade until the next mass movement occurs and the reflex is initiated again.

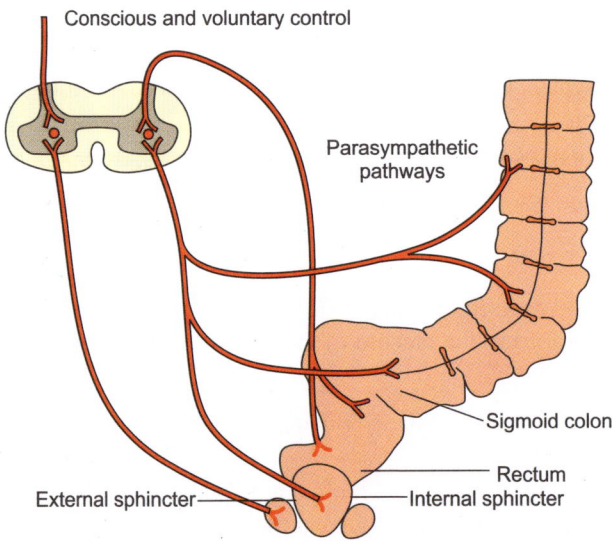

Figure 12.26 Defecation reflex.

Functions of the large intestine

The large intestine performs the following main functions:

1. **Absorptive function**: Large intestine plays an important role in the absorption of water, electrolytes and organic substances such as glucose, alcohol and certain drugs.

2. **Secretory function**: The large intestine secretes the intestinal juice that contains mucus and inorganic substances.

3. **Formation of faeces**: After absorption of nutrients, water and other electrolytes, the unwanted substances form faeces, which is excreted out.

4. **Synthetic function**: The bacterial flora of the large intestine synthesizes vitamins K and B_5 and biotin.

ACCESSORY ORGANS

LIVER

Liver is the heaviest gland in the body (weighing about 1.2–2.2 kg) located in the upper and right region of the abdominal cavity immediately beneath the diaphragm.

The portal vein, hepatic artery, parasympathetic and sympathetic nerves, hepatic ducts, lymph vessels enter and leave the liver at a point called *portal fissure*.

Liver is organized into the following four lobes (Fig. 12.27):

❑ Right lobe
❑ Left lobe

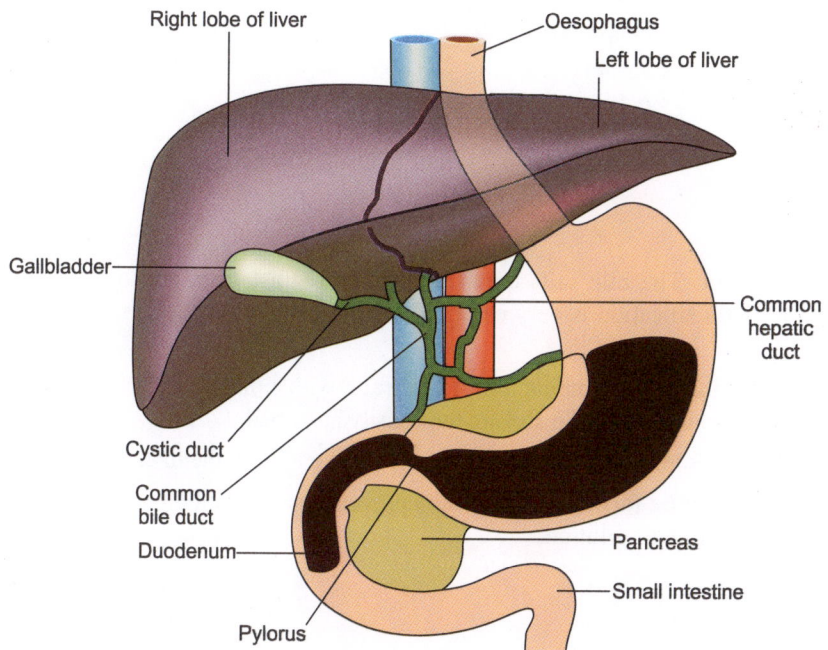

Figure 12.27 Overview of the liver and its anatomical location.

❑ Caudate lobe

❑ Quadrate lobe

Caudate and quadrate lobes are areas on the posterior surface.

Each lobe comprises hepatocytes, bile canaliculi and hepatic sinusoids.

Hepatocytes

The lobes of the liver are made of tiny functional units called *lobules* that consist of specialized epithelial cells called *hepatocytes*. These hepatocytes are arranged in irregular, branching, interconnected plates around a central vein.

These hepatocytes secrete bile, which is a yellow-brown-greenish viscid alkaline liquid having digestive function. For more details, see the section Digestion of Fats.

About 800–1000 mL of bile is secreted daily by hepatocytes.

The composition of bile is given in Table 12.7.

Table 12.7 Composition of bile

Bile salts: Sodium and potassium salts
Bile pigments: Bilirubin
Bile acids: Cholic acid and chenodeoxycholic acid
Phospholipids: Lecithin
Cholesterol
Ions
Water

Functions of bile

1. **Digestive function**: The bile salts emulsify the lipid substances and break them into minute particles. This emulsification is very essential for the digestion of lipids by various enzymes of the GI tract.
2. **Absorptive function**: The combination of bile salts with lipids leads to micelle formation. The lipids of micelle are water soluble and are thus easily absorbed.
3. **Antiseptic action**: Bile inhibits the growth of certain bacteria in the intestinal lumen.
4. **Prevention of gallstone formation**: Bile salts prevent the formation of gallstones by keeping the cholesterol and lecithin in solution.

Bile canaliculi

In between the hepatocytes, small ducts are present to receive the bile secreted by hepatocytes. These small ducts are called *bile canaliculi*. These join the common bile duct through the pathway explained in (Fig. 12.28).

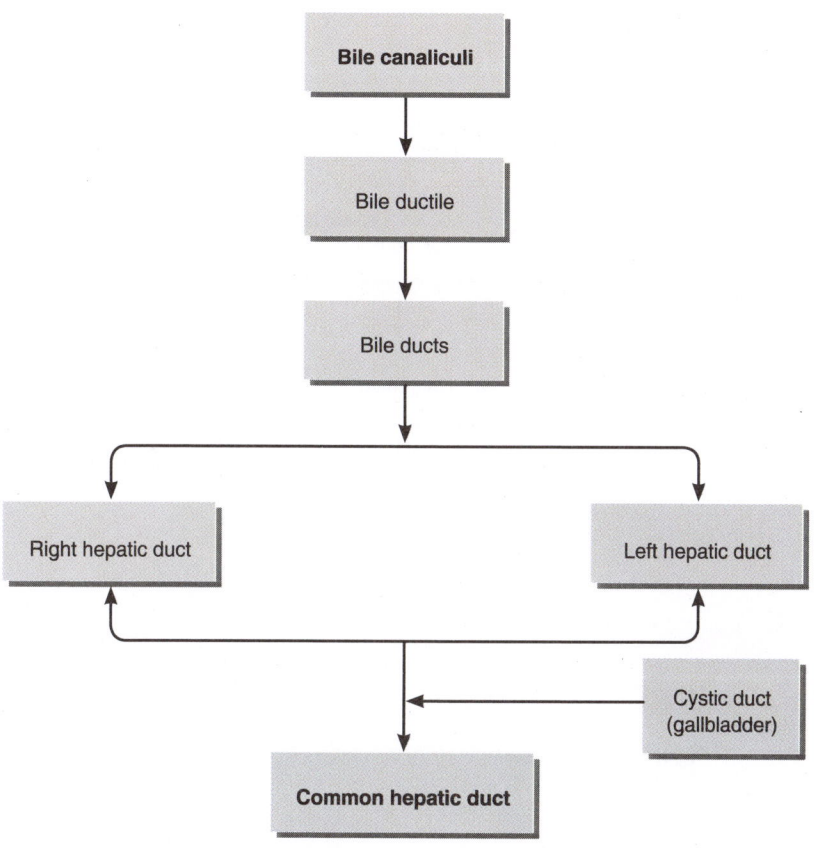

Figure 12.28 Pathway of bile from bile canaliculi to common bile duct.

Hepatic sinusoids

The blood capillaries that are highly permeable (due to incomplete walls) present between the hepatocytes are called hepatic sinusoids.

The blood from hepatic portal vein and branches of hepatic artery gets mixed up in sinusoids and then reaches the inferior vena cava (see Fig. 12.29).

The special types of cells are also present in between the hepatic sinusoids called *Kupffer cells* or *stellate reticuloendothelial cells*.

These cells cause the destruction of worn-out RBCs and WBCs and also any foreign matter present in the blood. Hence, these are known as *hepatic macrophages*.

Blood and nerve supply

❑ **Arterial**: Branches of hepatic artery
❑ **Venous**: Hepatic portal vein
❑ **Nervous supply**: Parasympathetic and sympathetic nerves

Chapter 12

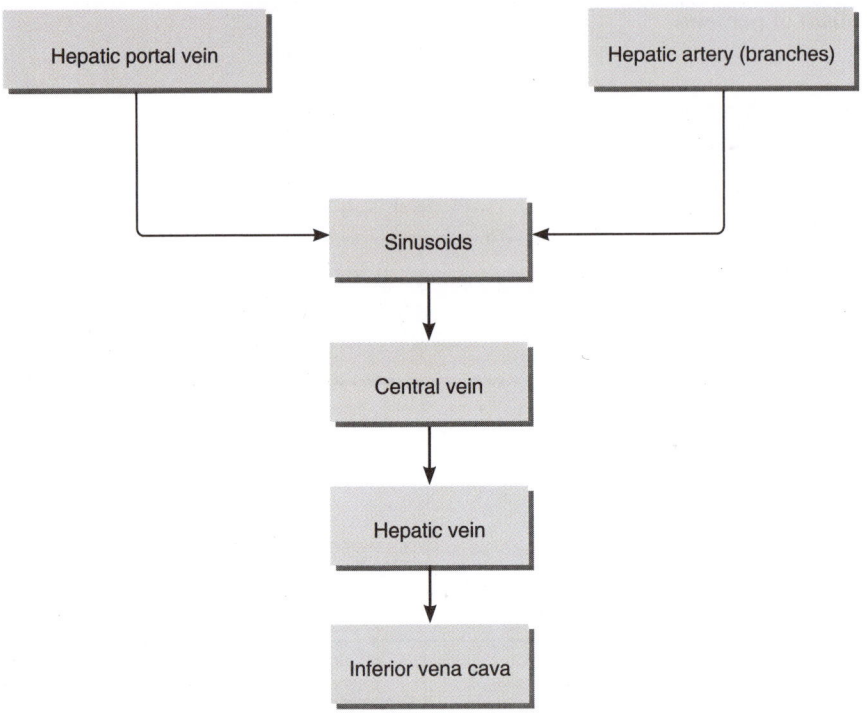

Figure 12.29 Blood flow from sinusoids to inferior vena cava.

Functions of the liver

The liver performs the following functions:

1. Metabolism of carbohydrates
2. Metabolism of proteins
3. Metabolism of fats
4. Secretion of bile
5. Phagocytosis

6. Detoxification of drug
7. Metabolism of alcohol
8. Processing of drug
9. Acts as a storehouse
10. Haemopoietic function

1. **Metabolism of carbohydrates**
   - ❑ The liver has an important role in maintaining plasma glucose levels.
   - ❑ Glucose, the final product of the metabolism of carbohydrate, is converted into glycogen under the influence of insulin and stored in the liver. Thus, it reduces the blood glucose level and when blood glucose level falls, the glycogen is converted back into glucose under the influence of glucagon.

Glucose (in blood)

Insulin ↓ ↑ *Glucagon*

Glycogen (stored in liver)

2. **Metabolism of proteins**
   - ❑ The hepatocytes cause the deamination of amino acids that can be utilized to produce ATP or converted into carbohydrates or fats.
   - ❑ The liberated ammonia, toxic in nature, is excreted in urine in the form of urea (harmless).
3. **Metabolism of fats**
   - ❑ The bile salts secreted by the hepatocytes play a vital role in fat metabolism.
   - ❑ These salts cause the emulsification of fats, which is an important step in the digestion of fat and also use the stored fat to generate energy in the form of ATP.
4. **Secretion of bile**: The hepatocytes secrete bile, which is required for the emulsification and absorption of fats in the intestine.
5. **Phagocytosis**: The Kupffer cells present in sinusoids of the liver phagocytose certain bacteria and worn-out RBCs and WBCs.
6. **Detoxification of drugs**: Various drugs such as penicillin and sulphonamides are detoxified by the liver and excreted in bile.
7. **Metabolism of alcohol**: Liver causes the metabolism of alcohol and excrete it in bile.
8. **Processing of hormones**: Various steroid and thyroid hormones are modified chemically by the liver.
9. **Acts as a storehouse**: Besides the storage of glycogen, liver acts as a storehouse for various vitamins such as A, D, E, K, niacin, riboflavin, B_{12} and folic acid.
10. **Haemopoietic function**: In the fetal stage, the blood cells are produced in liver. Liver also produces thrombopoietin that promotes the production of thrombocytes. Moreover, the liver manufactures the anticoagulant heparin and most of the other plasma proteins such as prothrombin and thrombin, which are involved in the blood-clotting mechanism.

GALLBLADDER

It is an important accessory organ (pear-shaped sac) of the digestive system, attached to the posterior surface of the liver by connective tissue (Fig. 12.30).

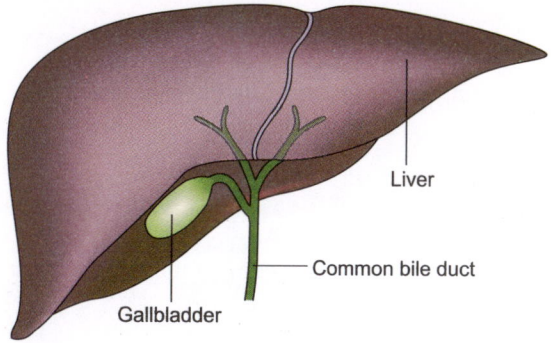

Figure 12.30 Anatomical location of the gallbladder.

Anatomically, it can be divided into three parts: fundus, body and neck.

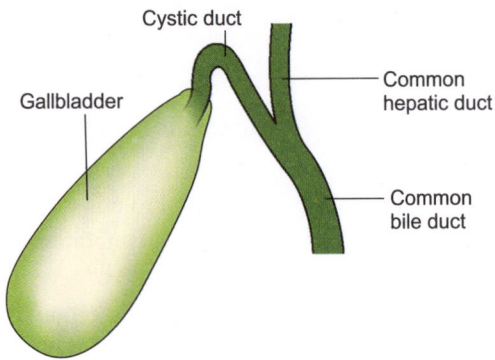

Figure 12.31 Gallbladder

The fundus is the expanded end of the gallbladder; the body constitutes the main part of gallbladder, while the part that is in continuation with cystic duct is called *neck* (Fig. 12.31).

All the four layers of the GI tract form the wall of the gallbladder. Similar to the stomach, it has extra oblique muscles and it is covered with adventitia on the inner side. The mucosa contains rugae, which smoothen up when it is distended due to the presence of bile.

Blood and nerve supply

- **Arterial**: Cystic artery
- **Venous**: Cystic vein (joins the portal vein)
- **Nervous supply**: Parasympathetic and sympathetic nerve fibres

Functions of the gallbladder

It performs the following functions:

- Storage of bile
- Concentration of bile
- Release of bile

Storage of bile

The bile secreted by hepatocytes in the liver is stored in the gallbladder. It acts as a storehouse of bile. It is released into the intestine only intermittently.

Concentration of bile

The stored bile is concentrated in the gallbladder.

The rapid absorption of water through the mucosa of gallbladder results in the concentration of the bile up to 12–15 folds.

Release of bile

The bile is released into the duodenum through the common bile duct upon the contraction of wall of the gallbladder.

The walls are contracted due to stimulation provided by the cholecystokinin secreted in the duodenum and presence of fats in the chyme in the intestine.

PANCREAS

Pancreas is an accessory organ located in the epigastric and hypochondriac (left) regions of the abdomen (Fig. 12.32).

It lies posterior to the stomach (greater curvature).

Anatomically, it can be divided into three parts: head, body and tail.

- ❑ The part that lies near the curve of duodenum is called *head*.
- ❑ The part superior to the head and lies behind the greater curvature of the stomach is called *body*.
- ❑ The tapering part almost reaching the spleen in front of the left kidney is called *tail*.
- ❑ Pancreas consists of two types of cells: exocrine cells and endocrine cells.

Exocrine cells

- ❑ These constitute about 99% of the total cells of pancreas.
- ❑ These are the glandular epithelial cells, called *acini,* that secrete the pancreatic juice.
- ❑ Pancreatic juice is a clear, watery fluid. The composition of pancreatic juice is given in Table 12.8.

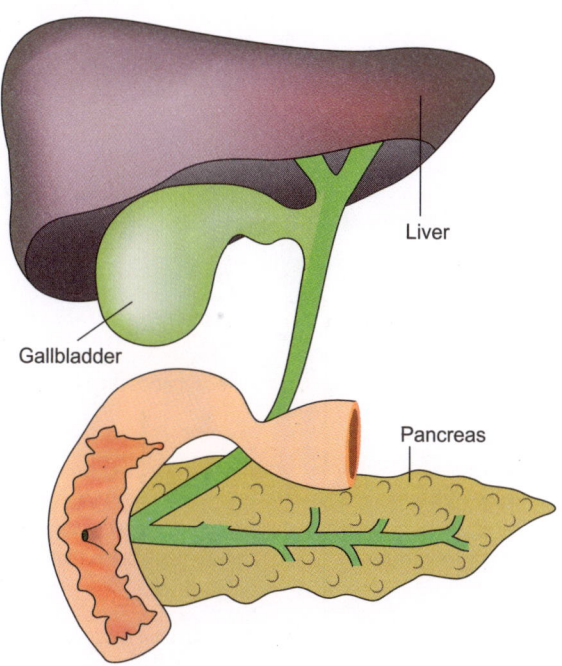

Figure 12.32 Anatomical location of the pancreas.

Chapter 12

Table 12.8 Composition of pancreatic juice

❏ Water
❏ Salts (sodium bicarbonate)
❏ Enzymes
    ➤ Pancreatic amylase
    ➤ Trypsin
    ➤ Chymotrypsin
    ➤ Elastase
    ➤ Pancreatic lipase
    ➤ Ribonuclease
    ➤ Deoxyribonuclease

❏ The pancreatic juice leaves the pancreas through a large main duct called *pancreatic duct* or *duct of Wirsung*. This pancreatic duct unites with the common bile duct of the liver to form ampulla of Vater or hepatopancreatic ampulla, which opens into the duodenum.

The functions of pancreatic juice are as follows:

1. **Digestive functions**: Pancreatic juice plays an important role in the digestion of proteins, lipids and carbohydrates.
   (a) *Digestion of proteins*: It happens by proteolytic enzymes—trypsin, chymotrypsin, carboxy-peptidases, elastase and collagenase (convert polypeptides to tripeptides, dipeptides and amino acids) (Fig. 12.33).

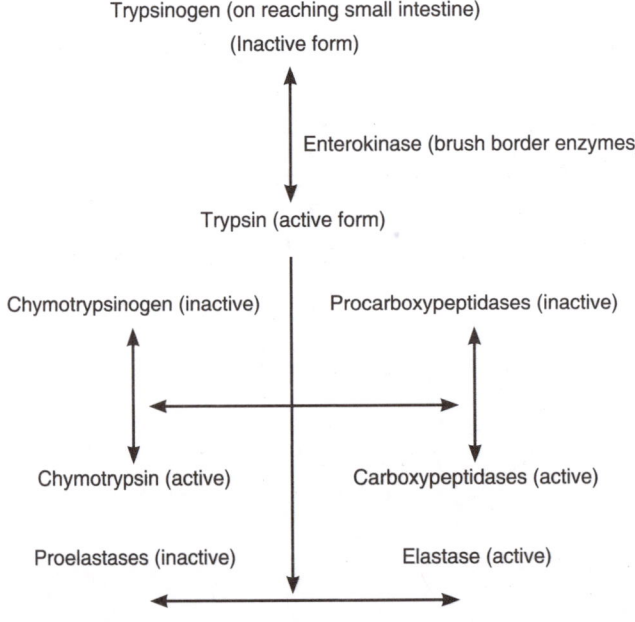

Figure 12.33 Activation of various pancreatic enzymes.

Note: Most of the pancreatic enzymes are secreted in inactive form. Hence, the pancreatic enzymes are unable to digest the pancreas itself. These are converted into the active forms, which have digestive functions.

    (b) *Digestion of lipids*: This is by lipolytic enzymes—pancreatic lipase, phospholipase A and B (convert fats to fatty acids and glycerol).

    (c) *Digestion of carbohydrates*: This is by amylolytic enzyme—pancreatic amylase (convert polysaccharides to disaccharides).

  2. The sodium bicarbonate salt present in pancreatic juice performs the following three functions:
  - Makes the acid chyme alkaline
  - Inhibits the activity of pepsin
  - Provides proper pH for optimum action of digestive enzymes

Phases of pancreatic secretion

There are three phases of pancreatic secretion, which are as follows:
- Cephalic phase
- Gastric phase
- Intestinal phase

Cephalic phase

This phase is solely under nervous control. In this phase, the secretion of pancreatic juice occurs before food reaches the intestine. When the food is placed in mouth, afferent impulses arise from taste buds and reach the appetite centre in amygdala and hypothalamus. From here, the efferent impulses pass through the vagus nerves that stimulate the acinar cells to secrete pancreatic juice by the release of acetylcholine.

The smell, sight, taste or thought of the food also stimulate the pancreatic secretion by sending the impulses to the cerebral cortex, which further activates vagus nerves and increases the secretions.

Gastric phase

This phase of gastric secretion occurs when the food enters the stomach.

The presence of the food in stomach stimulates the following:
- Vagal reflexes—release of acetylcholine—increased pancreatic secretion
- Gastrin secretion: This hormone is secreted from the stomach when food enters the stomach. The gastrin is transported by blood, and while reaching the pancreas, it causes release of pancreatic juice.

Intestinal phase

This occurs when the chyme reaches the duodenum.

In this phase, large amount of pancreatic juice is secreted due to release of the hormones secretin and cholecystokinin in the small intestine.

Endocrine cells

The endocrine cells (alpha and beta cells) secrete the hormone glucagon and insulin that regulate and control the blood glucose levels.

The endocrine function of the pancreas is discussed in detail in the chapter the Endocrine System.

Chapter 12

SALIVARY GLANDS

The salivary glands secrete the saliva, which serves the moistening and lubricating function.

These are present in the mucous membrane of the oral cavity and are made of numerous lobules. These lobules contain small acini, which are surrounded by secretory cells.

The secretion from the secretory cells is poured into small ductules that join to form the large ducts (collecting ducts). These ducts open in the oral cavity (Fig. 12.34).

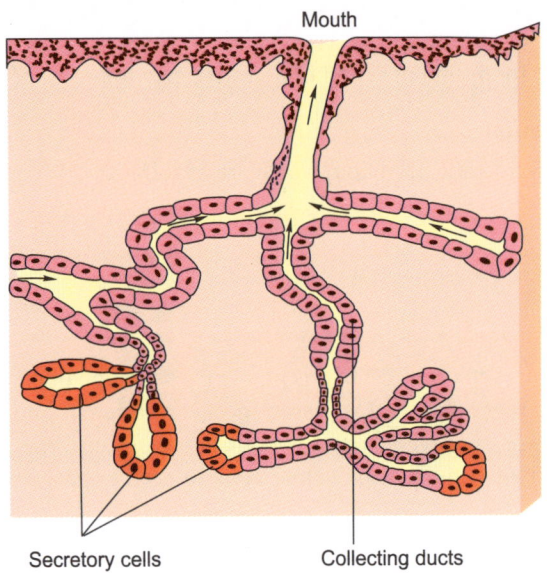

Figure 12.34 Opening of the salivary ducts in the mouth.

There are mainly three types of salivary glands:

❑ Parotid gland
❑ Submandibular glands or submaxillary glands
❑ Sublingual glands (Fig. 12.35)

Parotid glands

These are the largest of salivary glands. These are two glands present on each side of the face just below the external acoustic meatus.

These glands pour their secretion into the ducts called *parotid ducts* that open in the oral cavity at the level of the second upper molar teeth.

Submandibular glands

Each of the pair of submandibular glands is present on each side of the face near the jaw.

These glands pour their secretion into ducts called submandibular ducts that open in the mouth.

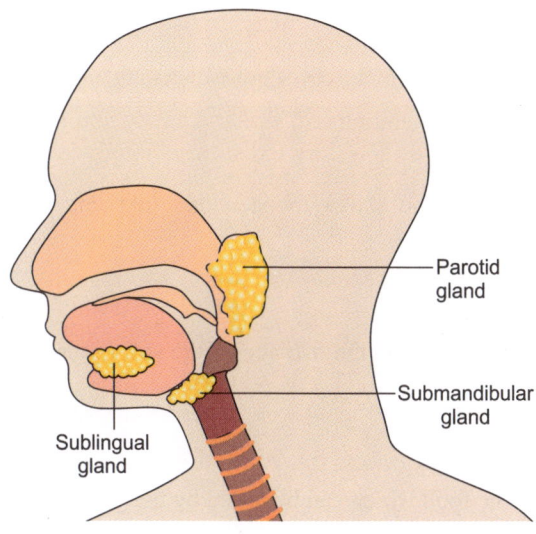

Figure 12.35 Anatomical location of salivary glands.

Sublingual glands

These are the smallest of the three major salivary glands. These glands are present under the mucous membrane of the floor of the mouth in front of the submandibular glands.

The composition of saliva is given in Table 12.9.

Table 12.9 Composition of saliva

Water
Solutes (mainly ions—Na^+, K^+, Cl^-, HCO^-, PO_4^-)
Urea
Uric acid
Mucous
Immunoglobulin
Lysozyme
Enzymes—salivary amylase/ptyalin and lingual lipase

Salivation

The secretion of saliva is called salivation and about 1–1.5 L of saliva is secreted daily.

The salivation is controlled by the parasympathetic nervous system. For more details, see chapter Nervous System.

Functions of saliva

❑ Lubrication of mouth and food
❑ Cleansing of mouth

❏ Taste
❏ Digestion of carbohydrates and fats
❏ Immune functions

Lubrication of mouth and food

The water and mucus present in the saliva moisten and lubricate the bolus and facilitates the swallowing.

Cleansing of mouth

The saliva cleans the mouth and prevents the damage of the soft tissues of oral cavity from rough or abrasive food.

Taste

The water in saliva dissolves the food which can be tasted by the gustatory receptors in the oral cavity.

Digestion of carbohydrates

The chloride ions present in the saliva activates the salivary amylase that acts on the starch (polysaccharides). The digestion of carbohydrates in the mouth accounts only 5% of the total carbohydrates ingested. The lingual lipase converts triglycerides into fatty acids and diacylglycerol.

Immune function

The presence of immunoglobulin A and the lysozyme present in saliva provides the nonspecific defence.

Regulation of salivary secretion

❏ Salivary glands are under the control of autonomic nervous system.
❏ Stimulation of parasympathetic nerves—Increased salivary secretion
❏ Stimulation of sympathetic nerves—Decreased salivary secretion

DIGESTION AND ABSORPTION OF NUTRIENTS IN THE GI TRACT

The food we eat cannot be digested as such in its crude form (complex form). This is converted into simpler forms by our digestive system through the process called *digestion*. The so-formed simpler forms of food molecules are rapidly taken up by body through a process called *absorption*.

BASIC MECHANISM OF DIGESTION

❏ The basic mechanism involved in the digestion of carbohydrates, proteins and fats is hydrolysis.
❏ The carbohydrates consist of polysaccharides, which are converted to monosaccharides by various digestive enzymes. These enzymes cause the hydrolysis of polysaccharides and the resultant monosaccharide (hydrolyzed product) is then absorbed in the GI tract.

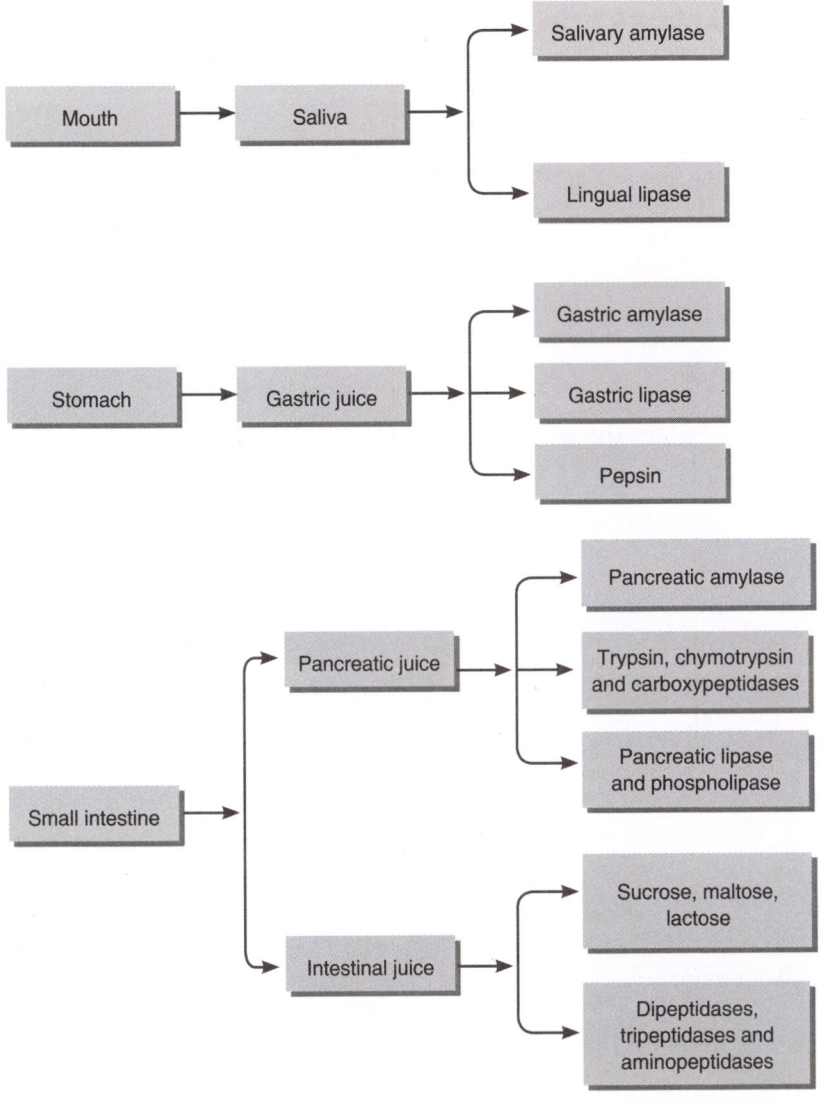

❏ Proteins are the long-chain amino acids linked together by peptide linkages. These linkages are broken through hydrolysis by various digestive enzymes into the final product amino acids that are absorbed in the GI tract.

❏ Fats are the condensation products of glycerol (one molecule) and fatty acids (three molecules). They are hydrolyzed by various digestive enzymes and bile salts to release the free fatty acids that are absorbed in the GI tract.

❏ The various digestive enzymes released from different parts of digestive system are summarized below.

DIGESTION AND ABSORPTION OF CARBOHYDRATES

Digestion

The major components of the carbohydrates in the human diet are sucrose, pectin, dextrin, lactose, starch, amylose, glycogen, pyruvic acid and lactic acid.

The digestion of carbohydrates is explained in (Fig. 12.36).

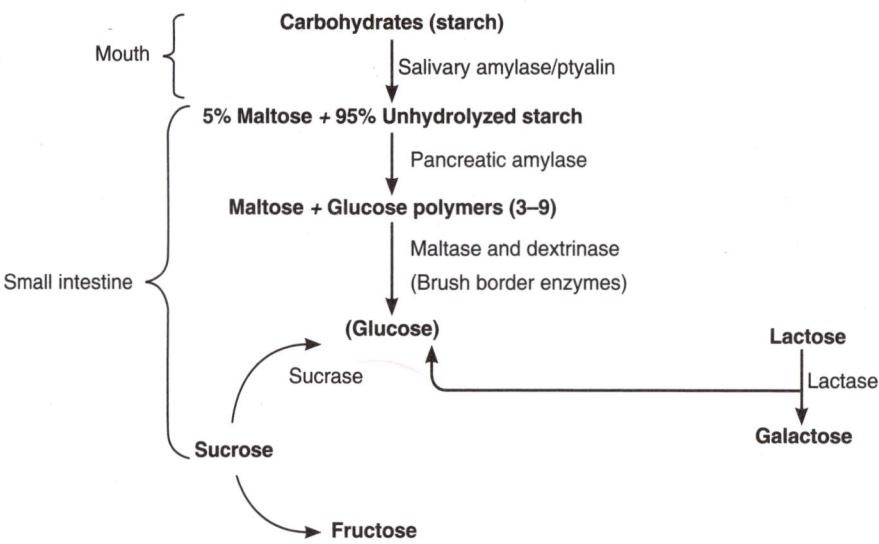

Figure 12.36 Digestion of carbohydrates.

Absorption

The carbohydrates are absorbed from the small intestine mainly as monosaccharides, namely glucose, galactose and fructose.

Glucose and galactose are absorbed into the portal blood through the sodium cotransport mechanism.

The fructose is absorbed by the facilitated diffusion all the way through the epithelium of the intestine.

DIGESTION AND ABSORPTION OF PROTEINS

Digestion

The digestion of protein is explained in (Fig. 12.37).

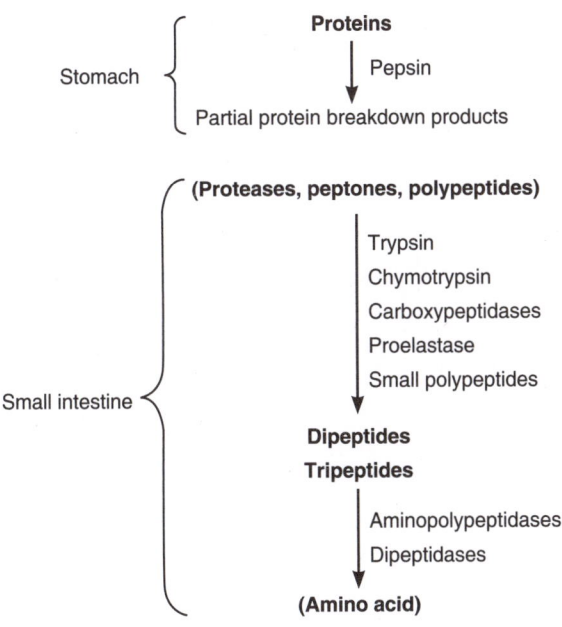

Figure 12.37 Digestion of proteins.

Absorption

Amino acids along with some small number of dipeptides and tripeptides are absorbed by numerous microvilli (brush border of the intestine) and transported to the cytoplasm of enterocytes, where these are further digested by some peptidases to form the amino acids of the indigested dipeptides and tripeptides and finally passed into blood circulation.

The levo amino acids are actively absorbed by the means of sodium cotransport, whereas the dextro amino acids by facilitated diffusion.

DIGESTION AND ABSORPTION OF FATS

Digestion

The human diet's fat content mainly consists of neutral fats called *triglycerides*. The other fats include phospholipids, cholesterol and cholesterol ester.

Cholesterol is derived from fats and metabolized like fats. Unlike phospholipids and cholesterol esters, cholesterols do not contain fatty acids.

The digestion of fats is explained in (Fig. 12.38).

Absorption

Fatty acids and monoglycerides diffuse through the membrane of microvilli to enter the interior of the epithelial cells in the membrane of which the lipids are soluble.

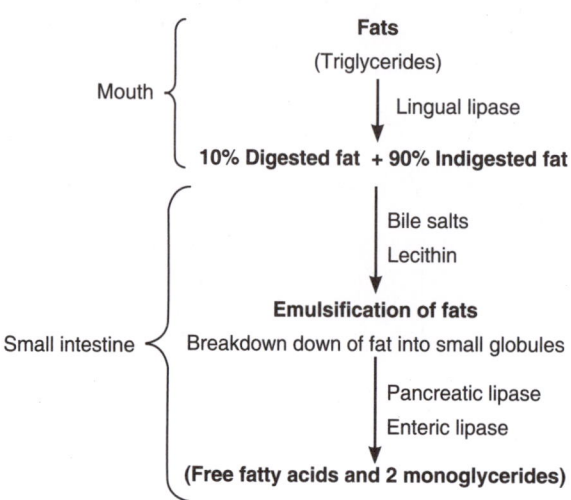

Figure 12.38 Digestion of fats.

From the epithelial cell membrane, these are taken up by the endoplasmic reticulum to form new triglycerides and cholesterol esters (chylomicrons). These enter the lymph as they cannot pass through the membrane of the blood capillaries due to large size and finally reach into the blood circulation.

The short-chain fatty acids directly enter the blood capillaries of villi on the intestinal epithelium.

DISEASES OF THE DIGESTIVE SYSTEM

DISEASES OF THE MOUTH

Cleft palate

It is the birth defect of lip and mouth.

Symptoms

- ❑ Split in the upper lip and upper palate—the roof of the mouth
- ❑ Difficulty in drinking and swallowing
- ❑ Speech defects

Dislocated jaw

It is a condition where the bones of the jaw are knocked out of place. This is often caused by a trauma or blow to the face but may also be occasionally caused by yawning or yelling. The condition is usually very painful.

Symptoms

❏ Mouth not closing properly, difficulty in moving jaw
❏ Swollen jaw, pain and redness in jaw

Dental caries

It is a destructive process causing decalcification of the tooth enamel, leading to cavitations of the tooth.

Symptoms

❏ Tooth pain, bad breath and foul taste
❏ Fever, chills

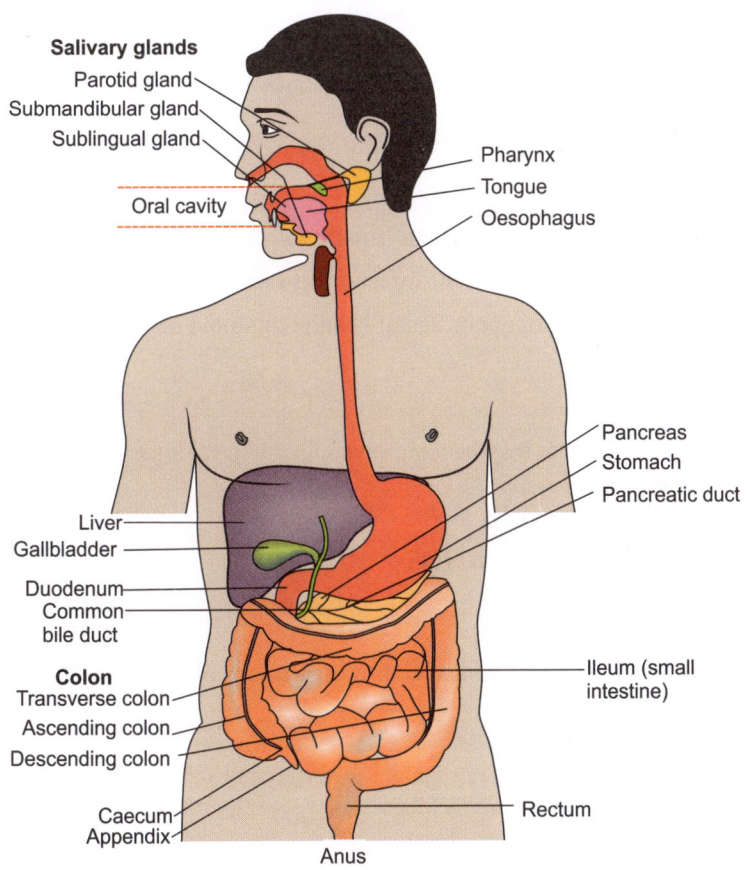

Figure 12.39 Various organs of the digestive system.

Gingivitis

It is the inflammation of the gums, which causes them to become swollen and tender.

The gums tend to bleed easily when the teeth are brushed. The condition is usually caused by food particles or plaque becoming trapped between the teeth and gums.

The resulting bacteria cause the gums to become inflamed and can lead to serious dental damage if left untreated.

Symptoms
❑ Red, swollen, tender and bleeding gums
❑ Bad breath

Oral cancer

It may include cancer (malignant) of the lips, tongue, pharynx, gums or mouth.

Symptoms

Nonhealing oral sores and lump in the lips, mouth or tongue. In some cases, it may cause bleeding in gums.

Tooth abscess

It is referred to as a pus-filled structure caused by a tooth infection.

An untreated tooth abscess can result in the infection spreading to other areas of the body.

Tooth abscesses usually result from poor dental health (e.g. tooth decay). The condition sometimes results in the tooth being removed.

Symptoms
❑ Mild toothache in early cases but may become severe in the later stages
❑ Loss of appetite and pain in chewing

DISEASES OF THE SALIVARY GLANDS

Salivary gland cancer

Salivary gland cancers are generally rare and occur mostly in one of the three larger glands such as the parotid gland.

Symptoms

Pain, facial paralysis and elevation in the ear lobe

Xerostomia (dry mouth)

When salivary glands fail to produce sufficient saliva, xerostomia occurs.

While everyone occasionally experiences a dry mouth, xerostomia can become a chronic condition.

Mumps

It is the acute viral infection that affects mostly the parotid glands. It is common in children who are not immunized but may affect adults also.

Symptoms

Swelling of parotid glands, sore throat and weakness

DISEASES OF THE OESOPHAGUS

Oesophagus cancer

It is the cancer of the oesophagus in the throat.

Symptoms

Pain in swallowing and severe weight loss

Types of cells affected by oesophageal cancer

❏ Squamous cell carcinoma (oesophagus)—affects the lining cells
❏ Adenocarcinoma (oesophagus)—affects the gland-like cells

Gastroesophageal reflux disease

Reflux refers to the stomach acid rising up the 'wrong way' back up the oesophagus and sometimes into the mouth. When this occurs chronically, it is probably caused by gastroesophageal reflux disease (GERD).

Symptoms

❏ Heartburn
❏ Persistent heartburn—twice a week or more; the most common GERD symptom, though surprisingly you can have GERD without heartburn
❏ Acid regurgitation and bitter taste in mouth

DISEASES OF THE STOMACH

Causes of stomach diseases and problems greatly vary, although many stomach diseases are associated with infections, especially *Helicobacter pylori* infection. Causes of stomach diseases can be generally divided into the following two factors:

❏ *Internal factors* such as too high (hyperchlorhydria) or too low levels (hypochlorhydria) of gastric acid and too slow emptying of the stomach.
❏ *External factors*, which are in most cases responsible for stomach disease—stress, unhealthy diet, excessive consumption of coffee, alcohol and tea, smoking, certain medications, especially nonsteroidal anti-inflammatory drugs and infection with *H. pylori*.

Chapter 12

Gastritis

Gastritis is a condition in which the stomach lining known as the mucosa is inflamed. When the stomach lining is inflamed, it produces less acid, enzymes and mucus.

Gastritis may be acute or chronic. Sudden, severe inflammation of the stomach lining is called *acute gastritis*. Inflammation that lasts for a long time is called *chronic gastritis*. If chronic gastritis is not treated, it may last for years or even a lifetime.

H. pylori infection causes most cases of chronic gastritis.

Symptoms

Many people with gastritis do not have any symptoms, but some people experience symptoms such as upper abdominal discomfort or pain, nausea and vomiting. These symptoms are also called *dyspepsia*. Erosive gastritis may cause ulcers or erosions in the stomach lining, which can lead to blood in the stool.

Peptic ulcer

A peptic ulcer is a sore that develops on the lining of the stomach or duodenum, which is exposed to acidic gastric juice. Less commonly, a peptic ulcer may develop just above the stomach in the oesophagus.

A peptic ulcer in the stomach is called a *gastric ulcer*. One that occurs in the duodenum is called a *duodenal ulcer*. People can have both gastric and duodenal ulcers at the same time. They also can develop peptic ulcers more than once in their lifetime.

A bacterium called *H. pylori* is a major cause of peptic ulcers. Nonsteroidal anti-inflammatory drugs (NSAIDs), such as aspirin and ibuprofen, are another common cause. Rarely, cancerous or noncancerous tumours in the stomach, duodenum, or pancreas cause ulcers.

Peptic ulcers are not caused by stress or eating spicy food, but both can make ulcer symptoms worse. Smoking and drinking alcohol also can worsen ulcers and prevent healing.

Symptoms

Abdominal discomfort is the most common symptom of both duodenal and gastric ulcers. Other symptoms include weight loss, poor appetite, bloating, burping, nausea and vomiting. The severe symptoms may include sharp, sudden, persistent and severe stomach pain and bloody vomit.

DISEASES OF THE INTESTINE

Appendicitis

Appendicitis is a painful swelling and infection of the appendix.

An inflamed appendix may also burst if it is not removed. The bursting of appendix spreads infection throughout the abdomen and may result in a potentially dangerous condition called *peritonitis*.

Symptoms

The main symptom of appendicitis is abdominal pain, loss of appetite, abdominal swelling, constipation or diarrhoea, nausea and vomiting.

Crohn's disease

Crohn's disease is a disorder that causes inflammation of the digestive tract, also referred to as the GI tract. It can affect any area of the GI tract, from the mouth to the anus, but it most commonly affects the lower part of the small intestine, called the ileum.

The swelling extends deep into the lining of the affected organ. The swelling can cause pain and can make the intestines empty frequently, resulting in diarrhoea.

Symptoms

- ❑ The most common symptoms of Crohn's disease are abdominal pain, often in the lower right area, diarrhoea, rectal bleeding and weight loss.
- ❑ Bleeding may be serious and persistent, leading to anaemia.
- ❑ Children with Crohn's disease may suffer delayed development and stunted.

Ulcerative colitis

Ulcerative colitis is a disease that causes inflammation and sores, called *ulcers*, in the lining of the rectum and colon. Inflammation in the colon also causes the colon to empty frequently, causing diarrhoea.

The inflammation occurred in the rectum and lower part of the colon is called ulcerative proctitis. If the entire colon is affected, it is called *pancolitis*. If only the left side of the colon is affected, it is called *limited* or *distal colitis*.

Symptoms

The most common symptoms of ulcerative colitis are abdominal pain, bloody diarrhoea, anaemia, weight loss, fatigue, loss of appetite and growth failure (specifically in children).

Zollinger–Ellison syndrome (ZES)

ZES is a rare disorder characterized by one or more tumours in the pancreas, duodenum, or both. The tumours cause the stomach to make too much acid, leading to peptic ulcers in the duodenum. The tumours are sometimes cancerous and spread to other areas of the body.

Symptoms

ZES symptoms are similar to those of peptic ulcers and include burning abdominal pain, nausea and vomiting, weight loss, diarrhoea and severe gastroesophageal reflux.

Celiac disease

Celiac disease is a digestive disease that damages the small intestine and interferes with absorption of nutrients from food. People who have celiac disease cannot tolerate gluten, a protein in wheat, rye and barley.

When people with celiac disease eat foods or use products containing gluten, their immune system responds by damaging or destroying villi—the tiny, fingerlike protrusions lining the small intestine.

Celiac disease is both a disease of malabsorption (meaning nutrients are not absorbed properly) and an abnormal immune reaction to gluten. Celiac disease is also known as celiac sprue, nontropical sprue and gluten-sensitive enteropathy.

Chapter 12

Symptoms

Celiac disease symptoms are abdominal bloating and pain; chronic diarrhoea; vomiting; constipation; pale, foul smelling or fatty stool; and weight loss.

DISEASES OF THE PANCREAS

Pancreatitis

This condition occurs when the pancreas undergoes inflammation. The major causes are heavy alcohol ingestion, gallstones, trauma, drugs and heredity.

Symptoms

The main symptoms of pancreatitis are acute, severe pain in the upper abdomen, frequently accompanied by vomiting and fever.

Pancreatic tumours

The pancreas, like most organs of the body, can develop tumours. Some of these are benign and cause no problems. However, some benign tumours can secrete hormones, which when present in high levels have a detrimental effect. For example, insulin can be secreted in excessive amounts and result in dangerously low blood sugar levels (hypoglycaemia).

Another hormone, gastrin, can stimulate the stomach to secrete its strong hydrochloric acid causing recurrent stomach and peptic ulcers, with many complications.

Cancer of the pancreas is a serious malignancy, which is difficult to treat. The disorder occurs in middle- or older-aged people, with the first symptom often being dull pain in the upper abdomen that may radiate into the back.

Surgery is the only effective form of treatment for pancreas cancer.

DISEASES OF THE LIVER

The important liver diseases are summarized in Table 12.10.

Table 12.10 Diseases of the liver

Type of liver disease	Description	Examples of causes/conditions
Acute liver failure	Rapid decrease in liver function, which causes severe damage to liver. In majority of cases, there is widespread hepatocellular necrosis.	Drugs, toxins, various liver diseases
Cirrhosis	Scarring of liver tissue in which the hepatocytes are replaced by fibrous or adipose connective tissue. Symptoms include jaundice, uncontrolled bleeding and oedema in legs. This condition may result in decreased liver function	Can be caused by a variety of conditions but usually a result of chronic hepatitis, alcoholism, or chronic bile duct obstruction

Type of liver disease	Description	Examples of causes/conditions
Genetic	Gene mutations can lead to liver damage; relatively rare conditions. Symptoms include jaundice, abdominal pain, fever, nausea and vomiting.	Haemochromatosis, alpha-1 antitrypsin deficiency, Wilson's disease
Hepatitis	Acute or chronic liver inflammation. Symptoms include loss of appetite, nausea, diarrhoea and fever	Viruses, alcohol abuse, drugs, toxins, autoimmune, nonalcoholic fatty liver disease (NAFLD)
Liver cancer	A cancer that originates in the liver. The main symptoms include abdominal pain, jaundice, nausea, sweating and liver dysfunction. The major causes are autoimmune diseases, Hepatitis B and liver inflammation	Increased risk with cirrhosis and chronic hepatitis; hepatocellular carcinoma (HCC) is the most common primary liver tumour
Obstruction of bile ducts	Complete or partial blockage of bile ducts. Owing of this blockade, bile builds up in the liver and results in jaundice like condition. The major causes cyst, inflammation or tumour of bile duct. Symptoms include abdominal pain, fever, itching, nausea and vomiting.	Tumours, gallstones, inflammation, trauma

DISEASES OF THE GALLBLADDER AND BILE DUCTS

Cancer of the bile duct

Bile duct cancers, also called *cholangiocarcinomas*, may arise in many locations in and around the liver.

The only definitive treatment is the complete surgical removal of the tumour, which is not often possible.

Symptoms

Symptoms generally develop slowly and are often subtle. Jaundice (the skin turning yellow) and itching are the most common signs. Bloating, weight loss, decreased appetite, fever, nausea or an enlarging abdominal mass are all signs that may be attributable to bile duct cancer. Pain usually signifies advanced disease.

Cholecystitis

Cholecystitis is often caused by cholelithiasis (the presence of choleliths, or gallstones in the gallbladder), with choleliths most commonly blocking the cystic duct directly. This leads to inspissation (thickening) of bile, bile stasis and secondary infection by gut organisms, predominantly *Escherichia coli* and *Bacteroides* species.

Less commonly, in debilitated and trauma patients, the gallbladder may become inflamed and infected in the absence of cholelithiasis and is known as *acute acalculous cholecystitis*.

Stones in the gallbladder may cause obstruction and the accompanying acute attack. The patient might develop a chronic, low-level inflammation that leads to a *chronic cholecystitis*, where the gallbladder is fibrotic and calcified.

Symptoms

Cholecystitis usually presents as a pain in the right upper quadrant. This is usually a constant, severe pain and is usually accompanied by a low-grade fever, vomiting and nausea. More severe symptoms such as high fever, shock and jaundice indicate the development of complications such as abscess formation, perforation or ascending cholangitis.

Chronic cholecystitis manifests with nonspecific symptoms such as nausea, vague abdominal pain, belching and diarrhoea.

Gallstone

Gallstones (choleliths) are crystalline bodies formed within the body by accretion or concretion of normal or abnormal bile components.

Gallstones can occur anywhere within the biliary tree, including the gallbladder and the common bile duct. Obstruction of the common bile duct is choledocholithiasis, obstruction of the biliary tree can cause jaundice and obstruction of the outlet of the pancreatic exocrine system can cause pancreatitis.

Cholelithiasis is the presence of stones in the gallbladder or bile ducts (*chole* means bile, *lithia* means stone, and *-sis* means process).

Jaundice

Jaundice comes from the French word *Jaune*, meaning yellow.

Jaundice (also known as *icterus*, attributive adjective: *icteric*) is a yellowish pigmentation of the skin, the conjunctival membranes over the sclerae (whites of the eyes), and other mucous membranes caused by hyperbilirubinaemia (increased levels of bilirubin in the blood). This hyperbilirubinaemia subsequently causes increased levels of bilirubin in the ECF fluids.

It may occur due to excessive haemolysis of red blood cells, abnormal liver function or obstruction to the bile flow.

OTHER DISEASES OF DIGESTIVE SYSTEM

Diarrhoea

It is a condition of increased frequency and loose or liquid stools caused by increased motility and decrease in absorption by the intestines. Excessive fluid loss through diarrhoea can result in dehydration and electrolyte imbalance.

It may be caused by infection, stress, inflammatory bowel disease or irritable bowel syndrome.

Haemorrhoids or piles

It is an inflamed or swollen condition of the vascular structure in the anal canal. Symptoms include itching, rectal pain and rectal bleeding.

It is mainly caused by constipation.

Gastroenteritis

It is a condition characterized by inflammation and itching of the GI tract (stomach and intestine). It is mainly caused by viral or bacterial infection. Symptoms include diarrhoea, crampy abdominal pain, vomiting, headache and fever.

OVERVIEW OF THE DIGESTIVE SYSTEM

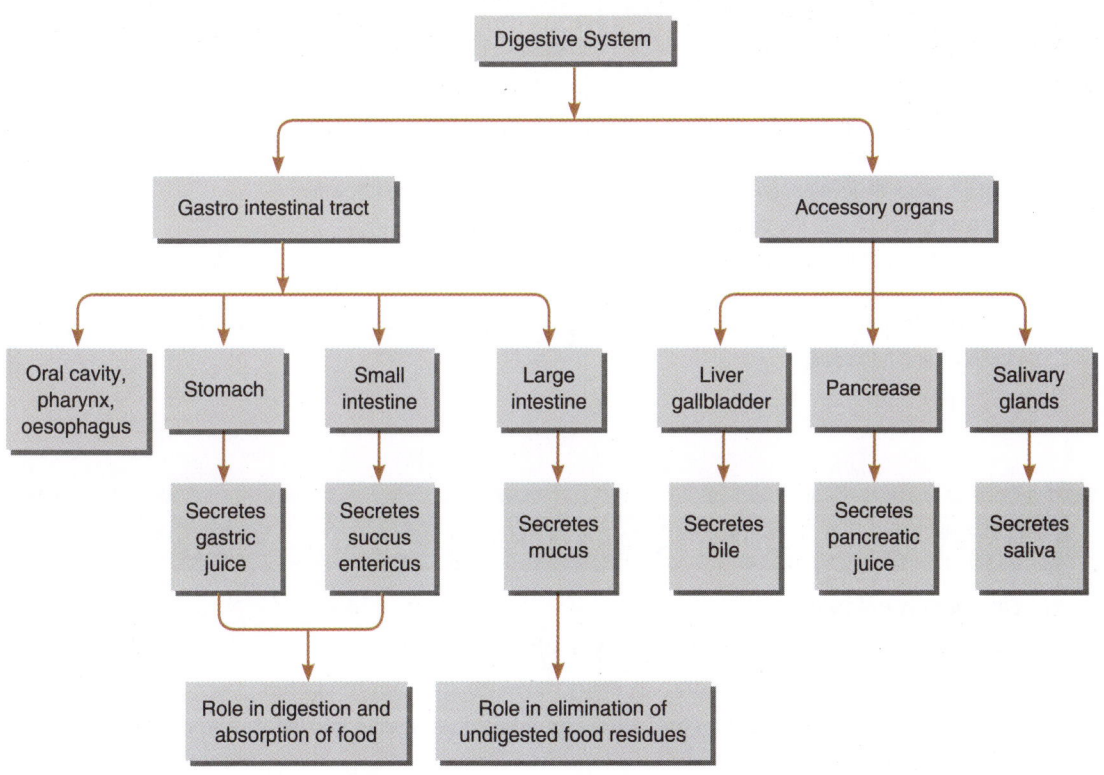

Ageing and the Digestive System

❑ With advancing age, the overall digestive system undergoes changes that include decreased peristalsis, loss of strength and tone of the muscular tissue, decreased enzymatic secretions, diminished sense of taste and decreased response to pain and internal sensations.

❑ The GI tract becomes less protected from toxic contaminants due to decrease in the protective connective tissue and mucous membrane lining.

❑ All these age-related factors make the elderly much more susceptible to infections, duodenal and peptic ulcers, maldigestion, malabsorption, gastritis and constipation. Moreover, the older adults have more chances to develop cancers and ulcerations of the tract, especially in the colon and rectum.

Embryonic Development of the Digestive System

❑ During 4th week of development, the endoderm forms the primitive gut.
➤ The endodermal layer forms glands and epithelial lining of the GI tract.
➤ The mesodermal layer forms smooth muscle and connective tissue.
❑ During 5th week of development, the primitive gut differentiates into the following:
➤ Foregut develops into the pharynx, oesophagus and stomach.
➤ Midgut develops into the small intestine.
➤ Hindgut develops into the large intestine.
❑ During later stages, the endoderm develops into some buds that differentiate to form salivary glands, liver, gallbladder and pancreas.

DIETARY GUIDELINES TO MAINTAIN HEALTHY BODY

1. Eat a variety of foods.
2. Maintain weight by balancing the food with physical activity.
3. Eat a rainbow of fruits and vegetables every day—the brighter the better.
4. Eat more healthy carbohydrates and whole grains and select diet low in fats and cholesterol with moderate sugar and salt.
5. Get a yearly medical check-up.

Review Questions

Long Answer Questions

1. Describe the anatomy of the oral cavity, pharynx and oesophagus, and state the digestive events that take place in these regions of the GI tract.
2. Describe the structure and function of the stomach.
3. What is gastric juice? Describe the various phases of gastric secretion.
4. List the digestive enzymes secreted by the intestinal glands and describe their actions.
5. Discuss about gallbladder and explain the function of bile.
6. Discuss the anatomy and physiology of stomach.
7. Describe the major and accessory organs of the digestive system.
8. Describe the mechanism for the absorption of carbohydrates in human beings.
9. What is defecation? Describe about defecation reflex.
10. Differentiate between succus entericus and saliva.

Multiple Choice Questions

1. The hepatic flexure of the large intestine occurs between
   (a) The transverse colon and descending colon
   (b) The cecum and ascending colon
   (c) The ascending colon and transverse colon
   (d) The descending colon and rectum
   (e) The descending colon and sigmoid colon
2. Obstruction of the common bile duct by gallstones would most likely affect the digestion of
   (a) Carbohydrates   (b) Fats
   (c) Proteins   (d) Nucleic acids
   (e) None of the preceding
3. Formation of gallstones is referred to as
   (a) Jaundice   (b) Cirrhosis
   (c) Hepatitis   (d) Cholelithiasis
4. Which of the following is *not* a function of saliva?
   (a) To initiate protein digestion
   (b) To aid in cleansing the teeth
   (c) To lubricate the pharynx
   (d) To assist in the formation of a bolus

Chapter 12

5. Peristalsis moves food material

   (a) In the stomach and small intestine only

   (b) In the intestines only

   (c) In the stomach and intestines only

   (d) From the pharynx to the anal canal

6. Most enzymes involved in protein digestion are

   (a) Secreted by the pancreas

   (b) Activated by hydrochloric acid (HCl)

   (c) Present in the stomach

   (d) Secreted in an inactive form

   (e) Stimulated by enterokinase

7. The terminal portion of the small intestine is

   (a) The ileum   (b) The cecum

   (c) The duodenum   (d) The jejunum

   (e) The colon

8. Amylase in saliva initiates digestion of

   (a) Lipids   (b) Proteins

   (c) Carbohydrates   (d) Fats

9. Pancreatic juice contains a protein-splitting enzyme called

   (a) Trypsin   (b) Zymogen

   (c) Pepsin   (d) Amylase

   (e) Nuclease

10. Secretin is a hormone that

    (a) Stimulates the release of pancreatic juice

    (b) Converts trypsinogen into trypsin

    (c) Activates chymotrypsin

    (d) Inhibits the action of pancreatic lipase

11. Which of the following ducts is *not* associated with the digestive system?

    (a) Cystic duct   (b) Parotid duct

    (c) Pancreatic duct   (d) Hepatic duct

    (e) Lacrimal duct

12. The salivary gland located in front and slightly below the auricle of the ear is

    (a) The buccal gland   (b) The parotid gland

    (c) The submandibular gland   (d) The sublingual gland

State True or False

1. The principal function of the digestive system is to prepare food for cellular utilization.
2. The GI tract has both sympathetic and parasympathetic innervations.
3. Parasympathetic impulses to the GI tract decrease the peristaltic activity.
4. Jaundice is a liver disease.
5. Pancreatic juice is secreted from acinar cells of the pancreas.
6. The spleen is an accessory digestive organ.
7. Deglutition is the process by which bile causes the breakdown of fat globules into smaller droplets.
8. Intestinal rugae are folds of the mucosa within the small intestine that greatly increase the surface area for absorption.
9. Cirrhosis is a chronic disease of the liver in which fibrous tissue replaces functional hepatic cells.

Fill in the Blanks

1. The _____ is the serous membrane that lines the wall of the abdominal cavity and covers visceral organs.

2. Food and fluid in the stomach are consolidated into a pasty material called _____.

3. Capillaries within the _____ of the small intestine are sites where nutrients and fluids are absorbed into the circulatory system.

4. Hepatic plates within a liver lobule are separated from each other by spaces called hepatic _____, which permit passage of blood.

5. _____ from the duodenum stimulates the release of pancreatic juice.

Match the Following

1. Gastrin	(a)	Emulsifies fats
2. Bile	(b)	Converts pepsinogen to pepsin
3. Peptidase	(c)	Converts proteins into amino acids
4. Sucrase	(d)	Stimulates secretion of HCl and pepsin
5. Nuclease	(e)	Converts fats into fatty acids and glycerol
6. HCl	(f)	Converts disaccharides into monosaccharides
7. Amylase	(g)	Activates trypsin secreted from the pancreas
8. Enterokinase	(h)	Converts nucleic acids into nucleotides
9. Lipase	(i)	Converts starch and glycogen into disaccharides

Chapter 12

Careers in Digestive System and Nutrition

✓ Dentists are qualified and trained professionals who specialize in the diagnosis and treatment of abnormalities of the teeth, gums and underlying bones.

✓ Nutritionists are professionals who monitor and prepare nutritional menus. They are employed in nursing homes, hospitals, schools and other public service agencies.

✓ Dieticians are the professionals who manage food and diets and provide nutritional care services.

✓ Gastroenterologists are specialized in the diagnosis and treatment of diseases that affect the gastrointestinal tract.

✓ Proctologists are specialized in the diagnosis and treatment of the disorders of the colon, rectum and anus.

✓ Hepatologists are the physicians specialized in the diseases related to liver.

13 The Urinary System

CHAPTER OUTLINE

- Introduction
- Organs of the Urinary System
- Micturition
- Disorders of the Urinary System

STUDY OBJECTIVES

- ✓ To describe the various organs of the urinary system.
- ✓ To discuss the anatomy of kidney.
- ✓ To explain the process of urine formation.
- ✓ To explain the role of kidney in homeostasis.

- ✓ To describe the anatomy and physiology of ureters, urinary bladder and urethra.
- ✓ To understand the process of micturition.
- ✓ To give a brief idea about the various disorders of the urinary system.

INTRODUCTION

The organs associated with the production and excretion of the urine from the body constitute a system called the *urinary system.*

The urinary system maintains the water and electrolyte balance, fluid volume and blood pressure and regulates the pH of the body. All these functions contribute to the homeostasis of the body.

ORGANS OF THE URINARY SYSTEM

The urinary system consists of the following organs:

- ❏ Two kidneys
- ❏ Two ureters
- ❏ One urinary bladder
- ❏ One urethra

The urine is produced by the kidneys, conveyed by the ureters, collected and stored in the urinary bladder and eliminated out of the body by the urethra (Fig. 13.1).

FUNCTIONS OF THE URINARY SYSTEM

The majority of work in the urinary system is performed by the kidneys, which maintains homeostasis by performing the following functions:

1. **Excretion of wastes and foreign substances**: Kidneys excrete the waste products formed during metabolism such as urea, creatinine, uric acid and bilirubin. Kidneys also excrete toxins, drugs, heavy metals, and so on.

2. **Maintenance of water and electrolyte balance**: Kidneys maintain the water balance

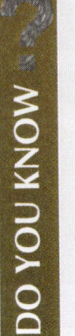

DO YOU KNOW?

- In a healthy adult, almost 440 gallons of blood is passed through the kidneys daily.
- Though we keep describing kidneys as bean-shaped organs, the beans were named after the organ and not vice versa.
- Urine is almost odourless when it leaves a healthy body.
- Have you heard of urine therapy? Well, urine therapy involves application of urine for medical or cosmetic purposes. People apply urine on the skin and even drink urine for medicinal benefits.

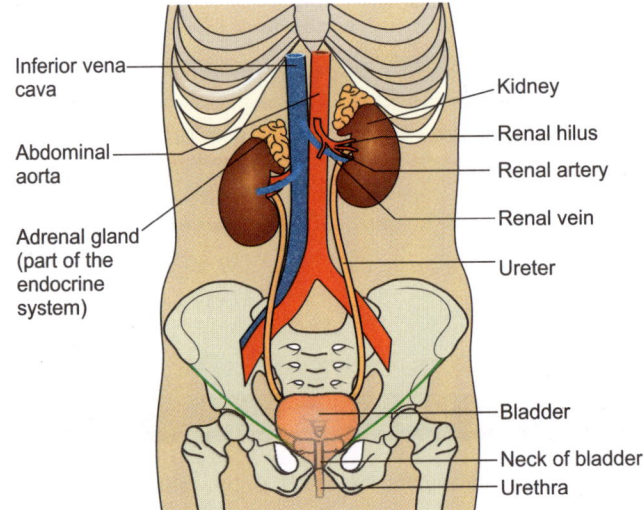

Inferior vena cava — Kidney — Renal hilus — Renal artery — Renal vein — Abdominal aorta — Adrenal gland (part of the endocrine system) — Ureter — Bladder — Neck of bladder — Urethra

Figure 13.1 Components of the urinary system.

MEDICAL TERMINOLOGY

- **Osmosis**: It is the diffusion of fluid through a semipermeable membrane from a solution with a low-solute concentration to a solution with a higher-solute concentration until there is an equal concentration of fluid on both sides of the membrane.
- **Passive diffusion**: It is the passive movement of molecules or particles along a concentration gradient.
- **Peristalsis**: It is the coordinated, rhythmic serial contraction of smooth muscle that forces food through the digestive tract, bile through the bile duct and urine through the ureters.

by conserving water (when decreased) and excreting water (when excess). Kidneys also regulate the concentration of ions such as sodium, chloride, potassium, calcium and phosphate ions in body fluids and blood.

3. **Regulation of pH**: The pH of blood and body fluids is maintained within a narrow range by the kidneys, lungs and buffers in the blood. Among these, kidneys play a major role in regulating pH by excreting H^+ and conserving bicarbonate ions.

4. **Endocrine function**: Kidneys secrete many hormones that include the following:
   - ❏ *Erythropoietin*: It stimulates red blood cell (RBC) production.
   - ❏ *Thrombopoietin*: It stimulates platelets production.
   - ❏ *Renin*: It regulates blood pressure.
   - ❏ *Prostaglandins*

5. **Regulation of the blood calcium level**: Kidneys play a major role in regulating blood calcium level by activating 1,25-dihydroxycholecalciferol to vitamin D. Vitamin D is essential for the absorption of calcium from the intestine.

KIDNEY

Anatomy of the kidney

Kidneys are dark red, bean-shaped organs about 10–11 cm in length, 5–6 cm in width and 2–3 cm in thickness. Each kidney weighs about 150 g in adult male and about 135 g in adult female.

These are present on either side of the vertebral column behind the peritoneum just below the diaphragm extending from the level of the XII thoracic vertebra to the III lumbar vertebra. Because they are situated posterior to the peritoneum of the abdominal cavity, kidneys are also referred to as *retroperitoneal organs*.

The left kidney is slightly larger than the right one, and also, the liver present above the right kidney pushes down the right kidney a little lower than the left kidney.

External anatomy

The medial portion of the concave border of each kidney presents a notch called *hilum* where the blood vessels, lymph vessels, nerves and ureters enter and leave the kidney.

Externally, the kidneys are enclosed by the following three layers of tissue:
- ❏ Renal capsule
- ❏ Adipose capsule
- ❏ Renal fascia

The *renal fascia* is the outer layer made of fibrous connective tissue that fixes the kidney to the abdominal wall and to the surrounding structures.

The *adipose capsule* is the middle layer of fat that holds the kidneys in the upright position in the abdominal cavity.

The *renal capsule* is the inner layer made of transparent, fibrous connective tissues that enclose the kidneys.

Chapter 13

Internal anatomy

Internally, kidneys can be divided into following two regions:

❑ Renal cortex
❑ Renal medulla

Renal cortex is the outer, light red, smooth-textured region of the kidney. It can be further subdivided into the following two different zones: cortical zone (outer) and juxtamedullary zone (inner).

Renal medulla is the inner, dark red–coloured region of the kidney. It consists of cone-*shaped wedges called renal pyramids that give a striated* appearance to the renal medulla. The pyramids have a broad base towards the cortex and a narrow end called *renal papilla* towards the hilum.

The renal cortex extends in between the space of renal pyramids in the form of columns, called *renal columns* or *columns of Bertin*. Renal columns along with the renal pyramid and superimposed area of the renal cortex constitute a *renal lobe*.

The hilum expands into a cavity within the kidney called the *renal sinus*, which consists of part of renal pelvis (the upper expanded part of ureter), subdivisions of pelvis (major and minor calyx), branches of renal blood vessels and fats.

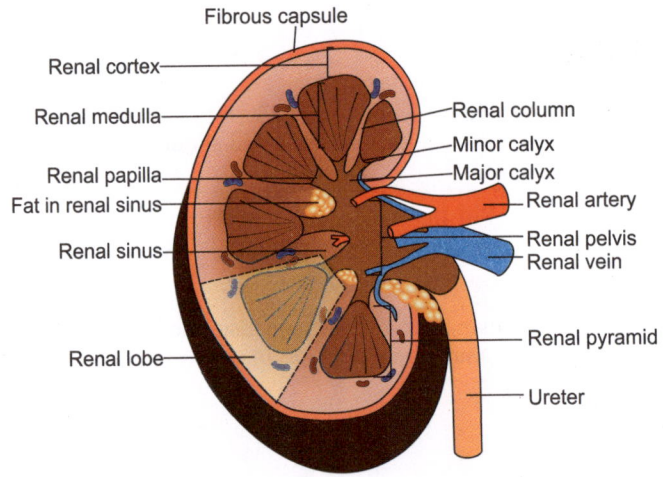

Figure 13.2 Internal structure of the kidney.

Urine formed in the kidney passes through renal papilla, which drains it into the cuplike structures called *minor calyx* (8–10 in each kidney) through the papillary ducts. The minor calyces join to form 2–3 *major calyces* that deliver the urine into a large cavity called the *renal pelvis*, which leads into the ureter. The urine finally reaches the urinary bladder through the ureters (Fig. 13.2).

Microscopic structure of the kidney

The kidney is composed of numerous microscopic coiled tubules called *nephrons* or *uriniferous tubules*. The nephrons are the structural and functional units of the kidney.

About 1.2 million nephrons are present in each kidney.

Types of nephron: Nephrons are of two types: *cortical* and *juxtamedullary*, based on their location in the kidney.

❑ The cortical nephrons have their renal corpuscles in the outer cortex of the kidney and have a very short loop of Henle, which penetrates only the outer zone of the medulla. In human kidneys, the cortical nephrons comprise about 80% of the total nephrons.

❑ The juxtamedullary neurons (*juxta*: near) have their corpuscles in the inner cortex near the corticomedullary junction. These nephrons have very long loop of Henle, which extends deep into the medulla.

A nephron consists of the following parts (Fig. 13.3):

❑ Glomerulus (Bowman's) capsule } Renal corpuscle
❑ Glomerulus

❑ Proximal convoluted tubule ⎫
❑ Loop of Henle   ⎬ Renal tubule
❑ Distal convoluted tubule   ⎪
❑ Collecting ducts   ⎭

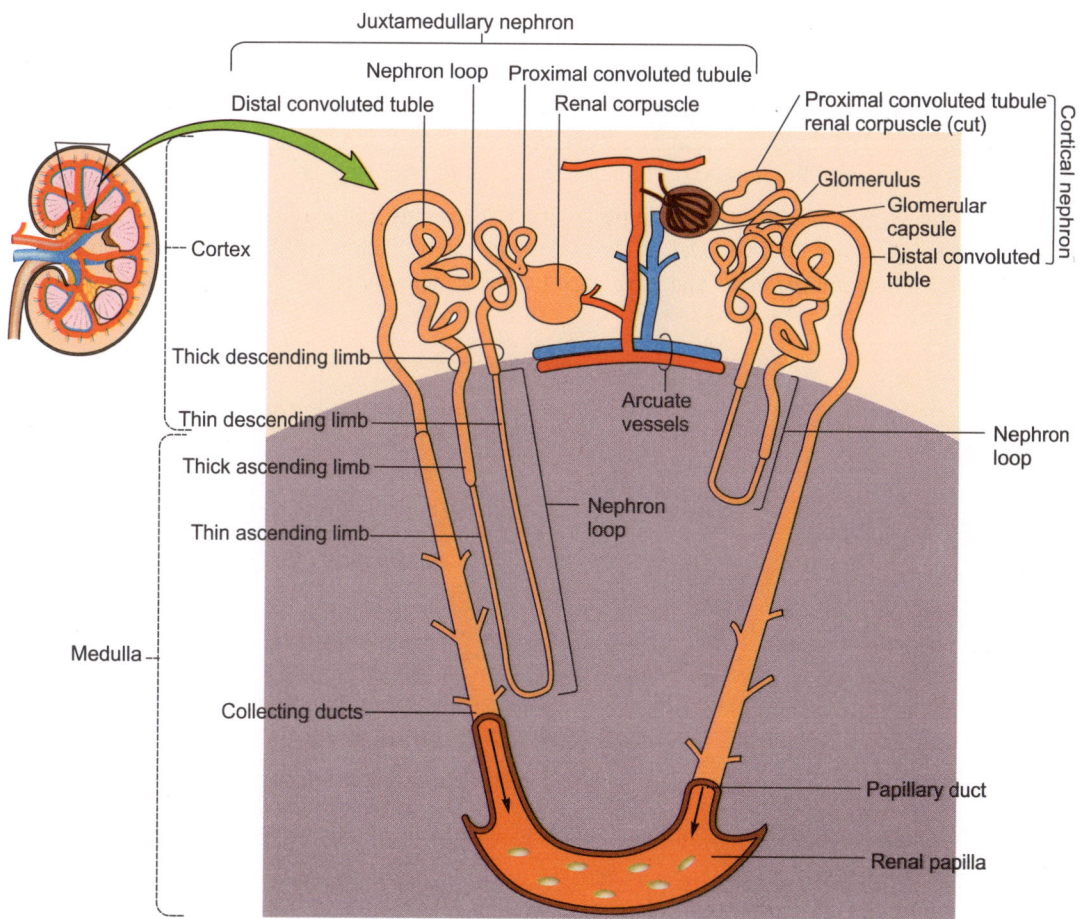

Figure 13.3 Parts of nephron.

The different parts of the nephron (see Fig. 13.3) are discussed in the sections that follow.

Glomerulus

Glomerulus consists of the bunch of fine network of capillaries called glomerular capillaries.

The afferent arteriole from the renal artery enters the glomerulus and divides into four or five large capillaries. Each large capillary subdivides into a cluster of fine capillaries called *glomerular capillaries*, which rejoin to form efferent arteriole through which a reduced volume of blood leaves the glomerulus. Thus, the vascular system in the glomerulus is purely arterial.

The glomerular capillaries are made of a single layer of endothelial cells that rest on a basement membrane. The endothelial cells have many pores between them called *fenestrations* that facilitate the filtration process.

Glomerulus (Bowman's) capsule

It is a cup-shaped structure present in the renal cortex that forms the beginning of the nephron.

The Bowman's capsule encloses the glomerulus and it is formed by the following two layers:

❑ Visceral layer: inner
❑ Parietal layer: outer

The visceral layer covers the glomerular capillaries and the parietal layer is continuous with the tubular portion of the nephron. The space between the two layers is known as the *capsular space*, which is continuous as lumen of the tubular portion.

Both the layers are composed of a single layer of squamous epithelial cells, and the cells of the visceral (inner) layer are called *podocytes*. The podocytes subdivide into primary, secondary and tertiary branches to terminate into *pedicels* and have gaps between them called *filtration slits* that facilitate the ultrafiltration process (Fig. 13.4).

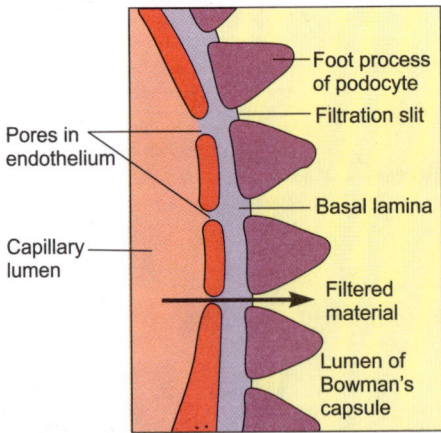

Figure 13.4 Passage of filtered substances through pores and filtration slits.

The structure of the glomerular capsule is explained in Figure 13.5.

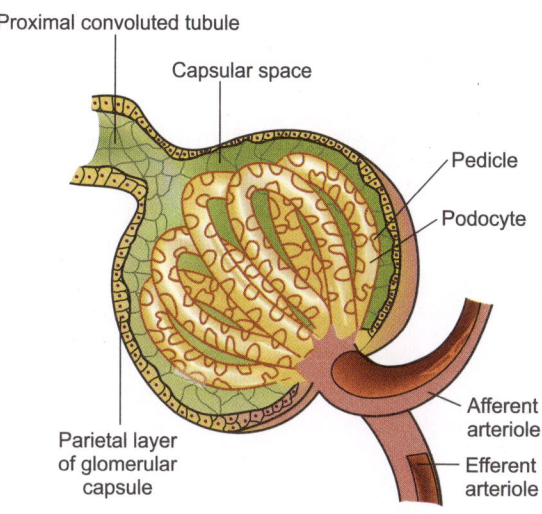

Proximal convoluted tubule

Capsular space

Pedicle

Podocyte

Afferent arteriole

Efferent arteriole

Parietal layer of glomerular capsule

Figure 13.5 Structure of the glomerular capsule.

Proximal convoluted tubule

Proximal convoluted tubule (PCT) (*proximal*: near; *convoluted*: tightly coiled) is the coiled tubule arising from the Bowman's capsule and located in the cortex of kidney.

Its wall consists of a single layer of cuboidal epithelial cells bearing microvilli (hair-like projections) on the surface. Because of these microvilli, the epithelial cells are called *brush-bordered cells*, and they serve to increase the luminal surface for secretion and reabsorption.

Loop of Henle

The loop of Henle is the U-shaped segment of nephron that extends into the renal medulla, makes a hairpin turn (loop) and then returns to the renal cortex. It is continuous with PCT and has three parts: descending limb, loop and ascending limb.

Both the ascending and the descending limbs have a thick region towards the cortex and a thin region on the other side. The thick regions are walled by *brush-bordered cuboidal* epithelial cells and the thin regions by flat cells.

In the final part of the ascending limb, which lies close to the afferent arteriole (as shown in Fig. 13.6), the cuboidal cells are closely packed and this zone is known as *macula densa* (*macula*: spot; *densa*: dense).

The wall of the afferent arteriole alongside the macula densa is composed of modified smooth muscle fibres called *juxtaglomerular (JG) cells* (Fig. 13.6).

JG cells along with macula densa constitute the *juxtaglomerular apparatus*, which helps regulate blood pressure within the kidneys by renin secretion (discussed later in detail).

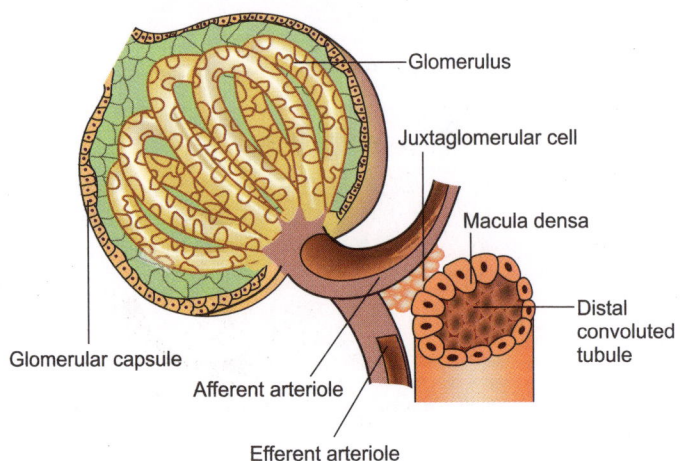

Figure 13.6 Juxtaglomerular apparatus.

Distal convoluted tubule

The distal convoluted tubule (DCT) is tightly coiled and lies in the renal cortex. A short terminal part of the DCT that collects urine is called the *collecting tubule*, which further opens into the collecting ducts.

The wall of DCT is mainly composed of principal cells (contain receptors for antidiuretic hormone (ADH) and aldosterone) and intercalated cells.

Collecting ducts

These are large tubes present in the renal medulla that receive the collecting tubules of several nephrons.

The collecting tubules further join many large collecting tubules in renal pyramids to form *ducts of Bellini* that open into calyces through renal papilla. It then joins the ureters at the renal pelvis.

Renal blood flow

The renal blood flow in an adult kidney is about 1200 mL/min. The renal artery supplies the blood to the kidney, whereas the blood from kidney is drained out by the renal vein.

The renal artery is divided into several arteries: segmental arteries, interlobular arteries, arcuate arteries, interlobular arteries and afferent arterioles. The efferent arterioles from the glomerulus, peritubular capillaries, vasa recta, interlobular veins, arcuate veins and interlobular veins join to form one single vein, the renal vein, to drain the blood out of the kidneys.

Renal blood flow is explained in Figure 13.7.

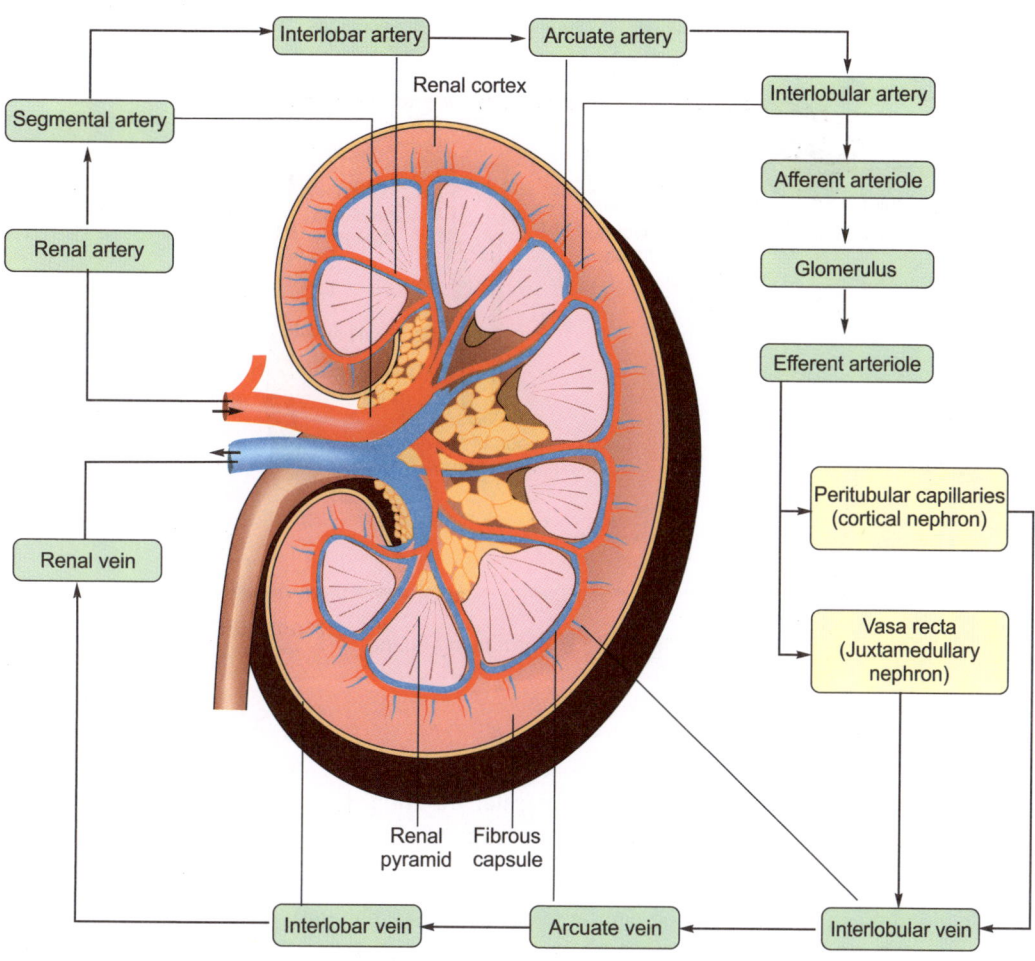

Figure 13.7 Renal blood flow.

Note: The network of *peritubular capillaries* supplies the tubular portion of cortical nephrons only, whereas the tubular portion of juxtamedullary nephrons is supplied by *vasa recta*.

Renal physiology (formation of urine)

The physiology of the formation of urine involves the following three processes:

❏ Glomerular filtration
❏ Tubular reabsorption
❏ Tubular secretion

It is described in Figure 13.8.

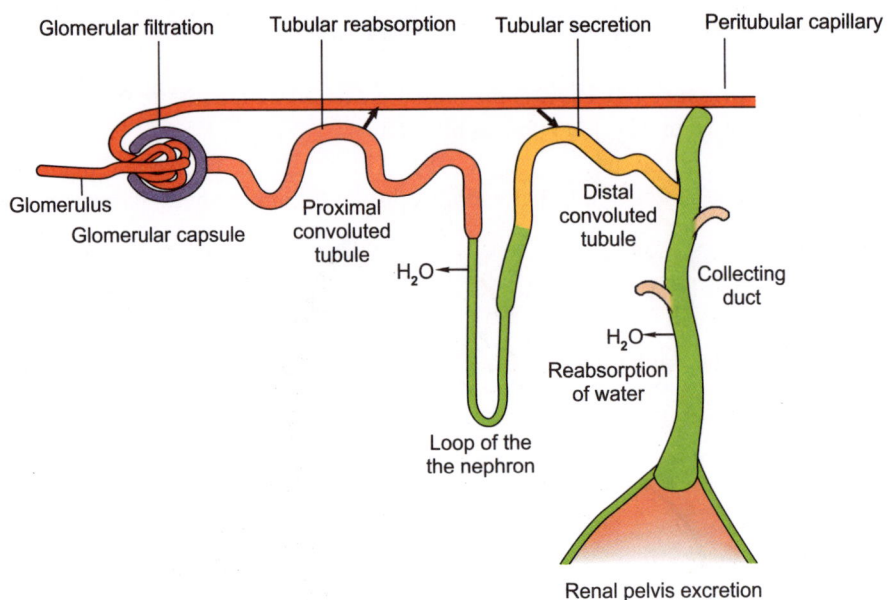

Figure 13.8 Formation of urine.

Glomerular filtration

The first step in the formation of urine is glomerular filtration. In this step, the glomerulus filters water and certain dissolved substances from the plasma of blood. The blood pressure in glomerular capillaries is very high as the efferent arteriole is smaller in diameter than the afferent arteriole.

Note: The blood pressure in glomerular capillaries is the highest capillary pressure in the body.

The high blood pressure forces the fluid to filter from the blood and pushes it out of the glomerular capillaries into the capsular space and subsequently into the Bowman's capsule. The filtered blood plasma is called the *glomerular filtrate* and it contains sodium, potassium and chloride ions, glucose, amino acids, urea, uric acid, creatinine, ketone bodies and a large amount of water.

Glomerular filtration is called ultrafiltration as even the minute particles are filtered when they pass through fenestrations in the endothelium of glomerular capillaries and filtration slits in the glomerular capsule. The plasma proteins, blood cells and other large molecules remain in the capillaries as they are too large to be filtered. Except the plasma proteins, the composition of the glomerular filtrate is very much similar to the blood plasma.

The rate at which the kidneys filter the blood plasma is called *glomerular filtration rate (GFR)*. The average GFR in an adult is about 180 L/day or 125 mL/day. The GFR is the measure of the kidney function, that is how efficiently the kidneys are able to filter.

The pressures that determine GFR are as follows:

- **Glomerular blood hydrostatic pressure (GBHP)**: It is the blood pressure in glomerular capillaries (about 60 mm Hg); it promotes filtration.
- **Bowman's capsule pressure (BCP)**: It is the pressure exerted by the filtrate in Bowman's capsule during filtration (about 18 mm Hg); it opposes filtration.
- **Glomerular colloid osmotic pressure (GCOP)**: This pressure is exerted due to increased concentration of plasma proteins in the glomerulus during filtration (about 32 mm Hg); it opposes filtration.

The net filtration pressure (NFP) can be calculated as follows:

$$NFP = (GBHP - BCP - GCOP) = (60 - 18 - 32) \text{ mm Hg} = 10 \text{ mm Hg}$$

Hence, the NFP required to filter the blood plasma from the glomerulus into the Bowman's capsule is 10 mm Hg (Fig. 13.9).

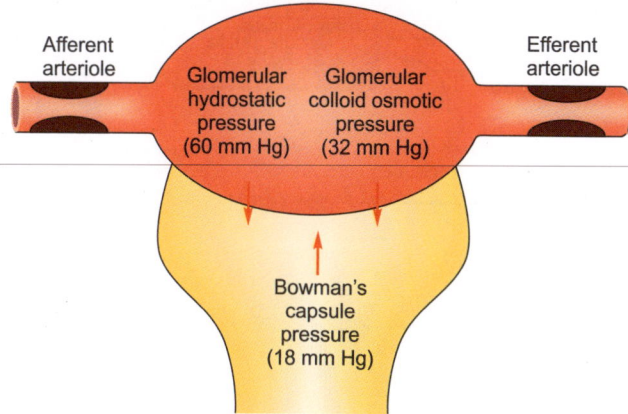

Figure 13.9 Pressures determining GFR.

Autoregulation of GFR

The kidneys help maintain a constant renal blood flow and GFR despite normal changes in blood pressure everyday. This capability is called autoregulation and the mechanism underlying is called *tubuloglomerular feedback* (i.e. part of renal tubules—macula densa—provides feedback to the glomerulus).

When the glomerular filtrate passes through the end portion of the loop of Henle, the macula densa detects the concentration of sodium chloride (NaCl) and accordingly changes GFR. Decreased blood pressure slows down the flow of filtered fluid along the tubules, which provides more time for reabsorption of sodium and chloride; consequently, NaCl concentration decreases, which is detected by macula densa. Macula densa increases renin secretion and constricts the efferent arteriole, thereby increasing GFR.

This process is explained in Figure 13.10.

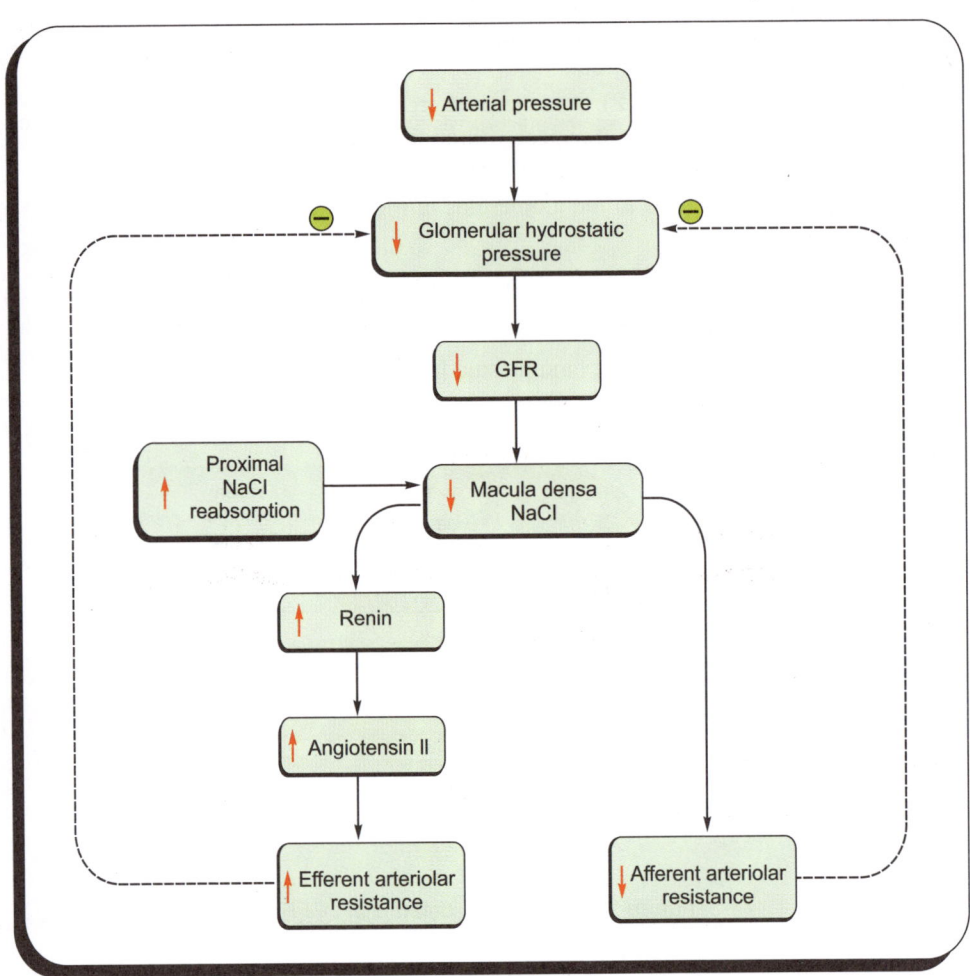

Figure 13.10 Autoregulation of glomerular filtration rate.

Tubular reabsorption

Tubular reabsorption refers to the qualitative and quantitative changes in the glomerular filtrate during its passage through the tubular portion of the nephron till the collecting duct.

Large quantity of water, electrolytes and other substances are selectively reabsorbed (according to the needs of the body) throughout the renal tubule, but the maximum reabsorption takes place in the PCT. The substances that are reabsorbed pass into the blood in peritubular capillaries.

The following two mechanisms are involved in tubular reabsorption:

1. **Active reabsorption**: It involves the movement of molecules against electrochemical gradient. This process needs energy, which is derived from ATP.

2. **Passive reabsorption**: It involves the movement of molecules along the electrochemical gradient. This process does not need energy.

The reabsorption of the substances occurs in almost all the segments of the tubular portion of the nephron.

1. PCT

- ❏ The cells lining PCT are well adapted for reabsorption of materials from filtrate as they bear numerous microvilli that increase the surface area for reabsorption.
- ❏ The cells of PCT reabsorb the following:
  - ➤ *Glucose*: 100% active reabsorption by sodium-glucose transport proteins and GLUT. The reabsorption of glucose is so efficient that appearance of only a trace of glucose in urine suggests diabetes mellitus. The condition in which glucose is not reabsorbed by the kidney is called glucosuria (glucose in urine).
  - ➤ *Oligopeptides, proteins and amino acids*: 95% active reabsorption; only 5% appears in urine.
  - ➤ Some urea is reabsorbed by diffusion and the rest remains in the filtrate for removal in urine.
  - ➤ *Electrolytes*: Sodium and potassium ions are reabsorbed actively by Na-H antiport, Na-glucose symport and sodium channels. The reabsorption of these ions from tubule reduces the concentration of filtrate, and an equivalent amount of water is passed into the peritubular capillaries by osmosis. The chloride ions are reabsorbed by passive diffusion.
  - ➤ *Bicarbonate ions*: 99.9% bicarbonate ions are reabsorbed, which play a role in the maintenance of the acid–base balance.

2. Loop of Henle

- ❏ The first wide part of the descending limb is impermeable to ions, water and urea, whereas the second part is freely permeable to water; thus, water is drawn out by osmosis, making the filtrate hypertonic as it reaches the ascending limb.
- ❏ The ascending limb is impermeable to water along its entire length while it is permeable to electrolytes (sodium, potassium, chloride) and urea. The electrolytes leave the filtrate by active transport as well as by diffusion, which makes the filtrate hypotonic to plasma as it passes into DCT.

3. DCT and collecting ducts

- ❏ The DCT and collecting ducts actively reabsorb sodium from the filtrate under the influence of the adrenal hormone *aldosterone*. The aldosterone makes the walls of DCT and collecting ducts permeable to ions, leading to reabsorption of sodium. This sodium reabsorption causes the uptake of an osmotically equivalent amount of water and thus plays a vital role in the maintenance of water and urine output.
- ❏ Bicarbonate ions are also reabsorbed in DCT.

Chapter 13

Tubular secretion

Some substances are not filtered during glomerular filtration due to either their large size or shorter contact time in the glomerulus. Such substances are secreted into the tubule from peritubular capillaries and thus get cleared from the body through urine.

These substances include the following:

❑ Some drugs (penicillin, aspirin) and foreign substances are actively secreted in PCT.
❑ Creatinine, ammonia, potassium and hydrogen ions are secreted in PCT and DCT.

The most important tubular secretion is the secretion of protons (H^+) and ammonia in the PCT and DCT as removal of hydrogen and ammonia plays a vital role in maintaining the normal blood pH (the acid–base balance).

The H^+ ions are secreted into PCT and DCT by the sodium-hydrogen antiport pump (secretion of H^+ in exchange for Na^+) and ATP-driven proton pump. The H^+ secreted into the renal tubule combines with the following buffers:

1. Bicarbonate to form carbonic acid ($H^+ + HCO_3^- \longrightarrow H_2CO_3$)
2. Ammonia to form ammonium ions ($H^+ + NH_3 \longrightarrow NH_4^+$)
3. Hydrogen phosphate to form dihydrogen phosphate
   ($H^+ + HPO_3^{2-} \longrightarrow H_2PO_3^-$)

Carbonic acid is converted to CO_2 and H_2O, and CO_2 is reabsorbed, which maintains the buffering capacity of blood. Hydrogen ions are excreted in the urine as ammonium salts and hydrogen phosphate. This mechanism maintains the acid–base balance of body fluids.

Tubular secretion has a minor role in the function of human kidneys in normal conditions. However, in pathological states such as decreased blood pressure when the filtration pressure drops below a certain level and filtration stops, the urine is formed only by tubular secretion.

Thus, by the processes of glomerular filtration, tubular reabsorption and tubular secretion, urine is formed in the nephron. The volume of urine is very less compared to the volume of glomerular filtrate because of tubular reabsorption and the countercurrent mechanism (discussed below) and ADH.

Urine

❑ A healthy adult passes about 1–1.8 L of urine per day. Excessive fluid intake and low temperature increases urine output and vice versa.
❑ Urine is clear and yellowish in colour due to the pigment urochrome derived from the breakdown of haemoglobin from the worn-out RBCs. It has a characteristic unpleasant odour.
❑ Its pH ranges around 6 (normal range is 4.5–8).
❑ The composition of urine includes the following:
  ➤ water: more than 95%, urea, uric acid, creatinine,
  ➤ salts: Sodium, potassium, chlorides, phosphates, oxalates, sulphates and ammonia. Urine also contains some epithelial cells, leukocytes, pigments and drugs.

COUNTERCURRENT MECHANISM OF URINE CONCENTRATION

- ❑ The countercurrent mechanism in kidney plays a vital role in conserving water and eliminating wastes and excess ions. Loop of Henle and vasa recta have an important role in this mechanism as the fluid flowing in one tube runs counter (opposite) to the fluid flowing in a nearby parallel tube and this arrangement is termed *countercurrent flow.*
- ❑ **Loop of Henle**: The descending limb is very permeable to water but impermeable to solutes except for urea. Thus, water moves out of the descending limb and makes the tubular fluid more concentrated (hypertonic). The ascending limb is impermeable to water but it causes reabsorption of the solutes, resulting in dilute (hypotonic) tubular fluid. The reabsorption of solutes leads to increased concentration of the solutes in interstitial fluid around the loop of Henle.
- ❑ **Vasa recta**: Similar to how tubular fluid flows in opposite directions in the loop of Henle, blood flows in opposite directions in the ascending and descending parts of the vasa recta. As the blood flows in the descending part of vasa rectum, solutes (Na^+ and Cl^-) and urea diffuse from the interstitial fluid into the blood. However, as the blood flows in the ascending part of vasa recta, the reverse occurs, that is, ions and urea diffuse from the blood into interstitial fluid and reabsorbed water diffuses from interstitial fluid into the vasa recta.
- ❑ Thus, the countercurrent mechanism in vasa recta prevents the loss of ions and helps conserve the body's water by concentrating the urine. The urine is four times more concentrated than blood plasma or the glomerular filtrate.

Role of kidneys in homeostasis

Maintenance of water level in the body

Kidneys play a pivotal role in maintaining the water balance in the body.

Decreased water level in plasma

↓

Stimulates posterior pituitary lobe to release *ADH*

↓

ADH increases the permeability of DCT and collecting ducts to water

↓

Leads to water reabsorption from the DCT and collecting ducts and production of a reduced amount of concentrated urine

This type of water reabsorption in the presence of ADH is called *facultative reabsorption.*

When the water level in plasma is normal, ADH is not secreted; thus, permeability of the DCT and collecting ducts to water decreases, leading to production of abundant dilute urine.

Maintenance of blood pressure and electrolyte balance (Renin-angiotensin-aldosterone system: RAAS):

The kidneys maintain the blood pressure and electrolyte balance in the body with the help of a system called *renin–angiotensin–aldosterone system (RAAS).*

RAAS plays a vital role in the regulation of blood pressure and comprises the following functional proteins:

❑ Renin
❑ Angiotensinogen
❑ Angiotensin I
❑ Angiotensin II

An enzyme known as *angiotensin-converting enzyme (ACE)* has a key role in the RAAS as it converts angiotensin I to form angiotensin II. *Aldosterone* is a steroid hormone released from the adrenal cortex that influences the water and electrolyte balance.

The activation of RAAS and its subsequent physiological effects is explained in Figure 13.11.

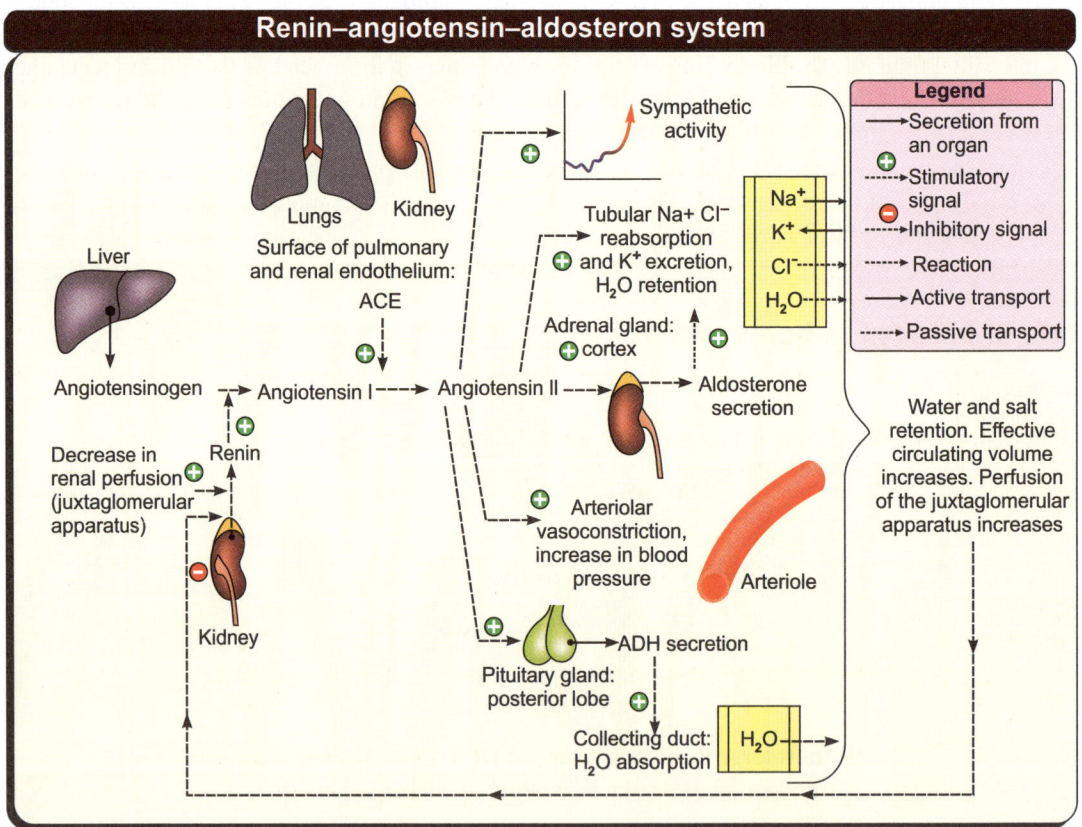

Figure 13.11 Activation of RAAS and its physiological effects.

When blood volume and blood pressure decrease, the juxtaglomerular (JG) cells secrete the enzyme renin into the blood. Renin stimulates the conversion of angiotensinogen (produced by liver) into angiotensin-I, and ACE (released by lungs) further converts angiotensin-I to angiotensin-II, which is the active form of the hormone.

Angiotensin-II maintains renal homeostasis by the following three principal ways:

1. It stimulates the reabsorption of Na⁺, Cl⁻ and water in the PCT.
2. It stimulates the adrenal cortex to release *aldosterone*, a hormone that acts on the renal tubule to reabsorb more Na⁺ and Cl⁻ and secrete more K⁺. The reabsorption of Na⁺ and Cl⁻, in turn, decreases the water excretion, which increases blood volume.
3. It is a powerful vasoconstrictor, thus increasing glomerular blood pressure, thereby regulating glomerular filtration rate.
4. Decreased blood volume also stimulates the posterior pituitary lobe to release ADH, which causes water reabsorption in the DCT and collecting ducts.

The various roles of kidney in the maintenance of homeostasis have been summarized in Figure 13.12.

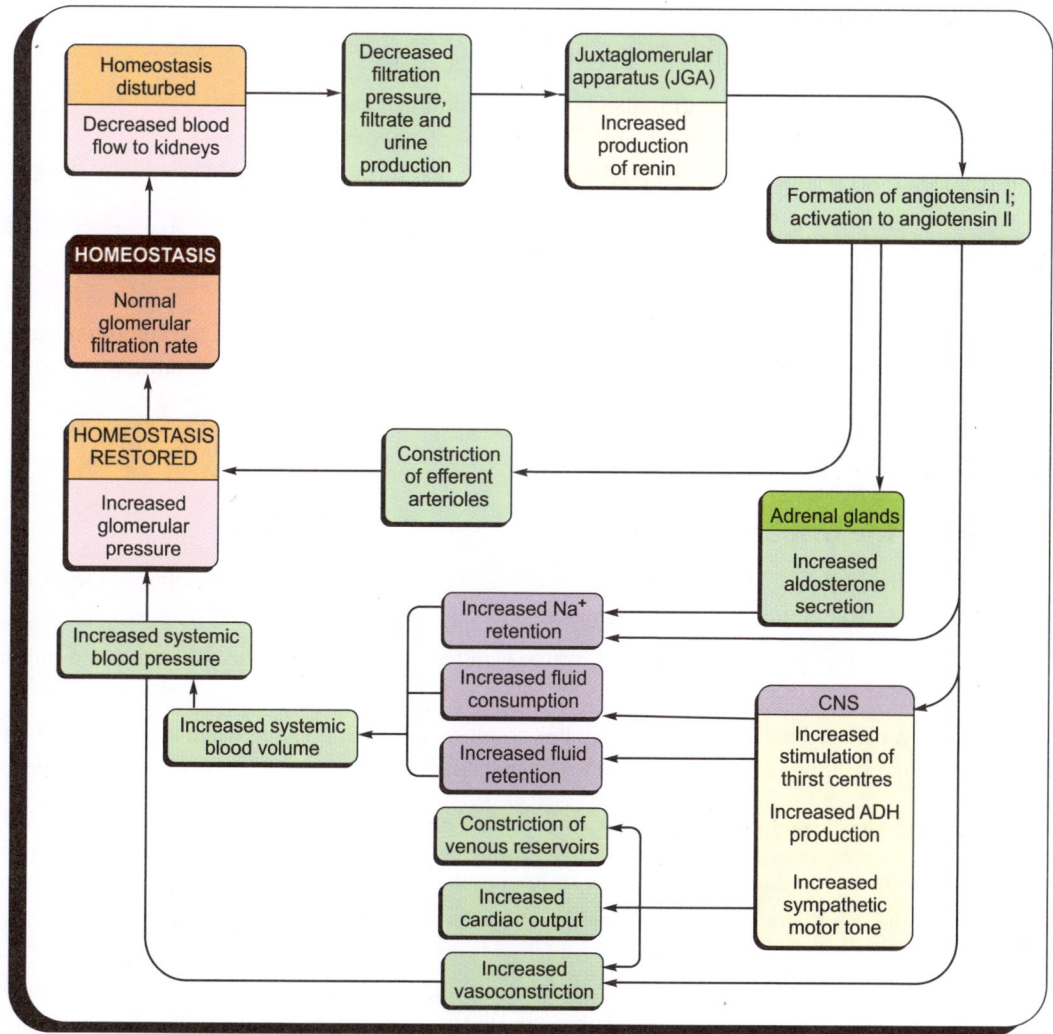

Figure 13.12 Role of kidney in the maintenance of homeostasis.

URETERS

Anatomy of ureters

The ureters are long tubular structures that extend from the renal pelvis of the kidney to connect to the posterior surface of the urinary bladder. Each ureter is about 10–12 in. (25–30 cm) long and 0.5 in. (0.3 cm) in diameter.

At the base of the urinary bladder, the ureters curve medially and pass obliquely through the posterior wall of the urinary bladder. When the urinary bladder fills with urine and pressure in the bladder increases, these oblique openings into ureters get compressed and serve as a valve to prevent the backflow of urine.

Histology of ureters

Each ureter is composed of the following three layers of the tissue:

- **Inner layer**: *Mucosa* is made up of transitional epithelium that can stretch.
- **Middle layer**: *Muscular layer* is made up of two layers of smooth muscle.
- **Outer layer**: *Fibrous layer* is made up of fibrous tissue that forms the outer covering of ureters.

Functions of ureters

The ureters serve to propel the urine from the kidney into the urinary bladder.

The urine is carried through the ureters primarily by peristaltic contractions of the smooth muscular walls of the ureters, but gravity and hydrostatic pressure also contribute. These peristaltic waves rise in the calyces of the kidney and pass to the urinary bladder about 1–5 times per minute.

URINARY BLADDER

Anatomy of the urinary bladder

It is a hollow, distensible (collapsible) pear-shaped sac located in the lower or pelvic region of the abdominal cavity, just behind the symphysis pubis.

In males it is directly anterior to the rectum, whereas in females it is anterior to the vagina and inferior to the uterus.

It resembles a deflated balloon when empty but assumes a spherical shape when slightly filled with urine. As the urine volume increases, it becomes pear shaped and the average capacity is 700–800 mL.

Histology of the urinary bladder

The wall of the urinary bladder consists of the following three tissue layers:

- Inner layer (mucosa) is composed of transitional epithelium; it consists of rugae (folds in mucosa) that help in the distension of the wall.
- Middle layer (muscular layer) is also called *detrusor muscles*. It consists of three layers of smooth muscle fibres: inner and outer longitudinal fibres and the middle layer of circular fibres. The contraction of these detrusor muscles results in the emptying of the bladder.
- Outer layer is composed of connective tissues; it contains blood vessels and nerves.

The interior of the urinary bladder has three openings: the two posterior openings from two ureters (ureter orifices) and the single anterior opening to the urethra (urethral orifice guarded by internal urethral sphincter). These three orifices form a small triangular area called the *trigone*. The internal urethral sphincter is made up of detrusor muscle (smooth muscle fibres) and is present at the junction of urinary bladder and urethra. This sphincter is not under voluntary control (Fig. 13.13).

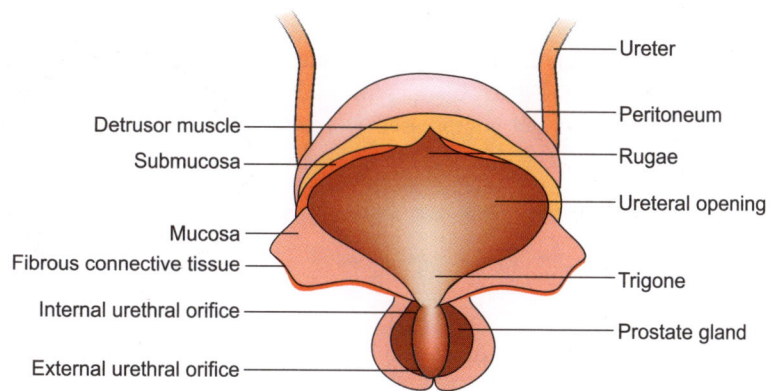

Figure 13.13 Structure of the urinary bladder.

Functions of the urinary bladder

It serves as the reservoir for urine, that is, it stores the urine prior to its excretion out of the body.

It helps expel the urine out of the body through the urethra.

URETHRA

Anatomy of the urethra

Urethra is a small tubular structure leading from the floor of the urinary bladder (internal urethral orifice) to the exterior of the body.

In females, the urethra lies behind the symphysis pubis and opens at the external urethral orifice between the clitoris and the vagina. It is quite short, (only about 3–5 cm long in females) and carries only urine. In males, urethra (about 20 cm) courses through the prostate gland and opens at the tip of the penis at the external urethral orifice (guarded by external urethral sphincter). It has a dual function in males: it carries urine and spermatic fluid. For further details, see the chapter The Reproductive System.

Histology of the urethra

In both males and females, the wall of urethra is composed of the following three tissue layers:

❑ **Mucosa**, which consists of stratified squamous epithelium that continues with the outer skin
❑ **Submucosa**, which consists of the spongy connective tissue that contains blood vessels and nerves
❑ **Muscle layer**, which forms the internal and external urethral sphincter

Chapter 13

The internal urethral sphincter is composed of smooth muscle fibres and elastic tissue. It is under involuntary control. The external urethral sphincter is composed of skeletal muscles and is under voluntary control.

The urethra in male and female is shown in Figure 13.14.

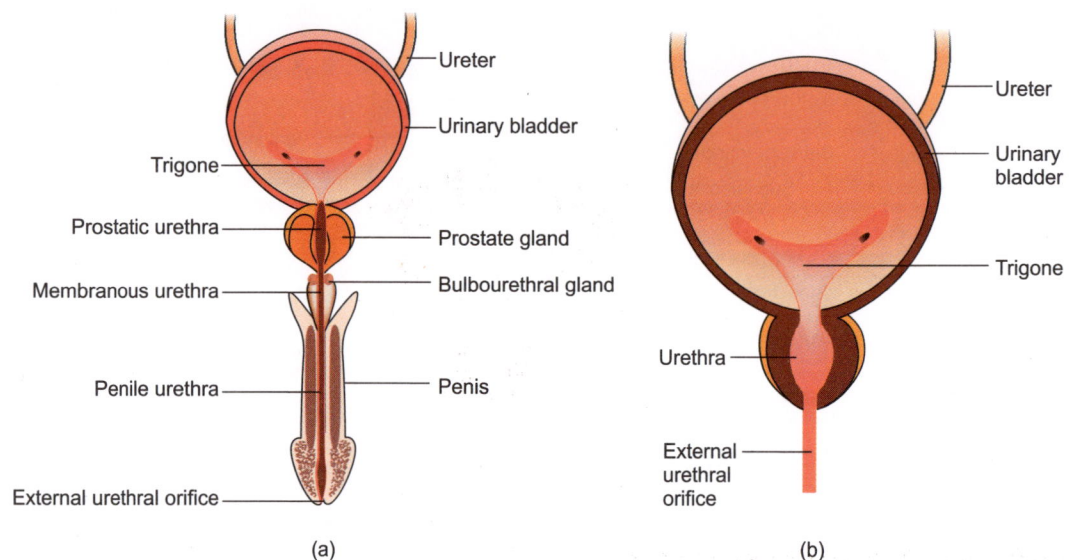

Figure 13.14 (a) Urethra in male; (b) Urethra in female.

Functions of the urethra

It serves as a channel through which the urine is expelled out of the body. In males, the urethra also serves as the channel through which semen is discharged out of the body.

MICTURITION

The process by which urine is voided from the urinary bladder is called *micturition* or *urination*. It is the result of the micturition reflex. In grown-up children and adults, it can be controlled voluntarily to some extent.

MICTURITION REFLEX

The impulses that initiate a conscious desire to expel urine by triggering a spinal reflex are called the *micturition reflex*.

The reflex starts when the urinary bladder is filled with about 300–400 mL of urine and pressure inside the bladder increases. The increase in pressure stimulates the stretch receptors situated on the walls of the urinary bladder and urethra (Fig. 13.15).

Now, the stretch receptors transmit sensory (afferent) impulses to the micturition centre located at S2 and S3 segments of the sacral spinal cord. This initiates a spinal reflex called *micturition reflex*. In this reflex arc, the micturition centre in the spinal cord sends the parasympathetic nerve impulses (via the pelvic nerve) towards the bladder and internal sphincter, resulting in the contraction of the detrusor muscle and relaxation of the internal sphincter so that urine enters the urethra from the bladder.

Once urine enters the urethra, the stretch receptors in the urethra are stimulated, which again send impulses towards the micturition centre, thereby inhibiting somatic motor neurons (pudendal nerve). Hence, the external sphincter relaxes and micturition takes place.

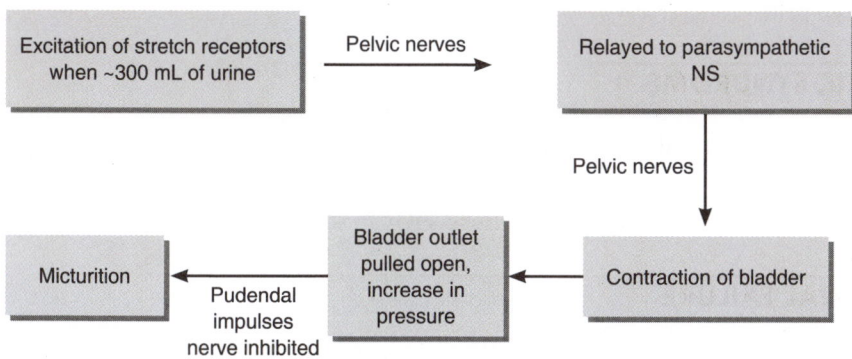

Figure 13.15 Micturition reflex.

DISORDERS OF THE URINARY SYSTEM

URINARY TRACT INFECTIONS

These are the microbial infections that are more common in females due to the shorter length of urethra. Symptoms include painful urination, frequent urination, bed-wetting and low back pain. UTIs include inflammation of ureters (ureteritis), bladder (cystitis), urethra (urethritis) and kidney (pyelonephritis).

The susceptible microorganisms include *Streptococcus faecalis*, *Neisseria gonorrhoeae* and *E. coli*.

GLOMERULONEPHRITIS

The inflammation of glomerulus is called *glomerulonephritis*.

It is often associated with the allergic reaction to the toxins produced by streptococcal bacteria. This can be an acute response followed by streptococcal sore throat or can be a chronic condition resulting in kidney failure.

Symptoms include inflammation of glomerulus and haematuria.

POLYCYSTIC DISEASE

It is a genetic disorder characterized by the formation of cysts (fluid-filled cavities) at the junction of the DCT and collecting tubule.

Chapter 13

As the cysts gradually become large, they exert pressure on the walls of DCT and collecting tubules, resulting in ischaemia and necrosis and may eventually lead to renal failure.

Symptoms include urinary tract infections, haematuria and large abdominal masses.

PYELONEPHRITIS

It refers to the microbial infection of the renal pelvis of the kidney.

The spread of the infection results in the formation of abscesses, which is usually followed by malaise, fever and groin pain.

NEPHROTIC SYNDROME

Nephrotic syndrome is a condition characterized by hyperlipidaemia, proteinuria, oedema and hypoalbuminaemia.

It affects both adults and children and is associated with several glomerular diseases.

ACUTE RENAL FAILURE

It refers to the condition in which the kidney function is dented reversibly, characterized by decreased glomerular filtration.

The reasons associated with acute renal failure may include decreased blood flow due to severe shock, glomerulonephritis, tubular necrosis, tumour of urinary bladder and tumour of uterus.

Symptoms include oliguria (decreased urine output) or anuria (urine output of less than 50 mL).

CHRONIC RENAL FAILURE

It is a condition in which the kidney function is dented irreversibly, characterized by irreversible decline in glomerular filtration rate (GFR).

More than 75% of the kidney function is lost due to chronic pyelonephritis, glomerulonephritis, hypertension or diabetes mellitus.

Patients with end-stage renal failure require haemodialysis and have to undergo kidney transplant.

RENAL CALCULI

These are also known as *stones* (*calculi*).

The precipitation of various substances such as oxalates, urates, phosphates and uric acid results in the formation of stones in the kidney and urinary bladder.

TUMOUR OF THE URINARY BLADDER

The development of tumour, both benign and malignant, is the major disease of the urinary bladder.

Often there are multiple tumours, which may lead to severe pathophysiological conditions.

NEPHROPTOSIS OR FLOATING KIDNEY

It is the inferior displacement or slipping of the kidney from its normal position. It mainly occurs when the kidneys are not held properly by the adjacent organs or its fat covering.

This condition can block the urine flow and put pressure on the kidneys. It is more common in thin people.

OTHER DISEASES OF URINARY SYSTEM

1. **Uraemia**: It is the condition of high level of urea in blood due to severe kidney malfunction.
2. **Polyuria**: It is characterized by excessive urine formation due to certain conditions such as diabetes mellitus and glomerulonephritis.
3. **Cystitis**: It is the inflammation of the urinary bladder and is caused mainly due to bacterial infection.
4. **Pyelitis**: It is the inflammation of the renal pelvis mainly caused by bacterial infection.

OVERVIEW OF THE URINARY SYSTEM

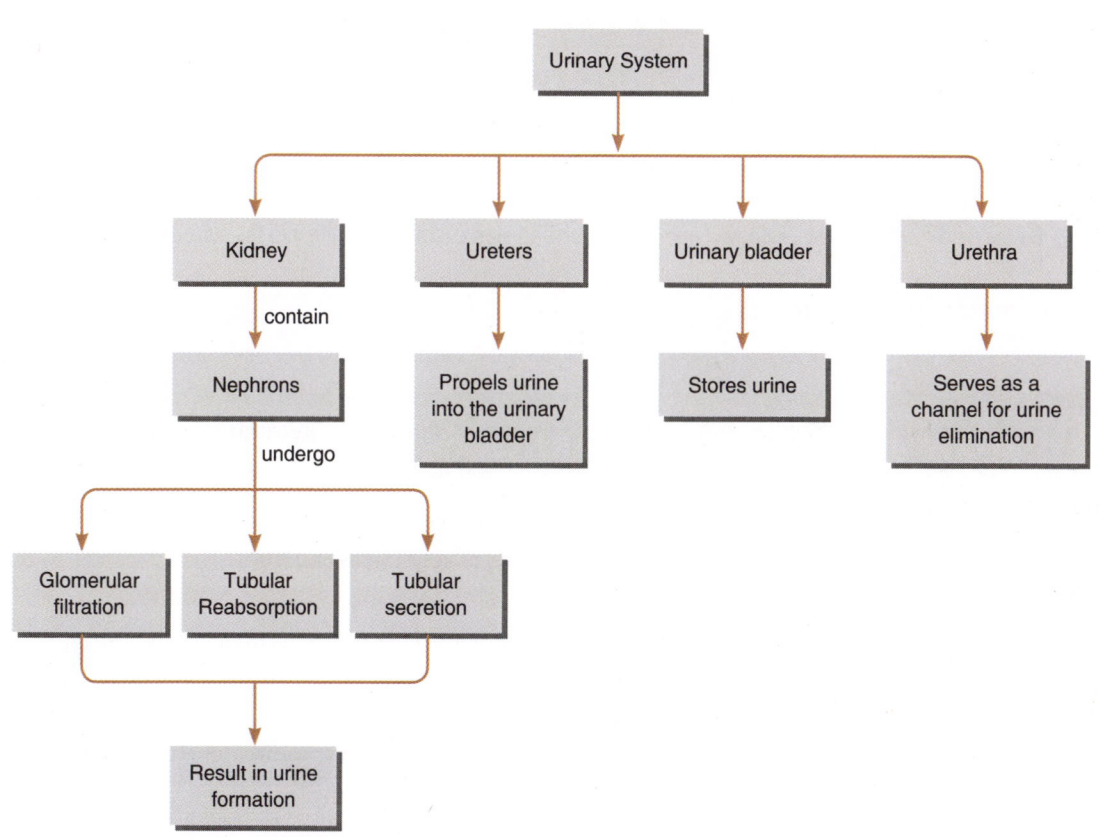

Ageing and the Urinary System

❑ With ageing, the urinary system undergoes various changes such as the following:
1. Decreased kidney size
2. Decreased blood flow to kidneys
3. Decreased glomerular filtration rate
❑ These changes result in the following:
1. Decreased capacity of kidney for absorption and tubular secretion
2. Decreased ability to eliminate urea, uric acid, toxins and creatinine from blood
❑ All these age-related factors make the elderly much more susceptible to kidney diseases such as urinary tract infections, kidney stones and inflammation of the kidneys. Thus, older adults often tend to experience nocturia (urination at night), polyuria (excessive urine production), increased frequency of urination, dysuria (painful urination) or even haematuria (blood in urine).

Embryonic Development of Urinary System

❑ During the third week of development, the mesoderm part differentiates into the kidneys.
❑ During the fifth week of development, the mesoderm develops an outgrowth called *ureteric bud* that differentiates to form collecting ducts, calyces, renal pelvis and ureter.
❑ By the third month, the fetal kidneys begin to function and start excretion of urine into the surrounding amniotic fluid.

HOW TO KEEP YOUR URINARY SYSTEM HEALTHY

1. Drink at least eight glasses of water daily as it helps in eliminating waste products.
2. Maintain a balanced diet, which should include lots of vegetables and fruits.
3. Avoid large intake of caffeine and salt.
4. Fresh pomegranate juice and cranberry juice limits urinary tract infections.
5. Avoid alcohol and spicy food to prevent urinary tract infection.
6. Maintain proper hygiene.

Kidney Transplantation

- ❏ Kidney transplantation or renal transplantation is the organ transplant of a kidney into a patient with end-stage renal disease.
- ❏ Kidney transplant may be recommended for patients with kidney failure caused by:
  - ➤ Severe, uncontrollable high blood pressure (hypertension)
  - ➤ Infections, diabetes mellitus
  - ➤ Congenital abnormalities of the kidneys
  - ➤ Other diseases that cause renal failure, such as autoimmune disease
- ❏ Donor kidneys are obtained from either brain-dead organ donors, or from living relatives, or friends of the recipient.
- ❏ The new kidney is sutured into place. The vessels of the new kidney are connected to the vessels leading to the right leg (the iliac vessels) and the ureter is sutured to the bladder. In most cases, the recipient's native kidneys are left in place, and the transplanted kidney performs all the functions that both kidneys perform in healthy people. Kidney transplant recipients are required to take immunosuppressive medications for the rest of the lives to prevent immune rejection of the transplanted organ.

Haemodialysis

- ❏ Removal of waste materials and toxic substances with the help of a machine that filters the blood of a person whose kidneys are damaged is called haemodialysis.
- ❏ It works on the principle of dialysis, that is diffusion of small solute molecules through a semipermeable membrane.
- ❏ Patient's arterial blood is made to flow through the artificial kidney (haemodialyzer) and then back to the body through the vein. Heparin is used as an anticoagulant while passing the blood through the machine.

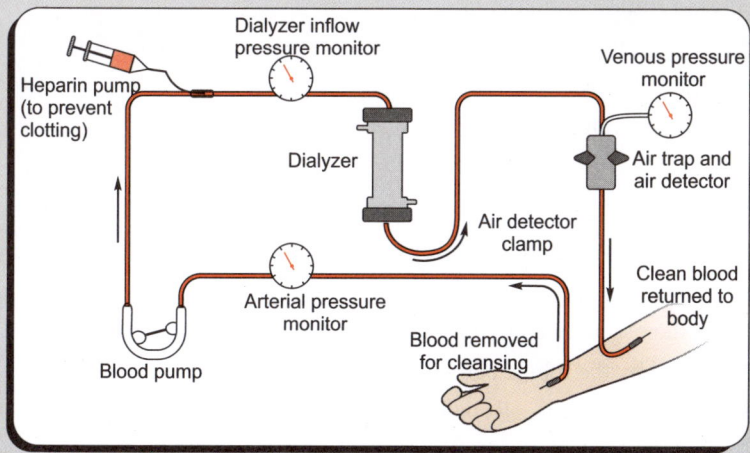

Chapter 13

Review Questions

Long Answer Questions

1. Describe the glomerulus and surrounding glomerular capsule. Describe the structural components of the tubular segments of the nephron.
2. What is meant by the juxtaglomerular apparatus?
3. How does ADH participate in regulating the final urine concentration? How does aldosterone modify the chemical composition of urine?
4. Discuss in detail the process of urine formation.
5. What is micturition? Describe the micturition reflex.
6. Explain the renin–angiotensin–aldosterone system.
7. Discuss the anatomy and physiology of kidneys.

Multiple Choice Questions

(Some questions have more than one correct answer. Select the best answer or answers from the choices given.)

1. The lowest blood concentration of nitrogenous waste occurs in
   - (a) Hepatic vein
   - (b) Inferior vena cava
   - (c) Renal artery
   - (d) Renal vein
2. The glomerular capillaries differ from other capillary networks in the body because they
   - (a) Have a larger area of anastomosis
   - (b) Are derived from and drain into arterioles
   - (c) Are not made of endothelium
   - (d) Are sites of filtrate formation
3. Damage to the renal medulla would interfere first with the functioning of the
   - (a) Glomerular capsules
   - (b) Distal convoluted tubules
   - (c) Collecting ducts
   - (d) Proximal convoluted tubules
4. Glucose is not normally found in the urine because it
   - (a) Does not pass through the walls of the glomerulus
   - (b) Is kept in the blood by colloid osmotic pressure
   - (c) Is reabsorbed by the tubule cells
   - (d) Is removed by the body cells before the blood reaches the kidney

5. Filtration at the glomerulus is inversely related to
   (a) Water reabsorption
   (b) Capsular hydrostatic pressure
   (c) Arterial blood pressure
   (d) Acidity of the urine

6. Transitional epithelium is characteristic of
   (a) The nephron
   (b) The glomerulus
   (c) The urinary bladder
   (d) The urethra

7. The trigone is
   (a) A urine-filled cavity within the kidney
   (b) A muscular sphincter at the neck of the urinary bladder
   (c) A smooth connective tissue region in the urinary bladder
   (d) A tunic of the ureter

8. Transport of urine through the ureter is by
   (a) Peristalsis
   (b) The effect of gravity
   (c) Fluid pressure
   (d) Passive transport

9. A glomerulus is
   (a) Located between a descending and ascending limb of a nephron
   (b) Composed of simple squamous epithelium
   (c) Located at the junctions of minute arteries and veins
   (d) Collapsed when not filtering urine

10. Podocytes are specialized cells found within
    (a) The nephron loop
    (b) The urinary bladder
    (c) The glomerulus
    (d) The urethra
    (e) The glomerular capsule

Chapter 13

Match the Following

1.	Glomerulonephritis	(a)	Inflammation of the renal pelvis mainly caused by bacterial infection
2.	Polycystic disease	(b)	Inflammation of the urinary bladder caused mainly due to bacterial infection
3.	Pyelonephritis	(c)	Inflammation of glomerulus
4.	Nephrotic syndrome	(d)	A genetic disorder characterized by the formation of cysts
5.	Acute renal failure	(e)	Microbial infection of the renal pelvis of the kidney
6.	Chronic renal failure	(f)	A condition characterized by hyperlipidaemia, proteinuria, oedema and hypoalbuminaemia
7.	Renal calculi	(g)	A condition in which the kidney function is dented reversibly, characterized by decreased glomerular filtration rate
8.	Nephroptosis	(h)	A condition in which the kidney function is dented irreversibly, characterized by irreversible decline in glomerular filtration rate
9.	Uraemia	(i)	Kidney stones
10.	Polyuria	(j)	Inferior displacement or slipping of the kidney from its normal position
11.	Cystitis	(k)	High level of urea in blood due to severe kidney malfunction
12.	Pyelitis	(l)	Excessive urine formation due to certain conditions such as diabetes mellitus and glomerulonephritis

State True or False

1. Bilirubin, a by-product of the destruction of erythrocytes, can be found in the urine.
2. Afferent arterioles bring arterial blood to the glomeruli.
3. Most water reabsorption occurs in the distal convoluted tubules.
4. The kidneys synthesize and secrete glucose during prolonged fasting.
5. The kidneys help counter alkalosis by reabsorbing excess HCO_3.
6. Aldosterone increases the permeability of the distal convoluted tubules to water only.
7. The kidneys regulate glucose levels by secreting any excess in the urine.
8. One symptom of diabetes is polyuria.
9. A difference in hydrostatic pressure is one of the mechanisms for pushing blood fluid through the glomerulus to form the filtrate.
10. ADH is necessary for the reabsorption of Na.

Chapter 13

Fill in the Blanks

1. The most primitive kidney, the _____, begins to develop during the fourth week of the embryonic period.

2. The _____ muscle within the wall of the urinary bladder forcefully contracts during micturition, forcing urine out of the urinary bladder.

3. The _____ is a network of about 50 capillaries surrounded by the glomerular capsule.

4. The inner visceral layer of the glomerular capsule is composed of specialized cells called _____.

5. Increased sodium stimulates the juxtaglomerular cells to secrete _____.

6. Approximately _____% of the filtrate is reabsorbed from the renal tubules and returned to the blood.

7. The condition of blood in the urine is called _____.

8. _____ refers to excessive blood nitrogen compounds.

9. _____ is the hormone that regulates water reabsorption in the distal convoluted tubule.

10. The _____ run parallel to the nephron loops and function as countercurrent exchangers.

Careers in Urinary System

- ✓ Urologists are physicians who specialize in the diagnosis and treatment of disorders of the urinary tract of both men and women.

- ✓ Dialysis technicians are allied health professionals who maintain and operate dialysis equipment to treat patients.

- ✓ Nephrologists are the physicians who specialize in the study and treatment of various kidney disorders.

14 | The Reproductive System

STUDY OBJECTIVES

- ✓ To describe the structure and functions of the organs of the male reproductive system.
- ✓ To discuss the process of spermatogenesis.
- ✓ To describe the location, structure and functions of the organs of the female reproductive system.
- ✓ To discuss the process of oogenesis.
- ✓ To explain the detailed events in menstrual cycle.

INTRODUCTION

Reproduction is the process by which the genetic material is passed onto the next generation. This process involves a special kind of cellular division called *meiosis* that produces specialized reproductive germ cells called *gametes*. The male gametes are called *spermatozoa* and the female gametes are called *ova*. The fusion of male gametes (sperms) and female gametes (secondary oocyte) by a process called *fertilization* gives rise to offspring.

The organs involved in human reproduction are called *reproductive organs*, and they constitute a system called the *reproductive system*. The major function of the reproductive system is to produce offspring and ensure the perpetuation of human species.

Males and females have anatomically distinct reproductive organs that are adapted for producing gametes and facilitating fertilization; in females, these organs are present to sustain the growth of embryo and fetus.

MALE REPRODUCTIVE SYSTEM

The male reproductive system consists of a number of organs (Fig. 14.1).

- ❑ Testes
- ❑ Ducts of testes
  - ➤ Epididymis
  - ➤ Ductus deferens/vas deferens
  - ➤ Ejaculatory ducts
  - ➤ Urethra
- ❑ Accessory glands
  - ➤ Seminal vesicles
  - ➤ Prostate gland
  - ➤ Bulbourethral glands/Cowper's gland
- ❑ Supporting structure
  - ➤ Penis
  - ➤ Scrotum

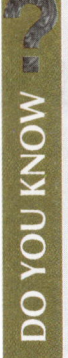

DO YOU KNOW

- ❑ The largest cell in the female body is the egg.
- ❑ Male sperms are significantly smaller than the female egg. While the sperm measures 2.5–3.5 µm across the head, the fully mature egg is 100–125 µm in diameter.
- ❑ A woman never runs out of eggs.
- ❑ At birth, a woman has between 1 and 2 million potential eggs (follicles), and by puberty she has 300,000–400,000 viable eggs (follicles) that can be fertilized.
- ❑ In the uterus, prior to birth, the baby's body is covered by a thin layer of hair. As soon as the baby is born that hair soon disappears. The hair is called *lanugo* (*lan-oo-go*).

TESTES

Testes are the reproductive glands of the male. They are paired oval-shaped glands housed in the scrotum and measure about 5 cm in length and 2.5 cm in diameter.

These are developed in the prenatal stage in the posterior portion of the abdomen, near the kidneys and descend down during the later part of pregnancy (often about 7 months of pregnancy).

Testes are covered by the following:

- ❑ The outer membrane called *tunica vaginalis* derived from the peritoneum. This is a double membrane that covers the testes partially.
- ❑ Beneath the tunica vaginalis, there is a layer of dense white fibrous connective tissue called *tunica albuginea*. The tunica albuginea extends inwards and divides the testis into a number of small, internal compartments known as *lobules*. Each of the 200–300 lobules contains 1–3 tightly coiled tubules, called the *seminiferous tubules*, where sperms are produced by a process called *spermatogenesis* (Fig. 14.2).

MEDICAL TERMINOLOGY

- ❑ **Antiflexed position:** It is the normal forward curvature of the uterus.
- ❑ **Capacitation:** It is the process by which spermatozoa in the ampullary portion of a uterine tube become capable of going through the acrosome reaction and fertilizing an oocyte.
- ❑ **Diploid**: It is a cell that contains two complete sets of chromosomes, one from each parent.
- ❑ **Dizygotic twins:** They are nonidentical twins formed when two different eggs are fertilized by two different sperm.
- ❑ **Monozygotic twins:** They are identical twins formed when one egg was fertilized by one sperm and somehow split and form two zygotes.
- ❑ **Pelvic cavity**: It is the space bounded by the bones of the pelvis and containing the pelvic viscera.
- ❑ **Pubic symphysis**: It is the fixed joint at the front of the pelvic girdle where the halves of the pubis meet.

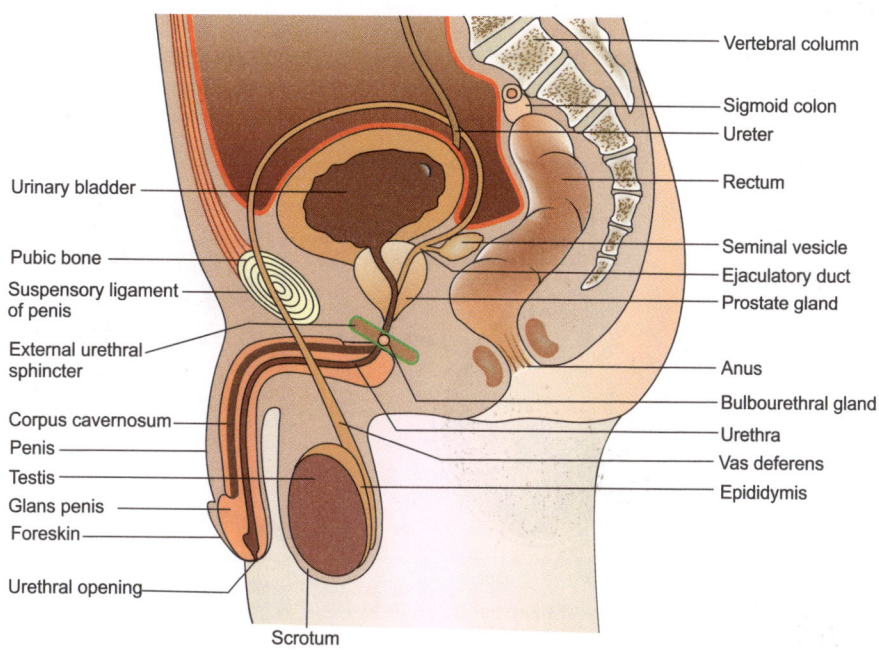

Figure 14.1 Organs of the male reproductive system.

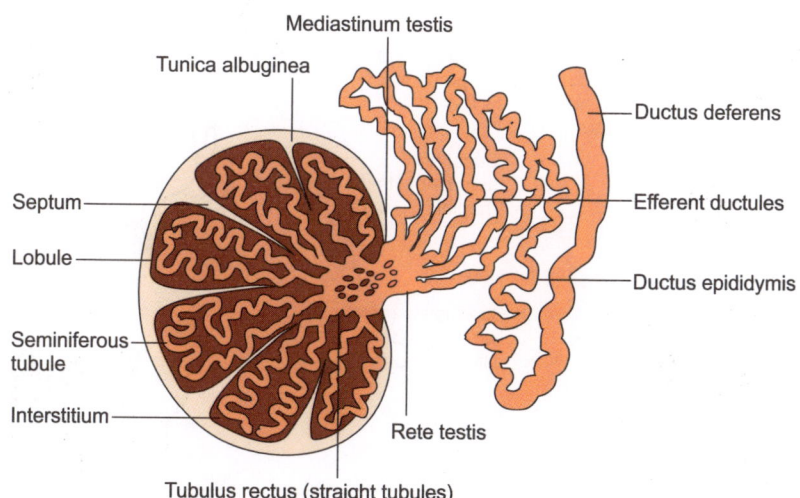

Figure 14.2 Testes.

The seminiferous tubules contain two types of cells: spermatogenic cells and Sertoli cells.

As indicated by the name, spermatogenic cells form sperms, whereas Sertoli cells play several supporting roles in spermatogenesis.

In the spaces between the adjacent seminiferous tubules, there are clusters of Leydig (interstitial) cells that secrete the male sex hormone testosterone (discussed later in the chapter).

Spermatogenesis

The process by which sperms are produced in the seminiferous tubules of the testes is called *spermatogenesis*. In humans, this process takes about 65–75 days.

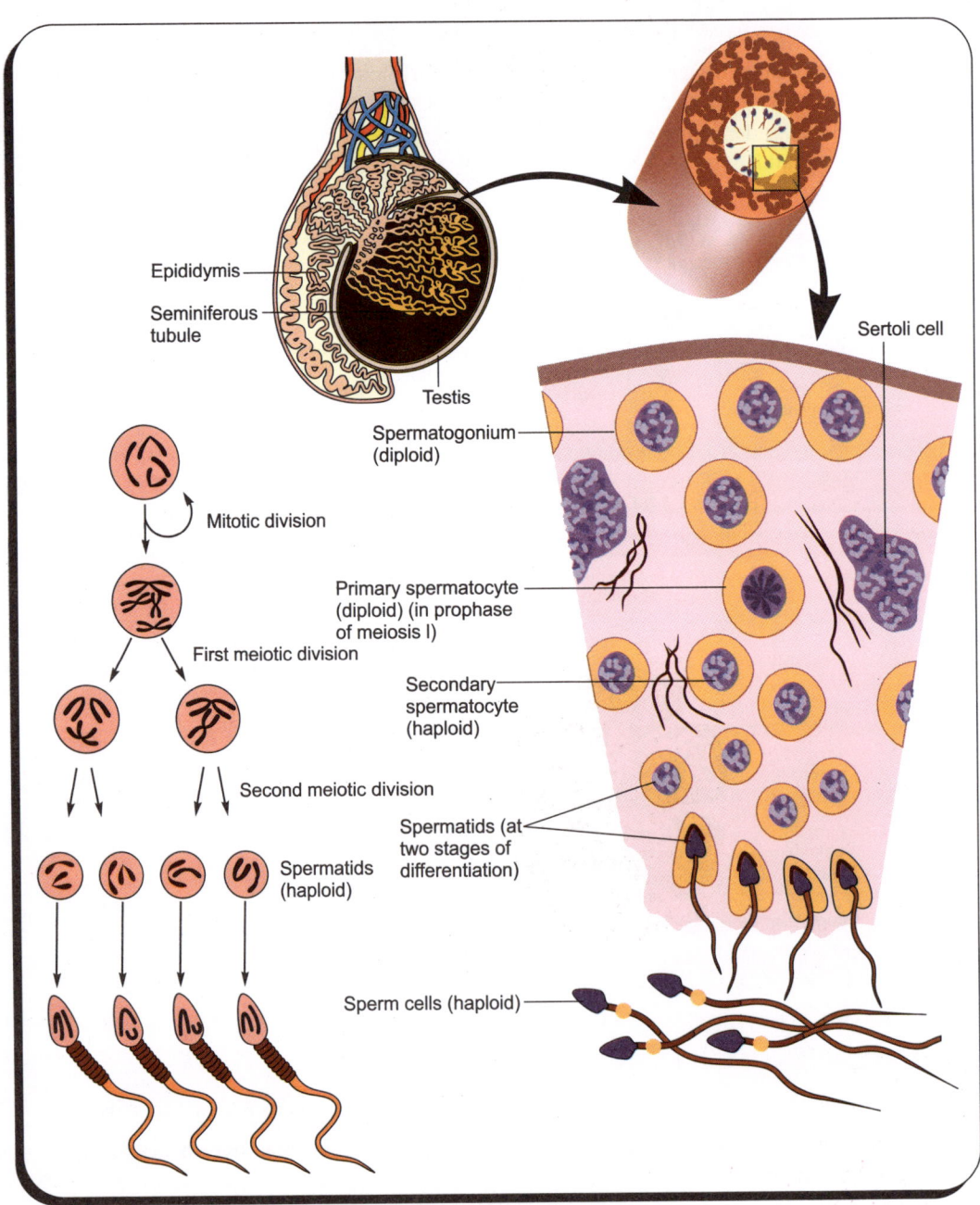

Figure 14.3 Spermatogenesis.

Normal sperm production requires a temperature of about 2–3°C below the normal body temperature, and this temperature is maintained within the scrotum that houses the testes because it is outside the abdominal cavity.

The sperm production begins in the stem cells called *spermatogonia* that line the periphery of the seminiferous tubules. The spermatogonia (diploid) undergo mitotic division to produce the daughter cells called *primary spermatocytes* (diploid) by a process called *spermatocytogenesis*.

The primary spermatocytes undergo first meiotic division (meiosis I) to form secondary spermatocytes (haploid). The secondary spermatocytes then undergo second meiotic division (meiosis II) to form *spermatids* (haploid), and this process is known as *spermatidogenesis*. A primary spermatocyte therefore produces four spermatids through two successive stages of meiosis (meiosis I and meiosis II).

Each spermatid eventually matures into a single sperm/spermatozoa (haploid) by a process called *spermiogenesis*. About 300 million sperm mature each day (Fig. 14.3).

Role of Sertoli cells

As Sertoli cells are in close contact with the developing sperm cells, they support and protect developing sperm cells. They provide and maintain the proper environment required for the development and maturation of the sperm cells.

They secrete testicular fluid (required for sperm transport), androgen-binding protein (required to concentrate testosterone) and secrete the hormone inhibin (a polypeptide hormone that regulates the pituitary gland control of spermatogenesis).

The developed and matured sperm cells are then released in the lumen of the seminiferous tubule by a process called *spermiation*. The fluid secreted by the Sertoli cells helps the sperms move towards ducts.

Sperm (spermatozoa)

Sperms are the male gametes. About 300 million matured sperms are produced every day in a man. Once ejaculated, they can survive only for 48 h in the female reproductive tract.

A human sperm is about 60 μm long and consists of head, middle piece and tail (Fig. 14.4).

❏ **Head** contains the *nucleus* with genetic material (23 chromosomes) and *acrosome*. Acrosome contains enzymes—hyaluronidase and proteinase—that aid the sperm cell in penetrating the secondary oocyte.

❏ **Middle piece** contains spirally arranged *mitochondria* that produce ATP (energy) required for sperm mobility.

❏ **Tail** of the sperm cell is a typical flagellum. The energy derived from ATP produced by the mitochondria helps the tail beat, which propels the sperms to swim up in the female reproductive tract.

Hormonal control of spermatogenesis

The feedback loop that includes the hypothalamus, pituitary gland and testes regulates spermatogenesis and testosterone (androgen) synthesis. Gonadotropin-releasing hormone (GnRH) secreted by the hypothalamus regulates the release of follicle-stimulating hormone (FSH) and luteinizing hormone (LH) from the pituitary, which in turn control the various functions of the testis.

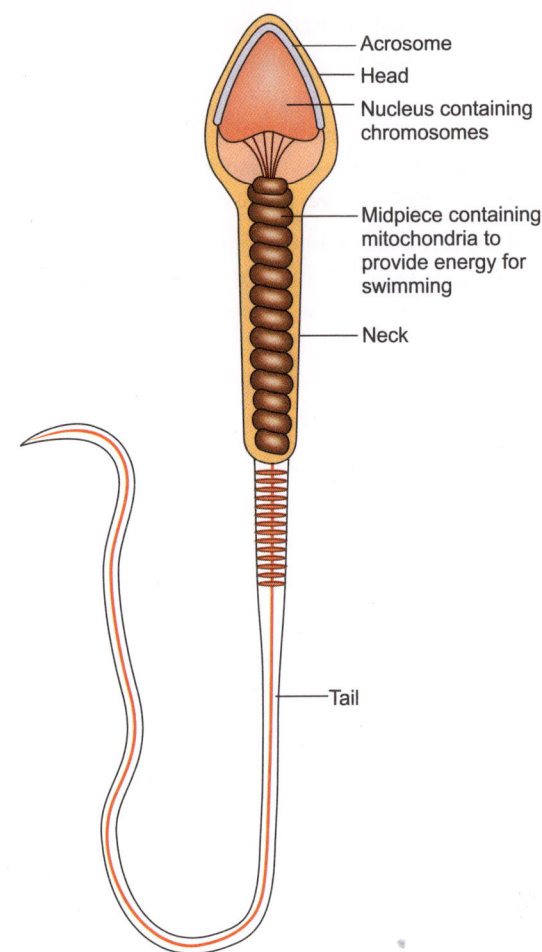

Figure 14.4 A human sperm.

GnRH levels become elevated at the time of puberty, which stimulate the anterior pituitary gland to increase its secretion of the gonadotropic hormones FSH and LH. FSH influences spermatogenesis by acting on Sertoli cells, whereas LH influences testosterone synthesis by stimulating Leydig cells.

A negative feedback system regulates testosterone production (see Fig. 14.5)

If testosterone concentration is very high, it inhibits GnRH production by its action on the hypothalamus, resulting in subsequent reduction in the LH and FSH levels that regulate the testosterone levels in blood.

Testosterone

Testosterone is the male sex hormone secreted by Leydig cells. In some cells such as in prostate gland and seminal vesicles, testosterone is converted to more potent dihydrotestosterone by the action of 5-α-reductase enzyme.

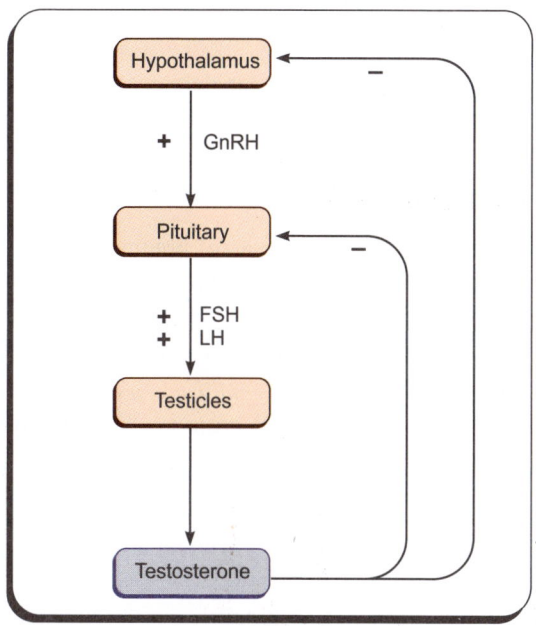

Figure 14.5 Negative feedback regulation of testosterone levels in blood.

Both testosterone and dihydrotestosterone bind to the androgen receptors present inside the nucleus of the target cells and form a *hormone–receptor complex* that regulates gene transcription and as a result, produces several effects.

The effects produced by androgens (testosterone and dihydrotestosterone) on males are as follows:

1. *Prenatal*
   - ❏ Before birth, they regulate the development and growth of male sex organs.
   - ❏ Just before birth, testosterone causes the descent of the testes from the abdominal cavity into the scrotal sac.

2. *Development of male sexual characteristics at puberty*
   - ❏ Promote the enlargement of male sex organs such as enlargement of penis, scrotum and prostate gland
   - ❏ Stimulates the maturation of seminiferous tubules and production of spermatozoa
   - ❏ Stimulates the development of male secondary sexual characteristics including broadening of shoulders; narrowing of hips; development of facial, chest, pubic and axillary hair; deepening of voice; enlargement of larynx; thickening of skin and increased sebaceous (oil) gland secretion.

3. *Development of sexual functions*: Contribute towards male sexual behaviour and stimulate spermatogenesis.

4. *Anabolic effects*: Testosterone promotes growth of muscles and bones and leads to increased muscle mass and strength. It also contributes towards bone density, linear growth of bone and its maturation and results in a marked increase in height and weight.

Chapter 14

DUCTS OF TESTIS

The ducts of testis include the epididymis, the ductus deferens, ejaculatory ducts and urethra. These glands store and transport the sperms.

Epididymis (*plural: epididymides*)

As the sperms are formed and released into the lumen of tightly coiled seminiferous tubules, they are propelled towards the straight tubules present at the tip of each lobule. The straight tubules lead to a network of ducts in the testes called the *rete testis*.

From the rete testis, the sperms are transferred out of the testes through a series of coiled efferent ducts that empty into a single tube known as *ductus epididymis* present in the epididymis. It is a comma-shaped structure about 4 cm in length, located on the posterior side of each testis (Fig. 14.6).

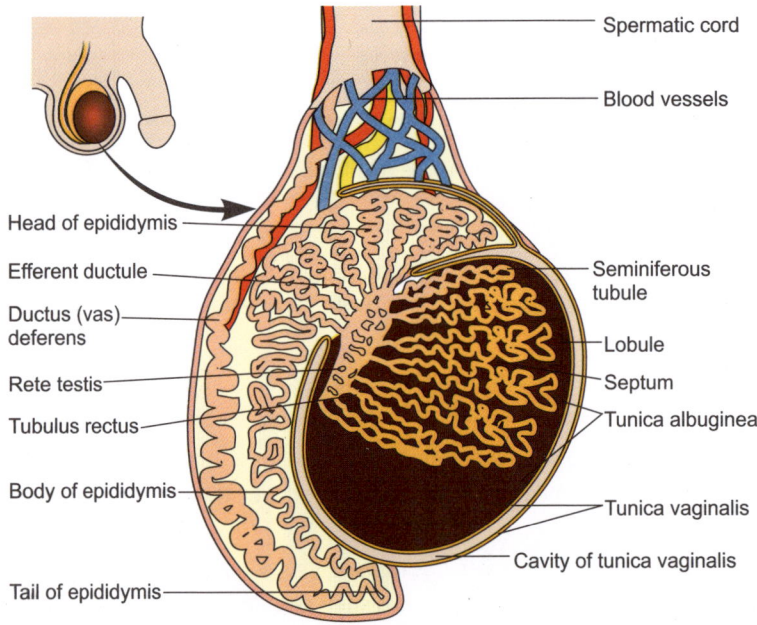

Figure 14.6 Ducts of testes.

Epididymis primarily consists of a tight coiled tube about 20-ft long called the *ductus epididymis* where the sperms continue to mature and acquire both mobility and ability to fertilize secondary oocyte. It takes the sperm about 20 days to move through this tube.

Ductus epididymis is composed of pseudostratified columnar epithelium, surrounded by smooth muscle layer and connective tissue. The sperms are stored in epididymis and the matured sperms are propelled into the vas deferens (ductus deferens) by the contraction of smooth muscles upon sexual stimulation.

Ductus deferens (vas deferens)

At the end of epididymis, the ductus epididymis becomes less convoluted and its diameter increases; at this point, it is referred to as *ductus deferens* or *vas deferens*; it is about 45 cm long.

The ductus deferens is enclosed in a connective tissue sheath along with nerves and blood vessels. This sheath is called *spermatic cord*.

It ascends along the posterior border of the testes, penetrates the inguinal canal and enters the pelvic cavity where it loops over the side and down the posterior surface of the urinary bladder. The end of the ductus deferens has a dilated terminal portion known as the *ampulla*.

Each ductus deferens empties into the ejaculatory duct during sexual stimulation; if not ejaculated, sperms are stored in the vas deferens and reabsorbed upon degeneration.

Ejaculatory ducts

Each ductus deferens joins its ejaculatory duct posterior to the urinary bladder. Each duct is about 2 cm in length.

The ejaculatory duct is formed by the union of the ductus deferens (vas deferens) and duct from seminal vesicles (discussed later).

The ejaculatory duct passes through the prostate gland and ejects sperms into the urethra.

Urethra

In males, the urethra serves as a common passage way for both urine coming from bladder and sperms coming from testes (Fig. 14.7).

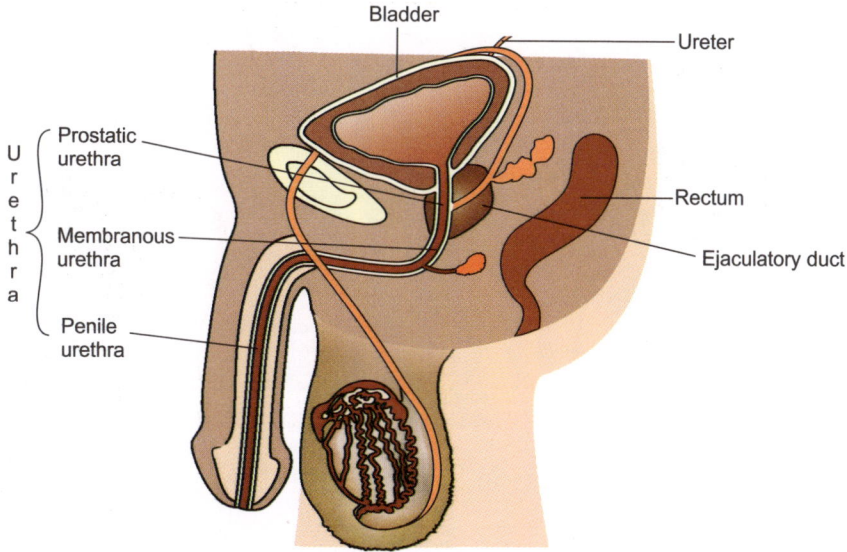

Figure 14.7 Urethra and ejaculatory duct.

It is about 20 cm long and is subdivided into three parts: the prostatic urethra, membranous urethra and spongy or penile urethra.

- ❑ The urethra that originates from the bladder and passes through the prostate gland is called *prostatic urethra*; it is about 2–3 cm long.
- ❑ The urethra that courses from the prostatic urethra to the penis is called *membranous urethra*; it is about 1 cm long.
- ❑ The urethra found in the penis is called *spongy urethra*; it is about 15–20 cm in length but varies according to the size of the penis.

The spongy urethra terminates at the external urethral orifice in the penis.

ACCESSORY GLANDS

The accessory glands include the two seminal vesicles, the prostate gland and the paired bulbourethral glands. These glands secrete the seminal fluid, that is the sperm-containing fluid (Fig. 14.8).

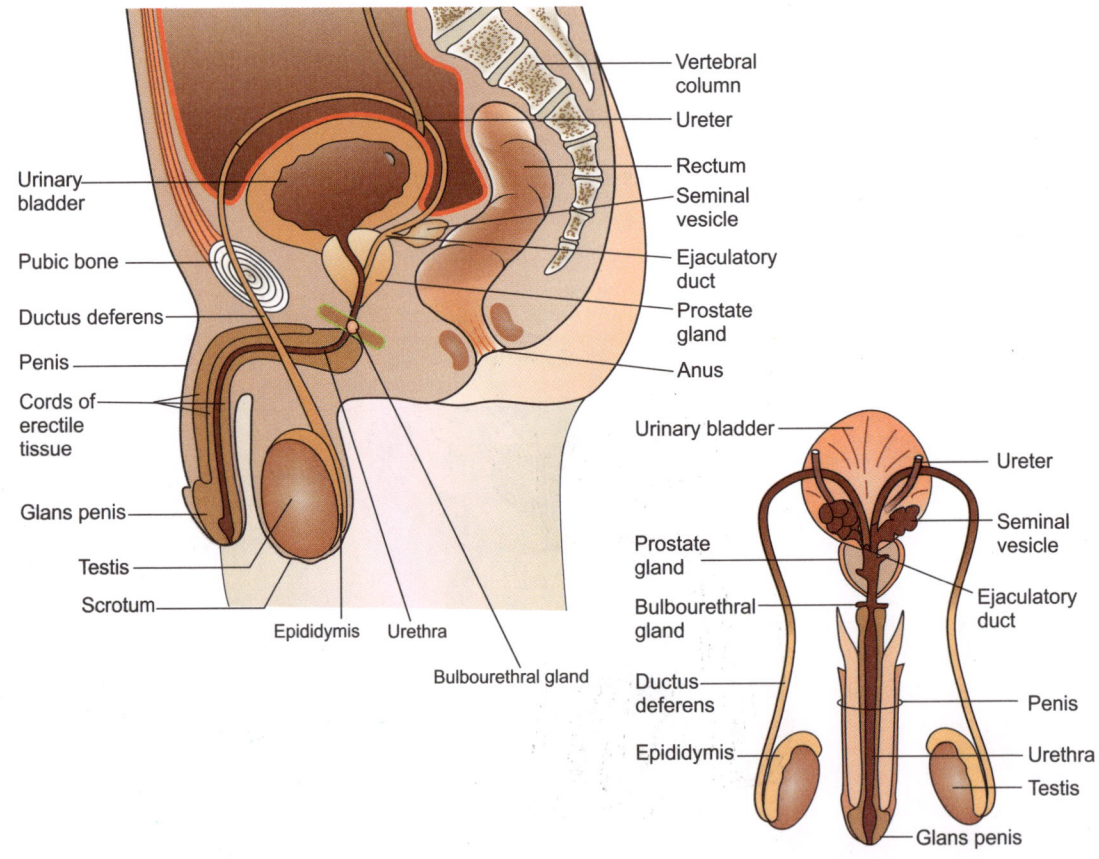

Figure 14.8 The accessory glands.

Seminal vesicles

These are the paired convoluted saclike structures approximately 5 cm in length. They are located posterior to and at the base of the urinary bladder anterior to the rectum.

The seminal vesicles secrete an alkaline, viscous fluid that consists of fructose (used by sperms to derive energy), prostaglandins (provides mobility and viability to sperm) and clotting proteins (coagulate sperms after ejaculation). The alkaline nature of the secretion helps neutralize the acidic environment in the male urethra and female reproductive tract and makes the surroundings amicable for the sperm to fertilize the secondary oocyte.

Fluid secreted by the seminal vesicles constitutes about 60% of the total volume of semen. The duct of seminal vesicle joins the ductus deferens to form the ejaculatory duct on each side; thus, both sperm and seminal fluid enter the urethra during ejaculation.

Prostate gland

Prostate gland is a single doughnut-shaped gland that surrounds the prostatic urethra. It is located inferior to the urinary bladder.

The secretion from the prostate gland is acidic in nature and contains various proteolytic enzymes such as pepsinogen, hyaluronidase, amylase and lysozyme (to break down the clotting proteins secreted by seminal vesicles), citric acid (for ATP production) and certain antibiotics (to kill the bacteria in semen and female reproductive tract).

This secretion constitutes about 25% of the total volume of semen and is responsible for its milky appearance. The secretion enters the prostatic urethra through several small ducts and activates the sperms to swim.

Bulbourethral glands or Cowper's gland

These are the paired pea-shaped glands present inferior to the prostate on either side of the membranous urethra. The ducts of these glands open into spongy urethra.

During sexual stimulation, they secrete an alkaline viscous fluid that neutralizes the traces of acidic urine present in the urethra and protects the sperms as they pass through the urethra. The secretion also acts as a lubricant for sexual intercourse.

Secretion from bulbourethral glands constitutes less than 1% of the total volume of semen.

Semen

Semen, also known as *seminal fluid*, is a mixture of sperms and secretions from seminal vesicles, prostate gland and bulbourethral glands.

It is translucent milky white in appearance and is sticky in nature. The prostrate secretions contribute to its milky appearance, whereas the secretions from Cowper's glands and seminal glands make it sticky in consistency.

The semen has slightly alkaline pH of 7.2–7.7. The volume of semen per ejaculation is about 2.5–5 mL containing about 50–150 millions sperms per millilitre. If the sperm count is below 20 millions/mL of semen, then the person is considered to be sterile.

Once ejaculated, the clotting proteins present in semen coagulate the semen immediately, but after about 10–20 min of ejaculation, the semen re-liquefies due to the action of various proteolytic enzymes present in the semen. The liquefaction of clotted semen makes the sperm free so that it can move upwards through the female reproductive tract.

SUPPORTING STRUCTURES

Penis

Penis is a pendulous structure hanging from the front that functions as a passage for the ejaculation of semen and the excretion of urine.

It is cylindrical in shape and consists of *body, glans penis* and *root*.

The body of penis is composed of three cylindrical masses of erectile tissue and smooth muscles. Each mass of erectile tissue is surrounded by fibrous tissue called *tunica albuginea* and has a rich blood supply. The two dorsolateral masses are called *corpora cavernosa*, whereas the mass between them is called *corpus spongiosum* (Fig. 14.9).

Corpus spongiosum constitutes most of the body of the penis and contains the spongy urethra that keeps urethra open during ejaculation.

The distal end of corpus spongiosum is slightly enlarged, tapered and expanded into a triangular structure called *glans penis*. The margin of glans penis is called *corona*.

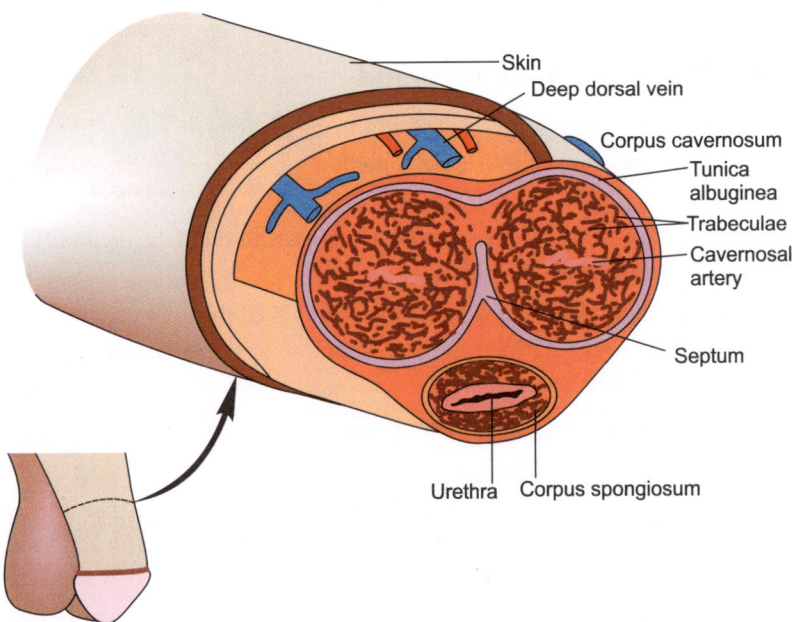

Figure 14.9 Internal structure of the penis.

The glans penis is covered by a loose foreskin called *prepuce*. The surgical removal of the prepuce is called *circumcision*.

The root of penis is triradiate in form and consists of *bulb of penis* and *crura of penis*. The bulb of penis is an expanded part of the base of the corpus spongiosum, whereas the tapered and separated parts of the corpora cavernosa are called crura of penis.

How does penis attain erection?

Upon sexual stimulation, arteries that supply the penis dilate and large quantities of blood begin to enter the blood sinuses (vascular spaces). Expansion of these blood sinuses compresses the veins, which normally drain the penis so that most of the blood is retained in the sinuses. This results in erection, a condition in which the penis becomes enlarged and rigid.

Erection of penis is necessary for coitus, during which the penis delivers the semen into the female reproductive tract (vagina). After the ejaculation, or upon the cessation of sexual stimulation, the arteries supplying the blood constrict and the blood is drained by veins. This results in a loss of erection and flaccid (relaxed) state of penis.

The smooth muscle sphincter present at the base of the urinary bladder remains closed during ejaculation to make sure that urine does not come out with semen and also prevents the entry of semen in the urinary bladder.

Scrotum

The scrotum houses the testes and consists of loose skin and superficial fascia. It appears externally as a single pouch divided into lateral portions by *raphe* (a median ridge), while internally it is divided into two sacs by a *scrotal septum*. Each sac contains a single testis.

As the scrotum lies outside the body cavity, the temperature of the scrotum is about 2–3°C lower than the normal body temperature. This temperature favours the normal production of sperms in testes.

The scrotal septum is composed of dartos muscle (bundles of smooth muscle fibres) and superficial fascia. A small strip of skeletal muscle called *cremaster muscle* is also associated with each testis housed in the scrotum. The temperature of the scrotum is regulated by the contraction of muscle fibres. In cold temperature, the cremaster and dartos muscles contract to bring the testes closer to the body so that they can absorb heat, whereas the reverse happens when exposed to high temperature.

FEMALE REPRODUCTIVE SYSTEM

The female reproductive system consists of the following organs (Fig. 14.10):
- ❏ Ovaries
- ❏ Fallopian/uterine tubes
- ❏ Uterus
- ❏ Vagina
- ❏ Vulva/pudendum/external female genitalia
- ❏ Mammary glands

Chapter 14

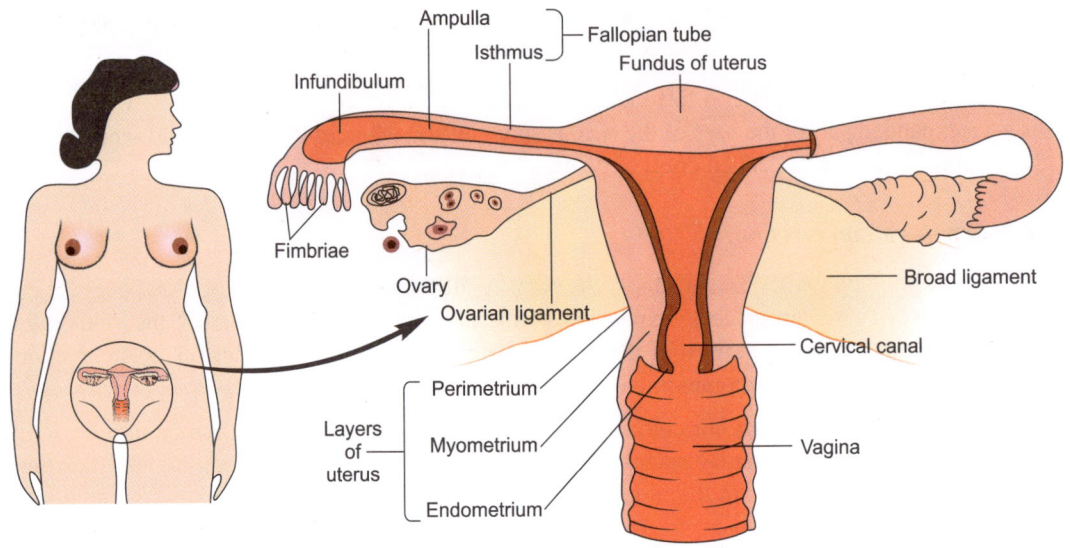

Figure 14.10 Organs of the female reproductive system.

OVARY

Ovaries are the paired oval-shaped structures that produce secondary oocyte (female gamete) and oestrogen and progesterone (female sex hormones).

Ovaries are present in the upper pelvic cavity, one on each side of the uterus. They are held in position by a series of ligaments. The ovarian ligament attaches ovaries to the upper part of the uterus, and the *suspensory ligament* anchors the ovaries to the lateral walls of the pelvis. The broad ligament of the uterus encloses the ovaries by a double-layered fold of peritoneum called the *mesovarium*.

Structure of the ovary

The surface of the ovary is covered by ovarian surface epithelium (previously called *germinal epithelium*). Beneath the germinal epithelium, there is a white capsule of dense irregular connective tissue called *tunica albuginea*. The tunica albuginea encloses an outer area called *ovarian cortex* that consists of ovarian follicles and dense connective tissue with several scattered smooth muscle cells. Beneath the ovarian cortex is the ovarian medulla that consists of connective tissues (loosely arranged), nerves, and blood and lymphatic vessels.

Ovarian follicles are the ova and surrounding tissues going through different stages of development. Each ovarian follicle contains an immature ovum (egg) called *primary follicle*. As the immature ovum gradually develops, it gains an increase in size and shape and develops a central region filled with fluid called *antrum*. At this stage, the follicle is called *secondary follicle* (Fig. 14.11).

When the secondary follicle becomes fully matured containing matured ovum (secondary oocyte), it is called *graafian follicle*. The formation of graafian follicle results in an increased secretion of oestrogen. As a result, the graafian follicle ruptures to release the matured ovum, a process called *ovulation*. During the childbearing years, about every 28 days, one graafian follicle matures, ruptures and releases its ovum into the peritoneal cavity.

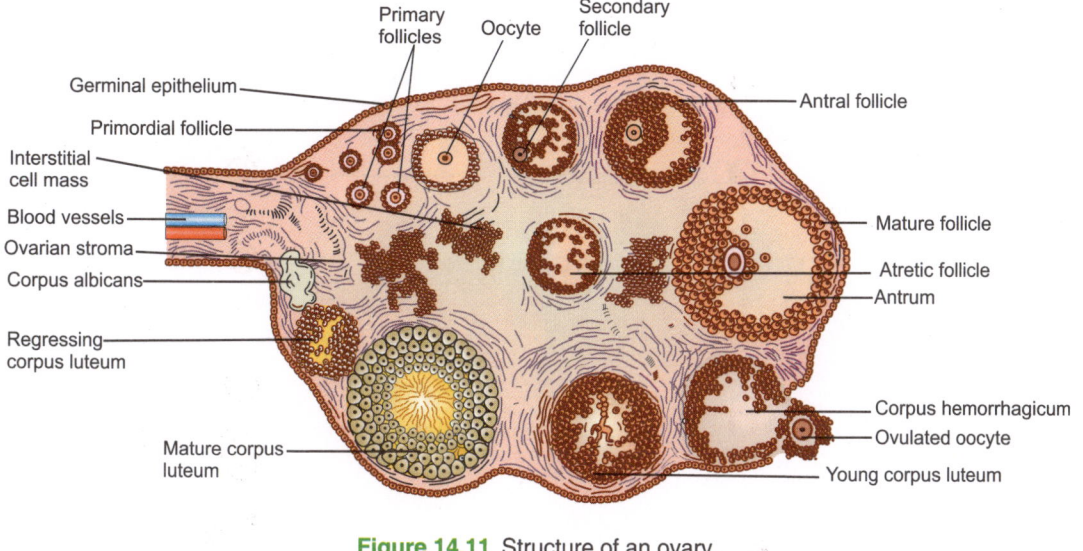

Figure 14.11 Structure of an ovary.

After the matured ovum ruptures out, the ruptured graafian follicle turns into corpus luteum, a yellow-coloured cyst that triggers oestrogen and progesterone secretion and eventually degenerates into corpus albicans, a white-coloured cyst.

Functions of ovary

❑ Production of secondary oocyte (female gamete).
❑ Secretion of oestrogen and progesterone (female sex hormones).

Oogenesis and follicular development

Oogenesis is the process of formation of female gamete (secondary oocyte) in the ovaries. Unlike spermatogenesis in males, which begins at puberty, oogenesis begins in the foetal period (see Fig. 14.12).

Before birth, the primordial germ cells from the yolk sac migrate towards the ovaries and begin to differentiate within the ovaries to form oogonia (diploid). The oogonia divide mitotically to form millions of germ cells, few of which develop into larger cells called *primary oocytes*.

Each primary oocyte is surrounded by a single layer of follicular cells and is called *primordial follicle*. The primary oocytes (diploid) undergo meiosis but remain in prophase I till puberty. Around 700,000 primary oocytes are produced at this time and represent the total number of eggs that a female can produce during her reproductive years.

At puberty, the primordial follicles begin to grow under the influence of FSH and LH and develop into *primary follicles*. Only a small number of primary follicles grow and develop further, and only about 450 eggs will be produced from the store of 700,000 primary oocytes through the process of meiosis.

Chapter 14

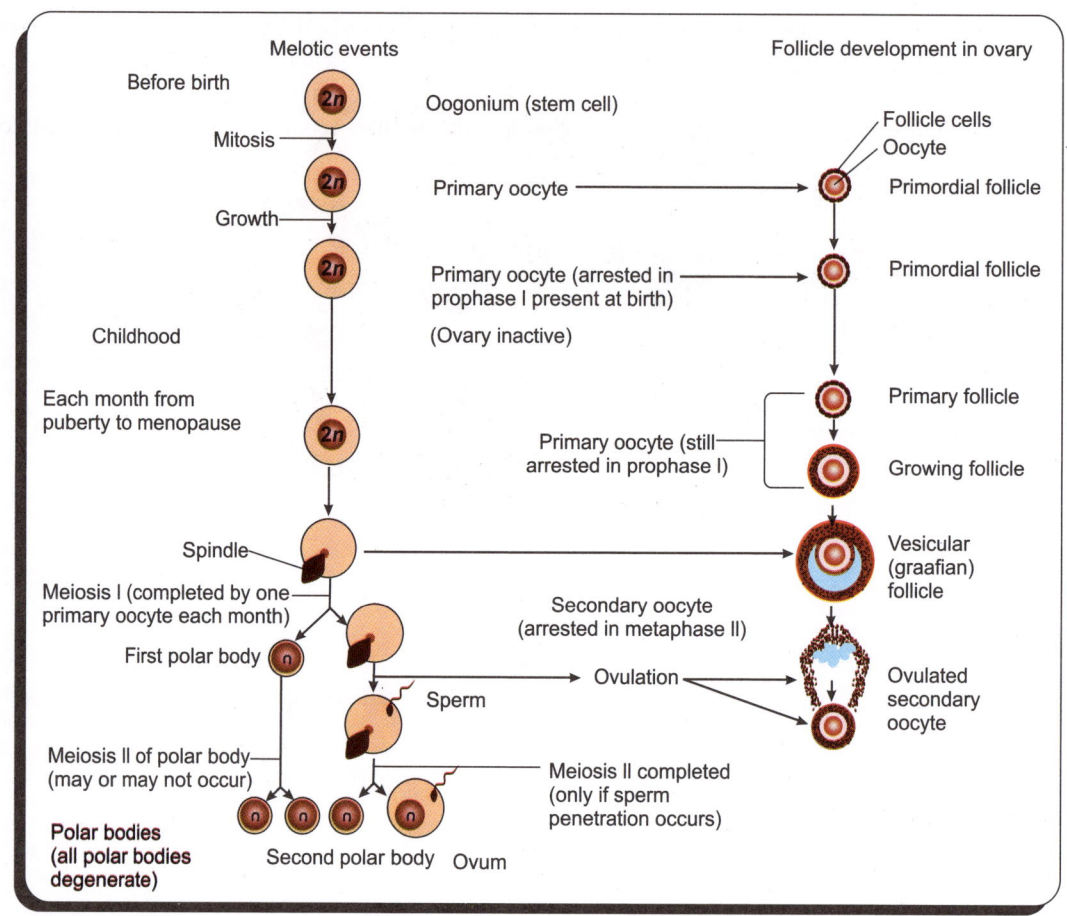

Figure 14.12 Oogenesis and follicular development.

As the primary follicles grow, the follicular cells surrounding the primary oocyte form several layers and are now referred to as *granulosa cells*. Furthermore, a layer of glycoproteins begins to appear between the granulosa cells and primary oocyte called as *zona pellucida* that eventually attaches to the innermost layer of granulosa cells and is called the *corona radiata*.

As the primary follicle continues to grow, a region called *theca folliculi* appears and encircles the outermost granulosa cells. Eventually, theca folliculi begins to differentiate into an internal thick layer, theca interna, and an outer layer of connective tissue cells, theca externa. At this stage, the granulosa cells start secreting the follicular fluid that develops into a cavity at the centre called *antrum* and this structure is now termed as the *secondary follicle*.

As the secondary follicle begins to turn into tertiary/matured/graafian follicle, the primary oocyte completes meiosis I to form the secondary oocyte (haploid) and first polar body (containing discarded nuclear material). If the first polar body undergoes another division, then the primary oocyte gives rise to three polar bodies and a haploid secondary oocyte.

As soon as the secondary oocyte is produced, it undergoes meiosis II but stops at the metaphase stage. At this stage, the theca interna and theca externa become crescent shaped and the secondary oocyte becomes eccentric within the graafian follicle. The granulosa cells protrude into cavity and form cumulus oophores. Eventually, the graafian follicle ruptures and the secondary oocyte is released into the pelvic cavity, a process known as *ovulation*.

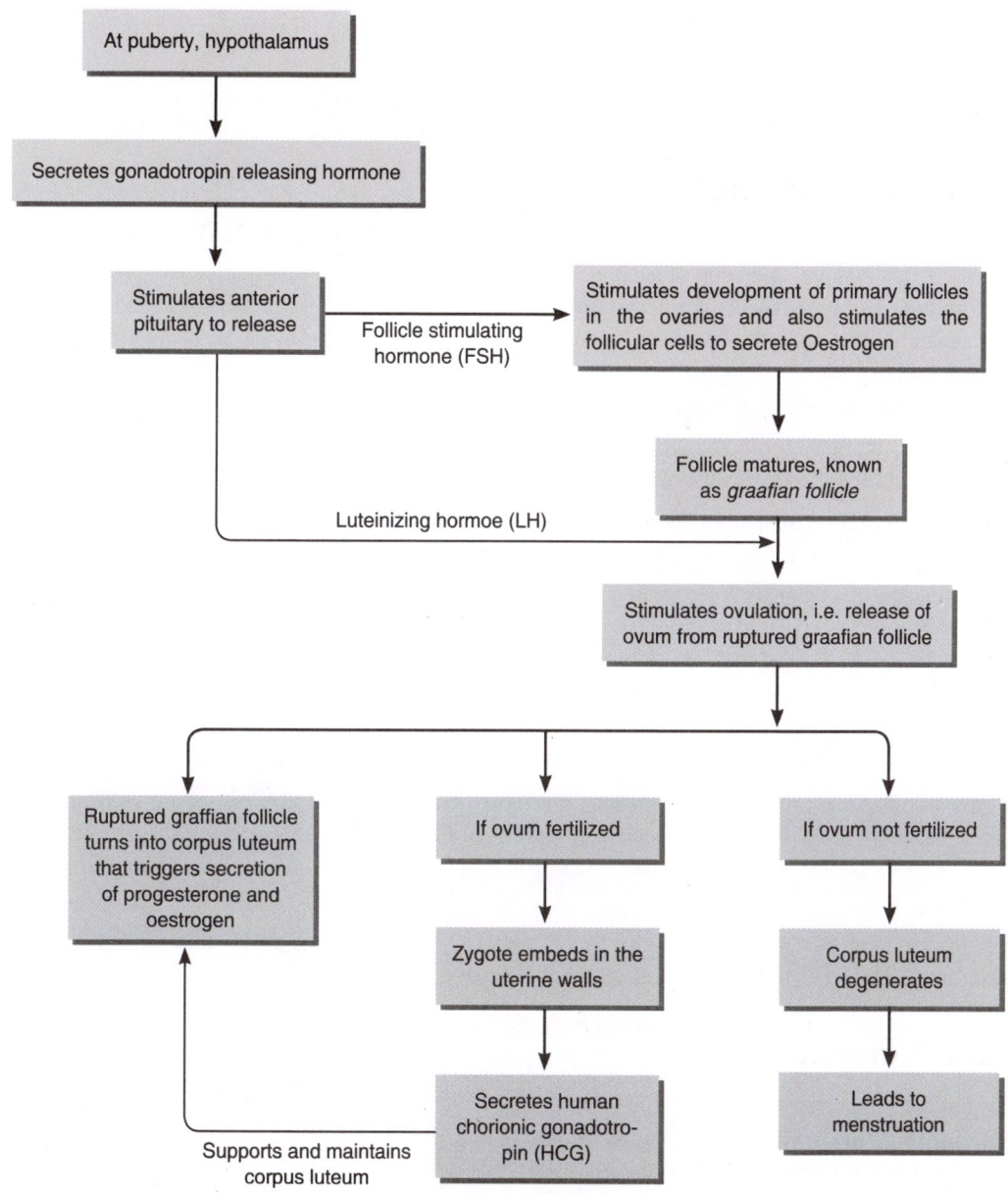

Figure 14.13 Hormonal changes that take place in ovary after puberty.

If the sperms are present in the uterine tube and one of them succeeds in penetrating the secondary oocyte, fertilization occurs. After fertilization the secondary oocyte resumes meiosis II and splits into two haploid cells:

❏ Mature egg or ovum is the larger one. The nuclei of ovum and sperm undergo fusion to form fertilized ovum/zygote.

❏ Second polar body (degenerates in the uterine tubes) is the smaller one.

Thus, one oogonium gives rise to a single gamete (ovum), a large cell whereas one spermatogonium produces four gametes (sperm).

Figure 14.13 shows the hormonal changes that take place in ovary after puberty.

FALLOPIAN/UTERINE TUBES

Uterine tubes are paired tubular structures about 10 cm long that extend from the sides of the uterus. There is a funnel-shaped open end of each uterine tube called *infundibulum*, lying close to the ovary. The infundibulum ends with finger-like projections called *fimbirae*, one of which is attached to the ovary. Approximately once a month, an ovum ruptures from the surface of an ovary near the infundibulum, a process called *ovulation*.

From the infundibulum, the uterine tube extends medially and then inferiorly to form the longest and widest part of the uterine tube called *ampulla*. From the ampulla, the uterine tube becomes thick and narrow and gets attached to the uterus by a portion called *isthmus*.

The walls of uterine tube are made of the following three layers of tissue: *mucosa*, which is the inner layer; *muscularis*, which is the middle layer; and *serosa*, which is the outer layer.

❏ The mucosal layer consists of ciliated and nonciliated columnar epithelial cells. The ciliated cells help transport the fertilized ovum through uterine tube to uterus, whereas the nonciliated cells having microvilli secrete a fluid that serves to provide nutrition to the fertilized ovum.

❏ The muscularis layer is composed of inner circular smooth muscles (thicker) and outer longitudinal smooth muscles (thinner).

❏ Serosa is the outermost layer.

The movements of the fimbriae around the ovary sweep the secondary oocyte into the uterine tubes. The secondary oocyte or fertilized ovum is then moved along the uterine tube by the contraction of the smooth muscles of muscularis along with the ciliary action of mucosa towards the uterus.

Fertilization can occur at any time up to 24 h after ovulation and usually occurs in the ampulla of uterine tubes. The fertilized ovum takes about 6–7 days to reach the uterus.

Functions of uterine tubes

❏ Sweep the secondary oocyte towards the uterus
❏ Provide route to sperms to reach the secondary oocyte and thus aid in fertilization
❏ Transport the fertilized ovum into the uterus

UTERUS OR WOMB

Uterus is a hollow muscular pear-shaped organ located in the pelvic cavity between the urinary bladder and the rectum. It measures about 7.5 cm × 5 cm × 2.5 cm in dimensions, if not pregnant. The uterus enlarges if the female is pregnant, whereas it becomes smaller after menopause.

The uterus is the implantation site of the fertilized ovum and also acts as the pathway for the sperm to reach the uterine tube. It also serves as site for the discharge of menstrual fluid during the female reproductive cycle.

Anatomically, the uterus can be divided into fundus, body and cervix.

❑ The dome-shaped part superior to the uterine tube forms the *fundus* of the uterus.
❑ The slightly tapered central portion forms the *body* of the uterus.
❑ The narrow inferior portion that opens into the vagina is called the *cervix* (Fig. 14.14).

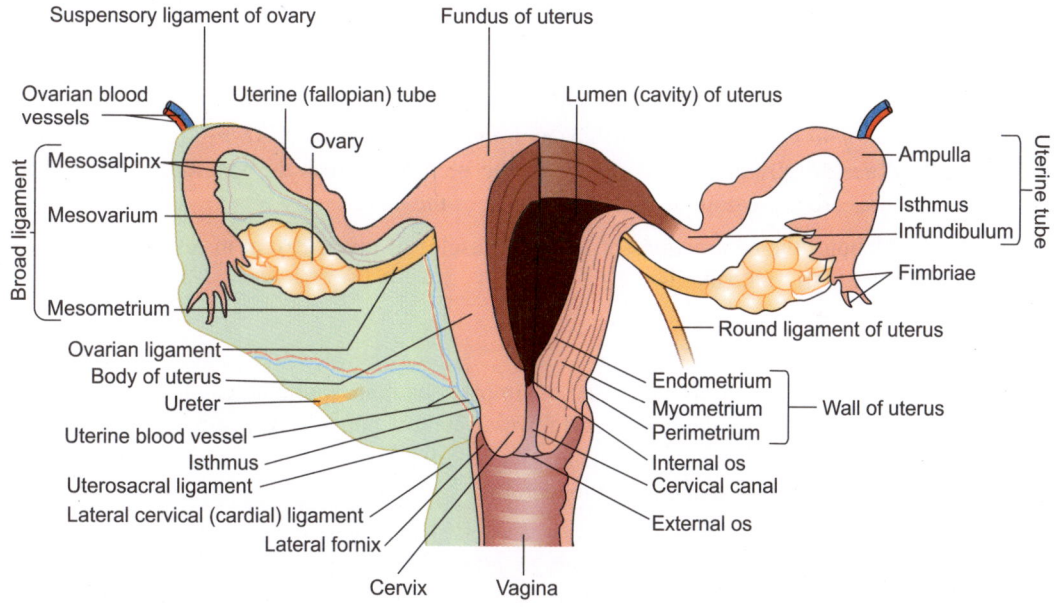

Figure 14.14 The uterus.

Between the body of the uterus and the cervix is the constricted portion called *isthmus*. The interior of the body of the uterus is known as the *uterine cavity*, whereas the interior of the cervix is known as the *cervical canal*. The junction of uterine cavity with the cervical canal is called the *internal os* and the opening of the cervix into the vagina is called the *external os*.

The uterus is held in position by a series of ligaments. It is attached to the either side of the pelvic cavity by *paired broad ligaments* and to the sacrum by the *uterosacral ligaments*. These ligaments serve to maintain uterus in the *anteflexed* position.

Histology of the uterus

The walls of uterus are composed of the three layers of tissue: *endometrium*, which is the inner layer; *myometrium*, which is the middle layer; and *perimetrium*, which is the outer layer.

Endometrium

It is the highly vascularized innermost layer. This layer is composed of the following:

❑ An innermost layer of *simple columnar epithelium* (composed of ciliated and secretory cells), followed by *lamina propria* (composed of areolar connective tissue) and the outermost *endometrial (uterine) glands* (formed as infolding of the luminal epithelium and present near the myometrium).

Endometrium can be functionally divided into two layers: *stratum functionalis* and *stratum basalis*. The stratum functionalis is the upper layer that forms the lining of the uterine cavity and this layer is shed during menstruation. The stratum basalis is the permanent basal layer that is not lost during menstruation. It is the layer from which the new stratum functionalis is formed after each menstruation.

Myometrium

It is the middle layer composed of three types of smooth muscle fibres: *circular smooth muscle fibres* (thick), *longitudinal smooth muscle fibres* (thin) and *oblique smooth muscle fibres* (thin). The circular smooth muscle fibres are present in the fundus of the uterus, whereas the longitudinal and oblique smooth muscle fibres are present in the body and cervix of the uterus.

At the time of labour, the contractions of smooth muscles of myometrium in response to oxytocin help expel out the fetus from the uterus.

Perimetrium

It is the outermost layer of the uterus composed of simple squamous epithelium and areolar connective tissue. Anteriorly, it extends over the fundus and forms a shallow pouch called *vesicouterine pouch* that covers the urinary bladder. Posteriorly, it extends over the fundus, body and cervix and forms a deep pouch called *rectouterine pouch* that covers the rectum.

The secretory cells of cervical mucosa secrete *cervical mucus*, which is a mixture of glycoproteins, lipids, inorganic salts, water and enzymes. About 20–60 mL of cervical mucus is secreted by a woman per day during her reproductive years. Cervical mucus provides the hospitable environment to the sperms at/near ovulation owing to its alkaline pH and also capacitates sperm to beat its tail more forcefully.

Functions of Uterus

❑ Serves as the implantation site of the fertilized egg
❑ Nourishes and protects the fertilized egg
❑ Powerful rhythmic contractions in the uterus help expel the baby during labour.

VAGINA

Vagina is a fibromuscular tube about 10-cm long present between the urinary bladder and the rectum. It acts as the receptacle for the penis during sexual intercourse and provides a passageway for menstrual flow and for childbirth.

Histologically, the vagina consists of three tissue layers: outer covering of *areolar connective tissue*, a middle layer of *smooth muscle* and an inner lining of *stratified squamous epithelium*. These tissue layers are present in the form of a series of transverse folds called *rugae* that contain large stores of glycogen. The glycogen produces organic acid on decomposition and thus is responsible for the acidic environment in the vagina. This acidic environment inhibits the growth of the microorganisms that may enter the vagina from the perineum.

There is a recess called *fornix* that surrounds the vaginal attachment to the cervix. The external vaginal opening is partially covered by a membrane called the *hymen*.

Functions of vagina

❏ Serves as the receptacle for the penis during sexual intercourse
❏ Provides a passageway for menstrual flow and for childbirth

VULVA OR EXTERNAL FEMALE GENITALIA

The external female genitalia comprises all the organs that are external to the vagina and includes mons pubis, labia majora, labia minora, clitoris, urethral orifice, vaginal orifice and vestibular glands.

Mons pubis

Mons pubis is an elevation of adipose tissue situated directly over the pubic symphysis. It becomes covered with pubic hair at puberty.

Labia majora

Labia majora are the two longitudinal folds of skin, extending posteriorly and exteriorly from the mons pubis. These folds are also covered with pubic hair and are composed of adipose tissue and a large number of sebaceous glands. It is homologous to the scrotum in males.

Labia minora

Labia minora are the two smaller folds of skin present between the labia majora. They do not have pubic hair but contain large number of sebaceous glands and few sudoriferous glands. It is homologous to the spongy urethra in males.

The region between the labia minora is the *vestibule*. The vagina, urethra and ducts of greater vestibular glands open into the vestibule.

Clitoris

Clitoris is a small, cylindrical mass of erectile tissue and sensory nerve endings present at the anterior junction of labia minora. A layer of skin called the *prepuce* or *foreskin* is formed at the point where labia minora join and cover the clitoris. It is homologous to the male penis.

Urethral and vaginal orifices

The *vaginal orifice* is the opening of the vagina to the exterior, whereas the *urethral orifice* is the opening of the urethra to the exterior. Both these orifices are located in the vestibule.

Vestibular glands

On either side of the urethral orifice are Skene's or lesser vestibular glands that secrete mucus that are homologous to the prostate glands in males. On either side of the vaginal orifice are the Bartholin's or greater vestibular glands, which are homologous to the Cowper's glands in males and also secrete mucus.

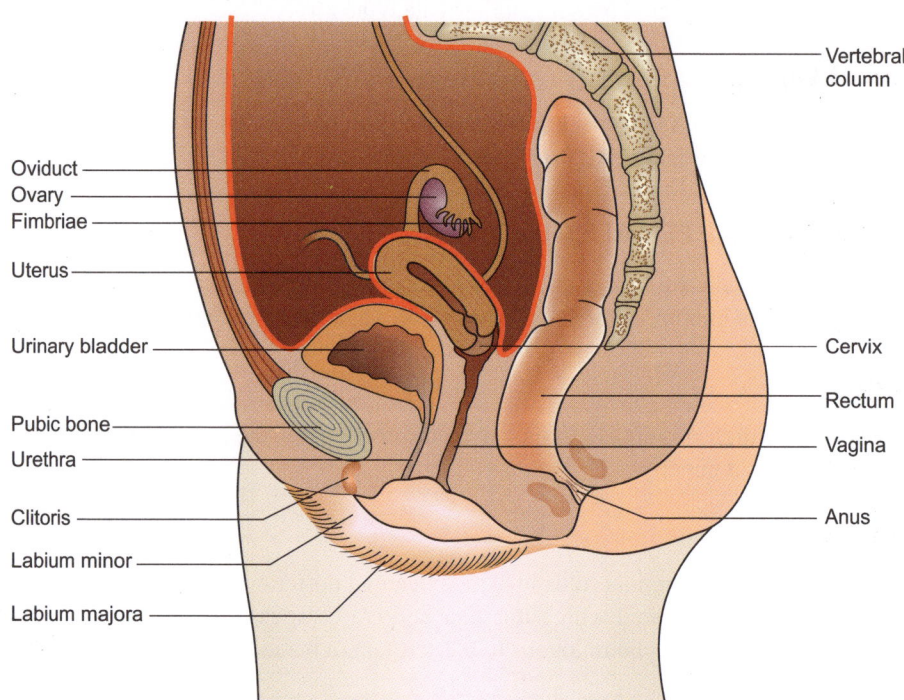

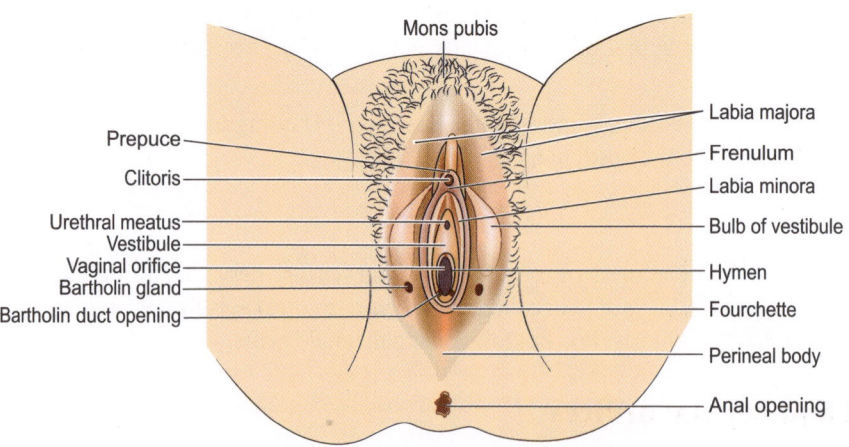

Figure 14.15 Vulva.

The mucus secreted by the vestibular gland provides lubrication at the time of sexual arousal and intercourse.

Perineum is the diamond-shaped region that covers the buttocks and thighs of both male and female and contains the external genitalia and anus. It can be divided into: anterior urogenital triangle that contains vulva and posterior anal triangle that contains the anus (Fig. 14.15).

MAMMARY GLANDS OR BREASTS

Mammary glands are modified sudoriferous glands present in both males and females, but these are functionally active only in females. They serve to produce milk for the nourishment of the infant.

In females, the breasts are small and immature till puberty. Thereafter, oestrogen and progesterone trigger an increase in the size of mammary glands, and during pregnancy, these hormones stimulate further growth of these glands.

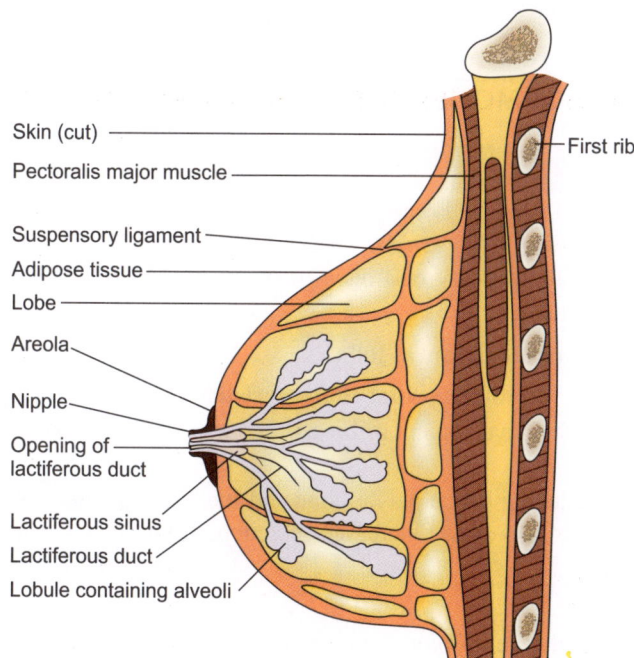

Figure 14.16 Mammary gland.

Structure of mammary glands

Each mammary gland comprises 15–20 *lobes* of glandular tissue separated by adipose tissue. In each lobe, there are several smaller compartments called *lobules* that contain milk-secreting glands called *alveoli glands*. These alveolar glands are surrounded by myoepithelial cells that undergo contraction to propel milk towards a series of secondary tubules and then into the mammary ducts. The mammary ducts expand near the nipple to form lactiferous sinuses where the milk is stored. These sinuses continue as lactiferous ducts that terminate in the nipple (Fig. 14.16).

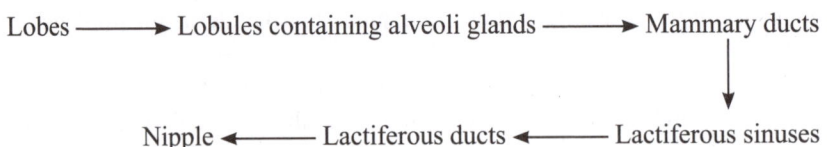

The circular pigmented projection of the breast is called nipple. The circular pigmented area around the nipple is known as areola. The breasts are supported by suspensory ligaments of the breast (Cooper's ligament) that are present between the skin and the deep fascia.

Functions of mammary glands

❑ They serve to synthesize, secrete and eject the milk—a process called *lactation*. Prolactin along with oestrogen and progesterone stimulates the milk production.

❑ The milk ejection is related to pregnancy and childbirth and is stimulated by oxytocin, released in response of sucking of nipple by infant.

ROLE OF DIFFERENT HORMONES IN THE FEMALE REPRODUCTIVE SYSTEM

Oestrogen

Oestrogen is the primary female sex hormone. Human female contains three different oestrogens in significant quantities: *estrone (E1)*, *estradiol (E2)* and *estriol (E3)*. Estrone is produced during menopause, while estriol is the primary oestrogen of pregnancy. Estradiol is the predominant form produced in nonpregnant females.

The different functions of oestrogen are as follows:

1. **Development of female secondary sexual characteristics**
   ❑ Oestrogen promotes the development of breasts and appearance of pubic hair and axillary hair at puberty.
   ❑ Oestrogen causes widening of the pelvic bone and increased adipose tissue deposition around the breasts and hips. It also causes increased secretions from oil and sweat glands that result in acne and body odour.

2. **Other functions**
   ❑ Oestrogen promotes the development and maintenance of female reproductive structures. It stimulates the endometrium growth of the uterus, causing the thickening of the vaginal wall. It also increases the vaginal lubrication during sexual intercourse.
   ❑ It increases protein anabolism and lowers blood cholesterol level.

3. **Role of oestrogen in the menstrual cycle**: It is discussed in the section Menstrual Cycle.

Progesterone

Progesterone is an important female sex hormone involved in the female menstrual cycle, pregnancy (supports gestation) and embryogenesis.

Progesterone is also known as the *hormone of pregnancy* as it plays the following important roles related to gestation:

❏ It turns the endometrium to its secretory stage, thus preparing the uterus for implantation. During implantation and gestation, it reduces the maternal immune response so as to allow the acceptance of pregnancy and also causes a decrease in the contraction of the uterine smooth muscles.

❏ During pregnancy, it prepares the breasts to secrete milk but inhibits lactation. Decrease in the levels of progesterone facilitates the onset of labour and also triggers milk production post delivery.

❏ In case pregnancy does not occur, the level of progesterone falls, leading to menstruation.

Relaxin

In both pregnant and nonpregnant females, relaxin is produced during each menstrual cycle by the corpus luteum. It relaxes the uterus and inhibits the contraction of uterine smooth muscles that facilitates implantation of the fertilized ovum if pregnancy occurs.

During pregnancy, relaxin is produced by the placenta, which continues to relax the uterus. During labour, it softens the symphysis pubis and dilates the cervix to ease delivery.

Inhibin

Inhibin is secreted by granulosa cells of the ovarian follicles and by the corpus luteum of the ovary. It suppresses FSH secretion.

MENSTRUAL CYCLE

The menstrual cycle refers to the series of events or physiological changes that occur in the ovaries and uterine walls of females during their reproductive years. The average duration of menstrual cycle is about 28 days, but it may vary from 24 to 35 days depending on the individual.

The first menstruation of a woman is called *menarche*, and it occurs between 10 and 14 years. The cessation of the menstrual cycle of a woman is called the *menopause* and this occurs between the ages of 45 and 55 years.

The menstrual cycle is divided into the following four different phases (Fig. 14.17):

❏ Menstrual phase
❏ Preovulatory phase
❏ Ovulation
❏ Luteal/postovulatory phase

Menstrual phase

Menstrual phase is also called as *menstruation* or *menses*, and it usually occupies the first five days of the cycle.

This phase occurs if fertilization does not occur and the corpus luteum starts to degenerate. The degeneration of the corpus luteum results in decreased levels of oestrogen and progesterone, and thus the uterine lining, which is dependent on high levels of these hormones, is shed during menstruation. (If fertilization occurs, the developing embryo secretes *human chorionic gonadotropin (hCG)* that protects the corpus luteum from degeneration and sustains its secretion of progesterone and oestrogen. These hormones maintain the uterine lining and prevent menstruation).

Chapter 14

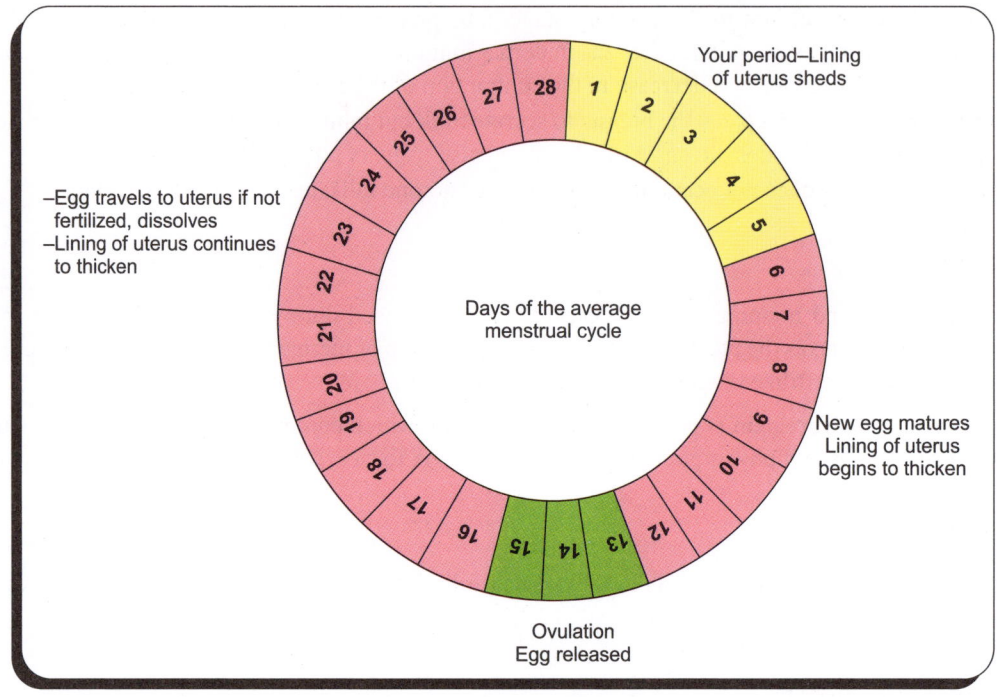

Figure 14.17 Menstrual cycle.

In this phase, stratum functionalis, which is the thickened uterine lining formed in the anticipation of the implantation of the fertilized ovum, sloughs off and discharges in the form of menstrual fluid from the vagina. The menstrual fluid contains blood (50–150 mL), endometrial cells, mucus and tissue fluid.

After degeneration of the corpus luteum, the declining levels of oestrogen and progesterone stimulate the release of GnRH from the hypothalamus. GnRH signals the pituitary gland to release FSH that stimulates the development of follicles in the ovary. This development begins from the first day of this phase (i.e. the first day of bleeding).

Preovulatory phase

Preovulatory phase is the phase between menstruation and ovulation. It is more variable in length and lasts from day 6 to day 14 in a 28-day cycle.

During this phase, about 5–20 follicles, each containing an immature ovum (egg), continue to develop and begin to secrete oestrogen. Although a number of follicles begin to develop during each cycle, only one attains maturity and becomes the mature or Graafian follicle. The Graafian follicle continues to secrete oestrogen that stimulates the thickening of the uterine lining (formation of the new stratum functionalis) and signals the pituitary to decrease the secretion of FSH (Fig. 14.18).

Oestrogen continues to rise till it triggers the release of LH from the anterior pituitary gland.

The menstrual phase and the preovulatory phase are collectively termed as the *follicular phase* because the follicles grow and develop in these phases.

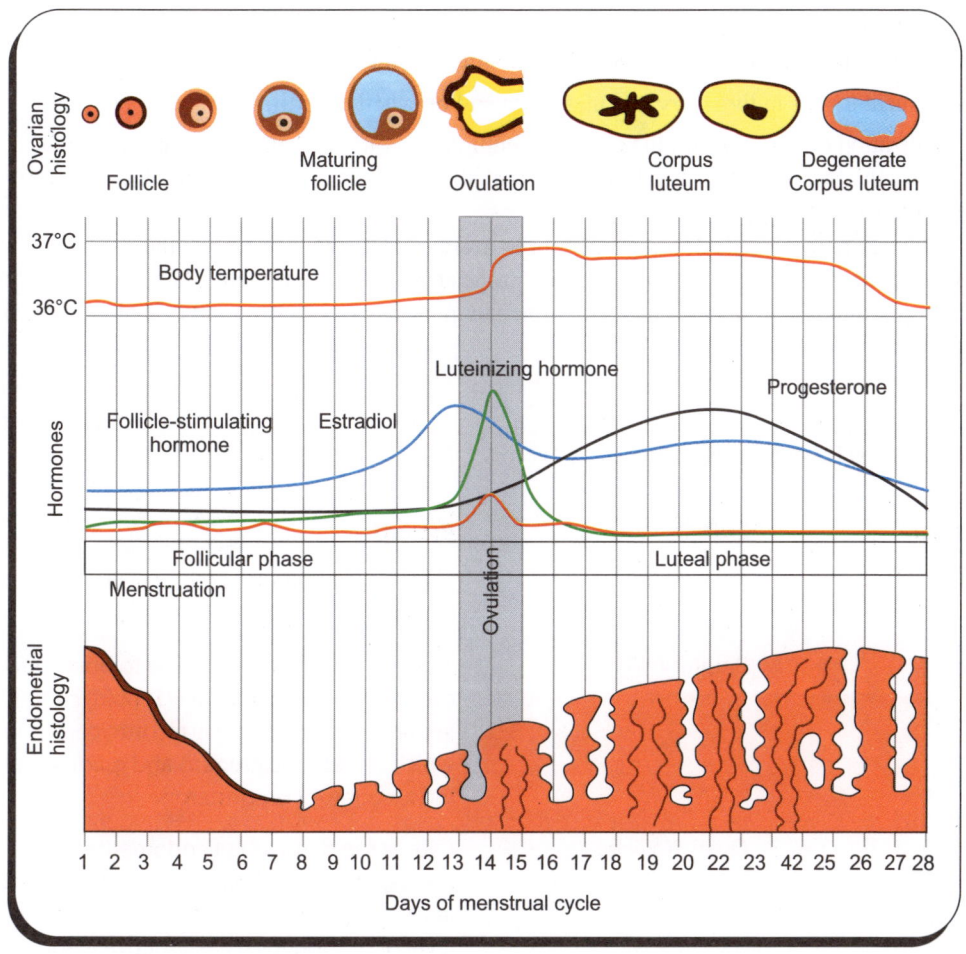

Figure 14.18 Levels of various female hormones during different stages of the menstrual cycle.

Ovulation

Ovulation usually occurs on the 14th day of the 28-day menstrual cycle. The LH surge produced in the preovulatory phase ruptures the Graafian follicle. This releases the secondary oocyte from the ovary, a process called *ovulation*.

Luteal/postovulatory phase

The postovulatory phase is the most constant phase in duration. It lasts for 14 days, from day 15 to day 28 in the 28-day menstrual cycle. It represents the time between ovulation and beginning of a new menstrual cycle.

During this phase, the continued secretion of LH stimulates the ruptured Graafian follicle to develop into a yellow-coloured cyst called the corpus luteum, which begins to secrete progesterone and some oestrogen. The progesterone prepares the endometrium to receive a fertilized ovum by developing glandular structures and blood vessels and thickening the endometrium.

Subsequent events in the ovary and uterus depend on whether fertilization occurs or not.

❑ If fertilization does not occur, the corpus luteum degenerates into the corpus albicans after 2 weeks. As a result, the hormonal levels decline and this initiates a new menstrual cycle starting with menstruation.

❑ If fertilization occurs, the developing embryo secretes hCG, which protects the corpus luteum from degeneration and sustains its secretion of progesterone and oestrogen. These hormones maintain the uterine lining and prevent menstruation. The presence of hCG in mother's blood or urine is an indicator of pregnancy (Table 14.1).

Table 14.1 Effect of hormones on menstrual cycle

Hormone	Source	Actions
GnRH	Hypothalamus	Stimulates pituitary to secrete FSH and LH above a basal level
LH	Pituitary	Surge of LH stimulates follicle to break open and discharge ovum and follicular fluid (containing estrogens); follicle converted into corpus luteum, which secretes oestrogens and gradually increasing amounts of progesterone
Oestrogens	Ovary (follicle)	Causes rapid growth of endomentrium of uterus; causes the breast sensitivity that often accompanies menstrual flow to disappear; rising level of oestrogens have negative feedback effect on hypothalamus and GnRH; GnRH output reduced, and secretion of FSH and LH inhibited; very high level of oestrogens reverses effect on hypothalamus, stimulating it to suddenly release large dose of GnRH; GnRH causes pituitary to release sudden surge of FSH and LH
Progesterone	Ovary (corpus luteum)	Causes endometrium to become thick, spongy, glandular, and receptive to a fertilized ovum (zygote); causes breast engorgement (may be sensitive or painful); has a negative feedback on pituitary; causing a drop in LH production, which results in the degeneration of the corpus luteum and a drop in progesterone and oestrogen production; lack of progesterone initiates menstrual flow

PREGNANCY, EMBRYONIC DEVELOPMENT AND PARTURITION

Pregnancy is a sequence of events that includes fertilization, implantation, embryonic development (first 8 weeks), fetal development (9th week till birth) and parturition.

Fertilization

A secondary oocyte is viable for about 24 hours after ovulation, whereas the sperms remain viable in the vagina for about 48 hours after ejaculation. For fertilization to occur, sexual intercourse must occur between a 3-day window, that is from 2 days before ovulation to 1 day after ovulation.

The process leading to fertilization begins when the sperm cells swim upwards through the vagina and uterine tube by movements of their tails. Although hundreds of sperms surround the ovum and undergo acrosomal reaction (i.e. release the enzymes to penetrate the ovum), only the first sperm cell to penetrate the plasma membrane of the ovum fuses with it to produce a fertilized ovum or *zygote*. This process is called fertilization and it normally occurs in the upper portion of the uterine tube. The time span from fertilization to birth is termed as the gestation period (Fig. 14.19).

As the zygote moves down the uterine tube towards the uterine cavity, it undergoes a series of rapid mitotic divisions, resulting in a hollow ball-like mass of cells called *blastula* or *blastocyst*. The blastocyst has an outer covering of cells called the *trophoblast*, an *inner cell mass* and an internal fluid-filled cavity called the *blastocele*.

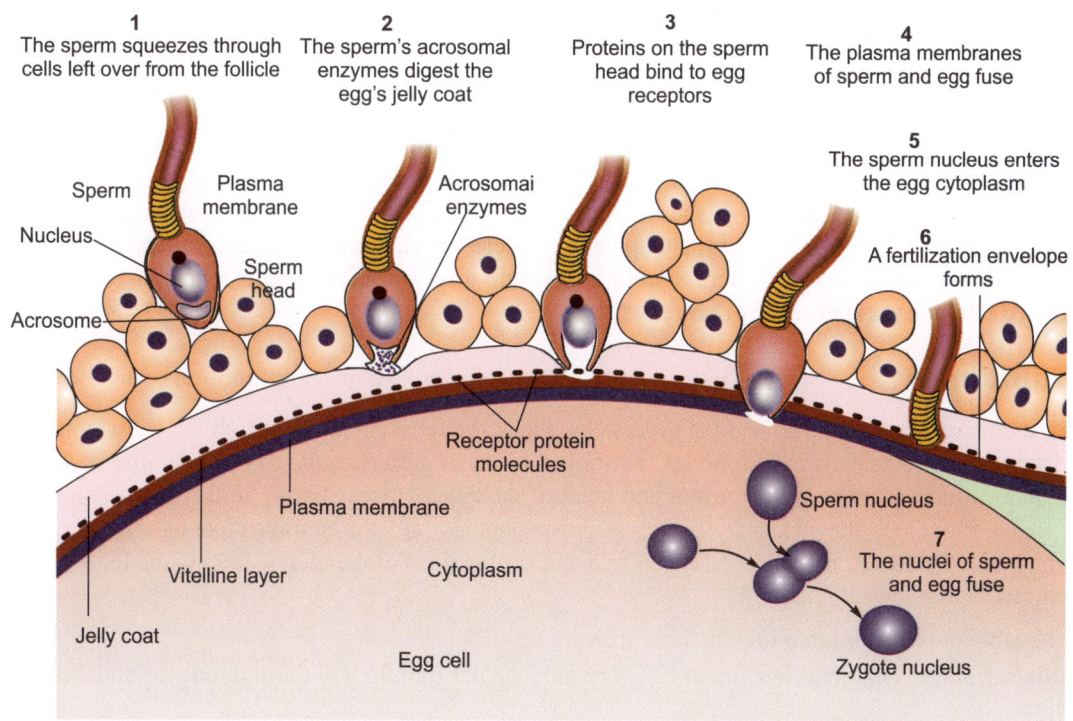

Figure 14.19 Process of fertilization.

Implantation

About 6 days after fertilization, the blastocyst attaches to the endometrial lining of the uterus and eventually gets embedded in it, a process called *implantation*. At this stage, the trophoblast secretes hCG, whose actions are similar to those of LH. hCG prevents the degeneration of corpus luteum and sustains its secretion of progesterone and oestrogen, thereby preventing menstruation.

Embryonic and fetal development

For the first two months after fertilization, the developing baby is called embryo and this is the phase of embryological development. After two months (or 9 weeks), the developing baby is called fetus and this phase is called *fetal development*.

The first major event of the embryonic period is the differentiation of the inner cell mass of blastocyst into three *primary germ layers*: ectoderm, endoderm and mesoderm, a process called *gastrulation*. As the embryo develops, the ectoderm develops into the skin and the nervous system; the endoderm forms the epithelial lining of gastrointestinal, respiratory tracts and several other internal organs and glands; and the mesoderm forms muscles, bones and other connective tissues.

The second major event in the embryonic period is the formation of *embryonic membranes*: amnion, chorion and allantois that surround and protect the embryo, and later the fetus.

During the third month of pregnancy, the chorion of the embryo and a portion of the endometrium of the mother form connections and develop into placenta. Placenta serves as the site of exchange of nutrients and wastes between the mother and fetus. It also acts as a protective barrier and prevents most of the microorganisms from passing through it. At this stage, the umbilical cord also develops, which serves as a vascular connection between the mother and the fetus.

In the later stages of fetal development, the placenta acts as an endocrine organ that secretes oestrogen and progesterone to maintain pregnancy and the umbilical cord allows the exchange of nutrients and wastes between the mother and the fetus. As pregnancy progresses, the uterus enlarges to accommodate the developing fetus. It eventually pushes up into the abdominal cavity and occupies most of this area. The abdominal organs push against the diaphragm muscle, causing the ribs to expand and the thorax to widen. In the pelvic cavity, compression of ureters and urinary bladder occurs, which may produce increased frequency and urgency of urination.

Parturition

Parturition means giving birth, and the process by which the fetus is expelled from the uterus through the vagina to the outside is called *labour*. Towards the end of gestation, the oxytocin hormone causes contractions of the uterine myometrium and level of oestrogens rises sharply in the mother's blood. Oestrogen stimulates the placenta to release prostaglandins and the combination of oxytocin and prostaglandins produces more powerful and frequent contractions of the uterus, forcing the fetus out of the uterus.

The labour occurs in the following three stages:
- **Dilation stage**: This stage lasts up to 12 hours and includes rupturing of the amniotic sac and dilation of the cervix.
- **Expulsion stage**: The child moves through the cervix and vagina to the outside world. Usually, the head of the child emerges first and this stage may take 10 minutes to several hours.

❑ **Placental stage**: Within 15 minutes after birth, the placenta detaches from the uterus and is expelled by powerful uterine contractions. The placenta and its attached fetal membranes are called the afterbirth.

DISEASES ASSOCIATED WITH THE REPRODUCTIVE SYSTEM

FUNCTIONAL PROBLEMS

❑ **Impotence**: It is a condition in which a man is unable to attain or maintain an erection.
❑ **Premature ejaculation**: It is a condition in which ejaculation occurs too early either during foreplay or shortly after penetration. It may occur due to lack of voluntary control over ejaculation.
❑ **Hypogonadism**: It refers to the lack of function of the gonads, with regard to either hormones or gamete production.
❑ **Female sexual arousal disorder**: It refers to the condition of decreased, insufficient or absent lubrication in females during sexual activity.

CANCERS OF REPRODUCTIVE ORGANS

❑ **Penile cancer**: It is the cancer of penis.
❑ **Testicular cancer**: It is the cancer of the testicles.
❑ **Prostate cancer**: It is the cancer of the prostate gland.
❑ **Breast cancer**: It is the cancer of the mammary gland. It causes retraction of the nipple and necrosis and ulceration of the overlying skin.
❑ **Uterine cancer**: It is the cancer of the uterus.
❑ **Cervical cancer**: It is the cancer of the cervix.
❑ **Ovarian cancer**: It is the cancer of the ovary. Risk factors include age (more than 50 years), family history of ovarian cancer and prolonged exposure to asbestos and talc. The initial symptoms include abdominal discomfort, nausea, loss of appetite and flatulence. In severe conditions, it may result in abdominal or pelvic pain, gastrointestinal disturbances, urinary complications, menstrual irregularities and heavy menstrual bleeding.

INFECTIONS IN THE REPRODUCTIVE SYSTEM

❑ **AIDS**: It is an *acquired immune deficiency syndrome* caused by the human immunodeficiency virus (HIV).
❑ **Herpes simplex**: It is a sexually transmitted infection caused by a virus called *Herpes simplex* virus (HSV) Type II. The symptoms include painful urination and formation of painful blisters at the site of infection.
❑ **Gonorrhoea**: It is a common sexually transmitted disease caused by the bacterium *Neisseria gonorrhoeae*. The bacterium invades the epithelial lining of the reproductive and urinary tracts, resulting in pus discharge. In severe conditions, it may lead to pelvic inflammatory disease.
❑ **Syphilis**: It is a sexually transmitted infection caused by the bacterium *Treponema pallidum*. The symptoms include development of a painless sore called chancre at the site of infection, fever, skin rashes and muscle aches. In severe conditions, it may cause extensive damage to nervous tissue, paralysis and eventually death.

- **Genital warts**: It is a sexually transmitted infection caused by *human papillomavirus* (HPV). It results in the formation of painless warts that may result in painful intercourse and bleeding.
- **Yeast infection**: It is the vaginal infection caused by any species of the fungus genus *Candida*.
- **Pelvic inflammatory disease**: It is the infection of the female uterus, fallopian tubes and/or ovaries that results in the formation of painful scars, vaginal discharges and pelvic pain.
- **Trichomoniasis**: It is a sexually transmitted infection caused by the protozoan parasite *Trichomonas vaginalis*.

CONGENITAL ABNORMALITIES

- **Cryptorchidism**: It is the absence of one or both testes from the scrotum.
- **Intersexuality**: It is a condition in which a person has genitalia and/or other sexual traits that are not clearly male or female.
- **Androgen insensitivity syndrome**: A genetic disorder in which people who are genetically male (i.e. XY chromosome pair) develop sexually as a female due to an inability to utilize androgen.

OTHER DISEASES OF THE REPRODUCTIVE SYSTEM

- **Hydrocele**: It is the collection of serous fluid in tunica vaginalis of the testes. It may be caused by injury to testes or inflammation of epididymis.
- **Varicocele**: It is a condition in which the scrotum gets swollen.
- **Ovarian cyst**: It is a fluid-filled sac in the ovary. It may cause pain, pressure in the abdomen, irregular menstrual periods and/or vaginal bleeding.
- **Endometriosis**: It is the growth of endometrial tissue outside the uterus. Symptoms include premenstrual pain or severe menstrual pain. It may result in inflammation, pain or infertility.
- **Fibroids**: These are the noncancerous tumours in the uterus composed of muscular and fibrous tissues. Symptoms include abnormal menstrual bleeding and pain in the pelvic area.
- **Leukorrhoea**: It is the whitish vaginal discharge containing mucus and pus cells.
- **Dysmenorrhoea**: It is the condition of painful menstruation. This may be due to uterine tumour, ovarian cyst or pelvic inflammatory disease.
- **Amenorrhoea**: It is the absence of menstruation. This may be due to pregnancy, menopause or reduced secretion of GnRH.
- **Menorrhagia**: It is the condition of excessively prolonged menstrual period. This may be due to disturbance in hormonal regulation, fibroids, intrauterine devices or pelvic infection.
- **Dyspareunia**: It is the condition of pain during sexual intercourse. This may be due to infection, inflammation, pelvic inflammatory disease or pelvic tumour.
- **Epididymorchitis**: It is the inflammation of epididymis or testis, which may be due to urine infection or sexually transmitted infection.
- **Mastitis**: It is the inflammation of breast tissue due to bacterial infection. This may cause pain and lumps in the infected breast.
- **Vaginitis**: It is the inflammation of the vagina due to bacterial infection or sexually transmitted infection. Symptoms include itching, inflammation and irritation of the genital area and vaginal discharge.

OVERVIEW OF THE MALE REPRODUCTIVE SYSTEM

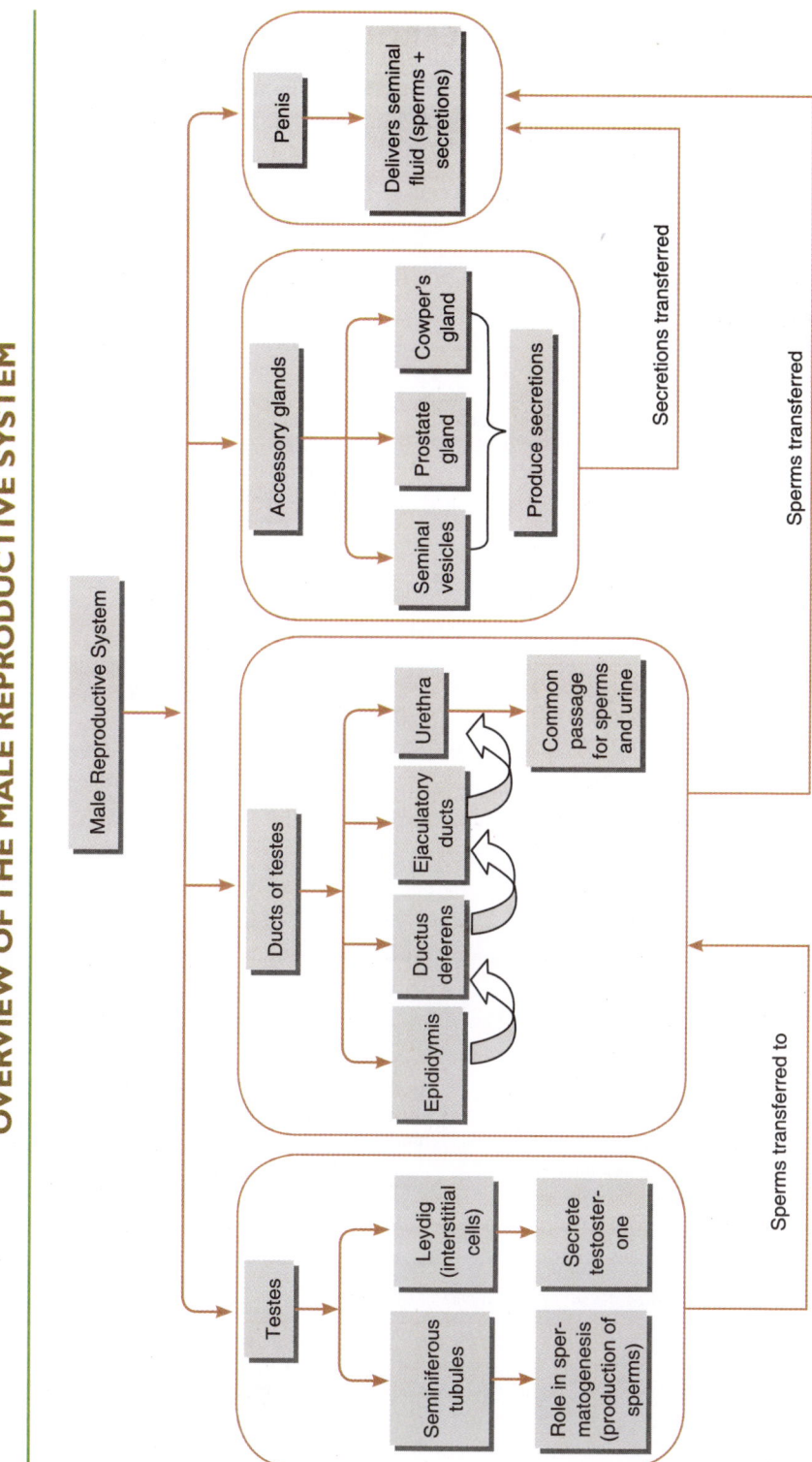

OVERVIEW OF THE FEMALE REPRODUCTIVE SYSTEM

Female Reproductive System
Ovaries
Fallopian/ uterine tubes
Uterus
Vagina
External genitalia
Produce oocyte and female sex hormones (oestrogen and progesterone)
Transports oocyte (or zygote if fertilization occurs) towards uterus
Implantation site of zygote
Receives sperms and acts as passageway for menstrual flow and childbirth
Contains glands that provide lubrication during sexual intercourse

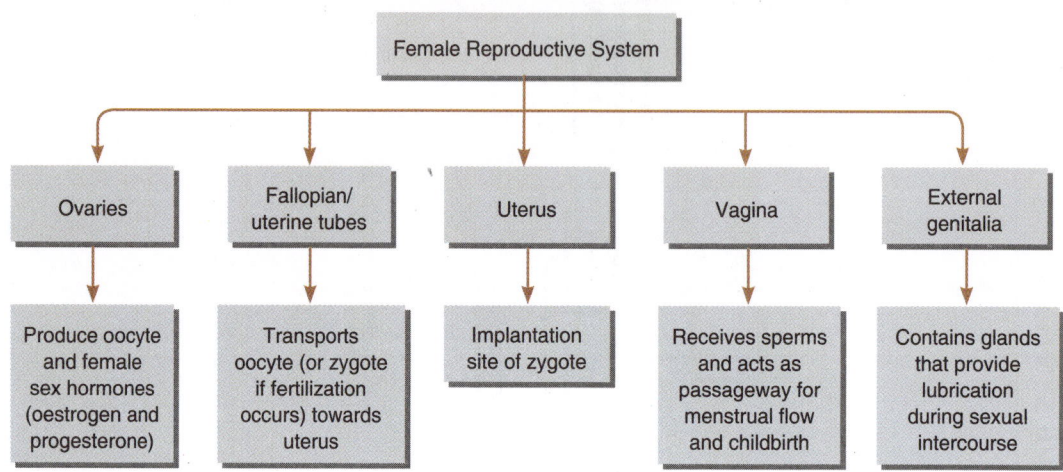

MENSTRUAL CYCLE

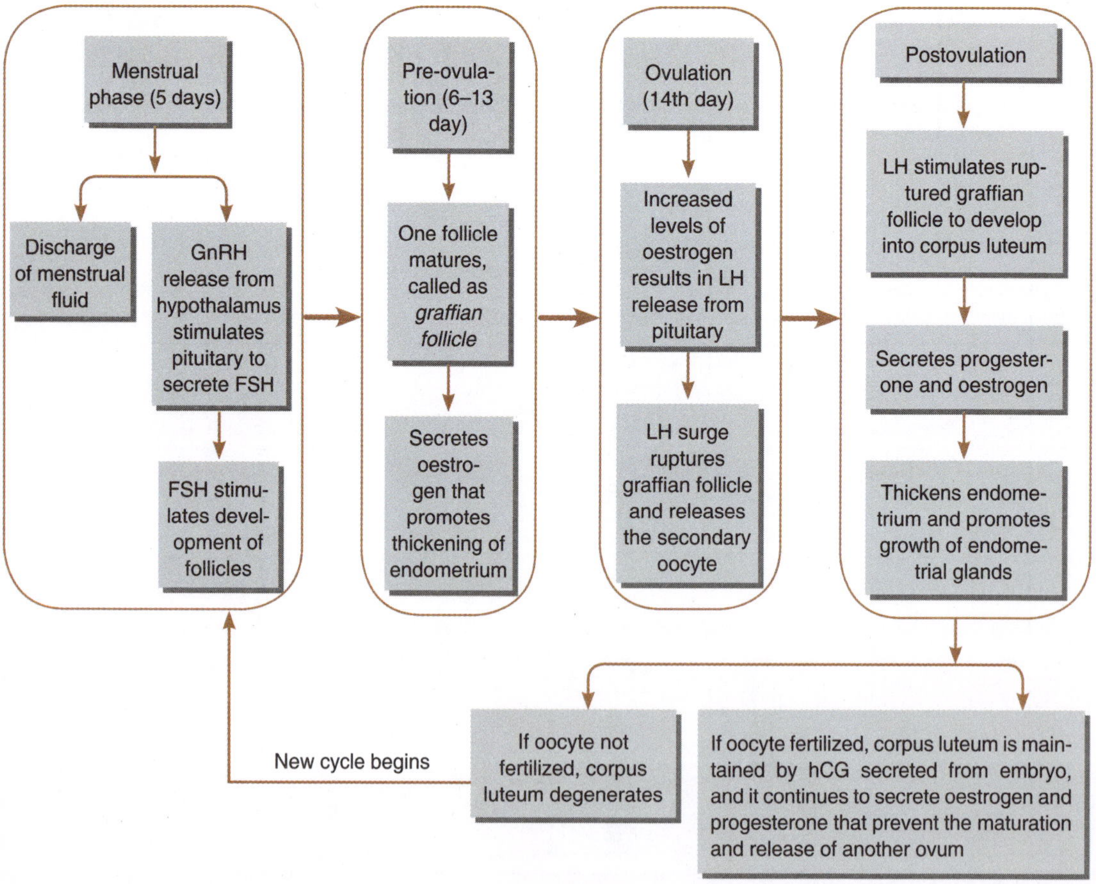

Menstrual phase (5 days)
Discharge of menstrual fluid
GnRH release from hypothalamus stimulates pituitary to secrete FSH
FSH stimulates development of follicles
Pre-ovulation (6–13 day)
One follicle matures, called as *graffian follicle*
Secretes oestrogen that promotes thickening of endometrium
Ovulation (14th day)
Increased levels of oestrogen results in LH release from pituitary
LH surge ruptures graffian follicle and releases the secondary oocyte
Postovulation
LH stimulates ruptured graffian follicle to develop into corpus luteum
Secretes progesterone and oestrogen
Thickens endometrium and promotes growth of endometrial glands
If oocyte not fertilized, corpus luteum degenerates
New cycle begins
If oocyte fertilized, corpus luteum is maintained by hCG secreted from embryo, and it continues to secrete oestrogen and progesterone that prevent the maturation and release of another ovum

Embryonic Development of Reproductive System

- ❑ By the 6th week of gestation, mesoderm forms bulges and develops into gonads.
  - ➤ Adjacent to gonads are mesonephric (Wolffian) ducts that develop into male reproductive organs.
  - ➤ Lateral to mesonephric ducts are paramesonephric (Mullerian) ducts that develop into female reproductive organs.
- ❑ Early embryo (till 8 weeks) can follow either male or female developmental pattern as it contains both ducts.
- ❑ Cells of male embryo:
  - ➤ Sertoli cells secrete Mullerian-inhibiting substance (MIS) that causes death of cells within the Mullerian duct.
  - ➤ During the 8th week of gestation, Leydig cells secrete testosterone that stimulates the development of epididymis, vas deferens, ejaculatory duct and seminal vesicle.
- ❑ Cells of female embryo:
  - ➤ Wolffian ducts form the uterus, vagina and fallopian tube.

Ageing and the Reproductive System

- ❑ *In females*, the reproductive cycle normally occurs once in each month from *menarche*, the first menses, to *menopause*, the permanent cessation of menses.
  - ➤ Between 40 and 50 years, oestrogen and progesterone production declines and ovaries become less responsive to hormonal stimulation.
  - ➤ After menopause, ovaries, uterine tubes, uterus, vagina and breasts undergo atrophy.
- ❑ *In males*
  - ➤ At around 55 years, testosterone synthesis declines, which leads to decreased muscle strength, decreased testes size, decreased sexual desire and fewer viable sperms.
  - ➤ After 60 years, approximately one-third of males experience enlargement of prostate gland, a condition known as benign prostatic hyperplasia (BPH).

TIPS TO MAINTAIN REPRODUCTIVE HEALTH

1. Avoid premarital sex and be faithful to your partner.
2. Avoid alcohol, drugs and smoking.
3. Eat a rainbow of fruits and vegetables every day—the brighter the better.
4. Maintain proper hygiene.
5. Get a yearly medical check-up.
6. Exercise regularly and stay away from stress.

Chapter 14

Birth Control Methods

- **Rhythm method**: It is abstinence from coitus for a few days before and a few days after ovulation.
- **Coitus interruptus**: It is the withdrawal of the penis prior to ejaculation.
- **Condom**: It is a rubber or latex sheath that covers the penis during coitus, preventing semen from being deposited in the vagina.
- **Diaphragm and spermicidal foams, gels and sponges**: These are the barriers that prevent spermatozoa from entering the cervix.
- **Oral contraceptives (the pill)**: These are drugs that inhibit the release of gonadotropins (LH and FSH) and therefore prevent ovulation.
- **Subdermal implants**: These are small (2 in.) rods filled with a hormonal contraceptive drug and implanted under the skin, usually on the upper arm.
- **Intrauterine devices (IUDs)**: These are contrivances that prevent implantation of the fertilized egg.
- **Vasectomy**: It is a surgical procedure for males that involves cutting and tying off the ductus deferentia, thus preventing sperms from becoming a component of the ejaculate.
- **Tubal ligation**: It is a surgical procedure for females that involves cutting and tying of the uterine tubes, thus preventing ova from contacting spermatozoa.

Review Questions

Long Answer Questions

1. Describe the processes of spermatogenesis and oogenesis.
2. Discuss the various organs of the male reproductive system.
3. Describe the structure and function of the testes.
4. Describe the structure of a mature spermatozoon.
5. Describe the organs of the female reproductive system.
6. Describe the structure of the uterus.
7. Describe the structure of an ovary and the cyclical development of the ovarian follicle, ovum and corpus luteum.
8. Discuss in detail the events of the menstrual cycle.
9. Describe the mechanisms of labour and parturition (childbirth).
10. What are the factors that initiate menstrual flow?

Multiple Choice Questions

1. Which of the following sex chromosome combinations causes a male fetus to develop?

   (a) XX

   (b) XY

   (c) YY

   (d) XO

   (e) YO

2. Which of the following is *not* an accessory male reproductive gland?

   (a) Prostate

   (b) Bulbourethral gland

   (c) Glans penis

   (d) Seminal vesicle

3. The penis is

   (a) The male primary sex organ

   (b) Composed of four longitudinal columns of erectile tissue

   (c) Homologous to the female labia majora

   (d) A copulatory organ

4. The portion of the female reproductive system that is homologous to the glans penis of the male is

   (a) The labia majora

   (b) The clitoris

   (c) The ovary

   (e) The vagina

5. The vascular mucosal lining of the uterus is

   (a) The peritoneum

   (b) The endometrium

   (c) The mediastinum

   (d) The synovial membrane

   (e) The mesentery

6. Fertilization normally occurs in

   (a) The uterine tube

   (b) The vagina

   (c) The uterus

   (d) The ovary

   (e) The peritoneal cavity

7. Which of the following is *not* part of the female external genitalia?

   (a) Clitoris

   (b) Vagina

   (c) Labia majora

   (d) Labia minora

8. Testosterone is responsible for the maintenance of

   (a) A functional male reproductive system

   (b) Regular ovulation

   (c) A mature endometrium

   (d) Cells of the interstitial spaces

   (e) All of the above

9. The function of the male secondary sex organs is to
   (a) Transfer spermatozoa to the female
   (b) Regulate sperm production
   (c) Produce sperm
   (d) Produce male sex hormones
   (e) Accomplish all of the above

10. The filling of venous sinuses under the influence of sexual stimulation is most closely associated with
    (a) Spermatogenesis   (b) Menstruation
    (c) Ovulation   (d) Erection

11. The number of gametes resulting from a single sequence of spermatogenesis is
    (a) 1   (b) 2
    (c) 4   (d) 8
    (e) over 100

12. The tightly convoluted tubule that lies along the posterior surface of the testis is
    (a) The seminiferous tubule (b) The rete testis
    (c) The epididymis   (d) The ductus deferens
    (e) The seminal vesicle

13. Spermatozoa are discharged through the male genital ducts in the order
    (a) Epididymis, ductus deferens, ejaculatory duct, urethra
    (b) Ejaculatory duct, epididymis, ductus deferens, urethra
    (c) Epididymis, ductus deferens, urethra, ejaculatory duct
    (d) Ductus deferens, epididymis, ejaculatory duct, urethra

14. The development of the ovarian follicle is influenced by
    (a) Prolactin   (b) Follicle-stimulating hormone (FSH)
    (c) Testosterone,   (d) Insulin
    (e) None of the above

15. Which of the following secretes progesterone?
    (a) Anterior pituitary   (b) Corpus luteum
    (c) Corpus luteum and ovarian follicle   (d) Hypothalamus
    (e) Posterior pituitary

16. Formation and maintenance of the corpus luteum are mainly effected by
    (a) FSH   (b) Luteinizing hormone (LH)
    (c) Progesterone   (d) Oestrogens

17. Which of the following secretes oestrogen?
    (a) Anterior pituitary   (b) Corpus luteum and ovarian follicle
    (c) Ovarian follicle only   (d) Hypothalamus

18. Menstruation is initiated by
    (a) A sudden release of FSH from the anterior pituitary
    (b) A lack of oestrogen and progesterone due to degeneration of the corpus luteum
    (c) An increased release of oestrogen and progesterone from the corpus luteum
    (d) A sudden drop in LH

19. Which hormone stimulates testosterone secretion?
    (a) LH
    (b) Progesterone
    (c) FSH
    (d) Adrenocorticotropic hormone (ACTH)

20. Spermatozoa are stored prior to ejaculation in
    (a) The prostatic urethra   (b) The prostate
    (c) The epididymides   (d) The seminal vesicles
    (e) The ejaculatory ducts

21. An embryo with XX chromosomes develops female secondary sex organs because of
    (a) Oestrogen   (b) Androgens
    (c) Absence of androgens   (d) Absence of oestrogen

22. The milk ejection reflex is stimulated by
    (a) Oxytocin   (b) Oestrogen
    (c) Prolactin   (d) Progesterone

23. Once ejaculated into the vagina, spermatozoa have a life expectancy of
    (a) 10–12 h   (b) 1 day
    (c) 2–3 days   (d) up to 5 days

State True or False

1. Seminal vesicles, bulbourethral glands and the prostate are all accessory glands of the male reproductive system.
2. The labia majora of the female genitalia are homologous to the scrotum in the male.
3. Meiosis is peculiar to the gonads.
4. The ejaculatory ducts store spermatozoa and additives to produce semen prior to ejaculation.
5. Mammary glands are modified sebaceous glands.
6. Prolactin causes the breasts to enlarge and the mammary glands to mature during puberty.
7. The first menstrual discharge is referred to as menarche.
8. Located at the vaginal orifice, the vestibular glands maintain the acidic pH of the vagina.
9. Interstitial cells produce spermatozoa and secrete nutrients to developing spermatozoa within the testes.
10. The secretory phase of menstruation is characterized by discharge of the menses.

Fill in the Blanks

1. _____ is a condition in which one or both testes fail to descend into the scrotum.

2. _____ is the discharge of semen from the erect penis.

3. _____ cells are located between the seminiferous tubules of a testis, where they produce and secrete androgens.

4. The _____ is a thin remnant of mucous membrane that may partially cover the vaginal orifice.

5. Ejaculated spermatozoa can live up to _____ days, whereas an ovulated egg can survive only about _____ h.

6. The first menstrual period is called _____.

Careers in the Reproductive System

✓ Gynaecologists are physicians who specialize in diagnosis and treatment of the reproductive organs of women.

✓ Obstetricians are physicians who specialize in taking care of women during pregnancy and childbirth.

✓ Paediatricians are the physicians who specialize in the diagnosis and treatment of diseases in infants and children.

✓ Neonatalists are the physicians specialized in the diagnosis and treatment of diseases in new-borns.

15 The Sense Organs

CHAPTER OUTLINE

- Introduction
- Eyes (Organs of Sight)
- Ears—the Structures of Hearing and Equilibrium
- Sense of Smell
- Sense of Taste
- Disorders Associated with Sense Organs

STUDY OBJECTIVES

- ✓ To describe the structural components of the eye and discuss its accessory structures .
- ✓ To explain the image formation by refraction, accommodation and constriction of pupil.
- ✓ To describe the visual pathway.
- ✓ To describe the structure of the external, middle and internal parts of the ear.
- ✓ To discuss the physiology of hearing and explain the organs involved in equilibrium.
- ✓ To describe the auditory pathway.

INTRODUCTION

The special senses of hearing, sight, smell and taste have specialized sensory receptors (nerve endings) outside the brain. These sensory receptors are found in the ears, eyes, nose and mouth and enable us to detect changes in our own body and in objects and events in the world around us.

The receptor receives a particular stimulus and initiates a nerve impulse in the neuron, which carries these impulses to the brain. In the brain, the incoming nerve impulses undergo complex processes of integration and coordination that result in the perception of sensory information and various responses inside and outside the body.

The special senses of smell and taste are perceived by the interaction of the chemicals with sensory receptors on the tongue and in the nose. Vision occurs due to the interaction of light with sensory receptors in the eye. Hearing and balance functions are executed due to the interaction of mechanical stimuli (sound waves for hearing and movement for balance) with sensory receptors in the ear.

EYES (ORGANS OF SIGHT)

The eyes are the organs of sight located in the deep, protective bony cavities, called the *orbits* or *eye sockets* of the skull.

The eye is almost spherical in shape and measures about 2.5 cm in diameter. The space between the eye and the bony orbits is occupied by the adipose tissue, connective tissue, ligaments and muscles. The bony walls of the orbit and the adipose tissue help protect the eye from injury, and the ligaments suspend the eye in such a way that the muscles can move it to let one see up, down and on the sides. The study of the structure, functions and disorders of the eye is termed as *ophthalmology* (*ophthalmo*: eye; *logy*: study).

STRUCTURE OF THE EYE

Anatomically, the wall of the eyeball is composed of the following three layers:

1. **Outer fibrous layer or corneoscleral layer**: This layer includes the sclera and cornea.
2. **Middle vascular layer or uvea**: This layer includes choroid, ciliary body and iris.
3. **Inner nervous layer**: This layer includes the retina.

Structures inside the eyeball consist of the lens, aqueous fluid and vitreous body (Fig. 15.1).

Outer fibrous layer

It is the thick, superficial layer of the eyeball that consists of two regions: anterior cornea and posterior sclera.

Sclera

❑ The sclera or 'white of the eye' forms the outermost layer of the *posterior* and *lateral regions of the eyeball* and is continuous anteriorly with the transparent cornea. It is composed of a dense connective tissue made up of collagen fibres and fibroblasts.
❑ The sclera maintains the shape of the eye, protects its inner parts and gives attachment to the eye muscles.

DO YOU KNOW

❑ Your tongue is germ free only if it is pink. If it is white there is a thin film of bacteria on it.
❑ The pupil of the eye expands as much as 45% when a person looks at something pleasing.
❑ The only part of the body that has no blood supply is the cornea in the eye. It takes in oxygen directly from the air.
❑ In general, girls have more taste buds than boys do.
❑ Smoking, alcohol, caffeine, spicy and hot foods, onion and garlic dull the taste buds. It takes 24 h for taste buds to cleanse themselves after being exposed to these substances.
❑ A newborn baby sees the world upside down because it takes some time for the baby's brain to learn to turn the picture right-side up.

MEDICAL TERMINOLOGY

❑ **Cartilage**: It is a connective tissue that is present at ends of certain bones and joints and provides a smooth surface for adjacent bones to move against each other.
❑ **Ligaments**: Tough connective tissue structures that attaches bones to bones.
❑ **Photoreceptors**: Specialized cells present in the retina that process the light rays and convert them to nerve impulses.
❑ **Vitreous humor**: A gel-like fluid that fills the space between the lens and the retina.

Cornea

❏ Cornea is the transparent, anterior region of the eyeball composed of epithelial tissue. It lacks blood vessels; hence, corneal transplantation can be successfully performed because the blood-borne antibodies that might cause rejection do not enter the transplanted tissue and rejection rarely occurs.

❏ The cornea is convex (curved) anteriorly and is involved in *refracting (bending) light rays* that helps focus the light on the retina.

An opening, referred to as *canal of Schlemm* (sclera venous sinus), is present at the junction of sclera and cornea, which permits the drainage of aqueous humor (discussed later in detail).

The cornea and the exposed part of the sclera are covered externally by a thin, transparent membrane, called the *conjunctiva* (Fig. 15.2).

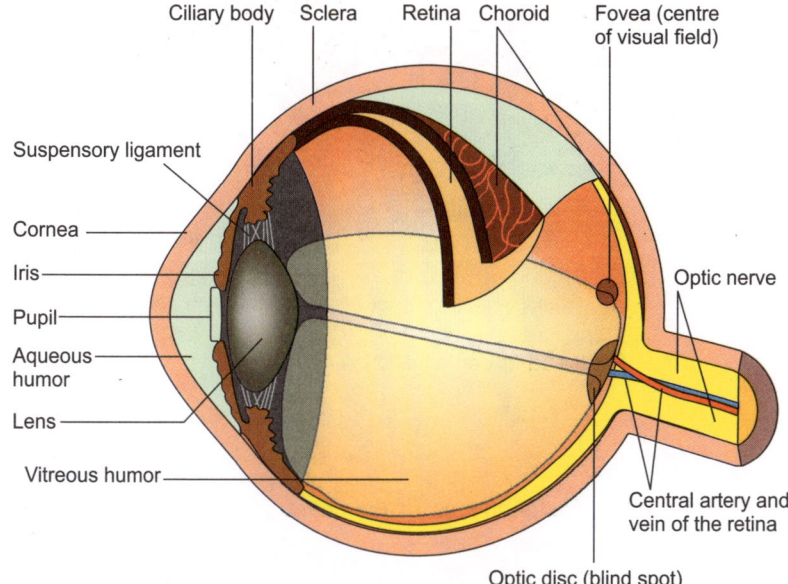

Figure 15.1 Structure of the eye.

Middle vascular layer

It is the middle layer of the eyeball that is composed of three regions: choroid, ciliary body and iris.

Choroid

❏ The choroid is the posterior portion of the middle layer that lines most of the internal surface of sclera. It contains numerous blood vessels and is composed of a soft connective tissue containing pigment cells, melanocytes that produce the melanin pigment.

❏ The melanin in the choroid is responsible for its dark brown colour. Melanin absorbs stray light and darkens the eyeball cavity, which prevents the internal reflection and scattering of light within the eyeball. As a result, the image remains sharp and clear.

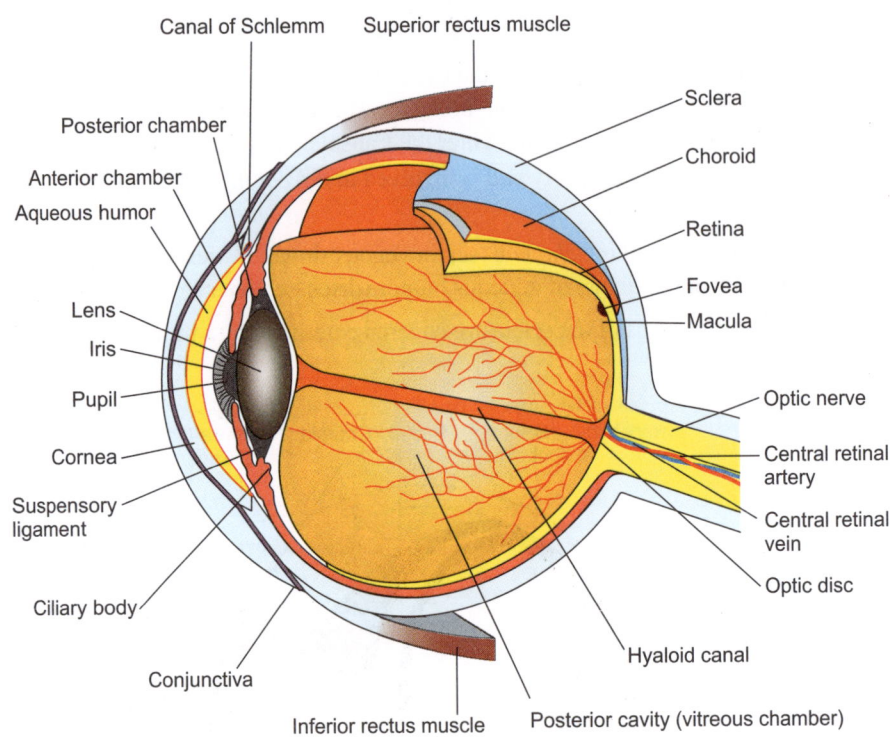

Figure 15.2 Vertical section of the right eye.

Ciliary body

❑ The ciliary body is the anterior continuation of the choroid consisting of ciliary muscle (smooth muscle fibres) and ciliary processes.

➤ The ciliary muscles are attached to the suspensory ligaments that hold the biconvex, transparent and flexible lens in place. The process of contraction and relaxation of the ciliary muscle changes the tightness of suspensory ligaments, which alters the shape of the lens and permits the adaptation for near or far vision (accommodation).

➤ The ciliary processes are the folds on the internal surface of ciliary body that contain secretory epithelial cells. The epithelial cells secrete *aqueous fluid* into the anterior segment of the eye (i.e. space anterior to the lens).

❑ The ciliary body appears dark brown in colour like the choroid as it also contains melanin-producing melanocytes.

Iris

❑ Iris is the coloured portion of the eyeball that extends anteriorly from the ciliary body and is suspended between the cornea and the lens. It consists of melanocytes and circular and radial smooth muscle fibres. The centre of the iris is perforated by an aperture (hole) called *pupil*.

❏ The amount of melanin in the iris determines the characteristic colour of the eyes (e.g. large melanin amount: brown to black eyes; moderate melanin amount: green eyes; less melanin amount: blue eyes).

❏ The principal function of the iris is to regulate the amount of light entering the eyeball by varying the diameter of pupil. This variation of pupil diameter in response to light levels is regulated by sympathetic and parasympathetic nerve fibres that innervate the iris.

➤ When we go out in bright light, the parasympathetic nerve fibres stimulate the circular muscles (sphincter pupillae) of the iris to contract and result in decreased size of the pupil (constriction), so that less light enters the pupil.

➤ In dim light, the sympathetic nerve fibres stimulate the radial muscles (dilator pupillae) of the iris to contract, resulting in the increased size of the pupil (dilation); this allows more light to enter the eyes.

❏ Thus, to summarize:

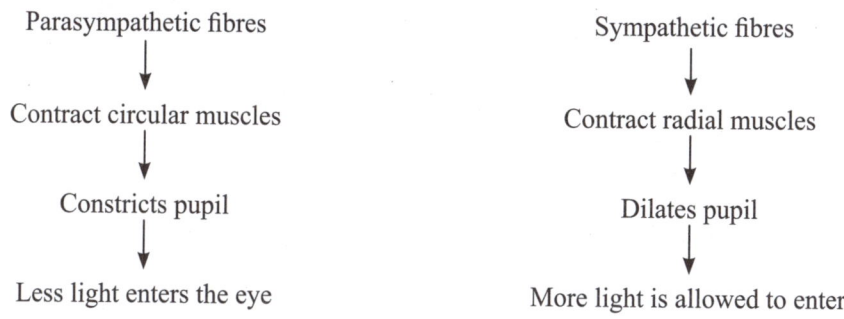

Inner nervous layer: the retina

The retina is the innermost layer of the eyeball. It is an extremely delicate structure and consists of a pigmented layer and a neural layer.

The *pigmented layer* consists of a sheet of melanin-containing epithelial cells that is attached to the choroid. The melanin in this layer reinforces the light-absorbing property of choroid and prevents the scattering of light within the eyeball.

The *neural layer* consists of three distinct layers of retinal neurons: the photoreceptor layer, the bipolar cell layer and the ganglion cell layer.

The photoreceptor layer lies on the pigmented layer and consists of specialized cells called *photoreceptors* that include *rods* and *cones*. The photoreceptor cells synapse with the bipolar cells, which in turn synapse with the ganglion cells. The axons of the ganglion cells form the optic nerve (Fig. 15.3).

Light rays pass through the ganglion cell layer and the bipolar cell layer to reach the photoreceptor layer where the visual data is extensively processed. The photoreceptor cells (i.e. rods and cones) contain photosensitive pigments that process the visual data and convert light rays into nerve impulses. The nerve impulses are then transmitted in the opposite direction through the bipolar cell layer towards the ganglion cell layer. The axons of the ganglion cells form the *optic nerve*, which carries these impulses to the brain for interpretation.

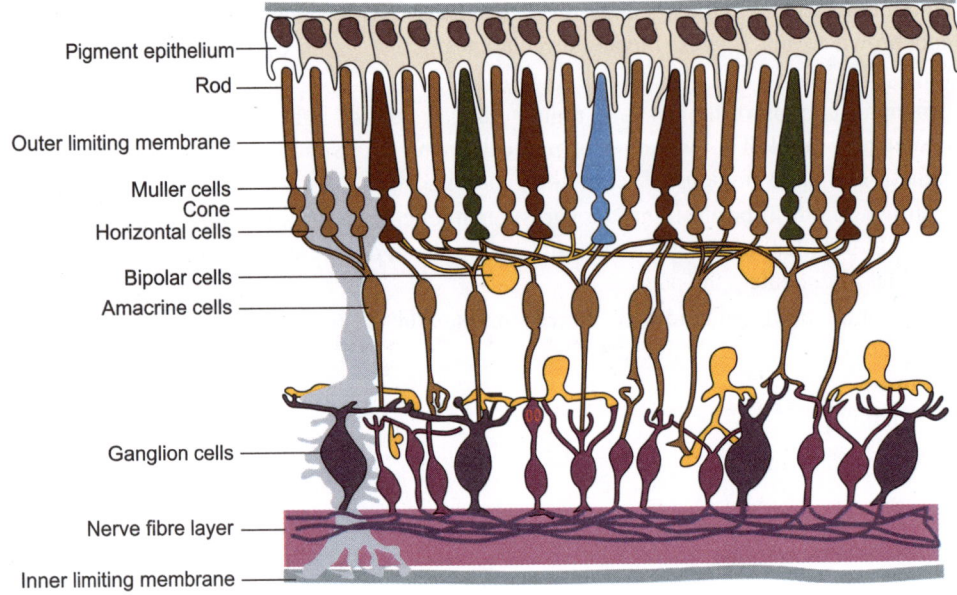

Pigment epithelium

Rod

Outer limiting membrane

Muller cells
Cone
Horizontal cells

Bipolar cells
Amacrine cells

Ganglion cells

Nerve fibre layer

Inner limiting membrane

Figure 15.3 The neural layer of retina.

Photoreceptors

As discussed previously, photoreceptors are the specialized cells present in the retina that process the light rays and ultimately convert them to nerve impulses. There are two types of photoreceptors: rods and cones. Each retina has about 6 million cones and 120 million rods.

❑ The outer segments of *rods* are cylindrical and rod shaped, and hence the name rods. The rod cells are stimulated by low-intensity light or dim light, allowing us to see in dim light. However, they do not produce colour vision, and therefore we can see only shades of grey in dim light. The photopigment present in the rods is rhodopsin.

❑ The outer segments of *cones* are tapered or cone shaped, and hence the name cones. The cone cells are sensitive to bright light and produce colour vision. The following three different types of cones are present in the retina:

1. Blue cones, which are sensitive to blue light
2. Green cones, which are sensitive to green light
3. Red cones, which are sensitive to red light

The stimulation of various combinations of the three types of cones by light of different wavelengths results in the perception of different colours. For example, yellow light stimulates the green and red cones to an approximately equal extent, and this is interpreted by the brain as yellow colour. Equal stimulation of all types of cones produces the colour sensation of white. Lack of one or more types of cone cells causes *colour blindness*.

Yellow spot or macula lutea

A small area of the retina present at the centre of its posterior part is called the *macula lutea* or *yellow spot*. In the centre of the macula lutea, there is a little depression called the *fovea centralis*, consisting of only cone cells. This region produces the sharpest vision and is considered the area of the highest visual acuity or resolution.

Away from the fovea, the rod and cone cells occur in equal numbers, and at the periphery of the retina, the rods are more numerous than the cones. This is why we see better in dim light by looking out of the corner of the eye.

Optic disc or blind spot

The optic nerve leaves the eyeball by piercing the eye coat at the back. The point on the retina from where the optic nerve leaves the eye is called the *optic disc* or *blind spot*. It is referred to as blind spot because it lacks the photoreceptor cells rods and cones, and therefore we cannot see an image that strikes the blind spot.

Lens

The lens is an elastic, perfectly transparent body present just behind the iris within the eyeball cavity. It is enclosed by a thin, elastic membrane, the lens capsule, and held in position by a firm, elastic, ring-like fibres, the suspensory ligament, which attach to the ciliary processes.

It is the only structure in the eye that changes its refractive power, and therefore light rays that enter the eyes are refracted by the lens that helps focus them on the retina to facilitate clear vision.

Interior of the eyeball

The lens divides the eye ball cavity into two chambers: the anterior small aqueous chamber and the posterior large vitreous chamber.

❑ The aqueous chamber (i.e. the space anterior to the lens) is divided into two chambers by the iris: large anterior chamber in front of the iris and small posterior chamber between the iris and the lens. Both the parts of the aqueous chamber are filled with a clear, watery fluid, the aqueous humor, secreted continuously by the ciliary processes of the ciliary body. The ciliary processes secrete aqueous humor in the posterior chamber, and from here, it flows forward through the pupil into the anterior chamber. From the anterior chamber,

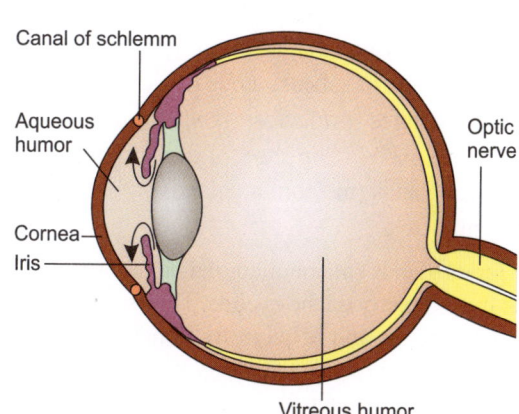

Figure 15.4 Flow of aqueous humor.

it is drained into the venous circulation through the *canal of Schlemm* (scleral venous sinus) (Fig. 15.4).

There is continuous production and drainage of aqueous humor, and normally, aqueous humor is completely replaced about every 90 min. The aqueous humor supplies nutrition, removes waste products from the lens and cornea and maintains pressure in the eyes (i.e. intraocular pressure, which is essential to maintain shape of the eyeball and prevent it from collapsing).

❑ The *vitreous chamber* lies between the lens and the retina and consists of a thick, transparent, jellylike substance, the vitreous body or the vitreous humor. The vitreous humor is secreted by the retina during development of the eye (embryonic life) and consists of water (90%), collagen fibres and hyaluronic acid. It does not flow, and thus is not replaced. It too helps maintain the intraocular pressure and the shape of the eyeball. It also supports and holds the retina and lens in place and helps refract or bend light rays.

ACCESSORY STRUCTURES OF THE EYE

The accessory structures of the eye include the eyebrows, eyelids and the lacrimal apparatus.

Eyebrows

The eyebrows contain numerous hairs that project obliquely from the surface of the skin. They protect the eyeballs from sweat, dust and other foreign objects.

Eyelids (palpebrae)

The eyelids are two movable folds of tissue situated above and below the front of each eye. On the free edges of the eyelids, there are short curved hairs, the *eyelashes*. The eyelids and eyelashes shade the eyes during sleep, protect the eyes from excessive light and foreign objects, and spread the lubricating secretions over the eyeballs.

The space between the upper and lower eyelids that exposes the eyeball is called the *palpebral fissure*. From superficial to deep, each eyelid consists of the following:

❏ A thin covering of skin (the epidermis and dermis)
❏ A thin sheet of subcutaneous tissue
❏ Muscle fibres (*orbicularis oculi muscle*: closes eye; and *levator palpebrae superioris*: opens eyes)
❏ A tarsal plate (a thin sheet of dense connective tissue that supports the eyelids)
❏ Tarsal glands (meibomian glands)
❏ Conjunctiva

Tarsal glands (meibomian glands) are modified sebaceous (oil) glands embedded in the tarsal plates that open directly on the eyelids. They secrete an oily substance that forms a film over the cornea to keep the latter moist and helps in frictionless blinking. Along the edges of the eyelids, there are numerous sebaceous (oil) glands (called *glands of Zeis*) and sudoriferous (sweat) glands (called *glands of Moll*) that open into the hair follicles of the eyelashes.

Conjunctiva is a thin, transparent mucous membrane that lines the inner portion of the eyelids and the front of the eyeball. It protects the delicate cornea and the front of the eye.

The lacrimal apparatus

The lacrimal apparatus (*lacrim*: tears) is a group of structures that produces and drains lacrimal fluid or tears (Fig 15.5).

The lacrimal apparatus consists of the following:

❏ **Lacrimal glands**: These are the exocrine glands situated in the upper outer part of each orbit and are about the size and shape of an almond. The lacrimal glands secrete the lacrimal fluid (tears) that is composed of water, mineral salts, some mucus and lysozyme, a protective bactericidal enzyme.

Each gland produces about 1 mL of lacrimal fluid per day.

❑ **Lacrimal ducts**: The lacrimal fluid (tears) leaves the lacrimal gland through 6–12 lacrimal ducts. The lacrimal ducts release the tears over the anterior surface of the eyeball, where it is spread medially over the surface of the eyeball by the blinking of eyelids. The fluid washes the cornea, kills the bacteria and moistens the surface of eyeball.

❑ **Lacrimal canals**: The excess of this fluid passes into the nasal chamber through superior and inferior lacrimal canals by two small openings called *lacrimal puncta*.

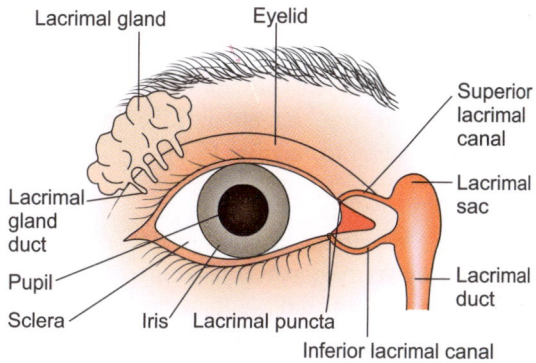

Figure 15.5 The lacrimal apparatus.

❑ **Nasolacrimal duct**: The fluid in the lacrimal canals drains into the lacrimal sac and then into the nasolacrimal duct, which carries the lacrimal fluid into the nasal cavity.

Normally, the rate of secretion of lacrimal fluid keeps pace with the rate of drainage. However, irritation by foreign particles, smoke or some gas and emotional stress stimulate the lacrimal glands to oversecrete, which floods the eyes with tears. The excessive lacrimal fluid then drains into the nasal cavity and thus produces a runny nose.

PHYSIOLOGY OF VISION

The eye resembles a camera in structure as well as in working. The optical elements of the eye (i.e. cornea and lens) focus the image of an object on the light-sensitive film, that is retina. The image formed on retina is inverted and small similar to that in a camera. This image is processed by the photoreceptor cells of the retina that convert the light rays into nerve impulses. The nerve impulses are then carried by the optic nerve to the visual areas of the cerebral hemisphere where the real perception of vision arises, allowing to see the objects upright.

Thus, it can be summarized that the human eye has two functional parts: the focusing part and the photoreceptor part.

Focusing part

Various processes are involved in focusing the light rays and producing a clear image on the retina. These processes are as follows:

1. Refraction or bending of light rays
2. Accommodation (i.e. change in the shape of lens)
3. Regulation of light entering the eyes by change in the pupil size

Refraction of light rays

When light rays travel from a medium of one density (such as air) to a medium of different density (such as water), they undergo refraction (bending). As the light rays reflected by the objects enter the eyes, they pass successively through the conjunctiva, cornea, aqueous humor, lens and vitreous humor. These parts are denser than air, refracting (bending) the light rays passing through the eye to bring them to a focus on the retina. Maximum (about 75%) refraction occurs at the cornea, which places the image approximately on the retina. The lens provides fine adjustments and further refraction (remaining 25%) to bring the image into a sharp focus (Fig. 15.6).

Accommodation

The light rays from distant objects need least refraction, but as the object comes closer, the degree of refraction should increase for a sharp focus. The degree of refraction cannot be varied at the corneal surface, but the lens being convex on both the anterior and the posterior surface can change its refractive power by changing its curvature.

The various adjustments in the eyes to see near or distant objects clearly are termed *accommodation*.

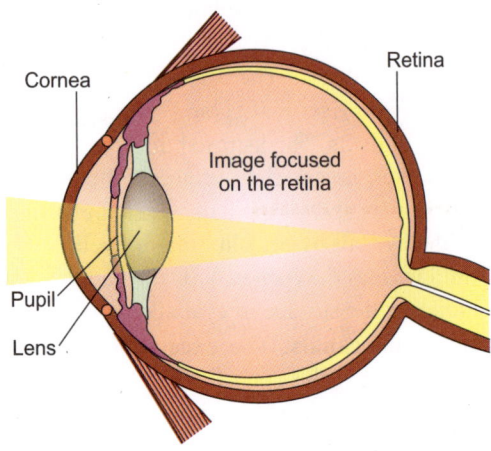

Figure 15.6 Refraction of light rays.

It is the process by which light rays from near or distant objects are brought to focus on the retina, and it is done with the help of ciliary muscles and suspensory ligament.

❑ **Accommodation for near vision**: The light rays from near objects (within 6 m) diverge when they strike the eye and thus need to be refracted more in order to be focused on the retina. To increase its refraction, the ciliary muscles contract, pulling the ciliary muscles and choroid forward towards the lens. This action shortens the radius of suspensory ligament, thus making it loose. Loosening of suspensory ligament allows the lens to bulge forward, which increases its convexity, resulting in greater refraction of light rays and enabling a sharp focus on the retina. Therefore, when we view near objects, it 'tires' the eyes more quickly due to the continuous use of the ciliary muscle (Fig. 15.7a).

❑ **Accommodation for distant objects**: The light rays from distant objects (beyond 6 m) are parallel when they strike the eye and thus are focused on the retina without adjustment of the lens. At this time, the ciliary muscles are fully relaxed, which increases their pull on the suspensory ligament. This flattens the lens and enables the light rays from distant objects to be focused on the retina. The eyes are said to be at rest while viewing distant objects (Fig. 15.7b).

Change in pupil size

Pupil size influences accommodation by controlling the amount of light entering the eyes. As discussed previously, the contraction of the circular muscles of the iris in bright light results in the constriction of pupil and prevents too much light from entering the eyes that may damage the sensitive retina. In addition, constriction of the pupil reduces the width of beam of light entering the eyes so that it passes through the lens appropriately, thus preventing blurred vision. In dim light, the contraction of radial muscles of the iris

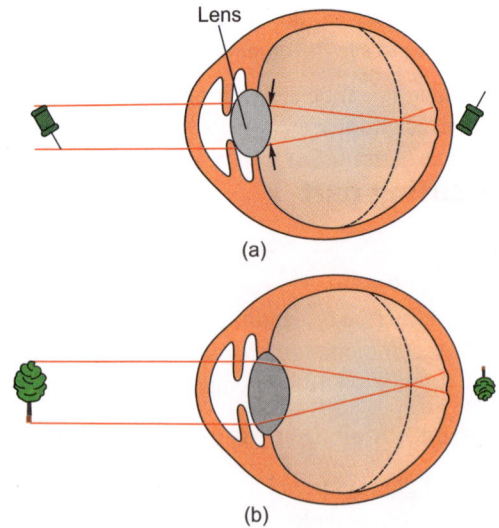

Figure 15.7 Accommodation for (a) near vision (b) distant objects.

results in dilation of the pupil and enables sufficient light to enter the eye, which can activate the photoreceptor cells.

Convergence

Humans have binocular vision, that is both the eyes focus on only one set of objects. This feature of our visual system provides depth to the images, that is gives the three-dimensional (3D) effect, and enables people to judge the distances correctly. This ability of binocular vision is possible when the light rays from an object stimulate the corresponding areas of the two retinas and is brought about by the movement of the eyeballs, referred to as *convergence*, so that both the eyeballs are directed towards the same object. The nearer the object, the greater the degree of convergence (eye rotation) needed to maintain binocular vision. For example, an individual focusing near the tip of his nose appears to be 'cross-eyed'.

Photoreceptor part

The retina consists of specialized cells called *photoreceptor cells* that include rods and cones. Both rods and cones contain light (photo)-sensitive pigments or photopigments. Light rays cause chemical changes in these photopigments and stimulates the photoreceptor cells to set up nerve impulses, which are transmitted to the occipital lobes of the cerebrum via the optic nerves for interpretation.

The single type of photopigment in rods is rhodopsin or visual purple (*rhod*: rose; *opsin*: related to vision). The cone cells contain three different photopigments, one in each of the three types of cones (blue cones: cyanopsin; green cones: iodopsin; red cones: porphyropsin). Different wavelengths of light selectively activate different cone photopigments and result in the perception of different colours.

The photopigments present in rods and cones consist of two parts: a glycoprotein called *opsin* and a derivative of vitamin A called *retinal*. Retinal is derived from food sources and is not synthesized in the body. It is derived from the carotenoid substances such as β-carotene present in carrots.

Thus, good vision depends on the adequate dietary intake of carotene-rich vegetables such as carrots and spinach.

Chemical basis of vision

As discussed previously, rods are extremely sensitive to light and have a low threshold. Therefore, the rods are responsible for dim light vision or night vision but they do not produce colour vision; hence, we can see only shades of grey in dim light. The cones are sensitive only to bright light and colour and have a high threshold for light stimulus. Therefore, the cones are responsible for bright light vision and colour vision.

The detailed explanation of the above facts is as follows:

❑ When an object is placed in front of a person in a dark room, he cannot see the object.
❑ When there is *slight illumination, rods being highly sensitive to light get stimulated* and thus the person can see the object but without colour.
❑ When illumination is increased, the threshold for cones is achieved and since the *cones are sensitive to only bright light, they get activated,* allowing the person to see the object along with colour vision.

The photopigments respond to light in the following cyclical process:

1. In darkness, retinal is present in the form of *cis*-retinal and is joined tightly with the opsin part of the photopigment.

2. When the *cis*-retinal absorbs a photon of light, it converts to the *trans*-retinal form. This *cis*-to-*trans* conversion is called *isomerization* and is the first step in visual process.
3. In about a minute, the photopigment splits and the *trans*-retinal completely separates from opsin. This process is called *bleaching* and these chemical changes lead to the production of a receptor potential (discussed later in detail).
4. The photopigment is quickly *regenerated by resynthesis process* in which the *trans*-retinal is converted back to the *cis*-retinal form by retinal isomerase enzyme. The *cis*-retinal form immediately combines to opsin, thus reforming the functional photopigment. This step is called *regeneration* and this process requires an adequate supply of vitamin A.

The cone photopigments regenerate much more quickly than the rhodopsin in rod cells. After complete bleaching of rods and cones, regeneration of half of the rhodopsin takes 5 min; while half of the cone photopigments regenerate only in 90 s.

Light and dark adaptation

Dark adaptation

When entering a darkened room (such as theatre, tunnel) after spending some time in a bright-lighted area, a person is unable to see anything for some time, but gradually the vision is established. The process by which a person is able to gradually see the objects in dim light after coming from a bright-lighted area is called *dark adaptation*. It occurs due to following changes in the eyes:

1. **Increased sensitivity of rod cells due to regeneration of rhodopsin**: In bright light, regeneration of rhodopsin (photopigment in rods) cannot keep up with the bleaching process, and thus much of the rhodopsin is broken down. Thus, when the person moves into a darkened area, where the light intensity is insufficient to stimulate the cones, temporary visual impairment occurs. However, gradually, regeneration of certain amount of rhodopsin occurs, allowing us to see in dim light after some time.
2. **Dilation of pupil**: The dilation of pupil during dark adaptation allows more light to enter the eye.

Aircraft pilots and radiologists, who need maximal visual sensitivity in dim light, wear red glasses before entering the dim lighted area, because the red of light spectrum allows the cones to function well and stimulates the rods very slightly. Thus, the person wearing red glasses can see well in bright lighted area as well as immediately when entering the dim-lighted area.

Light adaptation

On entering a bright lighted area from a dim lighted area, a person feels discomfort due to the dazzling effect of bright light. However, after sometime, the eyes become adapted to light by a process called *light adaptation*, allowing the person to see the objects without any discomfort. The reason for light adaptation is as follows:

1. **Reduced sensitivity to rod cells**: During light adaptation, the rhodopsin undergoes bleaching, decreasing the sensitivity of rod cells.
2. **Constriction of pupil**: The constriction of pupil reduces the quantity of light rays entering the eyes.

Production of receptor potential

As discussed previously, the absorption of light and splitting of the photopigment result in the chemical changes that lead to the production of a receptor potential. The process involved in the production of receptor potential in the photoreceptors is unique in nature. When other sensory receptors are stimulated, the electrical response is in the form of *depolarization*. However, in photoreceptors, the electrical response (receptor potential) is in the form of hyperpolarization.

The processes involved in the generation of receptor potential in photoreceptors are as follows (Fig. 15.8):

1. In darkness, sodium ions (Na^+) flow into the photoreceptor cells through the ligand-gated Na^+ channels. The ligand that keeps these sodium channels open is cyclic guanosine monophosphate (cGMP). The inflow of Na^+, called the *dark current,* partially depolarizes the photoreceptor and maintains the membrane potential to about -30 mV. This partial depolarization during darkness triggers the continual release of neurotransmitter *glutamate* at the synaptic terminals that inhibits bipolar cells.

2. When light falls on the retina and the photopigment splits, the enzyme cGMP phosphodiesterase gets activated, breaking down cGMP. Consequently, the ligand-gated Na^+ channels close, which prevents sodium ions from entering, leading to hyperpolarization, and the membrane potential reaches -70 mV. The hyperpolarization in photoreceptor decreases the release of neurotransmitter glutamate.

Hyperpolarization leads to the development of electrical response (receptor potential) that excites the bipolar cells. The excited bipolar cells subsequently stimulate the ganglion cells, and this action potential is transmitted to the occipital lobes of the cerebrum via the optic nerves.

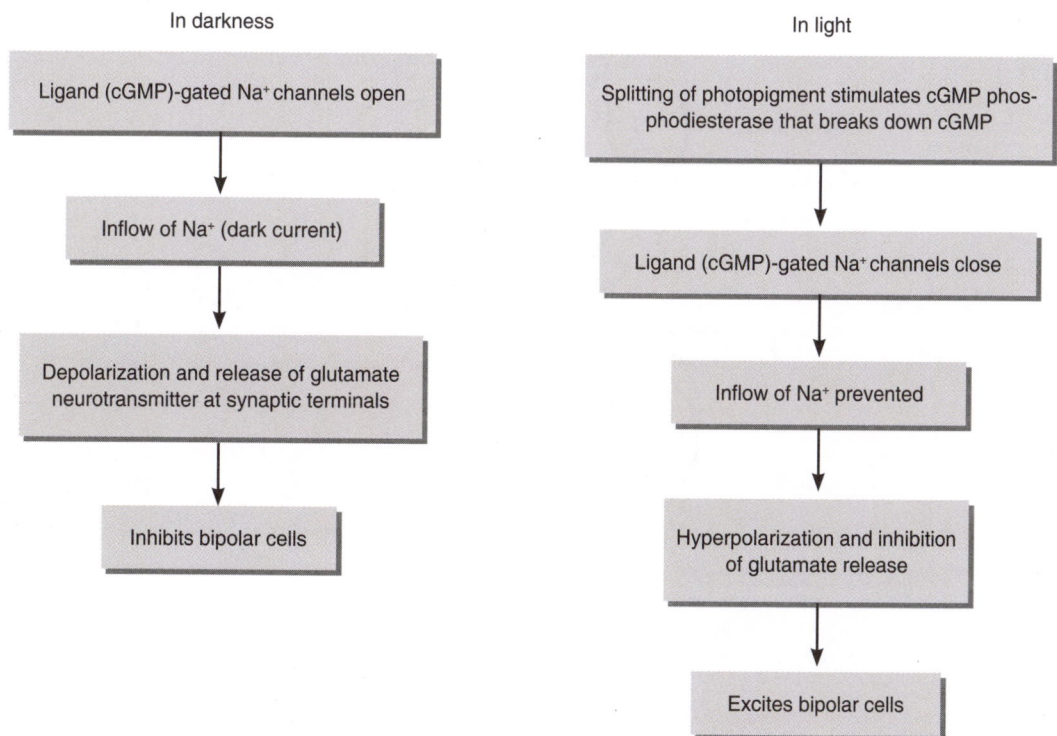

Figure 15.8 Operation of photoreceptors.

Visual pathway

The nerve impulses (action potential) generated in the photoreceptors is transmitted to the occipital lobe of the cerebrum by a nervous pathway, called the *visual pathway* or *optic pathway*.

The various steps of visual pathway are as follows:

1. The optic nerve is formed by the axons of ganglion cells. The excited ganglion cells transmit the action potential (electrical response) to the optic nerve, which leaves each eye through the optic disc or blind spot.

2. After leaving the eye, the axons within the optic nerve pass through the optic chiasm, a crossing point of the optic nerves present near the pituitary gland. In the optic chiasm, some axons cross to the opposite side, while others remain uncrossed at the same side.

3. After passing through the optic chiasm, the axons become part of the optic tract and enter the brain. The optic tracts then synapse with the nerve cells of the lateral geniculate bodies of the thalamus.

4. The nerve fibres of the lateral geniculate bodies of the thalamus then pass through the internal capsule and form the optic radiations that terminate in the visual area of the cerebral cortex in the occipital lobe of the cerebrum (Fig. 15.9).

5. The visual area of the cerebral cortex contains three areas, each with its own function. They are as follows:

    (a) **Primary visual area**: It is concerned with the perception of visual impulses.

    (b) **Visual association area**: It is concerned with the interpretation of visual impulses.

    (c) **Occipital eye field**: It is concerned with movement of eyes.

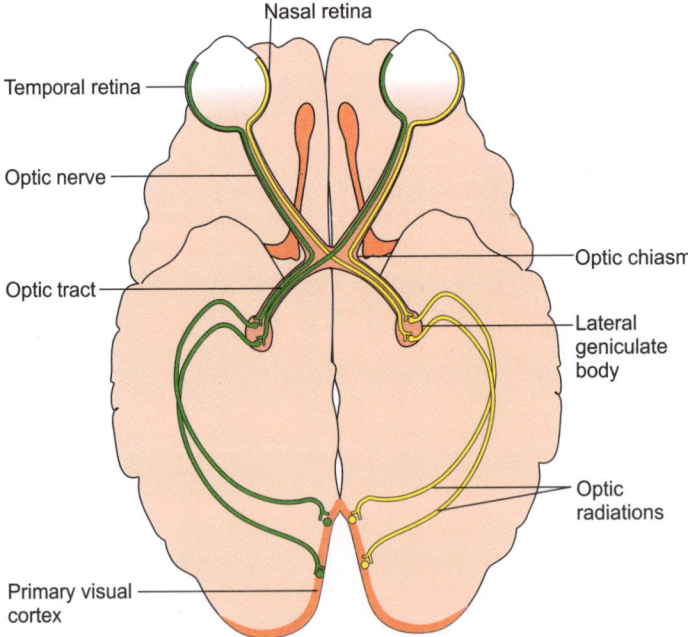

Figure 15.9 Visual pathway.

Visual pathway

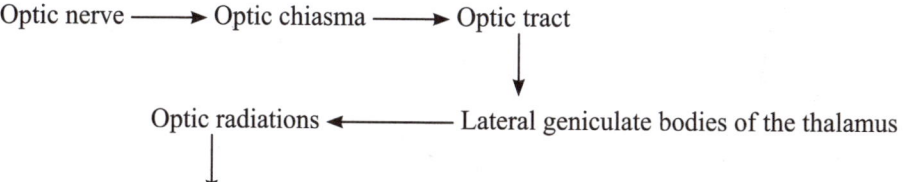

Optic nerve ⟶ Optic chiasma ⟶ Optic tract

Optic radiations ⟵ Lateral geniculate bodies of the thalamus

Visual area of the cerebral cortex

EARS: THE ORGANS OF HEARING AND EQUILIBRIUM

The ears are the organs of hearing and equilibrium that perform their functions by interaction of their sensory receptors with mechanical stimuli (i.e. sound waves for hearing and movement for balance). The study of structure, function and diseases of the ear is called *otology* (*oto*: ear; *logy*: study).

STRUCTURE OF THE EAR

The ear is divided into the following three distinct parts:

1. The external (outer) ear: It collects sound waves and directs them inwards.
2. The middle ear: It transmits the sound vibrations to the internal ear and amplifies them.
3. The internal (inner) ear: It contains receptors for hearing and equilibrium (Fig. 15.10).

External (outer) ear

The external (outer) ear consists of the auricle (pinna), external auditory meatus (auditory canal) and tympanic membrane (eardrum).

The auricle (pinna)

The auricle is the flexible, funnel-shaped, expanded portion that projects from the side of the head. It is composed of the fibroelastic cartilage covered by skin. It is deeply grooved and ridged; the most prominent outer ridge is the helix and the inferior soft part is the lobule.

The external auditory meatus (auditory canal)

The auditory canal is an S-shaped tube about 2.5-cm long, extending from the auricle to the tympanic membrane. Its curvature prevents hard objects from hitting the tympanic membrane directly. The canal is supported by the elastic cartilage in the outer side and by the temporal bone in the inner side. It is lined with the skin, continuous with that of the auricle.

The auditory canal is lined with hair follicles and modified sebaceous (oil) glands called *ceruminous glands* that secrete a brownish, semisolid, sticky substance, called the *cerumen* or *ear wax*. The hairs and cerumen prevent the foreign particles (e.g. dust, insects and microbes) from reaching the tympanic membrane. Movements of the temporomandibular joint during chewing and speaking help in moving the dried wax towards the exterior.

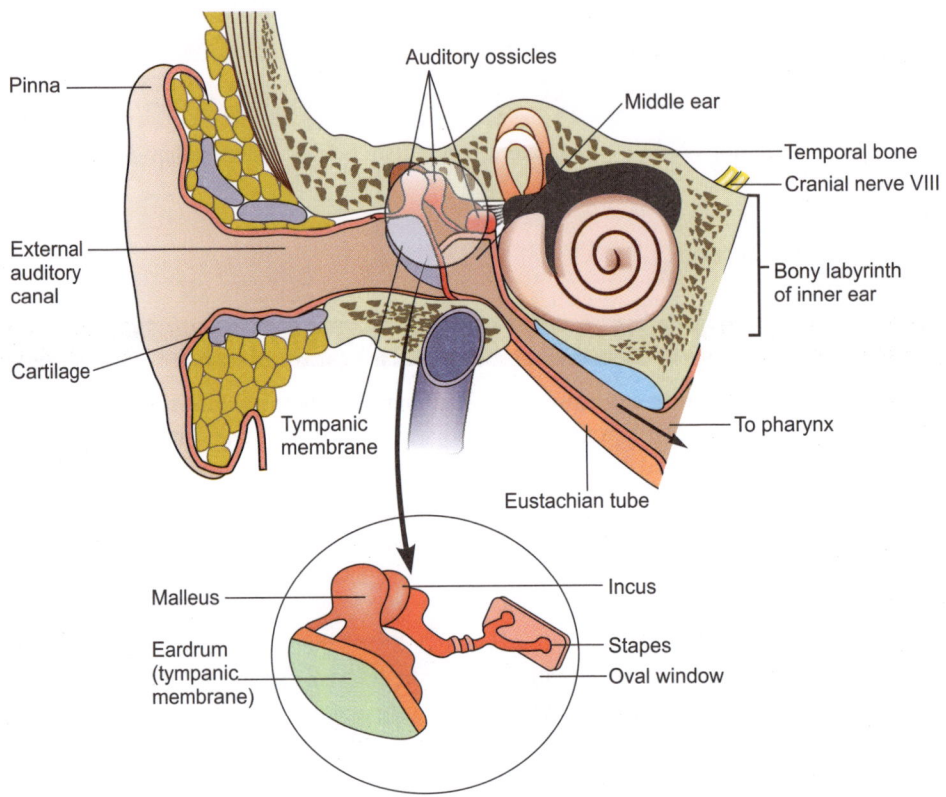

Figure 15.10 Structure of the ear.

Tympanic membrane (eardrum or tympanum)

The tympanic membrane is a thin, silvery grey, delicate membrane that completely separates the external auditory meatus from the middle ear. It is covered by three tissue layers: outer layer of the epidermis, middle layer of fibrous tissue and the inner lining of the mucous membrane.

The auricle allows the sound waves to enter the auditory canal, which directs those waves towards the delicate tympanic membrane and causes the membrane to vibrate.

Middle ear

The middle ear is an irregular-shaped, air-filled cavity enclosed in the temporal bone, and it is lined by the epithelium. It is separated from the external ear by the eardrum and from the internal ear by a thin bony partition that contains two small membrane-covered openings: the *oval window* (or fenestra ovalis) and the *round window* (or fenestra rotunda). The oval window is occluded by part of a small bone called the stapes and the round window by a fine sheet of fibrous tissue.

The middle ear communicates with the nasopharynx (upper portion of the throat) by the eustachian tube (auditory tube) that opens into the pharynx. The eustachian tube has a valve at its pharyngeal end that serves to equalize the air pressure on both sides of the tympanic membrane (i.e. between the external ear and middle ear) and thus enables the eardrum to vibrate freely when sound waves strike it.

This valve normally remains closed but opens during yawning, swallowing and during abrupt changes in altitude (ascent or descent in an airplane) to allow the air to enter or leave the middle ear until the pressure in the middle ear equals the atmospheric pressure. If the pressure is not equalized, intense pain and ringing in ears could develop. Sudden rise in air pressure may also lead to bursting of the eardrum, and this is prevented by the eustachian tube through the opening of its valve. This auditory tube also serves as a route for microorganisms to travel from the nose and throat to the middle ear.

Extending across the middle ear are the three smallest bones in the body, the auditory ossicles (ear bones), that extend from the tympanic membrane to the oval window. These bones are present in a series and are connected to each other by synovial joints. They are named according to their shapes: malleus (hammer shaped), incus (anvil shaped) and stapes (stirrup shaped).

❑ **Malleus**: The handle of malleus is attached to the internal surface of the tympanic membrane and the head forms a movable joint with the incus.
❑ **Incus**: The body of incus is joined to the malleus and the long process to the stapes.
❑ **Stapes**: The head of stapes is joined to the incus and its foot plate or base fits into the oval window.

The auditory ossicles transmit the vibrations from the tympanic membrane to the internal ear and also amplify them about 20 times.

Internal ear

The internal (inner) ear is also called the *labyrinth* (meaning: maze or network) due to its interconnected series of chambers and tunnels enclosed within the temporal bone. It contains the organs of hearing and balance.

Structurally, it consists of two main divisions: the bony labyrinth and the membranous labyrinth (Fig. 15.11).

Bony labyrinth

The bony labyrinth consists of a series of cavities lined with periosteum. It is larger than, and encloses, the membranous labyrinth of the same shape that fits into it, resembling a tube within a tube. Between the bony and the membranous labyrinth, there is a layer of watery fluid called *perilymph*, which closely resembles the cerebrospinal fluid in composition.

The bony labyrinth is divided into the following three areas:

1. **Vestibule**: This is the oval central portion of the bony labyrinth. It contains the oval and round windows in its lateral wall.
2. **The semicircular canals**: There are three semicircular canals in continuation with the vestibule: anterior, posterior and lateral, arranged in three mutually perpendicular planes. At one end of each canal, there is a swollen enlargement called the *ampulla of semicircular canal*.
3. **Cochlea**: It is a spiral canal present in continuation with the vestibule and resembles a snail's shell. It spirals around a central bony core called the *modiolus* (discussed in detail in the Membranous Labyrinth).

Membranous labyrinth

The membranous labyrinth has an almost similar shape as the bony labyrinth and consists of a series of sacs and tubes lying within the bony labyrinth. The membranous labyrinth is filled with the fluid, the *endolymph*, which resembles the intracellular fluid in composition.

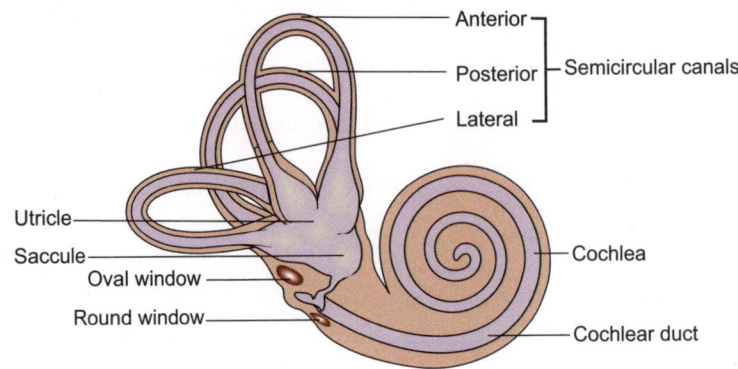

Figure 15.11 The internal ear.

The membranous labyrinth comprises of the following three areas:

1. *Vestibule*
   - ❏ The membranous labyrinth in the vestibule consists of two chambers: the larger chamber, *utricle*, and the smaller chamber, *saccule*. The utricle is connected to the saccule by a small duct.
   - ❏ The vestibule is the central portion; hence, it communicates with both the cochlea and the semicircular ducts. The utricle of the vestibule communicates with the semicircular ducts and saccule leads into the cochlear duct.

2. *Semicircular ducts*
   - ❏ The portion of the membranous labyrinth that is present inside the semicircular canals of bony labyrinth is called *semicircular ducts*. These ducts connect with the utricle of the vestibule. At one end of each duct, there is a swollen enlargement called the *ampulla of semicircular duct*.

3. *Cochlea*

The cross-section of the cochlea reveals that it contains the following three chambers:

1. The scala vestibuli (upper chamber)
2. The scala media or cochlear duct (middle chamber)
3. The scala tympani (lower chamber)

The scala vestibuli and scala tympani are part of the bony labyrinth of the cochlea; hence, these compartments are filled with perilymph. Both scala vestibuli and scala tympani communicate with each other at the distal end of the cochlea by a narrow passage, called the *helicotrema*. At the proximal end of the cochlea, the scala vestibuli and the scala tympani communicate with the oval and round windows, respectively, as shown in Figure 15.12.

The scala media, or the cochlear duct, continues from the saccule of the membranous labyrinth and it is filled with endolymph. The cochlear duct is triangular in shape and is present in the middle of scala vestibuli (upper chamber) and the scala tympani (lower chamber). The base of the scala media is called the *basilar membrane* and it separates the cochlear duct from the scala tympani. The roof of the scala media is called the *vestibular membrane*, or *Reissner's membrane*, and it separates the cochlear duct from the scala vestibuli (Fig. 15.12).

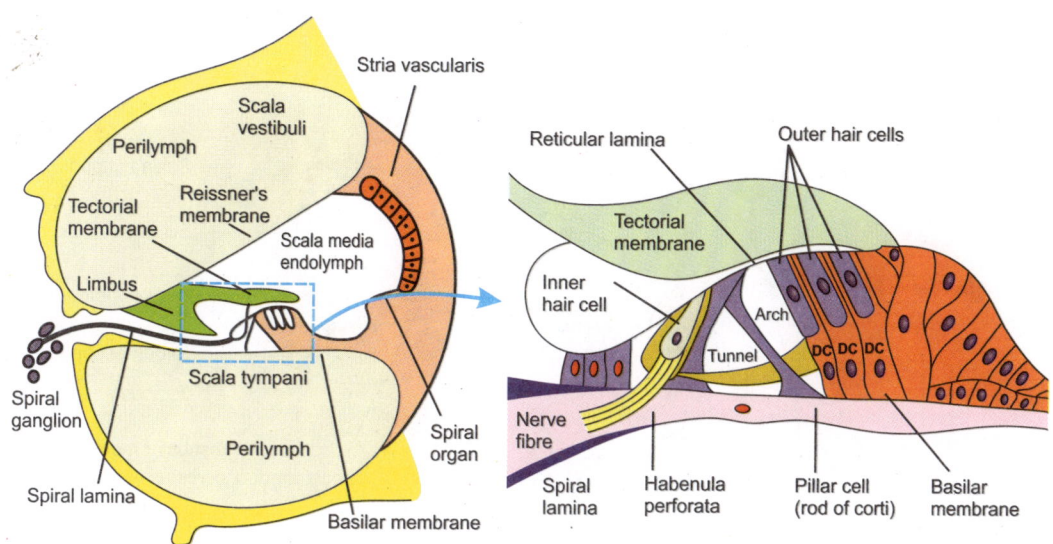

Figure 15.12 The cochlea.

The basilar membrane bears on it an organ of hearing called the *organ of Corti* or the *spiral organ*. The organ of Corti consists of supporting cells and about 16,000 specialized cochlear hair cells that contain auditory receptors. The specialized cochlear hair cells bear 'hair' (modified microvilli) at the free surface and have synaptic contacts with the dendrites of neurons at the bases. The dendrites of these neurons combine to form the cochlear branch of the vestibulocochlear (VIII) nerve. A flexible gelatinous membrane, called the *tectorial membrane*, covers the hair cells of organ of Corti.

The organ of Corti responds to the sound vibrations and produces action potential that ultimately leads to the generation of nerve impulses. These nerve impulses are carried to the hearing area in the temporal lobe of the cerebrum through the cochlear branch of vestibulocochlear nerve for interpretation.

PHYSIOLOGY OF HEARING

Every sound produces sound waves or vibrations in the air, which travel at about 332 m/s. Sound waves have the properties of pitch and intensity (volume). Pitch of sound is determined by the frequency of sound waves and is measured in Hertz (Hz). The audible range in humans extends from 20 to 20,000 Hz. The higher the frequency of vibration, the higher the pitch. The intensity of sound depends on the amplitude of the sound waves and is measured in decibels (dB). The larger the intensity of vibration, the louder the sound. An increase of 1 dB exhibits a 10-fold increase in sound intensity.

The ear not only detects sound but also notes its direction, judges its loudness and determines its pitch (frequency).

The various events that are involved in hearing are as follows (Fig. 15.13):

1. Sound waves are collected by the auricle and directed inwards through the external auditory canal.
2. When sound waves strike the eardrum, it begins to vibrate at the same frequency similar to that of sound waves. The low-frequency (low pitch) sound waves vibrate the eardrum slowly, while the high-frequency (high pitched) sound causes rapid vibrations of the eardrum.

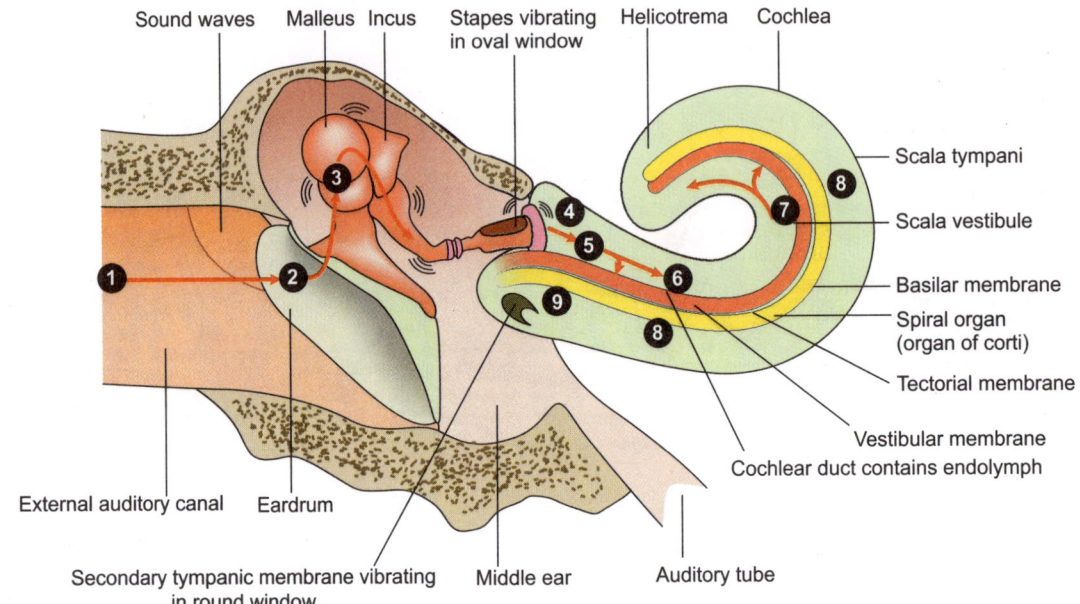

Figure 15.13 Various events involved in hearing.

3. The central area of the eardrum is attached to the malleus, which also starts to vibrate. The vibration is transmitted from the malleus to the incus and then to stapes.

4. As the stapes moves back and forth, the oval window that is fitted into the footplate of the stapes starts moving in and out 20 times more vigorously than the eardrum. The force of vibrations in the oval window is considerably increased due to the amplification of the vibrations as they move from large surface area (eardrum) to small surface area (oval window) by movement of the ossicles.

5. The movement of the oval window sets up fluid waves in the perilymph of the scala vestibule. The force of these fluid waves is then transmitted from the scala vestibule to the scala tympani and, eventually, to the round window, causing it to bulge outwards into the middle ear.

6. The force of fluid waves in the scala vestibule and the scala tympani also pushes the vestibular membrane (or Reissner's membrane) back and forth, creating pressure waves in the endolymph inside the cochlear duct.

7. The pressure waves in the endolymph of the cochlear duct result in vibration of the basilar membrane, which stimulates the auditory receptors in the specialized hair cells of the organ of Corti.

8. This stimulation of the auditory receptors causes depolarization of the receptor cells and produces receptor (action) potential that ultimately lead to the generation of nerve impulses. The nerve impulses are then transmitted to the temporal lobe of the cerebrum via the cochlear branch of vestibulocochlear nerve where it is interpreted as sound.

The receptor cells in different regions of the organ of Corti are sensitive to the sounds of different pitches. The receptor cells at the base of the cochlear duct (near the oval window) are stimulated by the sounds of high frequency and those towards the tip are stimulated by the sounds of low frequency.

Loudness of sound is determined by the intensity (amplitude) of sound waves. High-intensity sound waves cause larger vibrations of the basilar membrane, which results in the increased rate of nerve impulses reaching the brain. Excessive loudness may damage the sensitive hair cells of the organ of Corti and may cause hearing loss.

The auditory pathway

The nerve impulses (action potential) generated in the auditory receptors of organ of Corti are transmitted to the temporal lobe of the cerebrum by a nervous pathway called the *auditory pathway*.

The various steps of the auditory pathway are as follows:

1. The activated auditory receptors transmit the nerve impulses to the cochlear branch of each vestibulocochlear (VIII) nerve.
2. The vestibulocochlear nerve transmits the impulses to the auditory nuclei in the medulla, which then projects it towards the olivary nuclei in the pons on both the sides. Slight differences in the timing of impulses arriving from the two ears at the olivary nuclei allow in locating the source of a sound.
3. The nerve fibres of the olivary nuclei in the pons ascend towards the midbrain and transmit the nerve impulses to the medial geniculate nucleus of the thalamus.
4. From the thalamus, these impulses are conducted to the auditory area in the temporal lobe of the cerebrum where sound is perceived.

PHYSIOLOGY OF EQUILIBRIUM

Equilibrium (balance) is maintained by the organs collectively called the *vestibular apparatus*, which include the saccule, the utricle and the semicircular ducts.

There are two types of equilibrium (balance): static equilibrium and dynamic equilibrium.

Static equilibrium

It refers to the maintenance of the position of the body (mainly the head) relative to the force of gravity. Any change of the position of the head stimulates the *maculae* in the utricle and saccule, which are the receptors for static equilibrium.

The macula is a thickened region present in the walls of both the utricle and saccule. The macula consists of supporting cells and hair cells that contain the sensory receptors.

❏ The hair cells bear 'hair' (modified microvilli) at the free surface and have synaptic contacts with the dendrites of neurons at the bases. The dendrites of these neurons combine to form the vestibular branch of vestibulocochlear (VIII) nerve.
❏ The supporting cells secrete a thick, gelatinous, glycoprotein layer, called the *otolithic membrane*, that covers the hair cells. The otolithic membrane contains numerous minute, irregular particles, called *otoliths* or ear stones, composed of protein and calcium carbonate.

Any change in the position of body (or head) with respect to gravity (e.g. rapid forward movement) leads to the movement of the perilymph and endolymph. The otoliths, being heavier than the endolymph, lag behind and press upon the sensory hairs of the maculae and bend them. Bending of the hair cells produce receptor potential that lead to the generation of nerve impulses, which pass along the vestibular branch of vestibulocochlear (VIII) nerve.

Dynamic equilibrium

It refers to the maintenance of the body position (mainly the head) in response to sudden movements such as rotation, acceleration and deceleration. The three semicircular ducts play a role in the maintenance of dynamic equilibrium.

The three semicircular ducts—anterior, posterior and lateral—lie at right angles to one another in three planes. The anterior and posterior ducts are vertical and the lateral duct is horizontal in position. At one end of each duct, there is a swollen enlargement called the *ampulla*, and each ampulla has a small elevation called the *crista*, which detects turning or rotational movements of head. A crista resembles a macula in structure except that it lies on an elevation, and the gelatinous mass covering its hairs lacks otoliths and is called *cupula* (Fig. 15.14).

When the head is turned, the endolymph in the semicircular ducts due to its inertia does not move as fast as the head and the hair cells but continues to move after the head stops moving. Because of this difference in the rate of movement the sensory hairs of cristae are swept through the endolymph and therefore bend. Bending of the hair cells produces receptor (action) potential, which leads to the nerve impulses that pass along the vestibular branch of vestibulocochlear (VIII) nerve.

Equilibrium pathway

Most of the axons of the vestibular branch of vestibulocochlear (VIII) nerve enter the brain stem and terminate in vestibular nuclei in the medulla and pons. The remaining axons enter the cerebellum. Both the cerebellum and the vestibular nuclei are connected by bidirectional pathways and play a key role in maintaining equilibrium. The cerebellum continuously receives information from the vestibular

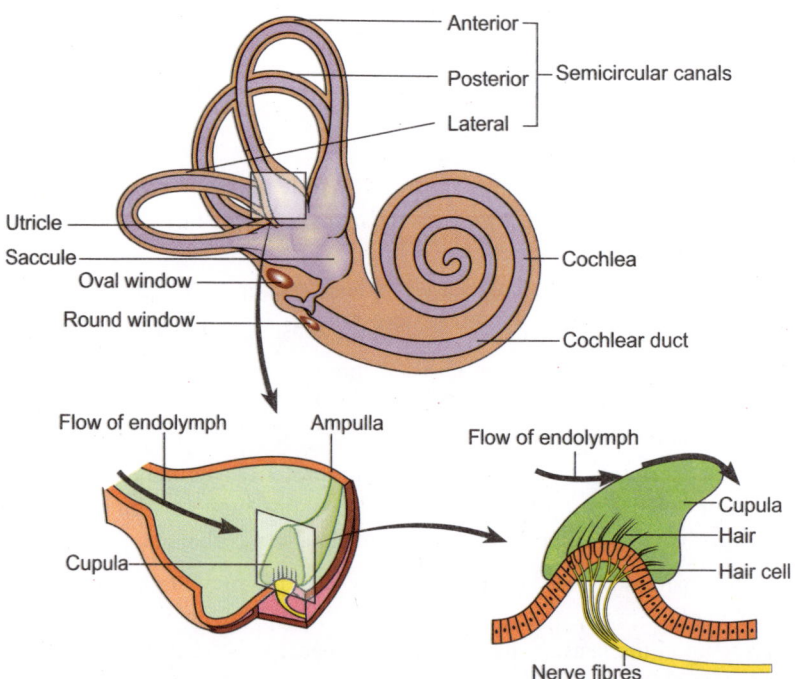

Figure 15.14 Physiology of equilibrium.

apparatus and then sends nerve impulses to motor areas of the cerebrum. The cerebrum then sends signals to specific skeletal muscles in order to maintain equilibrium.

SENSE OF SMELL

The sense of smell, or *olfaction*, is perceived due to interaction of the chemical molecules with sensory receptors in the nose. The nose contains 10–100 million olfactory receptors for the sense of smell in the mucus membrane that lines the upper part of the nostril.

OLFACTORY RECEPTORS

Olfactory receptors are spindle-shaped bipolar neurons with a knob-shaped dendrite and an axon that passes through the cribriform plate of the ethmoid bone. The odoriferous substances stimulate the olfactory receptors and result in the generation of receptor potential, thus initiating the olfactory response. We are able to recognize about 10,000 different odours due to the stimulation of many different combinations of olfactory receptors.

Along with olfactory receptors, the mucus membrane lining the nose contains the following:

1. **Supporting cells**: These are columnar epithelial cells that support and nourish olfactory receptors.
2. **Basal cells**: These are stem cells present between the supporting cells. They continually undergo cell division to produce new olfactory receptors, in order to replace the worn-out receptor cells that survive only for about a month.
3. **Bowman's glands**: These are the olfactory glands present beneath the mucus membrane. They secrete mucus that spreads over the mucus membrane and keeps it moist. The mucus also protects the cells from dust and bacteria.

PHYSIOLOGY OF OLFACTION (SMELL)

All odoriferous substances give off volatile molecules, which are carried into the nose with the inhaled air. Here, they dissolve in mucus covering the mucus membrane, bind to the olfactory receptors and stimulate them. The stimulated olfactory receptors produce receptor potential and lead to the generation of nerve impulse, which is carried by the olfactory nerve to the brain, where the sensation of smell is perceived.

'Sniffing' concentrates the volatile molecules in the roof of the nose and stimulates a large number of olfactory receptors, thus increasing the perception of smell.

Adaptation: When an individual is continuously exposed to an odour, perception of the odour decreases. The olfactory receptors adapt by about 50% in the first second and complete insensitivity occurs after about a minute of exposure.

OLFACTORY PATHWAY

The nerve impulses generated in the olfactory receptors are transmitted to the temporal lobe of the cerebrum by a nervous pathway called the *olfactory pathway* (Fig. 15.15). The various steps of olfactory pathway are as follows:

1. Olfactory receptors are present on the mucus membrane of the roof of the nasal cavity above the superior nasal conchae. The axons of the olfactory receptors extend through the cribriform plate of the ethmoid bone and join to form the right and left olfactory (I) nerves.

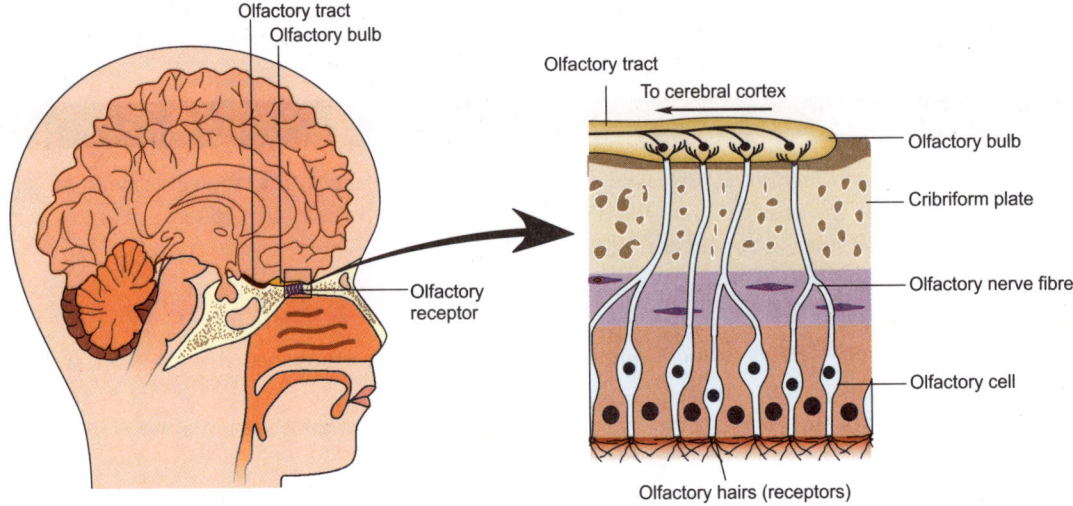

Figure 15.15 Olfactory receptors.

2. The olfactory nerves terminate in the olfactory bulb located below the frontal lobe of cerebrum. The axons of the olfactory bulb neurons extend posteriorly and form the olfactory tract.
3. The axons of the olfactory tract then move backwards and project towards the olfactory area in the temporal lobe of the cerebral cortex where the impulses are interpreted and odour is perceived.

SENSE OF TASTE

The sense of taste, or *gustation*, involves stimulation of the sensory receptors by dissolved chemicals. The sensory receptors for the taste sensation are located in the taste buds. There are about 10,000 taste buds in adults. The number of taste buds is more in children and it declines with age.

TASTE BUDS

Most of the taste buds are present in elevations on the tongue called *papillae*, but some are also found on the soft palate, epiglottis, pharynx and proximal part of the oesophagus.

The papillae on the tongue that contain taste buds are of the following three types:

1. Filiform papillae (*fili*: threadlike): These are small, conical-shaped structures present on the entire surface of the tongue. They contain very less number of taste buds.
2. Fungiform papillae (*fungi*: mushroom-like): These are round structures located mainly over the anterior surface of the tongue near the tip. Each papillae contains about 5–6 taste buds.
3. Circumvallate papillae (*vallate*: wall-like): They form an inverted V-shaped row at the back of the tongue. Each papilla contains about 100–300 taste buds.

Each taste bud is a spherical structure consisting of gustatory receptor cells that function as the receptor for gustation (taste). The taste buds have an opening called the *taste pore*. The gustatory receptor cells have long projections called *microvilli* that extend out of the taste pore and have synaptic contacts with the dendrites of neurons at the bases (Fig. 15.16).

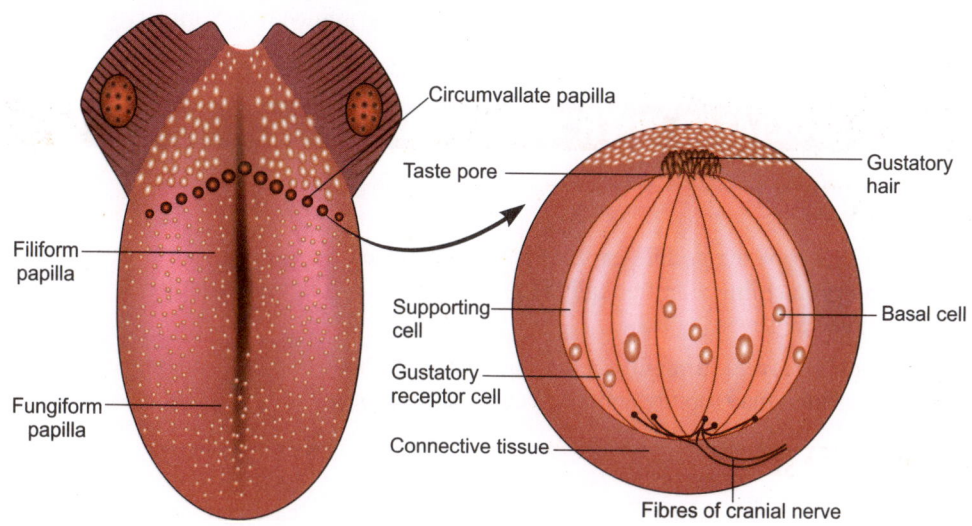

Figure 15.16 Taste buds.

PHYSIOLOGY OF GUSTATION (TASTE)

All the chemicals must first dissolve in fluid medium to activate the sensory receptors (e.g. like the odours in nose dissolve in mucus). The saliva produced by salivary glands provides this fluid medium for taste sensation. Once the chemical is dissolved in saliva, it acts on the microvilli of gustatory receptor cells and results in the development of receptor potential. This, in turn, generates nerve impulses that are transmitted to the brain for interpretation.

The primary or fundamental taste sensations are divided into four types: *sweet, sour, bitter* and *salt*. Although all taste buds can detect all the four sensations, some tastes consistently stimulate the taste buds in the following specific parts of the tongue:

❑ Sour and salty, mainly at the tip
❑ Sour at the sides
❑ Bitter at the back

The receptors of smell also play a role in tasting the food. The various forms of taste other than the four basic ones (sweet, salty, sour, bitter) are really due to the odours that reach the olfactory receptors through the throat. This is why we do not experience the characteristic flavour of food during cold.

Gustatory pathway

The nerve impulses generated in the gustatory receptors are transmitted to the brain by a nervous pathway called the ***gustatory pathway***. The various steps of gustatory pathway are as follows:

1. The gustatory receptor cells have synaptic contacts with the nerve fibres of facial (VII), glossopharyngeal (IX) and vagus (X) nerves. When the receptor cells are activated, nerve impulses are generated and conducted along the glossopharyngeal, facial and vagus nerves before they synapse in medulla and thalamus.

2. From the medulla and thalamus, the nerve impulses are transmitted to the primary gustatory (taste) area in the parietal lobe of the cerebral cortex where taste is perceived.

DISEASES ASSOCIATED WITH SENSE ORGANS

OTITIS MEDIA

It is an acute infection of the middle ear that is mainly caused by upward spread of microbes from an upper respiratory tract infection through the eustachian tube. It is very common in children and is usually accompanied by severe earache.

Symptoms include fever, irritability, pain and reddening and outward bulging of the eardrum. Sometimes, the eardrum may rupture and may cause loss of hearing.

MENIERE'S DISEASE

It is characterized by the accumulation of endolymph that results in increased pressure in the membranous labyrinth of the internal ear. The increased pressure may gradually cause destruction of the sensory cells in the ampulla and cochlea.

Symptoms include dizziness, nausea and vomiting, tinnitus (ringing of ears) and total hearing impairment over a period of years.

CONJUNCTIVITIS

It is the inflammation of the conjunctiva mainly caused by bacterial infection and irritants such as smoke, dust and pollutants in air.

It is very common in children and is highly contagious.

GLAUCOMA

It is a condition characterized by increased intraocular pressure in the anterior chamber due to impaired drainage of aqueous fluid through the canal of Schlemm. Persistently raised intraocular pressure results in irreversible destruction of retinal neurons and can damage the optic nerve, causing visual impairment.

Glaucoma is more common in people over 40 years and usually affects one eye.

CATARACT

It is characterized by loss of transparency (opacity) of lens due to changes in the structure of lens proteins.

It usually develops during older age and may also be caused by injury, excessive exposure to UV light, X-rays, cigarette smoke and diseases such as diabetes mellitus. The extent of visual impairment depends on the location and extent of loss of transparency.

REFRACTIVE ERRORS OF THE EYE

In the normal eye or *emetropic* state, light from near and distant objects is focused on the retina (Fig. 15.17).

In *myopia* or nearsightedness, the distant objects are focused in front of the retina as the eyeball is too long, and thus there is difficulty in viewing distant objects. Near objects are focused normally on the retina. The correction in myopia is achieved by using a biconcave lens.

In *hypermetropia* or *hyperopia* or farsightedness, the near image is focused behind the retina as the eyeball is too short. It can be corrected using a biconvex lens. The distant objects are focused normally.

Astigmatism results in blurred vision due to abnormal curvature of part of the cornea or lens that prevents focusing on the retina. It is corrected by using cylindrical lenses.

Figure 15.18 illustrates the different refractive errors of the eye.

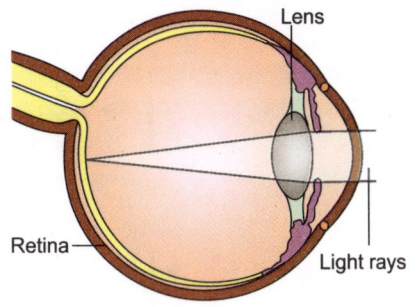

Figure 15.17 The normal vision.

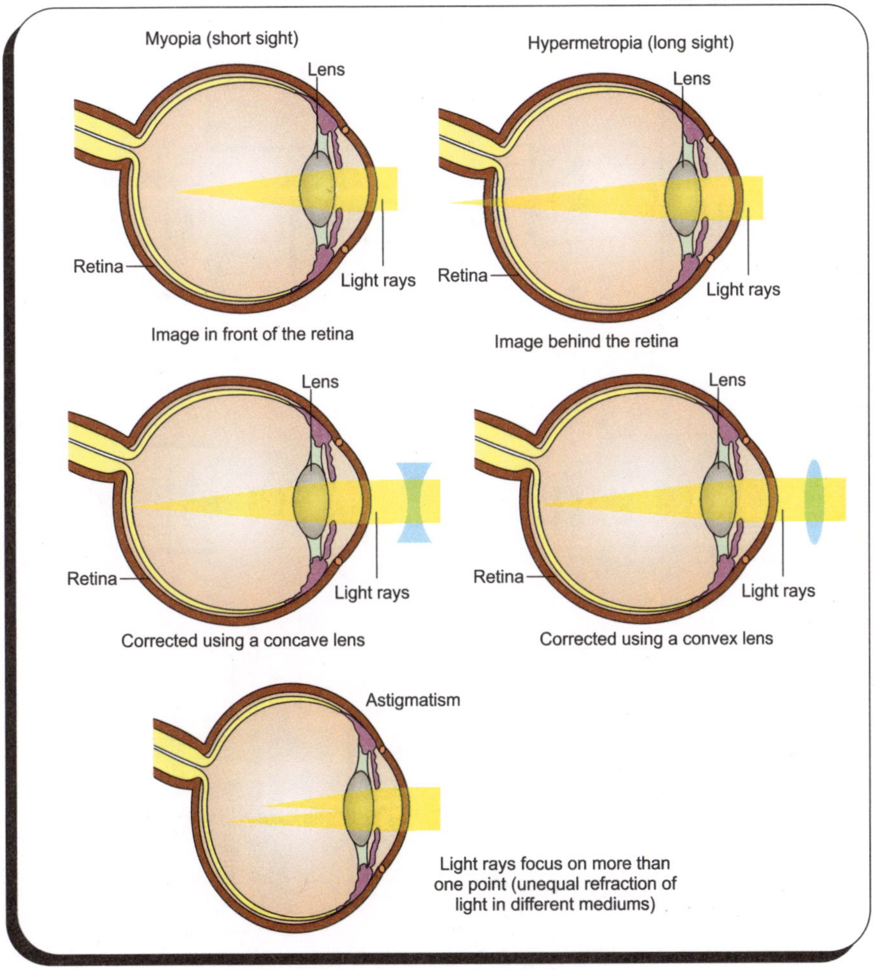

Myopia (short sight)
Lens
Retina
Light rays
Image in front of the retina

Hypermetropia (long sight)
Lens
Retina
Light rays
Image behind the retina

Lens
Retina
Light rays
Corrected using a concave lens

Lens
Retina
Light rays
Corrected using a convex lens

Astigmatism
Light rays focus on more than one point (unequal refraction of light in different mediums)

Figure 15.18 Refractive errors of the eye.

OVERVIEW OF SENSE ORGANS

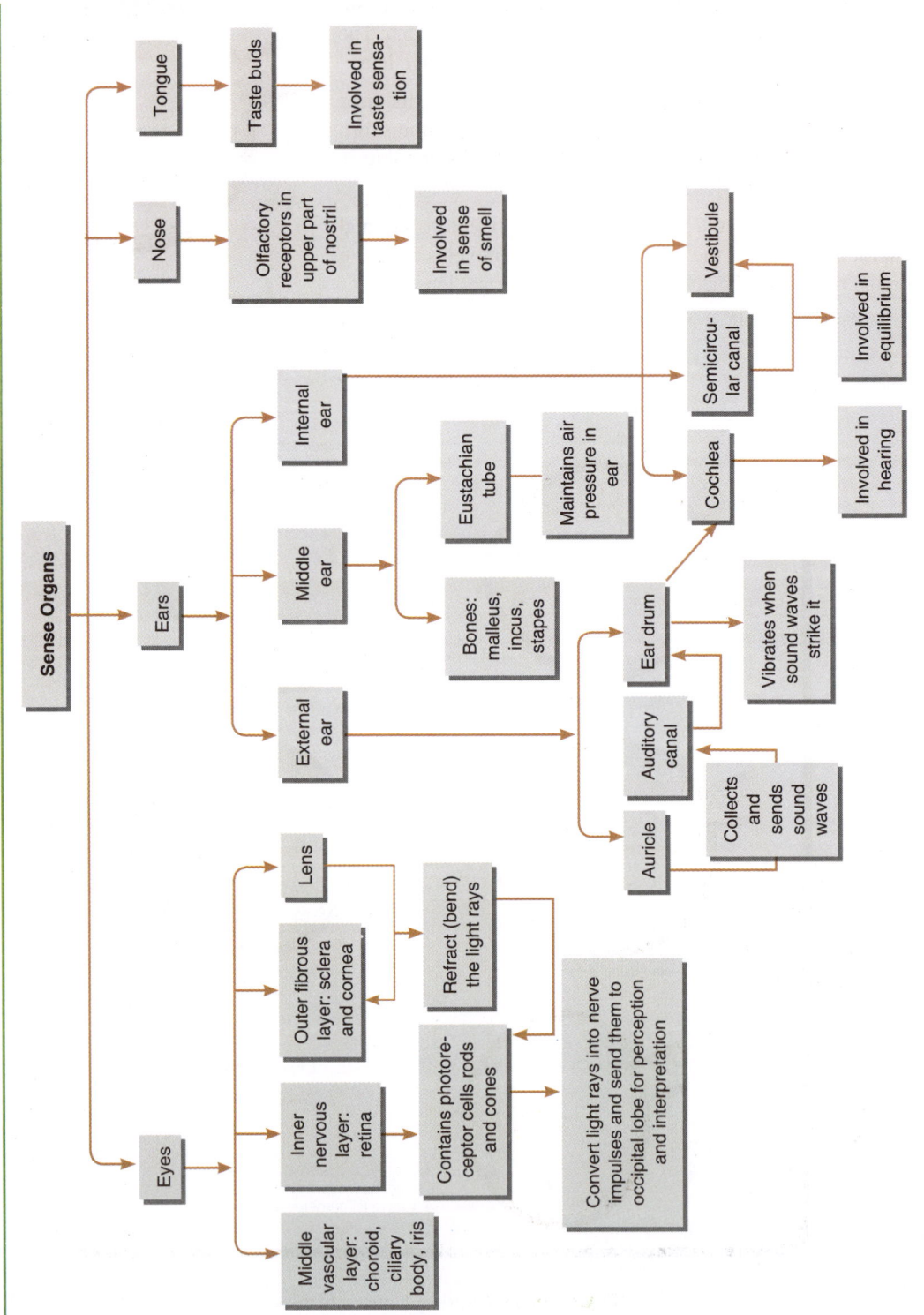

Embryonic Development of Eyes & Ears

Embryonic Development of Eyes

❏ *About 22 days after fertilization*

➤ The ectoderm bulges out to form the *optic grooves*. Within few days, optic grooves enlarge to form the *optic vesicles* and these vesicles reach the surface ectoderm.

➤ Surface ectoderm thickens to form the *lens placodes*, which eventually develops into the *lenses*.

➤ Distal portion of optic vesicle forms *optic cups*, which eventually develop into *optic part of the retina*. Optic cups remain attached to the ectoderm by structures called *optic stalks*; they eventually convert into *optic nerve*.

➤ Anterior portion of optic cup forms the epithelium of *ciliary body* and *iris*. Mesenchyme around the optic cup differentiates into an inner layer that forms *choroid* and an outer layer that develops into *sclera* and *cornea*.

➤ Mesenchyme between iris and cornea forms *anterior chamber*

➤ Mesenchyme between iris and lens forms *posterior chamber*

➤ Surface ectoderm and mesenchyme forms *eyelids* that remain closed until 26 weeks of development

Embryonic Development of Ears

❏ *About 22 weeks after fertilization*

➤ Surface ectoderm thickness to form *otic placodes*. The otic placodes quickly forms otic pits, which form otic vesicles at the surface ectoderm within mesenchyme of head.

➤ Otic vesicles eventually develop into *membranous labyrinth of the internal ear*.

➤ Mesenchyme around otic vesicle ossifies and forms *bony labyrinth of the internal ear*.

❏ Endoderm forms pharyngeal pouch that eventually forms the *middle ear.*

❏ Endoderm forms the first pharyngeal cleft that develops into the *external ear.*

Ageing and Sense Organs

❏ As we age, there is gradual loss of *olfactory receptors* and *gustatory receptor cells*.

❏ Several age-related changes occur in eyes:

➤ The lens loses some of its elasticity, sclera becomes thick and rigid, muscles that regulate pupil size weaken with age, and thus elderly people find difficulty in light and dark adjustments and have reduced colour and depth perception.

➤ Various eye-related diseases are more likely to occur in old age such as cataract, glaucoma and detached retina.

❏ Elderly people experience a noticeable hearing loss. The changes in the ears with age include loss of hair cells in organ of Corti and degeneration of nerve pathway; thus, elderly people experience tinnitus (ringing in ears) and vestibular imbalance more frequently.

TIPS FOR HEALTHY EYES AND EARS

Tips for Healthy Eyes and Ears

1. *Eat plenty of fruit and vegetables.* Broccoli, spinach, sweet corn, orange and yellow peppers, kiwi fruits, oranges and mangoes are all great sources of the substances lutein and zea xanthin, which may help protect against some eye conditions.

2. *Exercise your eyes at frequent intervals.* Eye exercise is simple. All you need to do is just blink several times, then close your eyes and role them in clockwise and anticlockwise direction.

3. *Give your eyes a rest.* If you spend a lot of time at the computer or focusing on any one thing, you sometimes forget to blink and your eyes can get fatigued. Try the 20–20–20 rule: Every 20 min, look away about 20 feet in front of you for 20 s. This can help reduce eyestrain.

4. *Drink more water.* You need to replenish the 8–10 cups of water your body uses every day. No other liquid provides the benefits of water.

5. *Quit smoking or never start.* Smoking is as bad for your eyes as it is for the rest of your body. Research has linked smoking to an increased risk of developing age-related macular degeneration, cataract and optic nerve damage, all of which can lead to blindness

6. *Have your eyes tested regularly.*

Tips for Healthy Ears

1. Never poke anything into your ears. The lining of the ear is delicate and can easily be damaged.

2. Do not use cotton buds to clean your ears. They can irritate the ear canal and push wax back inside, making it more difficult to remove.

3. Do not immerse your ears in your bath water; body bacteria may enter your ear canal and could cause an infection.

4. If you have an ear problem, do not ignore it. It would not improve without proper treatment. The longer an ear problem is neglected, the longer it may take to treat.

Review Questions

Long Answer Questions

1. Describe the receptors and the neural pathway for the sense of taste.
2. What are the three kinds of papillae, and where are they located?
3. Identify the receptors and neural pathway for the sense of smell.
4. Describe the accessory structures of the eye.
5. Describe the structure of the eye.
6. Describe the visual pathway.

7. Describe how the eye focuses on objects at various distances.

8. Describe the ear in general terms and elaborate on the structural components of the ear and their functions.

9. Describe the cochlea in detail.

10. Discuss the pathway of hearing and equilibrium.

Short Answer Questions

1. Why do you get a 'runny nose' when you cry?

2. Which cranial nerves conduct taste sensations to the brain?

3. Which of the cranial nerves innervate the olfactory mucosa?

4. Which are more numerous, rods or cones?

5. What are the layers of the retina?

Multiple Choice Questions

1. The structure that is in direct contact with the tympanic membrane is
   - (a) The stapes
   - (b) The incus
   - (c) The malleus
   - (d) The semicircular canals

2. In the central region of the retina there is a yellowish spot, the macula lutea, with a depression in its centre that produces the sharpest vision. This depression is called
   - (a) The optic disc
   - (b) The rods and cones
   - (c) The vitreous body
   - (d) The fovea centralis
   - (e) The ganglion cells

3. Which structure separates the external auditory canal from the middle ear chamber?
   - (a) Auditory membrane
   - (b) Vestibular membrane
   - (c) Tympanic membrane
   - (d) Acoustic membrane

4. Aqueous humor produced by the ciliary body is secreted into the posterior chamber and enters the anterior chamber through
   - (a) The pupil
   - (b) The scleral venous sinus
   - (c) The vitreous body
   - (d) The suspensory ligament
   - (e) The lens capsule

5. The basic functional unit of hearing is
   - (a) The utricle
   - (b) The auricle
   - (c) The spiral organ
   - (d) The semicircular canals

6. Identify the organ/innervation mismatch:
   - (a) Glossopharyngeal nerve–tongue
   - (b) Optic nerve–eye
   - (c) Facial nerve–olfactory epithelium
   - (d) Cochlear nerve–spiral organ
   - (e) Vestibular nerve–semicircular canals

7. Which portion of the cochlea responds to low-frequency sound waves?

    (a) The portion closest to the vestibular window

    (b) The middle portion

    (c) The portion closest to the cochlear nerve

    (d) The end portion

8. The hair cells in the spiral organ are supported by

    (a) The basilar membrane   (b) The vestibule

    (c) The tectorial membrane   (d) The utricle

    (e) The cochlear plate

9. Which of the following is the correct sequence for passage of sensory impulses through the cells of the retina?

    (a) Ganglion neurons, rods and cones, bipolar neurons

    (b) Rods and cones, bipolar neurons, ganglion neurons

    (c) Rods and cones, ganglion neurons, bipolar neurons

    (d) Ganglion neurons, bipolar neurons, rods and cones

10. Ceruminous glands secrete

    (a) Lacrimal fluid   (b) Mucus into the middle ear chamber

    (c) Aqueous humor   (d) Cerumen

    (e) Endolymph

State True or False

1. The special senses are localized in complex receptor organs and have extensive neural pathways.

2. Taste buds occur on the surface of the tongue, but they are also found in smaller number in the mucosa of the palate and pharynx.

3. The pitch of a sound is directly related to the wave frequency.

4. Lacrimal fluid (tears) contains the enzyme amylase.

5. The anterior chamber is located between the cornea and the iris and is filled with vitreous humor.

6. The malleus is the bone in the middle ear that is attached to the vestibular window.

7. Vibrations of the vestibular window set up compressional waves in the perilymph of the cochlea.

8. The saccule, semicircular canals and cochlea constitute the vestibular organs.

9. The auditory canal equalizes the pressure on the inside of the tympanic membrane to that on the outside of the membrane.

10. An awareness of the position of the head as it relates to gravity is due to stimulation of hair cells in the utricle.

Fill in the Blanks

1. The posterior eye cavity contains a transparent, jellylike substance called _____.

2. _____ is the condition resulting from an irregular curvature of the cornea.

3. True colour blindness is referred to as _____.

4. Movement of the thin _____ transmits sound waves from the outer to the middle ear.

5. The_____(oval) window is located at the footplate of the stapes, and the _____ (round) window is located at the end of the scala vestibuli.

6. The _____ organ (organ of Corti) is the functional unit of hearing.

7. The _____ organs are the functional units of balance and equilibrium.

Appendices: Health Education

HEALTH

World Health Organization (WHO) defined the term *health* as 'Health is a state of complete physical, mental and social well-being and not merely the absence of disease or infirmity'. Hence, there are four aspects of health: physical, mental, social and spiritual.

❑ **Physical health:** It refers to the normal functioning and growth of the body.
❑ **Mental health:** It refers to the state of balance between the individual and the surrounding world. A mentally healthy person is contented, has self-respect, is able to adjust with others and has firm determination and self-control.
❑ **Social health:** It refers to the ability of the individual to adjust with the society.
❑ **Spiritual health:** It refers to the integrity, principles and ethics; purpose in life; and serves as a connecting link between physiology and psychology.

DISEASE

Disease can be defined as any deviation from the normal state of complete physical, mental or social well-being. The end result or final outcome of the disease may be recovery, disability, illness or death. The various disease-causing agents may be broadly classified as follows:

❑ **Biological agents:** These are microorganisms such as bacteria, viruses, protozoa and fungi.
❑ **Physical agents:** These include heat, cold, pressure, electricity, radiation and humidity.
❑ **Chemical agents:** These may be exogenous (present outside the body) such as dust, fumes, gases and metals or endogenous (produced in the body) such as urea, uric acid, bilirubin and cholesterol.
❑ **Mechanical agents:** They include accidental exposure to mechanical forces or chronic friction that may lead to trauma, fracture, dislocation or death.

- ❏ **Social agents:** They include poverty, smoke, drug abuse, alcohol consumption and unhealthy lifestyle.
- ❏ **Absence or excess of health factors:** They include excess or lack of nutrients and hormones.

The prevention of disease can be done at three levels, which include primary, secondary and tertiary prevention.

- ❏ **Primary prevention:** These are the measures or actions taken before the onset of disease that eliminates the possibility of its occurrence. For example, immunization or lifestyle changes.
- ❏ **Secondary prevention:** These are the actions taken at the early stage of disease that halts the progress of disease and prevents complications.
- ❏ **Tertiary prevention:** These are the preventive measures taken during the advanced stage of a disease to reduce or limit the impairments and disabilities.

APPENDIX B: NUTRITION AND HEALTH

Balanced Diet: It is a diet that contains adequate amounts of all the necessary nutrients required for healthy growth and activity. It can also be defined as the diet containing foods that furnish all the nutritive factors in proper proportion for adequate nutrition.

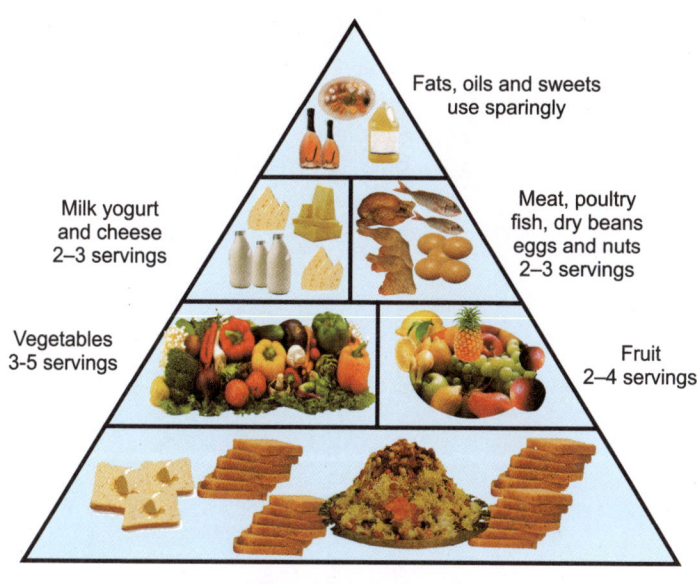

Balanced Diet

Details about vitamins

Vitamin	Chemical name	Year of discovery	Food source	Solu-bility	Recom-mended dietary allow-ance	Deficient disease	Upper intake level (UL/Day)*	Overdose disease
Vitamin A	Retinol, reti-nal, and four carotenoids including beta carotene	1913	Cod liver oil	Fat	900 µg	Night blindness, hyperkeratosis, and keratomala-cia	3,300 µg	Hypervitaminosis A
Vitamin B$_1$	Thiamine	1910	Rice bran	Water	1.2 mg	Beriberi, wernicke Korsadoff syndrome	Not de-termined	Drowsiness or muscle relation with large doses
Vitamin B$_2$	Riboflavin	1920	Meat, eggs	Water	1.3 mg	Ariboflavinosis	Not de-termined	
Vitamin B$_3$	Niacin, niacin-amide	1936	Meat, eggs, grains	Water	16.0 mg	Pellagra	35.0 mg	Liver damage (doses >2 gm/day)
Vitamin B$_5$	Pantothelic acid	1931	Meat, whole grains in many foods	Water	5.0 mg	Paraesthesia	Not de-termined	Diarrhoea; possible nausea and heartburn
Vitamin B$_6$	Pyridoxine, pyridoxamine, pyridoxal	1934	Meat, dairy products	Water	1.3* 1.7 mg	Anaemia periph-eral neuropathy	100 mg	Impairment of proprio-ception, nerve damage (doses > 100 mg/day)
Vitamin B$_7$	Biotin	1931	Meat, dairy products, eggs	Water	30.0 µg	Dermatitis, en-teritis	Not de-termined	
Vitamin B$_9$	Folic acid, folinic acid	1941	Leafy green vegetables	Water	400 µg	Megaloblast and deficiency during pregnancy is associated with birth defects, such as neural tube defects	1,000 µg	May mask symptoms of vitamin B$_{12}$ deficiency

Details about vitamins (*Contd...*)

Vitamin	Chemical name	Year of discovery	Food source	Solu-bility	Recom-mended dietary allow-ance	Deficient disease	Upper intake level (UL/Day)*	Overdose disease
Vitamin B$_{12}$	Cyanocobala-min, hydroxy-cobalamin, methylcoba-lamin	1926	Liver, eggs, ani-mal products	Water	2.4 µg	Megaloblastic anemia	Not de-termined	Acne-like rash (causal-ity is not conclusively established)
Vitamin C	Ascorbic acid	1920	Citrus, most fresh foods	Water	90.0 mg	Scurvy	2,000 mg	Vitamin C megadosage
Vitamin D	Cholecalcif-erol	1920	Cod liver oil	Fat	5.0 to 10 µg	Rickets and osteomalacia	50 µg	Hypervitaminosis D
Vitamin E	Tocopherols, tocotrienols	1922	Wheat germ oil, unrefined vegetable oils	Fat	15 mg	Deficiency is very rare, mild haemo-lytic anaemia in newborn infants	1,000 mg	Increased congestive heart failure seen in one large randomized study
Vitamin K	Phylloquino-ne, manaqui-nones	1931	Leafy green vegetables	Fat	120 µg	Bleeding diathesis	Not de-termined	Increased coagulation in patients in warfarin

* Male, age 19–70 years.

APPENDIX C: DEMOGRAPHY AND FAMILY PLANNING

DEMOGRAPHY

Demography is the scientific study of the size, distribution and composition of the human population. It uses birth and death rates and related statistics to determine the characteristics of a population.

FAMILY PLANNING

Family planning means to decide on the number and timings of children in the family. WHO defines family planning as 'a way of living and thinking that is adopted voluntarily, upon the basis of knowledge, attitudes and responsible decisions by individuals and couples in order to promote health and welfare of the family group, and thus contributes effectively to the social development of a country'.

The essential aims of family planning are as follows:

❑ Prevent unwanted pregnancies
❑ Limit the number of births
❑ Control the interval between birth

To attain these goals, eligible couples (married couples wherein the female is in reproductive age, i.e. 15–45 years) are advised to use preventive methods to avoid unwanted pregnancies. These methods are also called *contraceptive methods*.

The contraceptive methods are broadly grouped into the following two categories:

1. Temporary methods, which include the following:
   (a) Barrier methods: They include physical (condom, diaphragm, etc.), chemical (foam, cream) and combined methods.
   (b) Intrauterine devices
   (c) Hormonal methods: They include contraceptive pills, injectables and implants.
   (d) Post-conceptional methods (termination of pregnancy)
2. Permanent methods, which include male (vasectomy) and female sterilization (tubectomy).

Postconception Methods (Medical Termination of Pregnancy)

1. **Menstrual regulation**: It consists of aspiration of contents after 6–14 days of a missed period.
2. **Abortion**: *Abortion* is defined as termination of pregnancy before the fetus becomes capable of living independently (i.e., the time between conception and the 28th week of pregnancy). Abortions are categorized as spontaneous and induced. In India, 6 million abortions take place every year, of which 4 million are induced and 2 million are spontaneous.

Medical Termination of Pregnancy (MTP) Act, 1971

This act is a healthcare measure that helps reduce maternal morbidity and mortality resulting from illegal abortions. It also tries to motivate women to adopt some form of conception as repeated abortions are not safe for the health of women.

Important aspects of MTP Act, 1971

1. Conditions under which a pregnancy can be terminated:
   (a) **Medical**: If continuation of pregnancy is not safe for mother.
   (b) **Eugenic**: If there is any risk of child being born with serious abnormalities.
   (c) **Humanitarian**: If pregnancy is the result of rape.
   (d) **Failure of contraceptive device**: If pregnancy is caused by failure of contraception.
   (e) If the pregnant lady is **lunatic**.
2. Who can perform abortion: Only a registered medical practitioner having experience in obstetrics and gynaecology is authorized to perform MTP.
3. Where abortions can be done: MTPs can be done only in established hospitals or places approved by government under safe and hygienic conditions. The nongovernment institutions are supposed to obtain license from the chief medical officer of the district.

APPENDIX D: COMMUNICABLE DISEASES

The communicable or contagious diseases are those in which the causative agent may pass from one person to another, directly or indirectly. The Council for International Organizations of Medical Sciences defined *communicable diseases* in 1973 as 'an illness due to a specific infectious agent or its toxic products, capable of being transmitted from man to man, animal to animal or from environment (through air, dust, soil, water, etc.) to man or animal'.

Diseases such as cholera, typhoid and dysentery spread through food, fruits and water. Diseases such as dengue, malaria, filaria and plague spread through insects. Scabies and venereal diseases spread by direct contact, while leprosy spreads after prolonged contacts. Syphilis, gonorrhoea and AIDS spread by sexual contacts.

The causative agents, mode of transmission and the methods of prevention of some important communicable diseases are summarized below.

CHICKEN POX (VARICELLA)

Causative agent: Chicken pox is an acute, highly infectious disease caused by Varicella zoster (VZ) virus. The disease is mild and provides immunity for the rest of life.

Clinical features: It is characterized by vesicular rashes on the trunk, face and limbs. After 24 h, lesions become pustular (filled with pus), which dry up in few days to become scabs. Onset is associated with fever, pain in back, shivering and malaise. Fever subsides with the appearance of rashes, but may rise again in the pustular stage.

Mode of transmission:

1. This disease is transmitted by droplet infection and the virus usually enters the upper respiratory tract.
2. The disease may also spread by contamination from the discharge from skin lesions.

Incubation period: 14–16 days

Prevention: Varicella zoster immunoglobulin (VZ Ig) given within 72 h of exposure in a dose of 1.25–5 mL intramuscular has been recommended for prevention or modification of the disease. A live attenuated vaccine (OKA strain) developed in Japan is a safe and effective measure for prevention of the disease.

MEASLES OR RUBEOLA

Measles is a highly communicable, infectious viral disease that affects children. One attack confers high degree of immunity. Measles is associated with high morbidity and mortality in developing countries.

Causative agent: RNA paramyxovirus (rubeola virus).

Clinical features: The onset is characterized by sneezing, coughing, running nose, fever, redness of eyes, congested flushed face and *koplik spots* (small inflamed spots inside skin around the parotid glands). After 3–4 days of such symptoms, maculopapular rashes develop initially on the face and then all over the body. The rashes subside within 5–7 days, leaving a brownish pigmentation.

Mode of transmission: Transmission occurs directly from person to person mainly by droplet infection via the respiratory tract or rarely through conjunctiva.

Incubation period: 10 days from exposure to onset of fever and 14 days to appearance of rash.

Prevention: Measles is best prevented by active immunization. Only live attenuated, tissue-cultured, freeze-dried vaccine is used. A single dose of 0.5 mL of reconstituted vaccine is injected subcutaneously in children of age group 9–12 months.

INFLUENZA

Influenza is an acute respiratory tract infection.

Causative agent: Influenza viruses A, B and C.

Clinical features: The disease is characterized by the sudden onset of chills, malaise, headache, backache, pain in limbs and sometimes vomiting.

Mode of transmission: Transmission occurs directly from person to person mainly by droplet infection via the respiratory tract.

Incubation period: 1–2 days.

Prevention: Influenza is best prevented by prophylactic immunization. Killed chick embryo vaccine in aqueous or saline suspension in a single dose of 0.5 mL is given subcutaneously. Influenza is normally treated by antiviral drugs such as amantadine and rimantadine.

LEPROSY

Leprosy is a chronic infectious disease that mainly affects peripheral nerves and skin. The infection may also spread to muscles, bones, eyes, testes and internal organs. Leprosy is characterized by partial or total loss of cutaneous sensation in the affected area, thickening of nerves and hypopigmented patches.

Causative agent: *Mycobacterium leprae*, an acid-fast bacterium.

Clinical features: The disease is manifested in two forms: *lepromatous leprosy*, which affects the skin and mucous membrane, and *tuberculoid leprosy*, which causes infiltration of bacteria in nerves and results in subcutaneous nodules, bleaching of skin and may lead to deformities.

Mode of transmission: Transmission occurs from the nasal discharge of infected person mainly by droplet infection. It is also transmitted by close contact (direct or indirect) between the infectious patient and a healthy susceptible person.

Incubation period: 3–5 years.

Prevention: Immunoprophylaxis: Bacillus Calmette-Guérin (BCG) vaccine provides protection against clinical leprosy; several other vaccines are under the process of development.

Treatment: WHO has recommended multiple drug therapy for leprosy treatment. The bactericidal drugs used for the treatment include rifampicin, dapsone, clofazimine, ethionamide, quinolones, minocycline and clarithromycin.

SYPHILIS

Syphilis is a chronic infection that progresses in four stages, with a latent period between each phase during which the patient does not show any signs or symptoms of the disease.

Stage	Symptoms	Incubation Period
Primary stage	Lesions at the site of contact Painless hard sore called *chancre* on the penis of man or the cervix in woman	2–6 weeks
Secondary stage	Fever, malaise, headache and generalized lesions of skin, mucous membrane and eyes. Cutaneous rash, mucous patches, lymphadenopathy	6 weeks–6 months
Tertiary stage	Affects visceral organs such as the heart, liver, bones, testes and the CNS	2–3 years

Causative agent: *Treponema pallidum.*

Mode of transmission: Transmission occurs by sexual contact with infected person. Congenital syphilis is transmitted to the fetus from the infected mother through placenta.

Prevention: Syphilis can mainly be prevented by avoiding extramarital sex. The treatment is most effective during the first two stages and is treated by using penicillin.

GONORRHOEA

Gonorrhoea is the infection of the mucous membrane of the genitourinary tract.

Causative agent: *Neisseria gonorrhoeae*, Gram-negative diplococcus bacteria

Clinical features: Females: Yellowish vaginal discharge and dysuria; males: Dysuria, increased frequency of micturition and white discharge from urethra. At an advanced stage, infection may enter blood causing septicaemia, fever and chills.

Mode of transmission: Transmission occurs during sexual intercourse with infected person.

Incubation period: 3–10 days

Treatment: Procaine penicillin or penicillin with probenecid is the most efficient treatment.

DIPHTHERIA

Diphtheria is an acute infectious disease that mostly affects the upper respiratory tract.

Causative agent: Toxigenic strains of *Corynebacterium diphtheriae.*

Clinical features: The bacilli multiplies in the throat and produces powerful exotoxins that result in marked congestion, oedema, enlargement of lymph nodes and signs and symptoms of toxaemia.

Mode of transmission: Transmission occurs by droplet infection or from infected cutaneous lesions. The bacilli enter the body via the respiratory tract, middle ear, conjunctiva, genitalia or any cuts or wounds on skin.

Incubation period: 2–6 days.

Prevention:

❑ The only effective control is active immunization with combined vaccine called *DPT vaccine*. This vaccine contains toxoids of diphtheria, tetanus and killed organisms of pertussis. DPT is administered intramuscularly in three doses of 0.5 mL each at the age of 1.5, 2.5 and 3.5 months and, thereafter, two booster doses at 2.5 and 3.5 years.

❑ Diphtheria antitoxin prepared from horse serum is the mainstay of passive prophylaxis and for treatment.

WHOOPING COUGH (PERTUSSIS)

Whooping cough is an acute infection of respiratory tract usually occurring in young children.

Causative agent: *Bordetella pertussis*. In some cases, *B. parapertussis* is responsible for this disease.

Clinical features: Mild fever, whooping (loud crowing inspiration) cough, severe bronchitis, bronchopneumonia and haemoptysis, and in severe conditions it may also cause convulsions.

Mode of transmission: Transmission occurs by droplet infection or by direct contact. The bacillus enters the body through the respiratory tract and multiplies in its epithelium where it produces inflammation and necrosis of mucosa. Paroxymal attacks of cough mostly occur during night and may lead to cyanosis of face and injury to tongue.

Incubation period: 7–14 days.

Prevention: The active immunization with *DPT vaccine* (as discussed in Diphtheria) is best for prevention. Antibiotics such as erythromycin, ampicillin and cotrimoxazole are used to control secondary infections associated with pertussis.

TUBERCULOSIS (TB)

Tuberculosis is an infectious chronic disease that mainly affects lungs (pulmonary tuberculosis). It can also affect intestine, meninges, bones, joints, skin and lymph glands (extrapulmonary tuberculosis).

Causative agent: *Mycobacterium tuberculosis*, an acid-fast bacillus. Some atypical mycobacteria, namely *M. Kansasii*, M. intracellulare and M. scrofulaceum are also reported to cause tuberculosis in humans.

Clinical features: Prolonged cough, rise in temperature in the evening, loss of weight, loss of appetite, etc.

Mode of transmission: Transmission occurs mainly by infectious droplets. Coughing of infected patients generates a large number of droplet nuclei and these fresh droplets carry the viable organisms.

Incubation period: 3–6 weeks after receipt of infection. The *tuberculin test (Mantoux test)* is the only means for estimating the prevalence of infection.

Prevention:

❑ *BCG vaccination:* BCG vaccine consists of freeze-dried live attenuated bovine strain of tubercle bacilli. It is administered by an intradermal injection of 0.05–0.1 mL just after birth or with the first dose of DPT vaccine.

❑ The patients with a history of persistent cough, fever and haemoptysis are examined using sputum examination, mass miniature radiography and tuberculin test. If the tests are positive, the patients are isolated and treatment is started. The treatment is done with first line drugs (such as isoniazid, rifampicin, pyrazinamide, ethambutol and streptomycin) and second line drugs (such as thiacetazone, ciprofloxacin, clarithromycin and rifabutin).

❑ The most important part in the treatment of tuberculosis is patient compliance, that is adequate and complete intake of drugs because discontinuation of the treatment results in the development of drug resistance. Thus, to ensure patient compliance, *Directly observed treatment short course (DOTS) chemotherapy* is used, in which patients are asked to take the drugs in front of the physician or are asked to bring back the empty multiblister combipack.

POLIOMYELITIS

Poliomyelitis is an acute viral infection of the gastrointestinal tract. In severe cases, the virus can also infect the central nervous system and may cause paralysis or even death.

Causative agent: Poliovirus. This virus has three subtypes: I, II and III, and among them, type I virus is responsible for causing paralytic polio. Poliovirus is abundantly found in the faeces and oropharyngeal secretions of an infected person.

Clinical features: In 4–8% cases, mild illness is reported, and the patient may feel pain in the neck and back that subsides within 2–10 days, while 95% cases do not show any symptoms. In less than 1% cases, the virus invades the central nervous system and may cause asymmetrical flaccid paralysis (AFP).

Mode of transmission: The infection is spread mainly through the faecal–oral route, that is the ingestion of contaminated water, milk and food may cause infection. Transmission may also occur by droplet infection.

Incubation period: 7–14 days.

Prevention and Eradication:

❑ In India, oral polio vaccine (OPV) is used for active immunization. It is a live attenuated liquid vaccine that is required to be stored at 4°C. Three drops of OPV are given with each dose of DPT vaccine, while one dose is given along with BCG vaccine at birth (zero dose of polio vaccine).

❑ Eradication of polio: In India, a mass immunization program named *Pulse Polio Immunization (PPI)* was started in collaboration with WHO in December 1995, under which more than 80 million children have been immunized till date. Under this scheme, two doses of oral polio vaccine are given at specified intervals to children below 5 years of age, and the main principle behind PPI is 'All disease-causing virus strains are to be suppressed and replaced by vaccine virus strain'.

TETANUS

Tetanus is an acute disease characterized by muscular rigidity and painful spasms of muscles of the face, back, neck, lower limbs and abdomen.

Causative agent: *Clostridium tetani*, a Gram-positive spore-bearing bacteria. The causative bacteria mostly enters through open wounds and may invade the central nervous system and cause tonic convulsions, spasm and finally death due to asphyxia.

Mode of transmission: The infection is transmitted through open wounds and injuries such as abrasion, burn, human or animal bite, unsterile injections or puncture wounds when contaminated by soil containing tetanus spores. The spores germinate in the body and the organism produces an exotoxin called *tetanospasmin*, which is responsible for the disease.

Incubation period: 3–21 days.

Prevention:

❏ Cleaning of wounds with hydrogen peroxide is the first aid prophylaxis to prevent tetanus. The best way to prevent tetanus is active immunization by purified tetanus toxoid and passive immunization by human tetanus hyperimmune globulin (TETGLOB).
❏ Tetanus can be prevented in neonates by immunizing the mother during pregnancy by two doses of tetanus toxoid. Children are immunized against tetanus at the time of birth along with diphtheria and pertussis vaccination.

RABIES

Rabies is an acute and highly fatal viral disease. Dogs, foxes, jackals, wolves, cats and such other carnivores are the carriers of infection.

Causative agent: Lyssavirus Type I, a bullet-shaped RNA virus belonging to *Rhabdoviridae* family.

Clinical features: The symptoms of infection in human beings are horrifying and include hydrophobia, increased temperature, excessive salivation, muscle spasm (face) and the inability to drink water, resulting in aggression. The disease mainly affects the central nervous system and causes encephalomyelitis, which may lead to hydrophobia and death.

Mode of transmission: The virus is transmitted to man by saliva secreted from the bites or licks of the rabies-infected animals. Infected dogs usually die within 7 days of infection.

Incubation period: 4 days to many years.

Prevention:

❏ **Pre-exposure prophylaxis:** Persons at high risk of exposure (veterinaries, animal housekeepers, persons related to wildlife, laboratory staff working with rabies virus) should be protected by preexposure vaccination in which 0.1 mL of cell culture vaccine is administered intramuscularly on 0, 7 and 28 days.
❏ **Postexposure prophylaxis:** The wound is first cleaned by water and then antiseptics such as alcohol and tincture iodine followed by antirabies serum, applied locally over the washed wound. The patient is then vaccinated against tetanus (TET-VAC injection 0.5 mL intramuscular). The animal should be observed for the next 10 days, and if the animal remains healthy and alive for 10 days, there is no need for antirabies treatment; otherwise the person should be vaccinated with antirabic vaccine.
  ➤ **Antirabic Vaccine:** This vaccine is unique as it is the only vaccine that is given after exposure. This vaccine is derived from the nervous tissue of adult sheep or from suckling mouse brain. The dose of vaccine depends on the degree of exposure.
    – *Class I Exposure:* It includes licks on healthy skin and consumption of unboiled milk. In this case, there is slight risk.

- *Class II Exposure:* It includes licks on cuts, scratches with oozing of blood and licks on broken skin. In this case, there is moderate risk.
- *Class III Exposure:* It includes all bites or scratches with oozing of blood, lacerated wound and contamination of mucous membrane with saliva.

➤ **Cell culture vaccine**

- Human diploid cell vaccine (HDCV)
- Tissue culture vaccine

Both these vaccines are safe and effective. Six doses of 1 mL each on 0, 3, 7, 14 and 30 days and booster dose on 90 days is administered intramuscularly in the deltoid region.

TRACHOMA

Trachoma is a chronic infection of conjunctiva characterized by conjunctival scarring, inward deviation of eyelashes, corneal ulceration, and so on and is an important cause of blindness.

Causative agent: *Chlamydia trachomatis*

Mode of transmission: The infection is transmitted through ocular discharges of infected person, infected fingers or towels.

Incubation period: 5–12 days.

Treatment: Antibiotic treatment such as tetracycline, erythromycin and rifampicin is generally prescribed.

APPENDIX E: FIRST AID MEASURES

First aid is the process of carrying out essential emergency treatment of the accident victim or sudden illness quickly and correctly before medical help is made available.

SHOCK

Shock is defined as a condition of severe depression of vital functions of the body due to poor circulation of blood. It is a very serious condition and if not handled promptly and properly, it may lead to death.

Symptoms: Dry mouth, cold skin, dilated pupil, anxiety, difficulty in breathing, low blood pressure and temporary loss of consciousness.

Emergency treatment:

❑ Place the patient in supine position and elevate the legs to increase venous return to the heart.
❑ Loosen the clothing and keep the patient warm in a blanket.
❑ The patient should be shifted to hospital as early as possible. Dopamine is given by intravenous infusion to raise the blood pressure, oxygen inhalation to correct hypoxia and fluid replacement (blood plasma or saline) carried out, if required.

SNAKEBITE

There are more than 3500 species of snakes, out of which only 250 are poisonous. In case of snakebite, if the snake is identified to be poisonous, antivenom treatment is given; otherwise there is no need of treatment.

Signs and symptoms of poisonous snakebite: Two puncture wounds with or without scratches (only scratches are seen in nonpoisonous snakebite), burning pain at site of bite, swelling, nausea, rapid pulse, shortness of breath and dimmed vision. In case of severe poisoning, the patient feels sleepy and experiences excessive salivation, convulsions, paralysis and loss of consciousness.

Emergency treatment:

❑ Assure the patient, immobilize the bitten part and apply a broad firm bandage or tourniquet proximal to the site of bite to prevent the spread of poison to other parts of the body.
❑ Clean the wound with sterile saline or water.
❑ Make a sharp cut over the bitten area and allow it to bleed by squeezing the area. If possible, poison should be sucked out with a suction pump.
❑ The patient should be shifted to hospital as early as possible where antisnake venom serum should be given intravenously.

BURNS

Burns are the injuries caused by dry heat (fire, flame, hot metal), chemicals (strong acids such as sulphuric acid, hydrochloric acid; strong alkalis such as sodium hydroxide, ammonium hydroxide), electricity and radiation.

Effects of Burns: Reddening of skin, blister formation, loss of fluid from burnt tissue and destruction of skin and deeper tissues.

Emergency treatment:

❏ Cool the burnt area immediately by putting plenty of cold water or by placing a clean cloth soaked in cold water. This treatment removes residual heat from tissues and prevents further damage.

❏ Keep the patient in a lie-down position and remove the clothing of the patient by cutting it around.

❏ Do not apply antiseptic, lotion, oil, baking soda, ink or flour on the burn and the burnt area should not be touched. Immediately remove things like rings, bangles, belt and boots from the body as they may cause gangrene.

❏ In case of chemical burn, wash the area with plenty of water until all the chemical has been washed away.

❏ In case of extensive burn, wrap the patient in a clean cloth and transfer to a hospital immediately.

POISONING

A poison is a substance which, if introduced in the body or brought in contact with any part in sufficient quantity, will produce ill health or even death. Poison can be consumed accidentally, for suicidal purpose or may be administered for homicidal purpose.

Emergency treatment:

❏ The first treatment should be to remove the unabsorbed poison from the body. It can be done by inducing vomiting by administration of emetic drug or two tablespoonful of common salt in a glass of warm water. Vomiting is induced only when the patient is conscious.

❏ When the patient is unconscious or is suspected to have consumed strong acid or alkali, vomiting is not induced. Instead, administer sodium bicarbonate, milk of magnesia if patient has consumed strong acids and lemon juice, vinegar or butter milk for strong alkalies.

❏ If the poison is detected, specific antidote is given; otherwise universal antidote can be administered. The universal antidote consists of one part of magnesium oxide, two parts of tannic acid and two parts of activated charcoal.

❏ If the symptoms are serious, shift the patient immediately to hospital emergency room.

FRACTURE

A break or crack in a bone is called *fracture*. This may occur during an accident where bones may break due to direct force or indirect force.

Symptoms of fracture: Pain at or near the site of fracture, swelling, inability to move the affected part, peculiar sound called *crepitus* on movement of fractured bone and aggravation of pain on movement.

Emergency treatment:

❏ Immobilize the fractured part immediately using bandage or splint and support the injured tissue on some pillow or

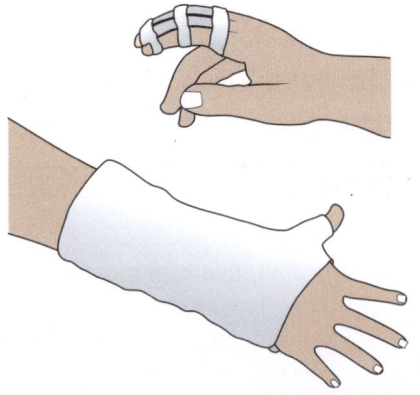

quilt. This immobilization is very essential to prevent pain and to prevent further damage to other parts by the broken ends.

❑ Do not give anything orally to the patient because emergency operation may be required.

❑ Transfer the patient to the hospital as early as possible for further treatment.

RESUSCITATION METHODS

Resuscitation is the most important first aid procedure to save the life of a patient. It is done when there is no breathing or inadequate circulation.

Commonly, when people see an unconscious person, they administer water to the person in order to revive him. But this is a very wrong practice as water given by mouth can enter the lungs and choke the respiratory passage, which may cause immediate death of the person.

The procedure to give artificial respiration and artificial circulation when the patient is unconscious and has no pulse is termed *Cardiopulmonary Resuscitation (CPR)*.

Procedure for CPR:

1. *Clean the airway:*
   ❑ The air passage should be opened and cleaned to allow free passage of air. This is done to remove any obstruction that may occur due to inhaled foreign body or rolling back of the tongue.
   ❑ For this, wrap a handkerchief or a clean cloth on the first two fingers and clean the victim's mouth thoroughly. During this process, the mouth of the patient should be turned to a side so that any particle does not fall in the respiratory tract.

2. *Artificial Breathing:*
   ❑ If breathing stops, artificial respiration should be given immediately because a person cannot survive for more than 3–4 min without air. Artificial respiration can be given by the following procedures:
   (a) *Mouth-to-mouth respiration*
      – The patient is placed horizontally on his back on a hard flat surface.
      – The head is tilted backwards with one hand and the neck is supported with the other hand. This lifts the tongue to normal position and the patient may start breathing on his/her own.
      – If breathing does not start, pinch the nose of the patient with one hand, seal the patient's mouth with your own mouth and breathe out the air forcefully into his lungs. Repeat this process rapidly a number of times till the patient starts breathing on its own.
   (b) *Mouth-to-nose respiration*
      – When mouth-to-mouth respiration is not possible due to the inability to open the mouth, mouth-to-nose respiration is given.
      – In this case, the mouth is first closed by the first aider's palm and the patient's nose is sealed with your mouth. The rest of the procedure is the same as in the case of mouth-to-mouth respiration.

3. Artificial Circulation
   ❑ This is done by cardiac massage in order to revive the functioning of the heart.

❏ For this, place the victim horizontally on a hard, flat surface. Kneel next to the victim's chest. Find the notch at the tip of the breastbone where the lower ribs meet the sternum, called the *xiphoid process*. Remember, if you push directly down on this puppy, you will likely rupture the vicitm's liver and perhaps a few other vital organs, and all the CPR in the world couldn't help. Place your middle finger on this notch, and place your index finger down next to your middle finger. That way, you are at least a good two fingers away from the xiphoid danger spot. Next, place the heel of your other hand on the victim's sternum next to your index finger. Place your other hand directly on top and interlace your fingers. Straighten your arms and lock your elbows. Your shoulders should be directly over your hands. Push the chest and each chest compression should push the sternum down 1.5–2 in.

❏ After four continuous cycles, check for a pulse. If there is no pulse, continue CPR, beginning with chest compressions and rechecking for a pulse every few minutes.

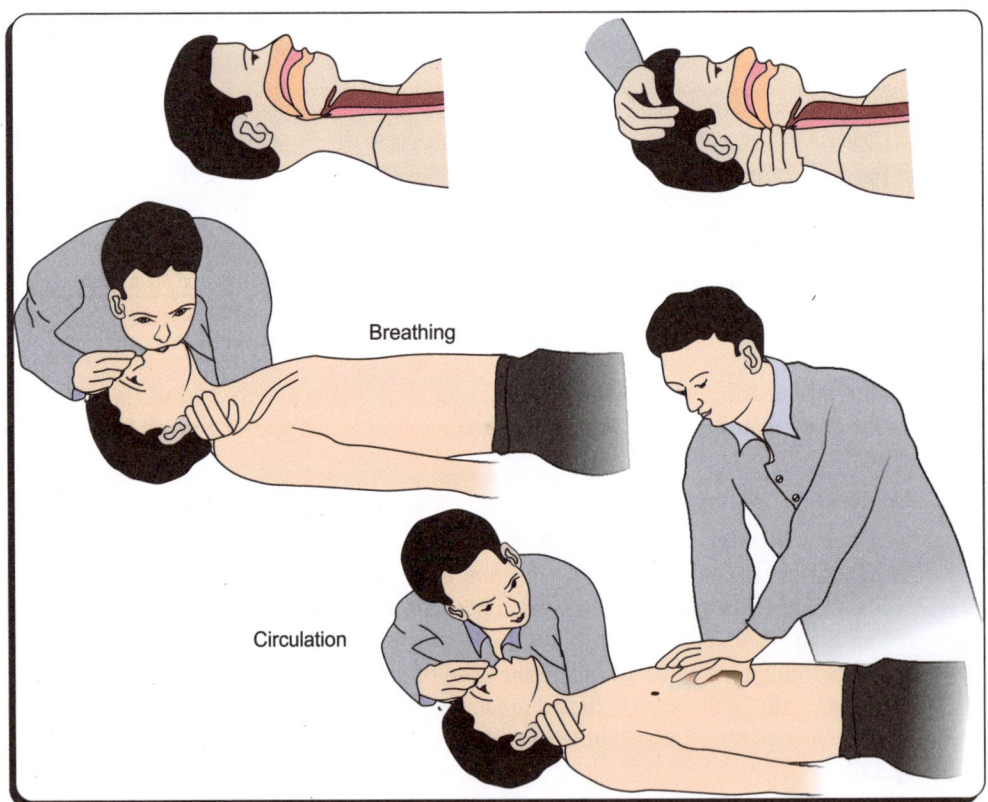

Breathing

Circulation

Cardiopulmonary Resuscitation

Index